MENTAL HEALTH EQUITY

Daniel E. Dawes, JD, DHL (Hon.), is a professor of health law, policy, and management, senior vice president of global health, and the founding dean of the School of Global Health at Meharry Medical College in Nashville, Tennessee. He is the author and editor of three health policy books on health equity, including *150 Years of ObamaCare* and *The Political Determinants of Health.* Dean Dawes is an elected member of the National Academy of Medicine, an elected fellow of the New York Academy of Medicine, and an elected presidential visiting fellow at Yale University. He has served as an advisor to the White House on health equity initiatives and was appointed by the U.S. Department of Health and Human Services to the Centers for Disease Control and Prevention's Advisory Committee to the Director and the National Institute of Health's National Advisory Council for Nursing Research. Among his many achievements, he was an instrumental figure in developing and negotiating the Mental Health Parity Act, the Genetic Information Nondiscrimination Act, and the Americans with Disabilities Act Amendments Act, and was an architect of the Affordable Care Act's health equity–focused provisions, among other landmark federal policies.

Nelson J. Dunlap, JD, is an assistant professor in the Department of Political Determinants of Health, vice president of public policy and external affairs, and the vice dean of the School of Global Health at Meharry Medical College. He has coauthored a number of health equity- and mental health–focused reports and peer-reviewed journal articles, including, but not limited to, *Economic Burden of Mental Health Inequities in the United States*, *Projected Cost and Economic Impact of Mental Health Inequities in the United States*, and *The Political Determinants of Health: A Global Panacea for Health Inequities.* Mr. Dunlap has served as the coprincipal investigator for grants such as the development of the first health equity tracker in the nation in partnership with Google, the creation of the American Medical Association's Medical Justice in Advocacy Fellowship, and the establishment of the Diverse Executive Leading in Public Health program at the Association of State and Territorial Health Officials. Given his contributions to the creation of new methodologies for health equity research, his noted scholarship on the political determinants of health, and in recognition of his commitment to the pursuit of health equity, he has recently been named to the de Beaumont Foundation's 40 Under 40 in Public Health.

Octavio N. Martinez, Jr., MD, MPH, MBA, DLFAPA, is senior associate vice president and executive director of the Hogg Foundation for Mental Health; professor of psychiatry and associate chair for faculty academic affairs, Department of Psychiatry and Behavioral Sciences, Dell Medical School; clinical professor, Steve Hicks School of Social Work; and faculty affiliate of the Rapoport Center for Human Rights and Justice, at the University of Texas at Austin. He was appointed by the White House to the Presidential COVID-19 Health Equity Taskforce and by the U.S. Department of Health and Human Services to the Centers for Disease Control and Prevention's Advisory Committee to the Director. Dr. Martinez serves as inaugural chair of the Yale University Pozen-Commonwealth Fund Fellowship in Health Equity Leadership's National Advisory Council, serves on the board of Trust for America's Health, is appointed a commissioner to the Texas Judicial Commission on Mental Health, and is an executive committee member of the Texas Child Mental Health Care Consortium.

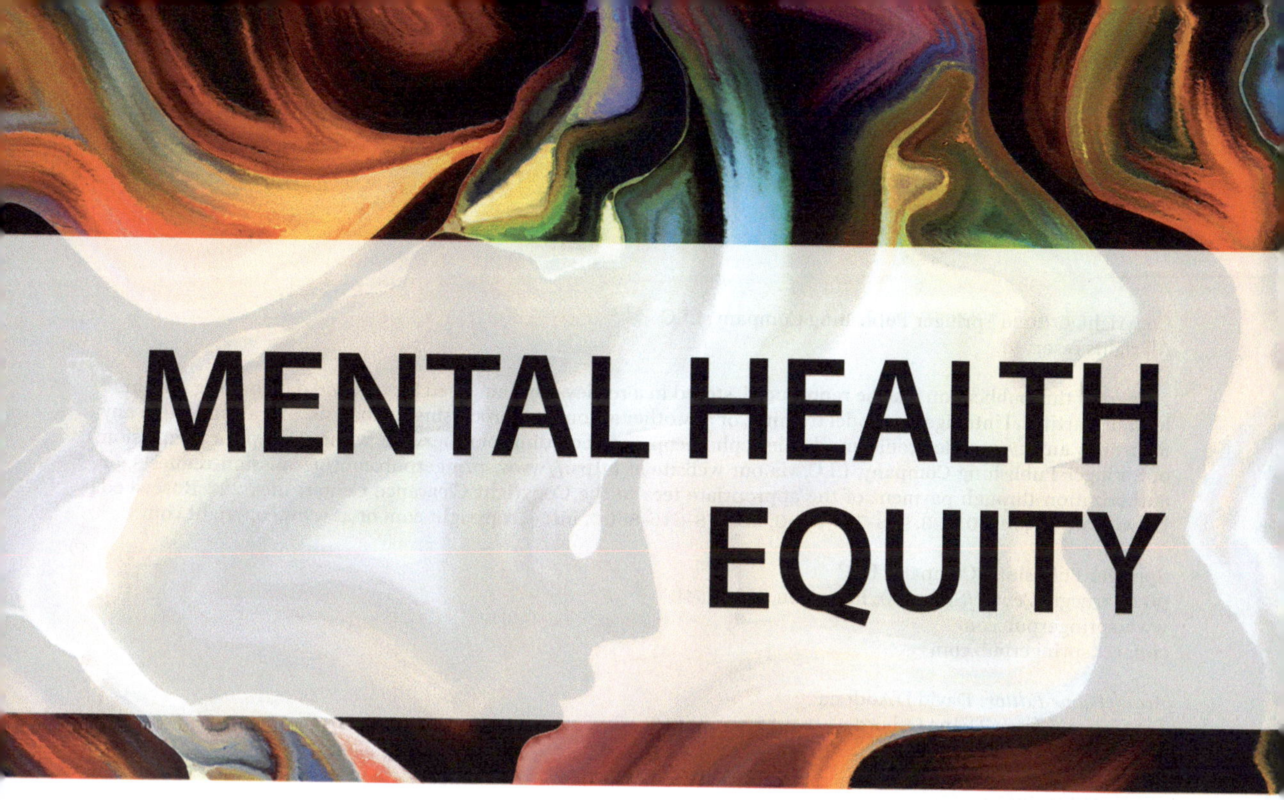

MENTAL HEALTH EQUITY

Editors

DANIEL E. DAWES, JD, DHL (HON.)

NELSON J. DUNLAP, JD

OCTAVIO N. MARTINEZ, JR., MD, MPH, MBA, DLFAPA

SPRINGER PUBLISHING

Springer Publishing Company, LLC
902 Carnegie Center/Suite 140, Princeton, NJ 08540
www.springerpub.com
connect.springerpub.com

Acquisitions Editor: David D'Addona
Production Editor: Diana Osborne
Compositor: Thomson Digital

ISBN: 978-0-8261-8055-1
e-book ISBN: 978-0-8261-8059-9
DOI: 10.1891/9780826180599

A robust set of instructor resources designed to supplement this text is located at http://connect.springerpub.com/content/book/978-0-8261-80599. Qualifying instructors may request access by emailing textbook@springerpub.com.

Instructor Materials:
LMS Common Cartridge—With All Instructor Resources ISBN: 978-0-8261-79883
Instructor's Manual ISBN: 978-0-8261-8056-8
Sample Syllabus ISBN: 978-0-8261-9372-8
Test Bank ISBN: 978-0-8261-8058-2
PowerPoint Slides ISBN: 978-0-8261-8057-5

25 26 27 28 / 5 4 3 2 1

Library of Congress Control Number: 2025018746

Publisher's Note: **New and used products purchased from third-party sellers are not guaranteed for quality, authenticity, or access to any included digital components.**

Printed in the United States of America.

For Nedeeka, my unwavering partner, and Marc and Raymond, my greatest inspirations—this book is a testament to the love and joy you all bring to my life.

DANIEL E. DAWES

For my loving wife, Erin, my greatest supporter and the staunchest mental health champion I've ever known.

NELSON J. DUNLAP

For my beloved wife, Clarissa, and my loving daughter, Sofia, who have been my shining stars.

OCTAVIO N. MARTINEZ, JR.

Contents

Contributors

Leslie Adams, PhD, MPH
Assistant Professor, Department of Psychiatry and Behavioral Sciences, Stanford University School of Medicine, Palo Alto, California

Sergio Aguilar-Gaxiola, MD, PhD
Professor of Clinical Internal Medicine, Director of the Center for Reducing Health Disparities, University of California, Davis Health, Sacramento, California

Christian M. Amador, MBA, MSc
Assistant Vice President of Strategic Initiatives, Meharry Medical College, Nashville, Tennessee

Juan Carlos Araque, PhD
Teaching Professor, Suzanne Dworak-Peck School of Social Work, University of Southern California, Los Angeles, California

Whitney Barnett, PhD, MPH
Assistant Professor, School of Global Health, Meharry Medical College, Nashville, Tennessee

Regina Benjamin, MD, MBA
18th United States Surgeon General

Prashasti Bhatnagar, JD, MPH
Law/Public Health Post Doctoral Scholar, Kirwan Institute, The Ohio State University, Columbus, Ohio

Dayna Bowen Matthew, JD, PhD
Dean and Harold H. Greene Professor of Law, George Washington University Law School, Washington, DC

Gail C. Christopher, DN
Executive Director, National Collaborative for Health Equity, Washington, DC, Senior Scholar, Center for the Advancement of Well-Being, George Mason University, Fairfax, Virginia

Walter D. Conwell, MD, MBA
Associate Professor of Medicine, Morehouse School of Medicine, Atlanta, Georgia

King E. Davis, PhD
Professor, The University of Texas at Austin, Austin, Texas

Daniel E. Dawes, JD, DHL (Hon.)
Professor of Health Law, Policy, and Management; Senior Vice President of Global Health; Founding Dean, School of Global Health, Meharry Medical College, Nashville, Tennessee

Fernando De Maio, PhD
Professor, Department of Sociology, DePaul University; Vice President, Health Equity Research and Data Use, American Medical Association, Chicago, Illinois

Nelson J. Dunlap, JD
Assistant Professor, Department of Political Determinants of Health; Vice President of Public Policy and External Affairs; Vice Dean, School of Global Health, Meharry Medical College, Nashville, Tennessee

Catherine K. Ettman, PhD
Assistant Professor, Department of Health Policy and Management, Johns Hopkins Bloomberg School of Public Health, Baltimore, Maryland

Carlos Fayard, PhD
Associate Professor of Psychiatry, Loma Linda University School of Medicine, Loma Linda, California

Shaakira A. Ford, DSW, LCSW
Assistant Professor, Morehouse School of Medicine, Atlanta, Georgia

Debra M. Furr-Holden, PhD
Dean and Professor, New York University School of Global Public Health, New York, New York

Casey Glasser, JD
The George Washington University Law School, Washington, DC

J.C. Gonzalez, Jr., MBA, PMP
Assistant Vice President of Strategic Planning, Meharry Medical College, Nashville, Tennessee

Kisha Braithwaite, PhD, MSCR
Professor and Psychologist, Morehouse School of Medicine, Atlanta, Georgia

Alicia Holloway, EdD, MBA
Associate Dean of Academic Affairs and Assistant Professor, Meharry Medical College, Nashville, Tennessee

Darrell Hudson, PhD, MPH
Professor and Chair, Department of Health Behavior and Health Equity, University of Michigan, Ann Arbor, Michigan

Vanessa Jackson, LCSW
President, Healing Circles, Inc., Atlanta, Georgia

Shaneeta M. Johnson, MD, MBA
Professor, Vice President Global Health Innovation, Associate Dean, Meharry School of Global Health, Nashville, Tennessee

Fazal Khan, MD, JD
Chair, Department of Population Health, Professor of Health Law, Policy and Management, School of Global Health, Meharry Medical College, Nashville, Tennessee

Wonha Kim, MD, MPH, CPH, FAAP
Director of the Institute for Health Policy and Leadership, Loma Linda University Health, Loma Linda, California

Sung-Jae Lee, PhD
Professor in Residence, Department of Psychiatry and Biobehavioral Sciences, David Geffen School of Medicine, University of California, Los Angeles, California

Pierluigi Mancini, PhD, MAC, CCS
President and CEO, Multicultural Development Institute, Inc., Atlanta, Georgia

Octavio N. Martinez, Jr., MD, MPH, MBA, DLFAPA
Senior Associate Vice President and Executive Director, Hogg Foundation for Mental Health; Professor of Psychiatry and Associate Chair for Faculty Academic Affairs, Department of Psychiatry and Behavioral Sciences, Dell Medical School; Clinical Professor, Steve Hicks School of Social Work; and Faculty Affiliate of the Rapoport Center for Human Rights and Justice, at the University of Texas at Austin, Austin, Texas

J. Lloyd Michener, MD
Emeritus Professor, Family Medicine and Community Health, Duke University School of Medicine, Durham, North Carolina

Margaret P. Moss, PhD, JD, RN, FAAN (Hidatsa/Dakhóta)
Professor, Associate Dean of Nursing and Health Policy, University of Minnesota, School of Nursing, Minneapolis, Minnesota

Ronjonette O'Bannon, PhD, LCSW
Dean, Well-Being and Strategic Planning, Spelman College, Atlanta, Georgia

Elizabeth Pendo, JD
Kellye Y. Testy Professor of Law, University of Washington School of Law, Seattle, Washington

Celeste M. Philip, MD, MPH
Associate Dean and Professor, Public Health Practice, School of Global Health, Meharry Medical College, Nashville, Tennessee

Joseph V. Sakran, MD, MPH, MPA, FACS
Executive Vice Chair of Surgery, Director of Clinical Operations, Johns Hopkins Medicine, Baltimore, Maryland

Karen A. Scott, MD, MPH, FACOG
Chief Black Feminist Physician Scientist, Founding CEO and Owner, Birthing Cultural Rigor, LLC, Nashville, Tennessee

Joshua M. Sharfstein, MD
Distinguished Professor of the Practice, Johns Hopkins Bloomberg School of Public Health, Baltimore, Maryland

Steven S. Sharfstein, MD, MPA
Associate in Health Policy and Management, Johns Hopkins Bloomberg School of Public Health, Baltimore, Maryland

Ruth S. Shim, MD, MPH
Luke and Grace Kim Professor in Cultural Psychiatry, University of California, Davis School of Medicine, Sacramento, California

Ife Shoyombo, MD, MS, MPH
House Staff Department of Surgery, Johns Hopkins Hospital, Baltimore, Maryland

Brian Smedley, PhD
Senior Fellow, Urban Institute, Washington, DC

Roland J. Thorpe, Jr., PhD, MS
Professor, Department of Health, Behavior, and Society, Johns Hopkins Bloomberg School of Public Health, Baltimore, Maryland

Sidney D. Watson, JD
Jane and Bruce Robert Professor of Law and Scholar in Residence, Saint Louis University School of Law Center for Health Law Studies, Saint Louis, Missouri

Britt Weinstock, PhD, MA
Associate Professor, Department of Population Health, School of Global Health, Meharry Medical College; and Principal and Chief Strategist, Health Equity Strategies Group, LLC, Washington, DC

Eugenia L. Weiss, PhD, PsyD, LCSW
Associate Professor and Associate Dean, School of Social Work, University of Nevada, Reno, Nevada

John M. Westfall, MD, MOH
Vice President of Medical Affairs, DARTNet Institute, Aurora, Colorado

Eboni C. Winford, PhD, MPH
Vice President of Research and Health Equity, Cherokee Health Systems, Knoxville, Tennessee

Shale L. Wong, MD, MSPH
Professor of Pediatrics, Executive Director, Eugene S. Farley, Jr. Health Policy Center, University of Colorado, Aurora, Colorado

Ruqaiijah Yearby, JD, MPH
Kara J. Trott Professor in Health Law, Moritz College of Law, The Ohio State University, Columbus, Ohio

Foreword

The pursuit of mental health equity has become one of the most pressing challenges of our time. As the first textbook to comprehensively examine the critical issues underpinning mental health equity, *Mental Health Equity* serves as an essential resource for students, scholars, practitioners, community leaders, and policy makers alike. This groundbreaking work synthesizes the latest evidence on the root causes of mental health inequities, highlighting the systemic factors that perpetuate disparities. It brings to the forefront the determinants and drivers that collectively shape mental health outcomes, presenting a holistic understanding of the multifaceted nature of equity in mental health and its connection to our overall health.

A cornerstone of this textbook is its commitment to addressing intersectional issues—those often overlooked yet profoundly impacting dimensions of identity, experience, and systemic barriers to mental health equity. By integrating discussions on race, socioeconomic status, gender, sexuality, disability, and other intersecting factors, this text challenges traditional, siloed approaches to mental health. It moves beyond the theoretical, bridging the gap between understanding and action. Readers will find themselves equipped not only with a deep appreciation for the complexity of mental health equity but also with the tools to transition from theory to tangible policy changes and operational strategies with solid grounding in the political determinants of health framework.

What sets this textbook apart is its emphasis on actionable insights and innovative approaches to actualizing health equity. With its blend of rigorous research, real-world examples, and practical frameworks, *Mental Health Equity* provides a more compelling road map for positive change. It empowers readers to envision and implement solutions that dismantle inequitable systems and develop interventions at the clinical, community, and structural levels, while fostering environments where mental health is a universal priority. This pioneering work is not merely a collection of knowledge, it is a call to action—a guiding light for those committed to creating a future where mental health equity is not an aspiration but a reality.

Regina Benjamin, MD, MBA
18th United States Surgeon General

Preface

To eliminate disparities in health, we need leaders who care enough, know enough, will do enough, and are persistent enough.

—David Satcher, MD, PhD

David Satcher, MD, PhD, who served as the 16th Surgeon General of the United States, the 11th U.S. Assistant Secretary for Health, and the 13th Director of the Centers for Disease Control and Prevention, recognized early on in his career that there were four distinct qualities that health leaders needed to successfully eliminate disparities in health: caring, knowledgeable, actionable, and persistent. He was speaking from experience and drawing upon a vast amount of knowledge with respect to developing and shaping leaders over the course of his tenure in academia and public service.

The past few years, in the wake of the COVID-19 pandemic, have made two things abundantly clear. First and foremost is that the link between our physical health and our mental health is as strong and as articulated as ever. Unless we take the necessary steps to truly elevate and prioritize addressing disparities and inequities in mental health, we will never be able to care for the whole person. Second, the interconnectedness of the global society that we all operate in requires that any solutions we conceive of today, for tomorrow's problems, include perspectives from a diversity of scholars, leaders, community members, and those with lived experiences from across all population groups.

Stated more succinctly, the types of leaders that Dr. Satcher envisioned are individuals who understand that not only is there no health without mental health, but there is no health equity without mental health equity, and that it is going to take a team effort of new and innovative approaches to old problems if we are to see a significant improvement in mental and behavioral health, as well as in our systemic health. The desire to properly equip those types of leaders with an innovative resource that bridges the latest research with evidence-based interventions, to effectively make the case for mental health equity, is precisely why the coeditors of this textbook joined forces.

DISTINGUISHING FEATURES

In every chapter of this first-of-its-kind textbook, readers will be guided through some of the most prescient themes in mental health equity by researchers, scholars, and luminaries from across the United States who have been working tirelessly to highlight and address the problems as well as develop and implement solutions to the mental health crisis affecting population groups. Further, each chapter includes thought-provoking discussion questions that will not only confirm the substance of the material but will charge the reader to consider their worldview and their role in achievement of mental health equity.

INTENDED AUDIENCE

Although the pursuit of mental health equity is a calling that all can respond to, this text is designed to serve as an introduction to the field of mental health equity for some, and to enhance the research considerations for others. For many undergraduate students, the history, concepts, and frameworks discussed in this text may be new information that will hopefully trigger a desire for deeper instruction. For graduate students and other professionals already familiar with the field, the groundbreaking research, frameworks, and models provided in this text should elucidate the continued importance and necessity of mental health equity while also serving as a springboard for novel research and collaborations.

CONTENT

This book proceeds in five parts to guide the reader along the path from novice to mental health equity champion. Beginning in Part I, readers will be introduced to concepts surrounding the history, design, and impact of public mental health. Part II serves to present and discuss the driving forces or determinants of mental health inequities and health equity, whereas Part III builds upon the determinants frameworks to highlight some pressing intersectional issues in the field. In Part IV, readers will begin to shift their focus toward actualization of mental health equity by grappling with policy implications, before delving into Part V, which illuminates current and future considerations to mental health equity.

Daniel E. Dawes
Nelson J. Dunlap
Octavio N. Martinez, Jr.

Acknowledgments

We want to thank the entire community of health equity scholars and researchers, past, present, and future, for their tireless commitment to expanding the boundaries of our collective knowledge on these pressing issues. By gathering the evidence and shining a light on some of the most critical equity concerns of our time, you continue to ensure that there is a path forward to a more equitable tomorrow.

To our colleagues Mr. David D'Addona, Ms. Kristen Mejia, Dr. Clarissa Moreno, Ms. Ayanna Smith, and Dr. Britt Weinstock, we sincerely thank you for your feedback, critiques, and guidance. Without your relentless dedication to excellence and the advancement of mental health equity, none of this would have come to fruition.

Instructor Resources

SPRINGER PUBLISHING CONNECT™ A robust set of instructor resources designed to supplement this text is located at http://connect.springerpub.com/content/book/978-0-8261-8059-9. Qualifying instructors may request access by emailing textbook@springerpub.com.

- **LMS Common Cartridge With All Instructor Resources**
- **Instructor's Manual**
  - Learning objectives
  - Chapter summaries
  - Learning activities
- **Sample Syllabus** featuring a course description, course objectives, and a course schedule
- **Test Bank** with 100 multiple-choice questions (including full rationales)
- **PowerPoint Slides** summarizing chapter content

SPRINGER PUBLISHING

Visit https://connect.springerpub.com/978-0-8261-8059-9 and look for the **"Show Supplementary"** button on the **book homepage.**

MENTAL HEALTH EQUITY

Part I

PUBLIC MENTAL HEALTH: EXAMINING THE ROOT CAUSES

1 AN INTRODUCTION TO MENTAL HEALTH EQUITY

WHITNEY BARNETT, NELSON J. DUNLAP, AND DANIEL E. DAWES

LEARNING OBJECTIVES

After reading this chapter, readers will be able to:

- Define mental health.
- Define mental health equity.
- Describe concepts related to mental health equity.
- Recognize the role of the political determinants of health in addressing mental health equity.
- Identify key gaps in their understanding of mental health equity concepts to further explore throughout the text.

INTRODUCTION

In today's world, there are two key concepts that work together to play a larger-than-life role in how our society functions. Whether we are aware of their impact, they are constantly intersecting and interacting with one another, often in the background, to shape how each of our lives is formed, progresses, and thrives. These oft-overlooked concepts are mental health equity and their determinants and drivers. Mental health includes our emotional, psychological, and social well-being and affects how we think, feel, and act, and helps determine how we handle stress, relate to others, and make choices (Substance Abuse and Mental Health Services Administration [SAMHSA], 2023). Mental health equity, on the other hand, is the right of all individuals, regardless of race, age, ethnicity, gender, disability, socioeconomic status, sexual orientation, or geographic location, to access high-quality and affordable mental health care services and addresses systemic factors driving health inequities (SAMHSA, 2023). For purposes of this volume, *mental health equity* is generally defined as the state in which everyone has a fair and just opportunity to reach their highest level of health or full health potential.

GLOBAL MENTAL HEALTH

Mental health disorders are a significant global concern, impacting millions and posing serious challenges to public health systems, individual well-being, and economies. Mental and substance use disorders (SUDs) have increased globally over the past 30 years and represent some of the leading causes of disability (GBD 2019 Mental Disorders Collaborators, 2022). A disability-adjusted life year (DALY) represents the loss of 1 year of full health, either because of premature mortality or years lived with a disability. Not only are mental health disorders increasing globally in terms of the number of people affected, the proportion of

DALYs attributable to mental disorders is increasing (GBD 2019 Mental Disorders Collaborators, 2022).

Mental disorders are not only debilitating but are also risk factors for fatal outcomes including suicide and all-cause mortality (Moitra et al., 2021; Walker et al., 2015). Individuals with mental health diagnoses have a lower life expectancy (14.6 years; Chan et al., 2023) relative to the general population, and approximately 8 million deaths each year globally are attributable to mental disorders (Walker et al., 2015). Moreover, mental health conditions increase one's risk of physical disease and illness and adversely affect access to adequate healthcare (e.g., through stigma, or impact on health-seeking behaviors; Hert et al., 2011; Scott et al., 2016). People with mental disorders are at higher risk for chronic physical health conditions, including HIV and diabetes, as well as gastrointestinal, cardiovascular, and respiratory diseases (Hert et al., 2011; Scott et al., 2016). Chronic physical conditions and mental health problems often co-occur, acting synergistically by reducing access to care, increasing medical costs, and decreasing health-seeking behavior (e.g., treatment adherence and attending routine healthcare visits; Katon, 2011; Naylor et al., 2012). Globally, the treatment gap for mental health disorders is enormous—an estimated 450 million people do not receive the treatment they need (Vigo et al., 2016).

Critically, both globally and in the United States, the burden of mental health conditions is not shared equally. As most recently highlighted by the global COVID-19 pandemic, it is well established that both physical and mental health are very much shaped by inequalities in our social and physical environment (Bambra et al., 2020). Location and community play a crucial role in shaping mental health outcomes, profoundly influencing the prevalence and severity of mental health conditions. Social determinants of health, such as access to healthcare, education, employment opportunities, and social support, are largely dictated by where we live. Communities with limited resources often experience higher rates of mental health challenges as residents face increased stressors alongside reduced access to mental health services (Marmot & Bell, 2012).

Although much of the discussion around mental health equity focuses on addressing mental health conditions, measuring and framing mental health in terms of illness or deficits, it is important to recognize mental health as a positive asset—a state of well-being that enables individuals to flourish and lead fulfilling, productive lives (Huppert & So, 2013). Positive mental health contributes to better physical health, stronger social relationships, and improved economic outcomes, serving as a critical resource that enhances overall quality of life (World Health Organization [WHO], 2004). Promoting mental well-being, therefore, is not just about preventing or treating mental illness, but requires a focus on improving the social and environmental conditions in which people live, recognizing that these factors are deeply intertwined with not only mental health conditions, but mental well-being. In this light, mental health equity must include efforts to cultivate positive mental health as a key component of a just and equitable society.

MENTAL HEALTH EQUITY

Equity describes a fair allocation of resources based on need. Evidence of an equitable community would be the absence of avoidable differences among different groups of people. Mental health equity would mean that everyone, regardless of race, gender, socioeconomic status, or geographic location, would have access to the resources, opportunities, and support needed to achieve optimal mental health. However, there are well-documented disparities in the prevalence of mental health conditions, in access to care, and in quality of treatment (Dawes et al., 2024). These disparities are often rooted in systemic inequalities and exacerbated by social determinants of health. Achieving mental health equity requires a multifaceted approach that addresses these underlying factors, ensuring that mental health services are available, accessible, and culturally appropriate for all individuals.

How we define and measure mental health outcomes and their drivers (socioeconomic status, geography, sex, social capital) is key. Trends in mental health conditions at both the global and national levels can mask inequity among groups. These trends, as discussed earlier, show that mental health issues are increasing globally, but they do not provide insight into which groups are experiencing specific issues and where disparities exist. For example, globally, females are at higher risk for both depression and anxiety, whereas SUDs are more common in males (GBD 2019 Mental Disorders Collaborators, 2022). Globally, LGBTQ+ individuals have a significantly elevated risk of poor mental health compared with cisgender and heterosexual individuals (Blondeel et al., 2016; Valentine & Shipherd, 2018). Refugees and those experiencing forced displacement from their homes have a well-documented increased risk of depression, anxiety, and posttraumatic stress disorder (PTSD) compared with the general population (Turrini et al., 2017), and this increased risk persists following resettlement. Compared with the general population, people who are incarcerated (i.e., living in prisons, jails, and juvenile detention facilities) disproportionately experience mental health problems, such as substance misuse, and have extremely high rates of comorbidity (Fazel et al., 2016; Kinner & Young, 2018). Indeed, a recent review found that half of individuals entering prison with a mental health disorder had a comorbid SUD (Favril et al., 2024). Lastly, marginalized racial and ethnic groups often face higher rates of mental health disorders, often alongside limited access to care. For example, studies have shown that individuals from minority ethnic groups in the United Kingdom and other parts of Europe are about twice as likely to experience poor mental health compared with the majority population (Bignall, 2019). Additionally, Indigenous populations globally face disproportionately higher suicide rates than the general population (Pollock et al., 2018). These disparities are exacerbated by systemic issues such as socioeconomic inequality, cultural stigma, and a lack of culturally sensitive mental health services.

These documented disparities in mental health outcomes for specific marginalized groups are the result of economic, environmental, social, and structural inequities predominantly affecting marginalized communities (Sheiham, 2008). They reflect differences in resource allocation, such as doctors per capita, money available for healthcare, and policies that fail to respond to need, and misallocate resources to those already well resourced. Individual identities such as race or ethnicity, sexual orientation, or gender are inextricably linked to social power, discrimination, and resource allocation, each impacting access to and quality of mental health care. Although the focus in this book is mental health, these drivers of mental health disparities are also critical drivers of poorer physical health outcomes and are related to educational attainment, long-term financial stability, and life expectancy. Equity strives to ensure access to and fair allocation of resources according to need rather than equal distribution of resources (Culyer & Wagstaff, 1993). Whereas health disparities describe differences in health outcomes, equity seeks to minimize these differences by addressing the drivers of those disparities.

ISSUES IMPACTING MENTAL HEALTH EQUITY IN THE UNITED STATES

Although mental health issues have increased globally following the COVID-19 pandemic, the United States has particularly had one of the highest rates of diagnosed depression and anxiety and the highest suicide rate among high-income countries (Tikkanen, 2020). In the United States, 57.8 million adults (one in five) experienced mental health conditions in the past year, and one third of those had a co-occurring SUD (National Alliance on Mental Illness [NAMI], 2021). Yet, despite spending more than any other country on healthcare per capita, individuals in the United States face large barriers to accessing care. In 2021, more than 50% of adults with mental health conditions (NAMI, 2021) and 74% of those with an SUD did not receive treatment (American Addiction Centers, 2022). Moreover, although research shows that minorities have a lower or equivalent prevalence of mental health conditions, mental health services are more likely to be used by those who are White, high income, and living in urban areas (SAMHSA, 2021). In 2020, 48% of White adults with any mental health conditions received mental health services, compared with 31% of Black adults and 31% of Latino adults (SAMHSA, 2020). Barriers to receiving mental health care are substantial. High cost and limited insurance coverage are the most commonly cited barriers to receiving mental health care (SAMHSA, 2021). Among racial minority groups in the United States, barriers include stigma, negative experiences with providers, perceived ineffectiveness of treatment, and structural barriers such as limited appointment availability and lack of transportation (Howell & McFeeters, 2008). For example, research has shown that Black, Latino, and Asian populations are more likely to report prejudice, discrimination, and a lack of confidence that the services would help as reasons for not seeking treatment (Leong & Kalibatseva, 2011).

There are several features of the U.S. system, many unique among high-income countries, that result in these disparities in access to mental health care. For example, the United States stands out among its high-income peers for not guaranteeing access to affordable and comprehensive healthcare, including mental health care. Approximately 8% or almost 30 million Americans do not have health insurance (Centers for Disease Control and Prevention, 2024). Although significant strides have been made toward increasing insurance coverage, namely through the Affordable Care Act (ACA) and Medicaid expansion, access issues related to lack of insurance coverage persist. Payers historically have reimbursed less for mental health and SUD services compared with physical health services, often mental health care providers do not accept insurance even if an individual is insured, and regulators have not appropriately monitored or enforced policies such as the Mental Health Parity and Addiction Equity Act (National Alliance on Mental Illness, 2015; Morales et al., 2020).

Gaps in insurance coverage are exacerbated by a scarcity of mental health professionals and unequal geographic distribution. Mental health provider shortages are present in every U.S. state. In 2023, over half (52.7%) of the U.S. population lived in counties that are designated as Mental Health Professional Shortage Areas (Davenport, 2023). This provider gap is comparatively worse in the United States relative to other high-income countries. Countries such as the Netherlands and Sweden more frequently include mental health providers on primary care teams. Whereas, just one third of U.S. primary care practices have mental health professionals on their team, more than 90% in the Netherlands and Sweden include mental health professionals (Tikkanen, 2020). Additionally, access to mental health care in the United States is unevenly distributed across the country, with rural areas facing severe shortages of mental health professionals. Rural Americans are more likely to experience mental health issues and less likely to receive treatment because of factors such as fewer providers and greater distances to access care (Morales et al., 2020).

Poverty is a major risk factor for mental health issues. The United States has among the highest rates of overall poverty and child poverty of all high-income countries (and many less affluent ones). The relative poverty rate, which is the proportion of the population with low incomes relative to the median income, has been higher in the United States than in other high-income countries since at least 1980 (National Research Council and Institute of Medicine, 2013). People living in poverty are 2 to 3 times more likely to develop mental health issues than those with higher incomes. Further, there is evidence that the relationship between financial resources and mental health is nonlinear such that the impact of increased resources in low-income households has a greater impact in reducing stress and depression (Joseph Rowntree Foundation, 2015). The implication is that for low-income households, policies that increase access to financial resources have a disproportionately large positive impact on mental health.

Lastly, the United States has the highest incarceration rate among high-income countries, and this has increased over time. The absolute number of people in prison in the United States has tripled since the 1980s (Wagner, 2020), and Black males are more than

6 times more likely than White males to be incarcerated, with implications for mental health care (Nellis, 2021). An estimated 44% of individuals in jails and prisons have been diagnosed with a mental health disorder (James, 2006). Furthermore, access to mental health care within the prison system is often inadequate, leaving many inmates without the necessary treatment and support (Fazel et al., 2016). The prison environment often exacerbates these conditions, leading to a cycle of worsening mental health and increased recidivism (Fazel et al., 2016).

Although access to mental health care and resources is most definitely a human right, there is also an economic case to be made: improving mental health and equitable access to care could save billions. Mental health care costs, including those related to equitable access to care, in the United States are enormous. A recent report led by Dawes et al. (2024) estimates that the United States spends $477.5 billion each year in avoidable and unnecessary expenses related to mental health inequities. Improved access to care and recognition and appropriate treatment of mental health conditions can decrease frequency of medical visits, reduce the likelihood of chronic disease, and improve both physical and mental health outcomes (Reeves et al., 2011). Conversely, not addressing mental health issues and equitable access to mental health care will both perpetuate poorer health outcomes in marginalized and vulnerable communities and cost the United States trillions. By 2040, the cost of not addressing mental health inequities is projected to rise to $1.26 trillion annually (Dawes et al., 2024).

A report by the National Research Council (2013) asked the question: If the United States spends so much more per capita on healthcare than any other country, why are our health outcomes so poor, specifically compared with other high-income countries? Although its focus was on physical health, the National Research Council identified four features that distinguish top-performing countries from the United States, with important lessons for mental health equity. Namely, they found that better performing countries (a) provide for universal coverage and remove cost barriers; (b) invest in primary care systems to ensure that high-value services are equitably available in all areas and to all people; (c) reduce administrative burdens that divert time, efforts, and spending from health improvement efforts; and (d) invest in social services, especially for children and working-age adults.

Social determinants of mental health, such as income, education, and social support, are crucial factors that shape mental health outcomes by influencing the conditions in which people live, work, and interact. However, although these determinants are foundational, the political determinants of health—such as voting, governance, policies, and laws—are the mechanisms through which meaningful change can be enacted. More specifically, the political determinants of health encompass the systematic process of structuring relationships, distributing resources, and administering power that collectively impact health equity (Dawes, 2020). It is by addressing political determinants, such as equitable health policies, funding for mental health services, and social welfare programs, that we can create the structural changes necessary to improve mental health outcomes. Thus, political action is essential for transforming the social conditions that drive mental health disparities.

EXAMPLES OF SUCCESSFULLY ADDRESSING MENTAL HEALTH EQUITY

Efforts to address mental health equity have seen success both in the United States and globally. In the United States, the ACA included major mental health reforms, such as significantly expanding access to mental health services by requiring health insurance plans to cover mental health and SUD services as essential benefits (Dawes, 2018; Sommers et al., 2015). The ACA significantly increased funding for community health centers (CHCs), which serve as a critical access point for low-income and minority populations. CHCs are required to provide care that is culturally competent and responsive to the needs of the communities they serve. The expansion of CHCs under the ACA has improved access to care for minority groups, reduced health disparities, and enhanced the quality of care by ensuring that providers are better equipped to meet the diverse needs of their patients (Shin et al., 2015).

Similarly, expansion of Medicaid increased access to mental health care among low-income adults, increasing insurance coverage and access to mental health services for underserved populations, and helped reduce disparities in care (Wen et al., 2015). Both the ACA and expansion of Medicaid has improved continuity of care by reducing gaps in coverage and enabling more consistent access to health services, ultimately preventing interruptions in treatment.

Community-based programs have also been effective. In the United States, the Mental Health First Aid (MHFA) program trains individuals to recognize and respond to signs of mental health issues in their communities. Since its inception in 2008, MHFA has trained more than 2.5 million Americans, helping to reduce stigma and increase early intervention (Forthal et al., 2022).

Globally, the WHO's Mental Health Gap Action Programme (mhGAP) aims to scale up services for mental, neurological, and substance use disorders in low- and middle-income countries. The program focuses on integrating mental health into primary care, training nonspecialist health workers, and ensuring medication availability. Dozens of countries have successfully implemented mhGAP since its launch in 2010, resulting in improved symptoms management and increased access to mental health care (Keynejad et al., 2021).

These notable successes, which have improved access to care, reduced stigma, and increased integration of mental health services into communities and primary care, reflect the significant efforts of mental health champions and policy makers. However, although these achievements mark an important start, continued commitment and action are necessary to fully realize mental health equity and address remaining gaps in access and support. Celebrating progress should inspire ongoing efforts to build a more inclusive and equitable mental health system.

SUMMARY

Despite increased attention to mental health issues, significant inequities in mental health outcomes and access to care, treatment, and supports remain. Racial and ethnic minorities, low-income individuals, and those living in rural areas often face significant barriers to accessing mental health services, treatment, and supports, including financial constraints, lack of providers, and cultural stigma. These groups are also more likely to receive lower quality care and experience worse outcomes, such as higher rates of depression, anxiety, and suicide. Understanding the current state of mental health inequities is crucial for identifying gaps in the system and areas where targeted interventions are needed.

Advancing mental health equity requires a comprehensive approach that includes both systemic changes and targeted interventions. Key strategies include expanding access to mental health services, particularly in underserved communities, through policies that increase funding, support workforce development, and integrate mental health care into primary care settings. Additionally, addressing social determinants of health through initiatives that improve education, housing, and economic opportunities can help reduce the underlying causes of mental health disparities. Collaboration among policy makers, healthcare providers, and community organizations is vital for implementing these strategies and achieving sustainable progress in mental health equity.

Critically, we need to change the way we view mental health. Specifically, mental health exists on a continuum and is much more than the absence of illness. Mental health is a resource that enables a positive state of well-being: it is an intrinsic part of our individual and collective health, allowing us to connect with others, function, cope with stress, and achieve our full potential (Patel et al., 2018). A majority of national indicators of mental health focus on clinical classifications such as the prevalence of depression or anxiety rather than measures of positive mental health, such as well-being. The framing of mental health as the absence of mental health conditions targets those with currently active disease or who meet a predefined threshold whereas the promotion of positive mental health targets all members of society. The predominant illness-centric model targets few people, intervenes only after illness has begun, and is fundamentally reactive (Westerhof & Keyes, 2010). Although this is shifting slowly, it is critical to reframe mental health by using indicators of positive mental health to drive evidence-based policy decisions (Organisation for Economic Co-operation and Development, 2013). In this way, we will address not only clinical solutions for illness, but upstream factors that will promote positive mental health and contribute to overall well-being.

A deeper understanding of mental health equity, the intersectional issues impacting it, and the ensuing frameworks, models, interventions, policies, and programs discussed in this volume provides the ideal canvas upon which solutions to some of society's most pressing and challenging problems can be envisioned, developed, and implemented.

DISCUSSION QUESTIONS

1. How can we ensure that everyone, regardless of their background, has a fair opportunity to achieve mental well-being?
2. In what ways do societal and systemic factors shape mental health outcomes in different communities?
3. How can policy interventions advance mental health equity for population groups?
4. Describe the community you grew up in. Do you think it provides equitable mental health services or supports? What services or programs would you prioritize to support mental health equity?
5. Can you think of examples of innovative approaches that have successfully addressed mental health disparities? What lessons can we learn from them?

REFERENCES

American Addiction Centers. (2022). *Alcohol and drug abuse statistics.* https://americanaddictioncenters.org/addiction-statistics

Bambra, C., Riordan, R., Ford, J., & Matthews, F. (2020). The COVID-19 pandemic and health inequalities. *Journal of Epidemiology and Community Health, 74*(11), 964–968. https://doi.org/10.1136/jech-2020-214401

Bignall, T. (2019). *Racial disparities in mental health.* Race Equity Foundation.

Blondeel, K., Say, L., Chou, D., Toskin, I., Khosla, R., Scolaro, E., & Temmerman, M. (2016). Evidence and knowledge gaps on the disease burden in sexual and gender minorities: A review of systematic reviews. *International Journal for Equity in Health, 15,* 16. https://doi.org/10.1186/s12939-016-0304-1

Centers for Disease Control and Prevention. (2024). *Health insurance coverage: Early release of quarterly estimates from the National Health Interview Survey, January 2023–March 2024.* https://www.cdc.gov/nchs/nhis/index.htm?CDC_AA_refVal(https%3A%2F%2Fwww.cdc.gov%2Fnchs%2Fnhis.htm

Chan, J. K. N., Correll, C. U., Wong, C. S. M., Chu, R. S. T., Fung, V. S. C., Wong, G. H. S., Lei, J. H. C., & Chang, W. C. (2023). Life expectancy and years of potential life lost in people with mental disorders: A systematic review and meta-analysis. *eClinicalMedicine, 65,* 102294. https://doi.org/10.1016/j.eclinm.2023.102294

Culyer, A. J., & Wagstaff, A. (1993). Equity and equality in health and health care. *Journal of Health Economics, 12*(4), 431–457. https://doi.org/10.1016/0167-6296(93)90004-x

Davenport, S., Darby, B., Gray, T.J., Spear, C. (2023). Access across America: State-by-state insights into the accessibility of care for mental health and substance use disorders. *Milliman Report, 2.* https://www.inseparable.us/AccessAcrossAmerica.pdf

Dawes, D. E., (2018). *150 Years of ObamaCare.* Johns Hopkins University Press. https://doi.org/10.56021/9781421419633

Dawes, D. E. (2020). *The political determinants of health.* Johns Hopkins University Press. https://doi.org/10.56021/9781421437903

Dawes, D., Bhatt, J., Dunlap, N., Amador, C., Gebreyes, K., Rush, B., Westfall, J. Fendrich, M., Davis, A., Keita Fakeye, M., Philip, C., Wade, N., Hernandez, D., & Dhar, A. (2024). *The projected cost and economic impact of mental health inequities in the United States*. Meharry School of Global Health.

Favril, L., Rich, J. D., Hard, J., & Fazel, S. (2024). Mental and physical health morbidity among people in prisons: An umbrella review. *The Lancet Public Health, 9*(4), e250–e260. https://doi.org/10.1016/S2468-2667(24)00023-9

Fazel, S., Hayes, A. J., Bartellas, K., Clerici, M., & Trestman, R. (2016). Mental health of prisoners: Prevalence, adverse outcomes, and interventions. *The Lancet. Psychiatry, 3*(9), 871–881. https://doi.org/10.1016/S2215-0366(16)30142-0

Forthal, S., Sadowska, K., Pike, K. M., Balachander, M., Jacobsson, K., & Hermosilla, S. (2022). Mental health first aid: A systematic review of trainee behavior and recipient mental health outcomes. *Psychiatric Services (Washington, D.C.), 73*(4), 439–446. https://doi.org/10.1176/appi.ps.202100027

GBD 2019 Mental Disorders Collaborators. (2022). Global, regional, and national burden of 12 mental disorders in 204 countries and territories, 1990–2019: A systematic analysis for the Global Burden of Disease Study 2019. *The Lancet Psychiatry, 9*(2), 137–150. https://doi.org/10.1016/S2215-0366(21)00395-3

Hert, M., Correll, C. U., Bobes, J., Cetkovich-Bakmas, M., Cohen, D., Asai, I., Detraux, J., Gautam, S., Möller, H.-J., Ndetei, D. M., Newcomer, J. W., Uwakwe, R., & Leucht, S. (2011). Physical illness in patients with severe mental disorders. I. Prevalence, impact of medications and disparities in health care. *World Psychiatry: Official Journal of the World Psychiatric Association (WPA), 10*(1), 52–77. https://doi.org/10.1002/j.2051-5545.2011.tb00014.x

Howell, E., & McFeeters, J. (2008). Children's mental health care: Differences by race/ethnicity in urban/rural areas. *Journal of Health Care for the Poor and Underserved, 19*(1), 237–247. https://doi.org/10.1353/hpu.2008.0008

Huppert, F. A., & So, T. T. C. (2013). Flourishing across Europe: Application of a new conceptual framework for defining well-being. *Social Indicators Research, 110*(3), 837–861. https://doi.org/10.1007/s11205-011-9966-7

James, D. J. (2006). *Mental health problems of prison and jail inmates*. Bureau of Justice Statistics Special Report.

Joseph Rowntree Foundation. (2015, January 26). *Does money in adulthood affect adult outcomes*? https://www.jrf.org.uk/work/does-money-in-adulthood-affect-adult-outcomes

Katon, W. J. (2011). Epidemiology and treatment of depression in patients with chronic medical illness. *Dialogues in Clinical Neuroscience, 13*(1), 7–23.

Keynejad, R., Spagnolo, J., & Thornicroft, G. (2021). WHO mental health gap action programme (mhGAP) intervention guide: Updated systematic review on evidence and impact. *BMJ Ment Health, 24*(3), 124–130. https://doi.org/10.1136/ebmental-2021-300254

Kinner, S. A., & Young, J. T. (2018). Understanding and improving the health of people who experience incarceration: An overview and synthesis. *Epidemiologic Reviews, 40*(1), 4–11. https://doi.org/10.1093/epirev/mxx018

Leong, F. T. L., & Kalibatseva, Z. (2011). Cross-cultural barriers to mental health services in the United States. *Cerebrum: The Dana Forum on Brain Science, 2011*, 5.

Marmot, M., & Bell, R. (2012). Fair society, healthy lives. *Public Health, 126*(Suppl 1), S4–S10. https://doi.org/10.1016/j.puhe.2012.05.014

Moitra, M., Santomauro, D., Degenhardt, L., Collins, P. Y., Whiteford, H., Vos, T., & Ferrari, A. (2021). Estimating the risk of suicide associated with mental disorders: A systematic review and meta-regression analysis. *Journal of Psychiatric Research, 137*, 242–249. https://doi.org/10.1016/j.jpsychires.2021.02.053

Morales, D. A., Barksdale, C. L., & Beckel-Mitchener, A. C. (2020). A call to action to address rural mental health disparities. *Journal of Clinical and Translational Science, 4*(5), 463–467. https://doi.org/10.1017/cts.2020.42

National Alliance on Mental Illness. (2015). *A long road ahead*. https://www.nami.org/wp-content/uploads/2023/08/2015-ALongRoadAhead.pdf

National Alliance on Mental Illness. (2021). *Mental health by the numbers*. https://www.nami.org/learn-more/mental-health-by-the-numbers

National Research Council & Institute of Medicine. (2013). In S. H. Woolf & L. Aron (Eds.), *U.S. health in international perspective: Shorter lives, poorer health*. National Academies Press (US). http://www.ncbi.nlm.nih.gov/books/NBK115854/

Naylor, C., Parsonage, M., McDaid, D., Knapp, M., Fossey, M., & Galea, A. (2012). *Long-term conditions and mental health: The cost of co-morbidities*. The Kings Fund.

Nellis, A. (2021, October 13). *The color of justice: Racial and ethnic disparity in state prisons*. The Sentencing Project. https://www.sentencingproject.org/reports/the-color-of-justice-racial-and-ethnic-disparity-in-state-prisons-the-sentencing-project/

Organisation for Economic Co-operation and Development. (2013). *OECD guidelines on measuring subjective well-being*. OECD Publishing. http://www.ncbi.nlm.nih.gov/books/NBK189560/

Patel, V., Saxena, S., Lund, C., Thornicroft, G., Baingana, F., Bolton, P., Chisholm, D., Collins, P. Y., Cooper, J. L., Eaton, J., Herrman, H., Herzallah, M. M., Huang, Y., Jordans, M. J. D., Kleinman, A., Medina-Mora, M. E., Morgan, E., Niaz, U., Omigbodun, O., ... UnÜtzer, Jü. (2018). The Lancet Commission on global mental health and sustainable development. *Lancet (London, England), 392*(10157), 1553–1598. https://doi.org/10.1016/S0140-6736(18)31612-X

Pollock, N. J., Naicker, K., Loro, A., Mulay, S., & Colman, I. (2018). Global incidence of suicide among Indigenous peoples: A systematic review. *BMC Medicine, 16*(1), 145. https://doi.org/10.1186/s12916-018-1115-6

Reeves, W. C., Strine, T. W., Pratt, L. A., Thompson, W., Ahluwalia, I., Dhingra, S. S., McKnight-Eily, L. R., Harrison, L., D'Angelo, D. V., Williams, L., Morrow, B., Gould, D., Safran, M. A., & Centers for Disease Control and Prevention (CDC). (2011). Mental illness surveillance among adults in the United States. *MMWR Supplements, 60*(3), 1–29.

Scott, K. M., Lim, C., Al-Hamzawi, A., Alonso, J., Bruffaerts, R., Caldas-de-Almeida, J. M., Florescu, S., de Girolamo, G., Hu, C., de Jonge, P., Kawakami, N., Medina-Mora, M. E., Moskalewicz, J., Navarro-Mateu, F., O'Neill, S., Piazza, M., Posada-Villa, J., Torres, Y., & Kessler, R. C. (2016). Association of mental disorders with subsequent chronic physical conditions: World mental health surveys from 17 countries. *JAMA Psychiatry, 73*(2), 150–158. https://doi.org/10.1001/jamapsychiatry.2015.2688

Sheiham, A. (2008). *A report of the World Health Organization Commission on Social Determinants of Health.* World Health Organization.

Shin, P., Sharac, J., Barber, Z., Rosenbaum, S., & Published, J. P. (2015, March 17). Community health centers: A 2013 profile and prospects as ACA implementation proceeds. *KFF.* https://www.kff.org/medicaid/issue-brief/community-health-centers-a-2013-profile-and-prospects-as-aca-implementation-proceeds/

Sommers, B. D., Gunja, M. Z., Finegold, K., & Musco, T. (2015). Changes in self-reported insurance coverage, access to care, and health under the Affordable Care Act. *JAMA, 314*(4), 366–374. https://doi.org/10.1001/jama.2015.8421

Substance Abuse and Mental Health Services Administration. (2020). *Key substance use and mental health indicators in the United States: Results from the 2019 National Survey on Drug Use and Health.* https://library.samhsa.gov/product/results-2019-national-survey-drug-use-and-health-nsduh-key-substance-use-and-mental-health

Substance Abuse and Mental Health Services Administration. (2021). *Key substance use and mental health indicators in the United States: Results from the 2020 National Survey on Drug Use and Health* (HHS Publication No. PEP21-07-01-003, NSDUH Series H-56). Center for Behavioral Health Statistics and Quality, Substance Abuse and Mental Health Services Administration.

Substance Abuse and Mental Health Services Administration. (2023). *Culturally, racially, and ethnically diverse communities.* https://www.samhsa.gov/communities/culturally-racially-ethnically-diverse.

Tikkanen, R. (2020). *Mental health conditions and substance use: Comparing U.S. needs and treatment capacity with those in other high-income countries.* The Commonwealth Fund.

Turrini, G., Purgato, M., Ballette, F., Nosè, M., Ostuzzi, G., & Barbui, C. (2017). Common mental disorders in asylum seekers and refugees: Umbrella review of prevalence and intervention studies. *International Journal of Mental Health Systems, 11*, 51. https://doi.org/10.1186/s13033-017-0156-0

Valentine, S. E., & Shipherd, J. C. (2018). A systematic review of social stress and mental health among transgender and gender non-conforming people in the United States. *Clinical Psychology Review, 66*, 24–38. https://doi.org/10.1016/j.cpr.2018.03.003

Vigo, D., Thornicroft, G., & Atun, R. (2016). Estimating the true global burden of mental illness. *The Lancet. Psychiatry, 3*(2), 171–178. https://doi.org/10.1016/S2215-0366(15)00505-2

Wagner, P. (2020). *Mass incarceration: The whole pie 2020.* Prison Policy Initiative.

Walker, E. R., McGee, R. E., & Druss, B. G. (2015). Mortality in mental disorders and global disease burden implications: A systematic review and meta-analysis. *JAMA Psychiatry, 72*(4), 334–341. https://doi.org/10.1001/jamapsychiatry.2014.2502

Wen, H., Druss, B. G., & Cummings, J. R. (2015). Effect of Medicaid expansions on health insurance coverage and access to care among low-income adults with behavioral health conditions. *Health Services Research, 50*(6), 1787–1809. https://doi.org/10.1111/1475-6773.12411

Westerhof, G. J., & Keyes, C. L. M. (2010). Mental illness and mental health: The two continua model across the lifespan. *Journal of Adult Development, 17*(2), 110–119. https://doi.org/10.1007/s10804-009-9082-y

World Health Organization. (2004). *Promoting mental health: Concepts, emerging evidence, practice.* https://www.who.int/publications/i/item/9241562943

2 THE HISTORIOGRAPHY OF AFRICAN AMERICAN EXPERIENCES IN RACE AND MENTAL HEALTH POLICY

KING E. DAVIS AND VANESSA JACKSON

LEARNING OBJECTIVES

After reading this chapter, readers will be able to:

- Understand how historical policies shaped mental health care for African Americans.
- Explore the impact of the 1840 census on mental health policies.
- Understand the three hypotheses that undergird the development of services for African Americans.
- Examine how segregation influenced mental health care and education for professionals.
- Reflect on the long-term effects of public mental health policies on racial equity.

INTRODUCTION

A review of the literature shows the intensity of policy interest in race and mental illness in the United States, starting in the 19th century following publication of the 1840 census (Little, 2019). Many publications focused on disproportionate admissions, diagnoses, and treatment services for Black Americans (U.S. Department of Health and Human Services [HHS], 2001; Hylton, 2024; Jackson, 1998; Lewis et al., 2010; Manderscheid & Sonnenschein, 1985; Neighbors, 1984; Neighbors et al., 1989; Segrest, 2020; Summers, 2019). However, there has been limited scholarly analysis focused on the historiography of state and federal laws and policy decisions that relied on biased hypotheses, theories, and data that established overt structural inequities that compounded the burden of mental illness for Black Americans (Cohen, 1982; Dain, 1964; Davis & Jung, 2012; HHS, 2001; Downs, 2012; Drewry, 1916; Fischer, 1969; Grob, 1994; Hurd et al., 1916; Jackson, 1998; Rothman, 1970; Schor, 2017; Segrest, 2020; Summers, 2019; Zwerling, 1986).

Virginia was the first state to openly debate and enact a series of public mental health policies in the 18th and 19th centuries to create and finance the country's first state hospitals (Act Prohibiting Importation of Slaves, 1807; Dain, 1968; Drewry, 1916; Galt, 1853; Gonaver, 2018; House Joint Resolution, 1877; House Joint Resolution No. 5, 1848; Jackson, 1998; Joshi, 1999; Rothstein, 2017; Segrest, 2020; Summers, 2019; Walker, 1869). However, these first state hospitals were created primarily to meet the needs of middle-class White males thought to be disproportionately at risk for lunacy (Galt, 1845). Free Blacks with modest economic means were infrequently admitted to one of two state-owned hospitals, but the enslaved with lunacy were banned from admission at both hospitals until permissive legislation was enacted in 1846 (Act Prohibiting Importation of Slaves, 1807; Jackson, 1998). Denial of the enslaved was based on the hypothetical belief in their situational immunity and innate characteristics (Davis, 2018b; Galt, 1845; Stribling, 1845).

After the 1840 census erroneously reported that high rates of severe mental illness correlated with freedom and northern migration of Blacks, the Virginia legislature required its hospital directors to develop prospective plans for treating the enslaved. But the legislative requirement gave the directors full discretion without further oversight as to whether to admit Blacks or force them to seek services elsewhere (Admission of Patients Into the Lunatic Asylums, 1846). However, denial of admission resulted in untreated illness, delayed help-seeking, self-medication, and an increased burden of care on families and churches. The only other public options to manage the enslaved were jail or sale (Segrest, 2020). The Virginia discourse on race and risk of illness was instrumental in creating a national organization of state hospital medical superintendents that evolved into the American Psychiatric Association, which limited its focus on the depth of overt racial issues in public mental health policies and practices (Davis, 2020; Geller, 2020).

Responses to the 1840 census by Virginia's medical directors were based on opposing hypothetical perspectives. Dr. Francis T. Stribling, superintendent of the Western Lunatic Asylum, announced that the census found a correlation between a high incidence of severe illness and freedom. Stribling did not challenge the accuracy of the census findings or the methods of the census. Furthermore, Stribling narrowly interpretated the census findings as indicative of a need for separate residential services for the Black population. He also proposed that a separate segregated institution for Blacks with lunacy should be the only policy solution acceptable in Virginia (Stribling, 1845). Stribling's position on admitting Blacks was based on his belief that the behaviors of Blacks were so abhorrent it would deter the affluent White patients and staff that he sought to recruit to his hospital. However, he indicated that if the state adopted a policy of integration, it should occur only at Eastern State Hospital in Williamsburg (Wood, 2004).

Dr. John Galt was the progressive director at Eastern State Hospital and had already admitted free Blacks without awaiting a legislative directive (Gonaver, 2018). Galt critically examined the implications of the 1840 census findings and concluded that there was an insufficient rate of illness, and the limited numbers of Blacks in the population did not justify opening a separate hospital. Galt also did not find a medically acceptable reason to segregate psychiatric patients by race (Galt, 1853).

Stribling shared his race-based rationale for segregated admissions in his 1845 annual report to his board and to the public, in which he noted:

> No provisions having been made here for the comfortable accommodation of this class of patients, we have never found it practicable to admit them, although occasional applications have been made to us on behalf of free blacks and frequently of slaves. We will simply remark that for many reasons it would be desirable that an institution for colored persons should be entirely distinct from those occupied by insane whites. (Stribling, 1845)

That same year, Stribling introduced criteria for the provision of treatment for the enslaved. He saw his criteria as compatible with the idiosyncratic behavior and lower mentality of the Black population. For example, Stribling's criteria concluded that heavy labor would be the most effective treatment approach for Black patients based on their prior history of servitude and heavy manual labor (Stribling, 1845; Wood, 2004). He rationalized that treatment of all patients, even among the higher income patients in his facility, should routinely engage in activities that were congruent with and reminiscent of their pre-hospital social class lifestyles, cultural interests, and occupations. Hard labor for Blacks met that perverse standard and was deemed therapeutic.

In 1869, the Commonwealth of Virginia and the federal government formally adopted Stribling's proposal to create a racially separate asylum following the Civil War. As part of its Reconstruction policy, the federal government agreed to provide financial support to open and operate the first stand-alone mental asylum in the United States exclusively for its Black population (An Act to Establish the Central Lunatic Asylum for Colored Insane, 1870; Canby, 1869). But without public explanation, the federal government did not require, financially support, or encourage any other state to open a separate hospital for "colored" lunatics as a requirement for reentry to the Union. This Virginia-specific policy eviscerated their preexisting 1846 policy decision that Eastern State Hospital open its admissions to Blacks and openly advocate for an integration policy exclusive of the enslaved (Gonaver, 2018). The potential economic losses created by admitting free Blacks with and without lunacy were at the base of the policy decision by the state to voluntarily support segregation in state hospitals until forced by federal law to change 100 years later (Drewry, 1916; Wood, 2004).

The federal–state collaborative policy to initiate and support segregated psychiatric care became the operational state hospital model adopted across the nation for more than 100 years, until passage of the Civil Rights Act of 1964, which required racial integration (Civil Rights Act, 1964). Before its passage, however, states used a variety of overt tactics to maintain segregation through separate wards and buildings or, in a few instances, opening underfinanced hospitals such as Taft State Hospital in Oklahoma and Crownsville in Maryland (Henry, 1941; Hylton, 2024; Jackson, 1998).

This influential series of 18th and 19th century Virginia laws, polices, and medical practices predicted a higher risk of disabling illness based on a series of untested hypotheses linking race, servitude, migration, and social class (Chapter 144 of the Virginia Code, 1853; House Joint Resolution No. 5, 1848; Walker, 1869). However, the reality was that dark skin color or previous servitude did not preclude or increase the occurrence of serious illnesses, and that impending or actual freedom would not create an exaggerated frequency of illness. This reality appears to have eluded critical legal, medical, or scholarly research attention until well into the 21st century (Davis, 1998b, 2018b, 2019b; Fischer, 1969; Galt, 1845; HHS, 2001; Jackson, 1998; Weaver, 1841; Whaley, 2005). Part of the tragic outcome of the application of these hypotheses was the reporting of excessive diagnoses of severe illness in Black populations and homelessness after discharge from mental health hospitals and facilities (Lawson et al., 1994; Lewis et al., 2006; Manderscheid & Sonnenschein, 1985; Snowden, 2000).

Passage of the Federal Slave Importation Act (Act Prohibiting Importation of Slaves, 1807), barring future involuntary labor, gave supporters of continued enslavement the impetus to introduce extralegal methods that generalized its application to mental illness. These methods included interpreting efforts by the enslaved to secure their freedom and exercise constitutional rights as a priori evidence of mental pathology. These views also reflected pronounced fears of impending physical danger from marauding Black men (Act Prohibiting Importation of Slaves, 1807; Davis, 1998b; Galt, 1853; Jefferson, 1806). Another of the most unsubstantiated and pernicious methods was interpreting the desire to escape slave status as a unique Black psychological disorder cured only by continued enslavement (Cartwright, 1851; Weaver, 1841). Without evidence, enslavement was viewed as therapeutic and rationalized as a preventive psychiatric strategy that would provide external control of Black bodies and reconstruction of Black minds (Gates, 1997, 2019; Kendi, 2016).

The predictions and the impending fears that all 500,000 enslaved Black persons in Virginia would soon be free citizens seems to have contributed to reversing the long-held caricatured persona of the enslaved as passive/docile/happy people who were simply grateful for a secondary place in the colonial economy. However, the reconstructed persona of "Free emancipated Negroes" transformed into mentally disturbed lunatics, rivals, agitators, vagrants, addicts, rapists, welfare cheats, and thieves that were considered dangerous, devious, and physically threatening (Gates, 2019; Gray, 1831).

This negative Black persona portrayed the formerly enslaved as inciting civil disturbance and disruptive legal challenges that needed to be externally controlled, lest they do harm to the extant sociopolitical order (Alexander, 2012; Gray, 1831; Martin, 2023; Pepper, 2016; Williams, 2013). Metzl alluded to this phenomenon when he noted the increase in severe psychiatric diagnoses and increased rates of incarceration of Black men associated with civil rights activities, demonstrations, civil disobedience, boycotts, and lawsuits (Metzl, 2009). As recently as 2023, efforts by progressive political groups to petition government to sustain affirmative action and protect the right to vote were labeled as pathological (Cole, 2020).

When formerly disenfranchised individuals sought to freely exercise their newly granted constitutional/civil rights, their actions were interpreted for over a century as being synonymous with pathology and illegality, and defined in public laws and in the media as lunacy, insanity, or the result of smaller cranial size (Boster, 2013; Cartwright, 1851; Coates, 2014; Joshi, 1999; Martin, 2023; Metzl, 2009; Miller, 1896; Neighbors & Jackson, 1996; Oates, 1982; Rothstein, 2017; Savitt, 1975, 2007). Disproportionate admission rates to state facilities for the developmentally disabled, criminal, and mentally ill reflect this racial bias that attributed causality to skin color (Alexander, 2012; Davis, 2018a; Davis et al., 2011; Manderscheid & Sonnenschein, 1987).

The perception of free Blacks as physically and mentally threatening was a major impediment to public acceptance of racial integration of state hospitals, schools, colleges, public office, workplaces, public transportation, and neighborhoods well into the 21st century (*Brown v. Board of Education*, 1954; Feagin & Feagin, 1978; Grossack, 1963; Hernton, 1965; Segrest, 2020). The Supreme Court decision in *Plessy v. Ferguson* (*Plessy v. Ferguson*, 1896) concluded that the Black population, whether enslaved or free, could never be citizens of the United States based on pernicious racial differences. Similar interpretations of color were found in the debates and publications of medical practitioners (Cartwright, 1851; Jarvis, 1852; Smith, 1851).

Our analysis of hundreds of primary source documents obtained from the Central Lunatic Asylum for Colored Insane archives helps to explain how the systemically biased political, religious, educational, cultural, economic, and medical pathways led to exaggerated diagnoses of severe mental illness and admissions of Blacks (Davis, 2019b; Hylton, 2024; Jackson, 1998; Segrest, 2020; Summers, 2019). We propose that long-term race-based mental health policies and unequal practices had their origins in the application of three sequential hypotheses that falsely and inconsistently ascribed a causal relationship to Blackness, freedom, urban residence, and the risk and danger of severe mental illness, particularly in relation to Black men (Lewis et al., 2006; Malzberg, 1963a; Metzl, 2009; Neighbors & Lumpkin, 1990; Pasamanick, 1963; Wilson, 1963). Identification, definition, and analysis of the immunity, disproportionality, and disparity hypotheses form the theoretical bases of this chapter.

THE IMMUNITY HYPOTHESIS, PRE-1860

> Slaves are immune from much of the mental excitement to which the free population of the Union is necessarily exposed in the daily routine of life. Again, they have not the anxious cares and anxieties relative to property, which tend to depress some of our free citizens. (Galt, 1845, p. 25)

The term *immunity* has several meanings when used in legal, civic, and biomedical contexts. In biomedicine, *immunity* is broadly defined as not being susceptible to a disease condition or being exempt or free from an illness. Immunologists attempt to identify and study known risk factors that produce an immunity in individuals, groups, populations, or regions so that methods can be developed to treat, prevent, or eradicate the disease condition and its causes.

Immunities can be innate, adaptive, or situational. An innate immunity means that the individuals possess an inborn or natural ability to defend against a condition, whereas an adaptive immunity suggests that it derives from inoculation, vaccination, avoidance of pathogens, or control of known risk factors. For example, at the outset of the COVID-19 pandemic, little was known about the causes or sources of the pathogen or the risk factors, so no immediate therapeutic or preventive intervention could be applied. Biomedical researchers were able to create a novel vaccine to reduce the overall rate of COVID infection. However, even after vaccines were widely available, mortality rates within elderly, disabled, medically compromised, racial and ethnic minority, and impoverished populations were among the highest in the nation (Foster, 2024; Mude, 2021). So, too, were the mortality rates among registered Republicans when compared with those among registered Democrats (Wallace, 2022). Part of the successful biomedical intervention was based on lowering transmission rates in various populations based on their willingness to wear masks, increase handwashing, and socially distance themselves. There is an assumption, however, that the factors or variables that cause a disease are identified or recognizable and can be used to formulate hypotheses for study (Rubin & Babbie, 2008).

A situational immunity derives its protectiveness from specialized circumstances or conditions in which the individual or group is found. Historically, such characteristics as skin color, racial background, gender, religion, sinfulness, legal status (free or enslaved), morality, intelligence, education, or ownership of property were hypothesized to either increase or decrease the risk of contracting lunacy. Initially, slavery was a situation that was hypothesized to offer the enslaved immunity from contracting lunacy, resulting in either lower frequency or total absence of the disorder. Hypothetically, slavery was thought to offer some unknown protective shield for the enslaved. In addition, the situational immunity was hypothesized to be a function of an absence of involvement of Blacks in situations and conditions that were believed to increase the risk of lunacy, at least in Whites. These included participation in commercial activities, political engagement, and ownership of the enslaved. However, this situational (non-enslaved) hypothesis suggests that the White male population was at a higher risk of developing lunacy compared with enslaved Blacks, who, by law, could not be owners or office holders.

De facto racial segregation was ubiquitous across almost all social institutions in the United States until well into the 20th century. The effects of this history of segregation remain in various segments of the society today (Conley, 1999; Stiglitz, 2012). The association of Blackness as a prime causal factor in mental illness seems to have evolved soon after the publication of the 1840 census, preceded by the legal end of slave importation. Before 1840, the primary hypothesis quoted by Galt held that Blacks, particularly the enslaved, were immune from the ravages of lunacy (**Figure 2.1**). As ludicrous as it appears, the enslaved were described by Galt as protected from stresses he identified as the hypothetical sources of lunacy. Conceptually, it was freedom—rather than slavery—and full participation in the nooks and crannies of colonial society that Galt hypothesized would wither the protective shield afforded through enslavement. Surprisingly, Galt countered Stribling's view that race was the determining factor in illness or recovery and unsuccessfully petitioned for a state policy that would have permitted providing treatment for Blacks and Whites in the same institutions as he demonstrated in his facility (Galt, 1853). Oddly, Galt failed to identify and define slavery as a major source of stress, trauma, and angst for Blacks. He seemed not to have considered the immense physical and emotional effects that slavery and enslavement posed to the individuals most affected. Because enslaved populations were legally a propertyless class unable to participate in ownership or civic affairs, it was assumed that they were less at risk for lunacy or insanity than the wealthier and free White men who held, owned,

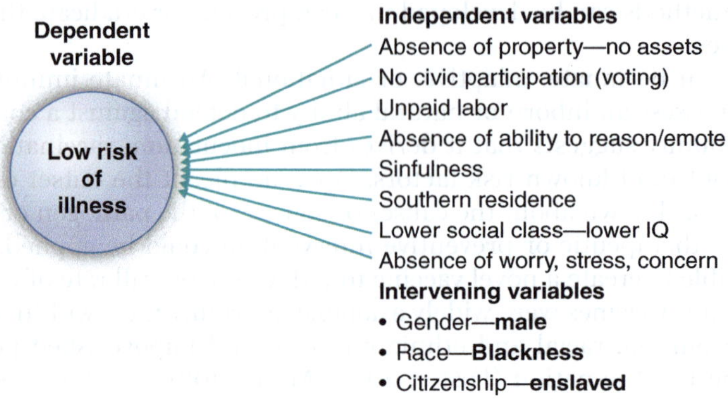

Figure 2.1 The immunity hypothesis, 1765–1865.

and managed them as human property. Galt's endorsement of immunity implied that the enslaved would become as vulnerable to lunacy as White men if slavery ended and they were free to engage in similar commercial and civic activities. Because of his stature, the conclusions reached by Galt had the potential to influence theory, practice, education, and policy for several decades (Davis, 2018a).

Clearly, Galt placed his psychiatric vision on socioeconomic determinants as the primary factors that gave rise to lunacy. As long as Blacks remained in the cocoon of slavery and free of civic and economic engagement, he believed they would remain free of lunacy while White men would be more vulnerable. However, the small numbers of Blacks affected could be easily accommodated and admitted—along with Whites—into either of Virginia's two institutions (Galt, 1845, 1846, 1853). The 1846 legislation that permitted conjoint admission of slaves affected only Eastern, reflecting the significant political dominance and influence wielded by Stribling as the more senior state psychiatrist (Act Prohibiting Importation of Slaves, 1807).

In addition to socioeconomic causes, Blacks were considered to lack the capacity for reason and were seen as at lower or no risk of developing lunacy. The concept of sin as causation also implied that the spread or distribution of lunacy was not universal and that some individuals and families escaped by not committing the sin, had no innate vulnerability, or were immune in some unknown way (Dain, 1964). The stigma of lunacy and efforts to banish the person affected was related to the fear that the misdeed and punishment or an unexpected harm might spread to others. Treatment often consisted of confinement, jailing, expulsion, bloodletting, or the use of strong purgatives to cleanse and remove the causes (Dain, 1980; Galt, 1846; Grob, 1973; Hinshaw, 2007). It was not until the latter part of the 18th century that mental and physical illness began to be viewed more as diseases that stem from identifiable pathogenic or environmental causes that could be controlled. The critical issue was the ability to identify causes, as did Koch in his discovery of the tuberculosis bacillus (Koch, 1882). Individuals who did not develop tuberculosis had either an innate or adaptable immunity from the bacillus.

This hypothetical, racially oriented reasoning could also have been used to unscientifically predict lower vulnerability and rates of mental illness in lower income Whites, Native Americans, women, and freedmen (Steen, 1991; Tasca 2012; Whaley, 2001). According to the flawed findings in and conclusions drawn from the 1840 census, the risk of lunacy was not spread universally or evenly in the population, which may have implied that vulnerability to lunacy might have been developed from unidentifiable determinants that were hidden and acquired from within the environment (e.g., migration) or that some populations were at higher risk because of their innate vulnerability.

Implications of Immunity

Before 1840, only a few free Blacks were allowed limited access to services in the first state mental hospital at Williamsburg, Virginia (Dain, 1968; Davis, 2022; Gonaver, 2018; Jackson, 1998). However, slaves were not allowed entry into the asylum until 1846 and only if the cost of their care was borne by their captors. Free Blacks could be admitted but not if by doing so, White Virginias were denied admission. Additionally, lunacy was viewed by physicians and politicians as a loss of reason. Enslaved African Americans were considered to lack an innate intellectual ability to reason or experience normative emotions, such as grief or sadness, thus further eliminating their risk of contracting lunacy (Fauquier, 1766).

The hypothesis that Blacks were immune from lunacy or insanity, despite abundant evidence to the contrary within the population, was easily used as justification throughout the South for failing to provide treatment services (Davis, 2018b; Drewry, 1900; Galt, 1853; Segrest, 2020). As early as 1800, however, South Carolina expected owners of the enslaved to be responsible for care of disabled slaves before the state or local community would intervene (History of the Ministry of Defence, 1998). Their intervention often involved forced residence in the workhouse. It seems probable that symptoms of serious illness were frequently ignored and easily interpreted as malingering as a means of avoiding labor. Diagnoses of serious illness in Blacks would have been missed, misinterpreted, and likely resulted in a high proportion of untreated individuals suffering from a plethora of mental disabilities. A third implication is that the absence of medical recognition of illness in the population could have the effect of encouraging reliance on informal culturally based approaches and excessive delays in help-seeking, as noted by Neighbors and others (Deutsch, 1944b; Hurd et al., 1916; Jackson, 1998; Neighbors, 1985).

THE DISPROPORTIONALITY HYPOTHESIS

> It has frequently been observed that prior to the war there were very few insane negroes, yet since then there has been a constant increase in their numbers ... A well-nourished, intelligent, thrifty negro, leading a correct life, is probably little more liable to become insane than a white person under similar conditions, except for the fact that the powers of resistance and endurance are weaker in his race than in the white race. In short, the negro is to-day an easier prey to constitutional diseases than the whites, succumbs more readily to strain, stress, and disease. (Drewry, 1916)

Dr. Francis Drewry introduced the disproportionality hypothesis to explain his dire prediction that the incidence of severe psychiatric illness in the Black population would markedly increase following the ending of the Civil War. He builds on the series of assumptions found in the 1840 census that freedom and migration were detrimental to the mental health of the enslaved Black population. Slavery, in his thesis, represented a healing salve for a defective Black mind.

Disproportionality is a statistical indicator in which the frequency of a disease or diagnosis significantly exceeds the expected frequency of occurrence within a group, population, or region. Until publication of the 1840 census, Black populations were hypothesized as having a situational or natural immunity from the risk for lunacy and/or insanity. At best, the observed rate of illness within this population was considered as significantly below expectations compared with White populations. Before 1840, the group considered as most at risk for lunacy were White men of wealth and influence. But as the Civil War ended, the disproportionate rate hypothesis that undergirded the 1840 census predicted that the rates of lunacy, mental disability, dependency, and crime in the newly freed Black population would increase exponentially, resulting in heightened demand for treatment and increased governmental policies and costs to provide inpatient hospital care that was historically denied for this segment of the population. Such a prediction raised trepidation and discomfort in the predominately White population amid increased calls to provide protection. The 500,000 Blacks who were on the cusp of freedom in Virginia at the close of the Civil War were seen by many as a source of imminent danger and dependency because of their vulnerability (Dain, 1964; Segrest, 2020; Wood, 2004).

In 1885, Dr. Randolph Barksdale, director of Central State Hospital (CSH), added to the application of disproportionate increases in lunacy and insanity of Blacks after the Civil War (**Figure 2.2**) by remarking, "the increase in insanity in this race is amazing....If the state intends to take proper care of insane colored people she will either have to enlarge here or build another institution somewhere else" to control the excess (Superintendent of Central Lunatic Asylum, 1885). Jarvis, a late opponent of the statistical descriptions in the 1840 census, also supported the thesis that slavery offered Blacks more psychological solace than freedom:

> Throughout the civilized world, the statement has gone forth, that, according to the experience of the United States, including a slave population of near two and a half millions, and a free coloured population in the northern States of near two hundred thousand, slavery is more than ten-fold more favorable to mental health than freedom. (Jarvis, 1844)

The following seven significant events reinforced adoption of the disproportionality hypothesis after the end of the Civil War that predicted and normalized exaggerated rates of lunacy fueled by impending and actual freedom of nearly 500,000 former slaves. These excess rates of admissions and diagnoses of severe illness continued throughout the 20th century (Barker et al., 1992; HHS, 1999, 2001; Manderscheid et al., 2009; Manderscheid & Sonnenschein, 1995; Neighbors & Lumpkin, 1990).

The 1840 Census of Population

The 1840 Census of Population was the first that enumerated the purported number of persons in each state mental institution by their race, gender, disability, and region (Cohen, 1982; Deutsch, 1944a; Little, 2019; Manderscheid et al., 1986; Weaver, 1841). However, the overt level of racial bias in the published document constituted a pro-slavery endorsement by falsely concluding there was a significant difference in the frequency of lunacy and insanity by race and region of the country. Enslaved Blacks in the southern states were reported to have had rates of lunacy 5 to 10 times lower than free Blacks in northern states (Weaver, 1841). Various historical and current reports implied or reinforced the perception that the structure and process of slavery was somehow therapeutic and emotionally beneficial to Blacks by preventing them from developing lunacy (Florida Department of Education, 2023; Kendi, 2016).

Methodologically, the 1840 census of persons in institutions relied on data drawn only from admissions to public mental hospitals. However, during the years the census gathered

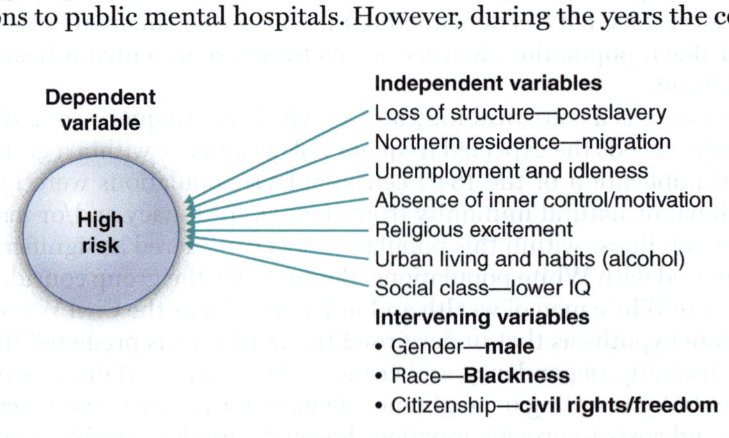

Figure 2.2 **The disproportionality hypothesis, 1865–1965.**

primary data, few public hospitals in northern states admitted Blacks as patients. Further, the census ascribed admission status to Blacks in cities where they were not part of the population (Jarvis, 1844). Additionally, there were no mental hospitals for Blacks exclusively in the highly segregated South, and only one hospital (Eastern Lunatic Asylum) in Virginia admitted both free Blacks (an average of one per year) and Whites (Davis, 2020; Drewry, 1916; Thomas & Sillen, 1972). The structural errors, unclear collection methods, inadequate data analysis, and absence of correlations were evident from published critiques of the census document (Cohen, 1982; Jarvis, 1852; Schor, 2017).

Absence of Medical Care

Enslaved Blacks were subjected to poor-quality, plantation-based medical care that prioritized maintenance of their ability to labor and breed (Blanton, 1931; Downs, 2012). However, once slaves were freed by the Union forces, Downs describes how the absence of basic medical care, food, shelter, clothing, and safety resulted in a rapid increase in excess morbidity and mortality rates as the former slaves were left economically, nutritionally, physically, and politically vulnerable following passage of the Emancipation Proclamation and rapid collapse of Reconstruction (Downs, 2012). Downs documented that postslavery government policies failed to provide adequate healthcare, resulting in high rates of morbidity and mortality (Downs, 2012). It was unclear whether the absence of mental health polices and services would result in similar behavioral outcomes. Enslaved Africans also were denied full access to the rudimentary psychiatric care offered in parishes, neighborhoods, churches, and state-sponsored mental hospitals between 1846 and 1870 (Breeden, 1976; Galt, 1853; Hurd et al., 1916; Randolph, 2003). Black families were the major source of care.

From 1770 to 1868, an average of only one Black person per year was allowed admission to Eastern Lunatic Asylum in Williamsburg (Davis, 2022; Jackson, 1998). The history of life within slave hovels suggests that the risk of harm was exceptional (Savitt, 1975, 1989). It could have been expected that the nature of enslavement, war, and postwar reactions might result in an increase in various mental disorders, particularly depression within the newly freed, yet still vulnerable Black population. However, there were no reasonable estimates of the extent that such illnesses were either present or on the cusp of occurring, except through the adoption of the disproportionality hypothesis that was more of a reactionary posture than the science of prediction.

American Psychiatric Association Commission on Race and Lunacy

Decades before the start of the Civil War, discussions about race and the need for hospital care of Blacks with mental illnesses took two divergent and conflicting perspectives. John Galt and Francis Stribling, superintendents of Virginia's first two mental asylums, held conflicting views on race and mental illness from 1844 to 1861. Throughout these years, Galt demonstrated that integrating mentally ill Blacks (free and enslaved) and Whites was a feasible practice in his asylum and proposed as the policy of the Commonwealth of Virginia. Of concern was that Galt and Stribling co-chaired the national superintendent's committee, which in 1845 sought to frame a policy that would guide the southern states in their efforts to recognize and treat mental illness in slaves. Stribling's position prevailed in the committee and provided the conceptual, medical, and political rationale for Virginia's subsequent race-based policy decision. Virginia adopted a policy of segregation despite Galt's successful, albeit numerically limited, experience in admitting and treating free Blacks (Galt, 1845, 1853).

The Virginia Asylum Commission

In 1846, the Virginia legislature considered a policy to allow for the admission of slaves into their two existing state hospitals in Williamsburg and Staunton. The language in the pending bill required the two hospital directors to assess the need for such admissions and propose how they could be provided services in their institutions. However, if the director concluded that it was not feasible to admit the enslaved, they were asked to provide an alternative. As noted, Dr. Galt suggested that his hospital would continue to accept Blacks as patients. However, the Virginia legislature passed a joint resolution in 1848 to study the long-term feasibility of developing separate wards, buildings, or a separate asylum based on Stribling's proposed policy of racially segregated care (Drewry, 1916; Hurd & Drewry, 1916).

General Canby's Order Creating Central Lunatic Asylum for Colored Insane

Virginia's post–Civil War readmission into the Union was predicated on the extent to which the state government adhered to the Freedman Bureau's requirements to accept and implement the Reconstruction Acts of 1866 and 1867 (Freedman's Bureau Acts, 1865). Specific features of Virginia's role in implementation were stipulated and driven by written military orders from Union Army General Edward Canby, who was appointed as Virginia's military governor by the Secretary of War in April 1869 (Canby, 1869).

One immediate challenge faced by Canby upon his arrival in Richmond was to find ways to reduce the exaggerated rates of morbidity and mortality within the newly freed Black population following cessation of the Civil War (Downs, 2012). The extent of psychological casualties was unknown but estimated as excessive by the newly appointed Asylum Commission chaired by Dr. Stribling (Wood, 2004)

As part of the Freedman Bureau's Reconstruction efforts, Canby hurriedly accepted consultation from the state's Asylum Commission to determine whether the primary medical mission of the hospital annex should continue or be expanded to include short-term subsidized housing, social welfare services, relocation assistance, family reconciliation, protection from physical harm, and psychiatric services to uprooted, displaced, traumatized, and economically vulnerable Blacks (Downs, 2012; Drewry, 1916; Whig, 1865). Based on its previous open admissions policy, the hospital's "colored annex" resembled and functioned as an all-purpose social service entity, available at least theoretically to admit and treat the medical and psychiatric needs of all 500,000 Black people from various small towns and larger cities across the state suffering from a variety of war-ravaged and postslavery trauma. Certainly, one could assume that the abruptness of freedom, without adequate resources or agency, would be followed by widespread and long-term trauma. The exceptionally limited Howard's Grove annex was the only source of inpatient medical and psychiatric care for Blacks in Virginia. Howard's Grove annex lacked adequate housing, heating, privacy, and safety for the patients. There was no adequate means of diverting water from flooding the grounds and contributing to infestation. Nor was there a dining hall where patients could eat or a health clinic where they could receive physical care (Drewry, 1916). Numerous modifications and improvements had to be made by the federal government to create a reasonable medical care environment.

Canby's agreement with Walker on the transformation of the Howard's Grove annex included five operational conditions to address Stribling's criteria: (a) all Black psychiatric patients housed anywhere in the state (jails, private hospitals, and Eastern Lunatic Asylum) would be transferred to the annex for admission and treatment; (b) the hospital annex could serve only Blacks with a primary diagnosis of insanity; (c) use of the Howard's Grove annex could be only temporary; (d) all existing equipment and supplies provided to Howard's Grove by the Freedman's Bureau would transfer without cost to the state; and (e) the federal government would provide additional funding in support of the unprecedented policy requirement to open a segregated asylum (Canby, 1869). One major effect of adopting these policy requirements was to maintain Stribling's refusal to accept Black patients at Western State Hospital. The second major issue was the elimination of access by race to the limited primary care provided at Howard's Grove.

Admissions to Central Lunatic Asylum for Colored Insane

From its 1870 origins, directors and board chairmen of CSH—in an effort to justify the opening of a segregated asylum for Blacks—agreed with Stribling's predictions that there would be an almost immediate postwar upsurge in rates of illness in the Black population. Dr. Hunter McGuire, a professor of medicine at the Medical College of Virginia, also served as chairman of the CSH board. He based his support on the innate and acquired differences between Blacks and Whites, noting:

> The necessity for a separate asylum for this unfortunate class is we think generally acknowledged by all who have seriously considered the subject. The disposition, temper, and habits of the colored race are so different from those of the white, and the management of the two classes so different that it would be impossible to keep and successfully treat them in the same institution. (McGuire, 1870)

McGuire's endorsement of the disproportionality hypothesis parallels the views of several directors of CSH throughout its history who predicted excessive rates of disease and incapability of joint treatment regimens. However, these predictions of excess rates of illness caused by freedom lacked data and research that did not materialize (Central Lunatic Asylum, 1870). Additionally, General Canby's agreement with Governor Walker was based on two of the criteria advocated by Stribling. First, he required a single statewide, standalone facility; second, it could accept only Black patients diagnosed with a psychiatric disorder. Both these requirements allowed Stribling's hospital to remain White (Wood, 2004).

The rate of hospitalization was continuously twice that of the Black proportion of the state's population as late as 1995. This disparate ratio in admissions by race also was found as recently as 2011 (Davis et al., 2011).

The Policy of Segregated Mental Health Care

Before 1840, physicians and politicians accepted the false belief that enslaved Black populations were situationally immune to developing lunacy. At the time, the risk of illness was hypothetically associated with the stress of civic engagement, quest for business profits, and overall management and management of personal property and family decision making (Galt, 1845). Because the enslaved were denied each of these, they were assumed to be free of stress. From 1765 to 1840, Virginia law and practice—based on the notion that slaves lacked the mental capacity to suffer from a psychiatric illness—denied any enslaved person access to a mental hospital bed (Drewry, 1916; Galt, 1853; Gonaver, 2018). Slaves whose behavior interfered with their ability to work would likely have been sent "farther south" or perhaps severely punished, abandoned, sold, jailed, or killed (Boster, 2013; Long, 2012). However, by 1846, the Commonwealth of Virginia reversed its early aversion to recognizing the risk of mental disability in the enslaved population and acceded to overtures to allow slaves entry to Eastern Lunatic Asylum, one of Virginia's two mental hospitals. From its opening in 1870 to 1968, Central Lunatic Asylum for Colored Insane (CLACI) functioned as a racially segregated hospital. Changes in federal laws in 1968 forced the Commonwealth of Virginia to accept integrated care despite continuation of the Stribling hypothesis and argument that Blacks and Whites could not be admitted and treated in the same institution.

From its origin in 1870 to 1967, CSH remained segregated by race and was the only hospital in the Commonwealth of Virginia that accepted African American mental patients from throughout the state. Black families, patients, and sheriff's officers had to travel hundreds of miles to reach CSH during segregation. Family visits were limited by the geographical barriers, and the archives show a correlation between distance from the hospital and sparse demand for service (Davis, 2015). Throughout its history, CSH has been an integral part of the city of Petersburg, Dinwiddie County, and central Virginia, offering accredited recovery, rehabilitative, and forensic evaluation and care to its citizens, extensive employment opportunities, and revenue through purchases of goods and services in the local economy (Davis, 2019a).

THE DISPARITY HYPOTHESIS

The term *disparity* originated in the 16th century in France and during that time, literally referred to measurable differences between two or more objects or people or to an absence of parity or equality (Plepys & Klein, 1995). *Disparity* has also been used in several different ways in the context of studying and addressing demographic inequities in the United States today. The National Cancer Institute defined the concept in relationship to disproportionate rates of mortality, diagnosis, and burden as evidenced by race, income, social class, or ethnicity (Center to Reduce Cancer Health Disparities, 2003). In his efforts to establish federal policy to reduce health disparities, former President Clinton defined such disparities as "differences in the incidence, prevalence, mortality, and burden of disease and other adverse health conditions that exist among specific population groups in the United States" (National Institutes of Health [NIH], 2002). These definitions emphasize the relationship between socioeconomic status and other social determinants and a variety of disparities in health.

"Health disparities are differences in the incidence, prevalence, mortality and burden of disease and other adverse health conditions that exist among specific population groups in the United States" (NIH, 2003). A related definition proposed that the concept of disparity refers "to the diminished health status of population subgroups as defined by demographic factors such as age and socioeconomic status" (National Institute of Dental and Craniofacial Research, 2002). This emphasis on equitable access to treatment reflects the IOM's policy proposal for reducing disparity in the prevalence and incidence of health problems. Anderson (2002) defines *prevalence* as a measure of the number of existing cases or health problems within a specified population, whereas *incidence* refers to the number of new cases or health problems. Despite the ubiquitous application of the term *disparity* in federal and academic reports, there is no universal agreement in the research literature or in the public policy sector about its operational definition (Atrash & Hunter, 2006; McGuire, 2006). In this chapter, therefore, *disparity* is defined simply as measurable differences in mental health diagnoses and services (quantity and quality) by race or between two or more groups, communities, organizations, or people, or an absence of parity or equity between the services available.

Additionally, the IOM describes disparities as a related train of events that are found in communities, systems, programs, policies, and organizations that increase the risk of illness (IOM, 2002). In behavioral health settings, significant racial disparities may exist in all areas of services, including design, delivery, access, diagnosis, treatment, models, location, staffing, utilization, and quality (IOM, 2002). Consumption of inpatient services ranges from underconsumption to overconsumption, with a disproportionate frequency of involuntary commitments and longer lengths of stay in residential settings (IOM, 2002). Populations of color are significantly underrepresented in almost all phases of research in mental health and clinical trials of treatment methods and medication (HHS, 2001).

Interest in understanding and reversing decades of disparities seemed to increase after the Civil Rights Act of 1964 (Civil Rights Act, 1964) required integration of previously segregated health services and the introduction of community mental health center concepts to support deinstitutionalization (Mental Retardation Facilities and Community Mental Health Centers Construction Act of 1963, 1963).

This new integrated policy direction was congruent with Fischer's research (1969). His research, and that of the Ecological Catchment Area (1978) and the National Co-morbidity Studies, (1990–1992) challenged decades of biased findings and theorizing by refuting that there were significant differences in rates of mental illness by race, ethnicity, culture, or language. Manderscheid's annual surveys on hospital admissions per 100,000 population in the 1980s also verified the relevancy of applying disparity theory. In his findings, he documented the extent that African American psychiatric admissions far exceeded not only the national average of admissions, but also those of all groups in the United States in all settings except private hospitals. **Table 2.1** shows the disproportionate admissions across types of facilities by race. However, the admission rate of African Americans to private hospitals slightly exceeded the national average by 0.3 and was only 0.5 less than the higher admission rate for Whites (Manderscheid & Sonnenschein, 1985). The Surgeon General's two critical reports, *Mental Health Culture, Race, and Ethnicity* and *Mental Health: A Report of the Surgeon General,* focused on numerous historical gaps in mental health service, education, and research disparities that were evident over decades (Davis, 2003; HSS, 1999, 2001). However, these earlier reports did not address the mortality rates of Blacks with serious mental illness, nor their post-deinstitutionalized struggles with unemployment and homelessness in large cities (Davis & Jung, 2012).

The prevailing hypotheses about mental illness ascribed causal significance to economic assets held throughout the colonial period in America, despite major changes in population and evidence of illness in populations of color and the poor (Dain, 1964; Drewry, 1916; Galt, 1845).

Although race and color have been volatile issues in American public policy, other factors have been instrumental in the conceptualization of mental illness. Poverty, mental illness, race, gender, and dependency were interdependent themes in early American philosophical and political thought (Day, 1989). To some extent, these themes underscored the powerful influence of the Elizabethan Poor Law and its religious emphasis on individual responsibility and self-sufficiency. When viewed as separate categories, the poor, mentally ill, Indians, Africans, and women were viewed as categorical economic burdens or barriers to the growth of American hegemony, independence, and democracy. However, when considered collectively, these groups were viewed as threats to the political integrity and economic survival of the nascent new world (Rothman, 1970). Rothman suggests that the negative perceptions of these populations as economically dependent threats resulted in a plethora of public policies that essentially segregated them from the inner workings of American society. Prisons, mental hospitals, poorhouses, tuberculosis sanatoria, and institutions of various kinds became their citadel. Popular science supported this policy direction for much of American history

Table 2.1 ADMISSIONS PER 100,000 BY RACE, ETHNICITY, AND FACILITY

POPULATION	TOTAL	STATE HOSPITAL	PRIVATE HOSPITAL	GENERAL HOSPITAL	VETERANS HOSPITAL
All groups	593.0	163.6	62.6	295.3	70.4
African American	931.0	364.2	62.9	386.6	118.2
American Indian	818.7	306.4	41.2	371.6	99.2
Asian American	268.1	75.4	25.0	161.0	6.6
Hispanic	452.3	146.0	34.4	227.0	44.1
White	550.0	136.8	63.4	284.9	67.9

Source: Manderscheid, R. W., & Sonnenschein, M. A. (1985). *Mental health, United States.* National Institute of Mental Health.

through its failure to offer hypotheses and epidemiological data that were counter to the false assumptions, bias, and distortions of data that supported race-based and asset-based public policy (Davis, 1998a; Metzl, 2009; Washington, 2006).

The historical disparity hypotheses linked mental health needs and disease risk to assets, race, and social class (**Figure 2.3**). These hypotheses formed the philosophical basis of much of American public mental health policy for over a century. As a result, many public mental health systems were structurally designed to meet the needs of a singular cultural group. Public laws from the Naturalization Act of 1790 to current state mental health policies excluded the cultural idiosyncrasies of racial and ethnic minority populations from guiding the creation of public policies and services. The hypotheses ranged from ideas that racial and ethnic minority individuals were immune from mental illness to those that predicted exaggerated demand for services (Davis, 2018b; Woods et al., 2012). It is proposed that disparities in both the design and delivery of mental health services were built into the fabric of American mental health care at all levels. The absence of valid epidemiological studies that provide data about the racial and ethnic differences in the needs or usage patterns of mental health care and services is congruent with long-held societal beliefs about mental health and race, color, gender, and social class. Societal beliefs, when combined with the prevailing scientific direction, resulted in an absence of relevant data, information, knowledge, skills, or evidence about racial and ethnic minority populations (HHS, 2001; Metzl, 2020). As a result of adverse policies toward racial and ethnic minority populations, a variety of disparities became prominent in health, welfare, unemployment, politics, economics, and mental health services (Manderscheid & Sonnenschein, 1985; Woods et al., 2012).

In the earliest years of the founding of the republic, two "minority" populations (Native Americans and Africans) were the primary targets of adverse public mental health policy. These two populations, along with the poor generally, were considered immune from mental illness. Because of this false assumption, public mental health policy was formulated on a dual race-based and asset-based ideology that excluded these populations from accessing available services. Science in mental health pursued hypotheses that were parallel to the dual ideological assumptions that undergird public mental health policy and politics generally. Historically, limited epidemiological data have been gathered on racial and ethnic minority individuals with mental illness (HSS, 2001). Most of the data that do exist have been primarily descriptive data on admissions to public mental hospitals (Pasamanick, 1963).

The historical disparity hypotheses linked mental health needs and access to services to a variety of social determinants, assets, race, and social class. These newer hypotheses formed the philosophical basis of much of American public mental health policy for over

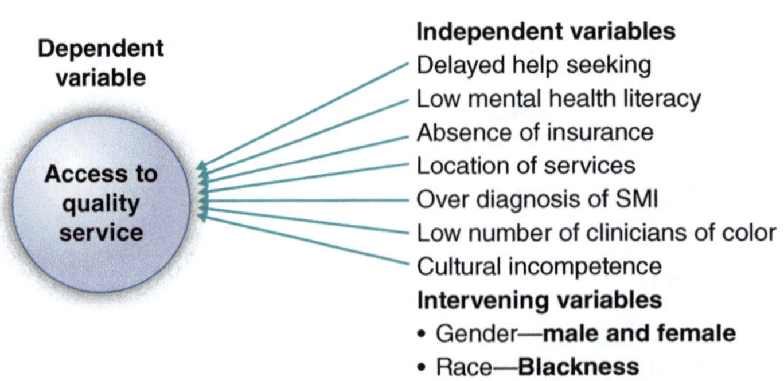

Figure 2.3 The disparity hypothesis (1965–2025).
SMI, serious mental illness.

a century. As a result, many public mental health systems were structurally designed to meet the needs of a singular cultural group rather than encompassing a racially and ethnically inclusive and more culturally competent orientation that would ensure that systems were designed to meet the mental health needs of an increasingly diverse population (Davis-Chambers, 1998).

SUMMARY

Beginning in 1868, nearly 54,000 Blacks were diagnosed and admitted to the first standalone state hospital from its Civil War–linked opening until its federally forced integration in 1967. Thousands more were admitted to similar segregated hospitals and wards that opened in almost every state through the great waves of segregation, institutionalization, deinstitutionalization, and integration policies and practices (Galt, 1853; Jackson, 1998; Malzberg, 1963b; Manderscheid & Sonnenschein, 1985; McCandless, 1996; Pasamanick, 1964; Segrest, 2020; Summers, 2019). In fact, the construction of hundreds of these segregated psychiatric hospitals in America and their increased involuntary admissions criteria resulted in a staggering 500,000 Black patients residing in state hospitals by 1955 (Foltz, 2015; Joint Commission on Mental Illness and Health, 1961). The number of individuals housed inhumanely in state hospitals alarmed public sentiment, resulting in a series of highly critical reports and policy proposals to shift the service burden from the state financial coffers to the federal government via President Kennedy's community-based care act (Gruenberg & Archer, 1979; Insel, 2022; Klerman, 1979; Mental Retardation Facilities and Community Mental Health Centers Construction Act, 1963). But it is unclear the extent to which these policy changes have improved the diagnosis and treatment of African Americans (Geller, 2020; Insel, 2022). In his 1985 report, Manderscheid confirmed that an unexplained and disproportionate number of state hospital patients were Blacks admitted across all types of psychiatric institutions, public, private, and federal, despite the availability of community mental health centers in some communities (Manderscheid & Sonnenschein, 1985).

We conclude that these racially disproportionate hospital admissions resulted from the historical acceptance and racial application of the tripartite hypotheses (immunity, disproportionality, and disparity) used to predict and justify excessive rates of illness and long-term hospitalization of the Black population. Historically, these contradictory explanations for the excess risk and incidence of psychiatric illness in Black populations often lacked underlying science and were also espoused by the medical directors of state hospitals based on the faulty 1840 census figures (Cartwright, 1851; Deutsch, 1948; Drewry, 1916; Jarvis, 1852; Stribling, 1845; Whaley, 2001).

But there were inherent deficiencies and risks associated with basing public policy decisions on unverified and untested hypotheses that drew a causal relationship between personal characteristics (e.g., skin color, race, and/or gender), social class, and previous servitude as putative causes of a dreaded disease. These hypotheses were ignited by the 1840 U.S. census that published faux data and unfounded conclusions that Blacks lacked the intellectual and moral capability to effectively manage their newly won freedom, citizenship, and northern migration without decompensating and flooding admissions to overcrowded state institutions (Deutsch, 1944a; Gates, 1997; Hinshaw, 2007; Jarvis, 1852; Schor, 2017). Although there were no state mental hospitals before 1870 that exclusively served Blacks, the 1840 census pronouncements made clear that Blacks were not the mental or emotional equals of Whites, but rather were riddled with inborn psychiatric vulnerabilities that made them irreversibly dangerous and unpredictable to others as they eventually became free, mobile, and urban dwellers. The flawed census data provided an erroneous statistical rationale for extending racial segregation to psychiatric hospital admissions as a precursor of what Whites should fear with the termination of slavery. Oddly, the persona created by the

1840 census converted the menial images of thousands of former Black servants, drivers, cooks, maids, gardeners, nurses, mechanics, carpenters, and tailors into lunatics. Without the constraints of slavery, overseers, owners, and police, the census forecast havoc and chaos (American Psychiatric Association Board, 2021; Finkelman, 2003; Jarvis, 1852). This emerging psychiatric persona was a total reversal in status emanating from the previous belief that Blacks were immune from lunacy and how they would become vulnerable with freedom and migration.

The exceptionally negative persona of the newly freed Black population justified strict and broad segregation throughout all societal structures, including state hospitals. Annual hospital reports in Virginia showed that 70% of patients were diagnosed with a form of mania (Davis, 2018a). In fact, Downs broadly identified the large number of individuals who simply were poor, physically ill, and/or homeless following the end of enslavement and the Civil War but could not count those who had psychiatric ailments. Others suffered from birth injuries or were otherwise developmentally delayed and unable to labor (Davis, 2018a). Downs questioned the extent to which there were significant numbers of former slaves who had become mentally ill. Predictions by supporters of slavery estimated that a significant proportion of the formerly enslaved would require mental health care (Walker, 1869). However, our preliminary analysis of data from the annual reports from CSH identify less than 1% of the newly freed Black population who evidenced psychiatric symptoms sufficient to require hospitalization (Davis, 2019b, 2024; Central State Hospital Superintendent, 1918).

These conditions of admission and treatment did not evaporate when racial integration was forced by federal law. Numerous publications illustrated the continued harmful effects of excess admissions and warehousing of persons seeking care under the constraints of untested hypotheses fueled by historical remnants of racial segregation (Randolph, 2003; Whaley & Hall, 2008; Woods et al., 2012).

Black families have historically been the primary providers of in-home care for their relatives with physical, developmental, *and* mental disabilities and illnesses (Neighbors & Jackson, 1984). Despite adverse symptoms, individuals with illness were maintained in their homes and communities well beyond the onset of symptoms and medical recommendations (Neighbors, 1985). Seeking and accepting external help was often delayed for decades but buttressed by friends, relatives, churches, pastors, and neighbors that formed supportive networks that kept individuals free of police arrest and appearances in court. This family- and community-based care is a strength in these communities that allows individuals with disabilities to remain in their communities for extended periods as the search for prevention, adequate treatment, cure, and recovery goes forward (Neighbors, 1985).

The use of these untested hypotheses appears to have spread broadly into psychiatric practice and education across the United States. This suggests that the connection between race and vulnerability to mental health became exceptionally broad in terms of application. Clear, too, was the potential for misdiagnosis of African Americans due in part to their persona within America as innately flawed, vulnerable, and unprotected (Whaley, 2001).

Harvard historian Henry Louis Gates wrote that the pathological persona of Blackness was fixated for over a century in public policy and thought. Those elements migrated and became embedded in psychiatry, psychology, sociology, religion, law, medicine, education, political science, social work, theater, art, economics, media, public law, and the American psyche (Gates, 2019). The persona was used to justify the less-than-stellar opportunities available to people of color. Jones concluded that these mal-perceptions became encased within the structure of all institutions within the American social system and have a deleterious effect on opportunities, safety, and life chances of people of color (Jones, 2021). Perception of African Americans as beings without soul, without feelings, or the capacity to think and reason or participate in the day-to-day activities of citizenship has been pervasive (*Dred Scott v. Sandford*, 1856). African Americans were seen as lesser beings than Whites and not exposed to the same stimuli. Africans were believed to be genetically idiotic, imbecilic, and generally unintelligent. These perspectives seem to reflect the emotional mystique and the long-term search for the existential meaning of Blackness.

DISCUSSION QUESTIONS

1. What are potential ways to address the growing issue of homelessness among mentally ill African Americans in major cities, especially as state psychiatric hospitals have few beds and short stays due to policy changes?
2. How do you think the 1840 census findings shaped societal views on race and mental health?
3. In what ways can current mental health policies address the inequities caused by segregation and historical biases?
4. How can African American community–led efforts, such as those by churches and local organizations, contribute to improving mental health literacy and access?
5. What role should education and training for mental health professionals play in addressing historical inequities in care?

REFERENCES

Act Prohibiting Importation of Slaves, Statutes of the United States, Pub. L. No. 9-22 § 10, 2 Stat. 426, Chap. 22 Stat. 426–430 (1807, March 2).

An Act Concerning the Admission of Patients Into the Lunatic Asylums of the Commonwealth, Developed in Response to the Census of 1840 and to Petitions by State Hospital Directors, Chapter 15, Acts of the Assembly Cong. Rec. § Public Buildings (1846).

Alexander, M. (2012). *The new Jim Crow: Mass incarceration in the age of colorblindness*. The New Press.

American Psychiatric Association Board. (2021). *APA's apology to Black, Indigenous and People of Color for its support of structural racism in psychiatry* [Press release].

An Act to Establish the Central Lunatic Asylum for Colored Insane, General Assembly, Chapter 146 Cong. Rec. 189 (1870).

Anderson, D. M. (2002). *Mosby's medical, nursing, and allied health dictionary* (6th ed.). Mosby.

Atrash, H. K., & Hunter, M. D. (2006). Healthcare disparities in the United States: A continuing challenge. In D. Satcher, R. J. Pamies, & N. N. Woelfl (Eds.), *Multicultural medicine and health disparities* (pp. 3–32). McGraw Hill.

Barker, P. R., Manderscheid, R. W., Hendershot, G. E., Jack, S. S., Schoenborn, C. A., & Goldstrom, I. (1992). Serious mental illness and disability in the adult household population: United States, 1989. *Advance Data, 218*, 1–11. https://doi.org/10.1037/e608882007-001

Blanton, W. B. (1931). *Medicine in Virginia in the eighteenth century*. Garett and Massie, Inc.

Boster, D. H. (2013). *African American slavery and disability: Bodies, property, and power in the Antebellum South, 1800–1860*. Routledge.

Breeden, J. O. (1976). States rights medicine in the old South. *Journal of Southern History, XXV*, 53–72.

Brown v. Board of Education, 347 U.S. 483 (1954). https://www.archives.gov/milestone-documents/brown-v-board-of-education

Canby, E. R. S. (1869). *General Order 136*. (General Order 136). 1st Military District.

Cartwright, S. (1851). Report on the diseases and physical peculiarities of the Negro Race. *New Orleans Medical Surgical Journal, 7*, 692–705.

Center to Reduce Cancer Health Disparities. (2003). *Researching and reducing cancer-related health disparities*. Government Publications Office.

Central State Hospital Superintendent. (1918). *Annual report number: 48 Central State Hospital*. State Printing Office

Chapter 144 of the Virginia Code, Virginia Legislature, page 126 Cong. Rec. (1853).

Civil Rights Act of 1964, Congressional Record, Pub. L. No. 88-352 § 11, 78 Stat. 241 Stat. (U.S. Congress 1964 July 2, 1964).

Coates, T.-N. (2014). Black pathology and the closing of the progressive mind. *The Atlantic*.

Cohen, P. C. (1982). *A calculating people: The spread of numeracy in early America*. Routledge.

Cole, B. (2020, July 2). *Tucker Carlson says black lives matter protests a "hysteria" pandemic*. https://www.newsweek.com/tucker-carlson-fox-news-black-lives-matter-statues-colombus-1514915

Conley, D. (1999). *Being black, living in the red: Race, wealth, and social policy in America.* Columbia University Press.

Dain, N. (1964). *Concepts of insanity in the United States 1789–1865.* Rutgers University Press.

Dain, N. (1968). *History of Eastern State Hospital.* Colonial Williamsburg Foundation.

Dain, N. (1980). The chronic mental patient in 19th century America. *Psychiatric Annals, 10*, 323–327.

Davis-Chambers, E. (1998). *Cultural competence performance measures.* New York State Office of Mental Health, The Research Foundation.

Davis, K. (1998a). Managed care, mental illness, and African Americans. In G. Schamess & A. Lightburn (Eds.), *Humane managed care?* (pp. 51–64). National Association of Social Workers Press.

Davis, K. (1998b). *Slaves don't get stress: The evolution of mental health policies and for African Americans: Implications for current and future public policy.* Center for Mental Health Services.

Davis, K. (2003). The policy implications of the surgeon general's report on mental health, race, culture, and ethnicity. In T. Bent-Goodley (Ed.), *African Amercian social workers and social policy* (pp. 93–122). Haworth.

Davis, K. (2015). *Final report on the Central State archives project for the Andrew W. Mellon Foundation.* School of Information, The University of Texas at Austin.

Davis, K. (2018a). *Analysis of admissions to psychiatric hospitals in Virginia, 1780–1970.* Research. School of Information, The University of Texas at Austin.

Davis, K. (2018b, May 18). Blacks are immune from mental illness. *Psychiatric News, 25*, 44.

Davis, K. (2019a). *Central Lunatic Asylum for Colored Insane final report.* Central Lunatic Asylum for Colored Insane. Research report. School of Information, The Andrew Mellow Foundation.

Davis, K. (2019b). Digital archive traces admissions to country's first mental hospital for Blacks. *Psychiatric News, 54*(8), 9–12. https://doi.org/10.1176/appi.pn.2019.4b26

Davis, K. (2020). America's first asylum for African Americans marks its 150th anniversary. *Psychiatric News, 55*(15), 3.

Davis, K. (2022). *The Central State Hospital archives.* Archival. School of Information, The School of Information, The University of Texas at Austin.

Davis, K. (2024, December). *Final report: Central State Hospital archives project on admissions 1840-1968.* School of Information, The University of Texas at Austin.

Davis, K., Lewis, A. N., Zhang, J., & Thompkins, A. L. (2011). Race and the policy of involuntary admissions to psychiatric hospitals. In J. H. Schiele (Ed.), *Social welfare policy: Regulation and resistance among people of color* (pp. 63–91). Sage.

Davis, K., & Jung, H. (2012). New federalism, new freedom, and states rights: The uncertain and fragmented direction of public mental health policy. In I. C. Colby (Ed.), *Comprehensive handbook of social work and social welfare* (Vol. 2). John Wiley and Sons.

Day, P. J. (1989). *A new history of social welfare.* Prentice Hall.

Deutsch, A. (1944a). The first IS Census of the Insane (1840) and its use as pro-slavery propaganda. *Bulletin of the History of Medicine, 15*(5), 14.

Deutsch, A. (1944b). The first U.S. census of the insane (1840) and its use as pro-slavery propaganda. *Bulletin of the History of Medicine, 15*, 469–482.

Deutsch, A. (1948). *The shame of the states.* Harcourt Brace.

Center to Reduce Cancer Health Disparities. (2003). *Researching and reducing cancer-related health disparities.* Government Publications Office.

Downs, J. (2012). *Sick from freedom.* Oxford University Press.

Dred Scott v. Sandford, 19 How. 393, 60 U.S. 393, 15 L.Ed. 691. (1856). https://www.archives.gov/milestone-documents/dred-scott-v-sandford

Drewry, W. F. (1900, July 16). To Virginia belongs the credit, medical. *The New York Times* (p. 1). https://www.nytimes.com/1900/07/16/archives/the-first-insane-asylum-to-virginia-belongs-the-credit-in-this.html

Drewry, W. F. (1916). Central State Hospital—Petersburg, Virginia. In H. M. Hurd & W. F. Drewry (Eds.), *The institutional care of the insane in the United States and Canada* (Vol. 3, Part 2, pp. 773–771). Johns Hopkins Press.

Fauquier, F. (1766, November 6). British Parliament Resolutions and Hospital for Lunatics. Presentation to the House of Burgesses, Williamsburg.

Feagin, J. R., & Feagin, C. B. (1978). *Discrimination American style: Institutional racism and sexism.* Prentice Hall.

Finkelman, P. (2003). *Defending slavery: Proslavery thought in the old South: A brief history with documents.* Bedford/St. Martins.

Fischer, J. (1969). Negroes, whites and rates of mental illness: Reconsideration of a myth. *Psychiatry, 32*, 438-446.

Florida Department of Education. (2023). *Florida state academic standards.* https://www.fldoe.org/academics/standards/

Foltz, C. D. (2015). *Race and mental illness at a Virginia hospital: A case study of Central Lunatic Asylum for the Colored Insane, 1869–1885* (Masters thesis). Virginia Commonwealth University.

Foster, T., Porter, S. R., & Pharris-Ciurej, N. (2024). *Black-White mortality gaps widened during pandemic, Hispanic mortality advantage disappeared.* https://www.census.gov/library/stories/2024/03/excess-mortality-during-covid-19.html

Freedman's Bureau Acts of 1865 and 1866, Chap. XC, United States Senate § 5 507–509 (1865, March 3).

Galt, J. M. (1845). *Annual report of the court of directors of the Eastern Lunatic Asylum, 1844–1860.* State Printing Office.

Galt, J. M. (1846). *The treatment of insanity.* Harper & Brothers.

Galt, J. (1853). Asylums for colored people. *American Psychological Journal,* 75–88.

Gates, H. L. (1997). *Thirteen ways of looking at a black man.* Random House.

Gates, H. L. (2019). *Stony the road: Reconstruction, white supremacy, and the rise of Jim Crow.* Penguin.

Geller, J. (2020). Structural racism in American psychiatry and APA: Part 6. *Psychiatric News,* 6.

Gonaver, W. (2018). *The peculiar institution and the making of modern psychiatry 1840-1880.* University of North Carolina.

Gray, T. R. (1831). *The confessions of Nat Turner the leader of the late insurrection in Southampton County Virginia.* Thomas R Gray Lucas and Deaver Printers.

Grob, G. N. (1973). *Mental institutions in America: Social policy to 1875.* The Free Press.

Grob, G. N. (1994). *The mad among us: A history of the care of America's mentally ill.* Harvard University Press.

Grossack, M. M. (1963). *Mental health and segregation.* Springer Publishing Company.

Gruenberg, E. M., & Archer, J. (1979). Abandonment of responsibility for the seriously mentally ill. *Milbank Memorial Fund Quarterly Health Society, 57*(4), 485–506,

Henry, E. P. (1941). State hospital for Negro Insane, Taft Oklahoma. *National Negro Health News, 10* (October–December), 41.

Hernton, C. (1965). *Sex and racism in America.* Grove Press.

Hinshaw, S. P. (2007). *The mark of shame: Stigma of mental illness and an agenda for change.* Oxford University Press.

History of the Ministry of Defence. (1998). Disability history enumeration and contents (1998–2023 ed., Archive). People Inc.

House Joint Resolution, Chapter 53 Cong. Rec. (1877).

House Joint Resolution No. 5, No. 5, page 354. Cong. Rec. (1848).

Hurd, H. M., Drewry, W. F., Dewey, R., Pilgrim, C. W., Blumer, G. A., & Burgess, T. J. W. (1916). *The institutional care of the insane in the United States and Canada.* Johns Hopkins Press.

Hylton, A. (2024). *Madness: Race and insanity in a Jim Crow asylum.* Legacy.

Insel, T. (2022). *Healing: Our path from mental illness to mental health.* Penguin.

Institute of Medicine. (2002). *Unequal treatment: Confronting racial and ethnic disparities in health care.* National Academies Press.

Jackson, V. (1998). *Separate and unequal: Legacy of racially segregated psychiatric hospitals.* http://www.healingcircles.org/uploads/2/1/4/8/2148953/sauweb.pdf

Jarvis, E. (1844). Insanity among the colored population of the free states. *American Journal of the Medical Sciences, 7,* 71–83.

Jarvis, E. (1852). Insanity among the coloured population of the free states. *American Journal of the Medical Sciences, VII,* 73–75.

Jefferson, T. (1806). Letter from Thomas Jefferson to the Senate and House, December 2, 1806. *Founders Online,* 5. https://founders.archives.gov/documents/Jefferson/99-01-02-4616.

Joint Commission on Mental Illness and Health. (1961). *Action for mental health.* Science Editions.

Jones, N. H. (2021). *The 1619 project: A new origin story.* One World.

Joshi, S. T. (1999). *Documents of American prejudice.* Basic Books.

Kendi, I. X. (2016). *Stamped from the beginning: The definitive history of racist ideas in America.* Nation Books.

Klerman, G. L. (1979). Patient reentry into the community: The federal viewpoint. *Journal of National Association of Private Psychiatric Hospitals, 11*(1 Fall), 5–11.

Koch, R. (1882). Die atiologic der tuberkulose. *Berliner Klinische Wochenschrift, 15,* 221–223.https://www.cdc.gov/mmwr/preview/mmwrhtml/00000222.htm

Lawson, W. B., Heplar, H., Holladay, J., & Cuffel, B. (1994). Race as a factor in inpatient and outpatient admissions and diagnosis. *Hospital and Community Psychiatry, 45*(1), 72–74. https://doi.org/10.1176/ps.45.1.72

Lewis, A., Davis, K., & Zang, N. (2010). Admissions of African American men to psychiatric hospitals: Historical and current statistical trends. *International Journal of Public Policy, 6*(34).

Lewis, A. N., Davis, King E., & Zhang, N. J. (2010). Admission of African Americans to state psychiatric hospitals. *International Journal of Public Policy, 6*(34), 17.

Little, B. (2019). The 1840 U.S. census was overly interested in American's mental health. *History,* 3. Retrieved from https://history.com/news/census-change-mental-illness-controversy

Long, G. (2012). *Doctoring freedom: The politics of African American medical care in slavery and emancipation.* University of North Carolina.

Malzberg, B. (1963a). Mental disease among Negroes. In M. M. Grossack (Ed.), *Mental health and segregation* (pp. 158–160). Springer Publishing Company.

Malzberg, B. (1963b). Mental disease among Negroes. In M. M. Grossack (Ed.), *Mental health and segregation* (p. 229). Springer Publishing Company.

Manderscheid, R. W., & Sonnenschein, M. A. (1985). *Mental health United States, 1985*. National Institute of Mental Health, U.S. Department of Health and Human Services.

Manderscheid, R. W., & Sonnenschein, M. A. (1987). *Mental health, United States, 1987*. National Institute of Mental Health, U.S. Department of Health and Human Services.

Manderscheid, R. W., & Sonnenschein, M. A. (1995). *Mental health United States, 1995*. National Institute of Mental Health, U.S. Department of Health and Human Services.

Manderscheid, R., Witkin, M. J., Rosenstein, M. Y., & Bass, R. D. (1986). *The national reporting program for mental health statistics: History and findings* (Vol. 5). National Institute of Mental Health.

Manderscheid, R. W., Atay, J. E, & Crider, R. A. (2009). Changing trends in state psychiatric use from 2002 to 2005. *Psychiatric Services, 60*(1), 29–34. https://doi.org/10.1176/ps.2009.60.1.29

Martin, L. A. (2023). *The gospel of J. Edgar Hoover: How the FBI aided and abetted the rise of white Christian nationalism*. Princenton University Press.

McCandless, P. (1996). *Moonlight, magnolias, & madness: Insanity in South Carolina from the colonial period to the progressive era*. University of North Carolina Press.

McGuire, H. (Chairman). (1870, November 10). *Annual Report of Central State Hospital* (p. 1). Richmond: Superintendent of Printing

McGuire, T. G., Alegria, M., Cook, B. L., Wells, K. B., & Zaslavsky, A. M. (2006). Health services research: Implementing the Institute of Medicine definition of disparities. *Health Services Research, 41*, 1979–2005.

Mental Retardation Facilities and Community Mental Health Centers Construction Act of 1963, Public Law 88-164 (U.S. Goverment Printing Office 1963).

Metzl, J. (2009). *The protest psychosis: When schizophrenia became a black disease*. Beacon Press.

Metzl, J. (2020). *Dying of whiteness: How the politics of racial resentment is killing America's heartland*. Basic Books.

Miller, J. F. (1896). *The effects of emancipation upon the mental and physical health of the Negro of the south*. Paper presented at the Southern Medico-Psychological Association, Ashville, North Carolina.

Mude, W., Oguoma, V. M., Nyanhanda, T., Mwanri, L., & Njue, C. (2021). Racial disparities in COVID-19 pandemic cases, hospitalisations, and deaths: A systematic review and meta-analysis. *Journal of Global Health, 11*(11), 05015. https://doi.org/10.7189/jogh.11.05015

National Institute of Dental and Craniofacial Research. (2002). *A plan to eliminate craniofacial, oral, and dental health disparities*. www.nidr.nih.gov/research/healthdisp/hdplan.pdf

National Institutes of Health. (2002). *Strategic plan and budget to reduce and ultimately eliminate health disparities*. http://www.healthequityks.org/download/NIH_Strategic_Plan_Health_Disparities_202.pdf

National Institutes of Health. (2003). *Addressing health disparities: What are health disparities?* http://healthdisparities.nih.gov/whatare.html

Neighbors, H. W. (1984). The distribution of psychiatric morbidity in Black Americans: A review and suggestions for research. *Community Mental Health Journal, 20*(3), 169–181. https://doi.org/10.1007/BF00808105

Neighbors, H. W. (1985). Seeking professional help for personal problems: Black Americans' use of health and mental health services. *Community Mental Health Journal, 21*(3), 156–166. https://doi.org/10.1007/BF00754731

Neighbors, H. W., & Jackson, J. (1984). The use of informal and formal help: Four patterns of illness behavior in the black community. *American Journal of Community Psychology, 12*(6), 629–644. https://doi.org/10.1007/BF00922616

Neighbors, H. W., & Jackson, J. S. (1996). *Mental health in black America*. Sage Publications.

Neighbors, H. W., Jackson, J., Campbell, L., & Williams, D. (1989). The influence of racial factors on psychiatric diagnosis: A review and suggestions for research. *Community Mental Health Journal, 25*(4), 301–311. https://doi.org/10.1007/BF00755677

Neighbors, H. W., & Lumpkin, S. (1990). The epidemiology of mental disorder in the black population. In D. S. Ruiz & J. P. Comer (Eds.), *Handbook of mental health and mental disorder among black Americans* (pp. 55–70). Greenwood Press.

Oates, S. B. (1982). *Let the trumpet sound: The life of Martin Luther King, Jr.* Harper and Row.

Pasamanick, B. A. (1963). Mental disease among Negroes. In M. M. Grossack (Ed.), *Mental health and segregation* (pp. 150–157). Springer Publishing Company.

Pasamanick, B. A. (1964). Myths regarding prevalence of mental disease in the American Negro. *Journal of the National Medical Association, 56*(1), 6–17.

Pepper, W. F. (2016). *The plot to kill King*. Skyhorse.

Plepys, C., & Klein, R. (1995). *Health status indicators: Differentials by race and Hispanic origin*. Centers for Disease Control and Prevention/National Center for Health Statistics.

Plessy v. Ferguson, U. S. Supreme Court, Rule Number 210. (1896).

Randolph, K. A. (2003). *Central Lunatic Asylum for the Colored Insane: A history of African Americans with mental disabilities, 1844–1885 (PhD thesis).* University of Pennsylvania History Department.

Rothman, D. (1970). *The discovery of the asylum.* Little, Brown.

Rothstein, R. (2017). *The color of law: A forgotten history of how our government segregated America.* Liveright Publishing.

Rubin, A., & Babbie, E. R. (2008). *Research methods for social work* (Vol. 6). Brooks/Cole.

Savitt, T. L. (1975). *Sound minds and sound bodies: The diseases and health care of blacks in antebellum Virginia* (PhD thesis). University of Virginia.

Savitt, T. L. (1989). Black health on the plantation: masters, slaves and physicians. In R. L. Numbers & T. L. Savitt (Eds.), *Science and medicine in the old South* (pp. 327–355). Louisiana State University Press.

Savitt, T. L. (2007). *Race & medicine in nineteenth and early twentieth century America.* Kent University Press.

Schor, P. (2017). *Counting Americans: How the US census classified the nation* (L. A. Weiss, Trans.). Oxford University.

Segrest, M. (2020). *Administrations of lunacy: Racism and the haunting of American psychiatry at the Milledgeville asylum.* The New Press.

Smith, J. T. (1851). Review of Dr. Cartwright's report on the disease and physical pecularities of the Negro race. *New Orleans Medical Surgical Journal, 8,* 230.

Snowden, L. R. (2000). Inpatient mental health use by members of ethnic minority groups. In J. M. Herrera, W. B. Lawson, & J. J. Smerck (Eds.), *Cross cultural psychiatry.* John Wiley.

Steen, S. (1991). Historical perspectives on women and mental illness and prevention of depression in women, using a feminist framework. *Issues in Mental Health Nursing, 12*(4), 359–374. https://doi.org/0.3109/01612849109010017

Stiglitz, J. E. (2012). *The price of inequality.* W.W. Norton.

Stribling, F. (1845). *Annual report of the Western Lunatic Asylum.* Superintendent Public Printing.

Summers, M. (2019). *Madness in the city of magnificient intentions: A history of race and mental illness in the nation's capital.* Oxford University.

Superintendent of Central Lunatic Asylum. (1870). *First annual report.* State Printing Office.

Superintendent of Central Lunatic Asylum. (1885). *Eighteenth annual report.* Richmond: State Printing Office.

Tasca, C. R., Mariangela, C., Giovanni M., & Bianca, F. (2012). Women and hysteria in the history of mental health. *Clinical Practice and Epidemiology in Mental Health, 8,* 110–119. https://doi.org/10.2174/1745017901208010110

Thomas, A., & Sillen, S. (1972). *Racism and psychiatry.* Brunneer/Mazel.

U.S. Department of Health and Human Services (1999). *Mental health: A report of the surgeon general.* U.S. Department of Health and Human Services, SAMHSA and NIMH.

U.S. Department of Health and Human Services. (2001). *Mental health: Culture, race, and ethnicity: A supplement to mental health: A report of the surgeon general.* U.S. Department of Health and Human Services, Substance Abuse and Mental Health Services Administration.

Walker, G. C. (1869). *Asylum for insane colored people.* James B. Goode's Steam Presses.

Wallace, J., Goldsmith-Pinkham, P., & Swartz, J. (2022). *Excess death rates for Republicans and Democrats during the COVID 19 pandemic* (30512). National Bureau of Economic Research.

Washington, H. A. (2006). *Medical apartheid.* Doubleday.

Weaver, W. A. (1841). *Sixth census or enumeration of the inhabitants of the United States as corrected at the Department of State.* Blair and Rives.

Whaley, A. L. (2001). Cultural mistrust: An important psychological construct for diagnosis and treatment of African Americans. *Professional Psychology: Research and Practice, 32*(6), 555–562. https://doi.org/10.1037/0735-7028.32.6.555

Whaley, A. L. (2005). *Cultural competence and evidence-based practice in mental health services: complementary not contradictory paradigms. American Psychology, 62*(6), 563–574. https://doi.org/10.1037/0003-066X.62.6.563. PMID: 17874897.

Whaley, A. L., & Hall, B. N. (2008). Cultural themes in the psychotic symptoms of African American psychiatric patients. *Professional Psychology: Research and Practice, 40*(1), 75–80.

Whig, R. (1865, April 10). All city hospitals taken by federal military. *Richmond Whig.* Retrieved from http://www.mdgorman.com/Written_Accounts/Whig/1865/richmond_whig_4101865a.htm

Williams, M. V. (2013). *Medgar Evers: Mississippi martyr.* University of Arkansas Press.

Wilson, D. C., & Lantz, E. M. (1963). Culture change and Negro state hospital admissions. In M. M. Grossack (Ed.), *Mental health and segregation* (p. 229). Springer Publishing Company.

Wood, A. D. (2004). *Dr. Francis T. Stribling and moral medicine: Curing the insane at Virginia's Western State Hospital, 1836–1874.* Gallileo.

Woods, D. V., King, N. J., Hanna, S. M., & Murray, C. (2012). *Pathways into the black population for eliminatlng mental health disparities.* Department of Mental Health.

Zwerling, S. S. (1986). *Quest for a cure: The public hospital in Williamsburg, Virginia 1773–1885.* Colonia Williamsburg Foundation.

3 INVISIBLE BY DESIGN

MARGARET P. MOSS

LEARNING OBJECTIVES

After reading this chapter, readers will be able to:

- Define who are American Indians and Alaska Natives in the eyes of the United States and why it matters (i.e., legal definition).
- Identify the major federal Indian policy periods and how they map onto the elements of genocide.
- Connect the impact of past and present federal Indian legislation on the mental health and well-being of Indigenous persons and communities.
- Describe the mental health status and disparities impacting American Indian and Alaska Native populations.
- Understand/use treatment modalities specific to this population in alleviating the stress of historical and contemporaneous traumas that have resulted in alarming substance abuse/misuse, suicide, homicide, depression, and other resulting disparities.

INTRODUCTION

In the United States, there are huge gaps in healthcare access, treatment, and outcomes between the various Indigenous, racial, and ethnic minority and dominant culture populations (National Center for Health Statistics, 2016; Williams et al., 2016). Nowhere is this gap more evident than between U.S. Indigenous perspectives and knowledge and Western perspectives and modalities (John & Baldridge, 1996; Warne & Lajimodiere, 2015). These disparities are in large part the result of purposeful, targeted, and sustained policies to "Get Rid of the Indian Problem" (Deloria, 1969; Jones, 2006) by the U.S. government, with the general population historically falling in line with the idea. At the very least, few Americans seem to notice what the government has visited upon the Indigenous people found within its borders for the past several hundred years. To truly understand the roots of today's poor health outcomes in the American Indian/Alaska Native (AI/AN) population, especially as it pertains to mental health disparities and inequities, we must note the impact of political, social, and structural determinants of health, along with the inadequate and insufficient provision of healthcare services and treatments for reservation, frontier, rural, and urban AI/AN individuals and communities.

The *Indian problem* began back to first contact in the 16th century.[1] "To understand the root causes of health inequities among [American Indians] it is important to understand the historical context in which this population has lived" (Warne & Lajimodiere, 2015, pp. 567–579). This includes the mental health of Indigenous peoples in northern North America. Of note is the "problem," which was that the Europeans, and later colonists and

[1] The 1492 reference to Columbus is not used here because he never stepped foot in what is now Canada or the United States. Therefore, this chapter references first contact as of 1500s.

settlers, not only wanted that land but deigned it to be theirs because of the Doctrine of Discovery. The Doctrine of Discovery was applied by Europeans coming into the Americas as the "lawful taking of Indigenous lands by any means (Miller, 2005). This taking was from the Indigenous people who had occupied, stewarded, and used the lands since time immemorial.

A purported legal basis stemmed from one of the so-named Marshall Trilogy cases from Chief Justice Marshall's court in the early 1800s (Geotting, 2008). The decision in *Johnson v. McIntosh* found that the Doctrine of Discovery held as law in America and that Natives no longer had complete sovereignty (Marshall J. & Supreme Court of the United States, 1823). Therein began America's goal to rid itself of this problem and begin expansion and the takeover of the land, its many bountiful resources, and geopolitical position. This all flew in the face of the Indigenous Nation's thousands of years of inherent sovereignty (Steele, 2016). "The United States has asserted vast powers over tribes yet has simultaneously proclaimed its respect for the principle that tribes retain inherent governing powers that predate the Constitution, and have never been extinguished" (Steele, 2016, pp. 666-675). Put another way, the sovereignty that American Indian tribes have predates the U.S. Constitution and Bill of Rights, in which the United States created its power. Therefore, this sovereignty is extraconstitutional (Wilkins & Lomawaima, 2001). "The relationship between American Indian tribes and the US federal government is an ongoing contest over sovereignty" (Wilkins & Lomawaima, 2001, p. 5).

This centuries-long, uneven contest and takeover of rights, land, and ultimately life have resulted in an Indigenous population today that is still coming back from near extinction (Thornton, 1987). Any gains in life expectancy, morbidity, and mortality have been slow. For example, the life expectancy for AI/AN persons born in 2021 is 65.2 years, or 11.2 years less than non-Hispanic Whites at 76.4 (Arias et al., 2022). On several reservations, life expectancies are at levels not seen in the U.S. overall population since 1900. On the Pine Ridge reservation in South Dakota, life expectancy is 48 years for males and 52 years for females, often the lowest in the Western Hemisphere (Smith, 2024). Further, the modest gains that have been made continue to be stifled by the backdrop of a colonialist structure often unaware of its own continued immovability and ongoing destruction. Wolfe contends in his treatment on settler colonialism that "Invasion is a structure not an event" (Wolfe, 1999, p. 3). Until these structures are seen, modified, or removed, little will change. This remains true even in 2025. American Indians must fit as individuals or as nations into the built U.S. structures that bear little resemblance to the reality, needs, and futures of the 7.1 million Natives—either of one race or in combination—who live in the United States today (U.S. Census Bureau, 2023b). Unfortunately, America's Indigenous peoples are often physically, mentally, emotionally, spiritually, environmentally, and politically lost, overlooked, and often ignored in a country of 333 million people (U.S. Census Bureau, 2023b).

This chapter provides a historical background that briefly touches on the major U.S. policy periods that were and are meant to rid the United States of the Indian problem by extermination, removal (1830–1850), reservations (1850–1891), allotment and assimilation (1887–1934), and relocation and/or termination (1953–1968; U.S. Department of the Interior, n.d.). These, in fact, *are* the policy periods that have been the most destructive to AI/AN individuals and communities (Helgesen, 2011). This is followed by a focus on how those and current policies have further created the health disparities and inequities that exist today. A discussion of health status, access to acceptable care and treatment, and outcomes is offered, with a spotlight on mental health. Finally, understanding health, care, and needs from the Indigenous point of view is offered. Legislators and practitioners must truly understand the concepts of historical trauma (HT); political, social, and structural determinants of health; and equity in order to meaningfully achieve positive steps forward. Change can occur only when armed with facts, truth, a desire to change, and a path forward.

AMERICAN INDIANS/ALASKA NATIVES

Practitioners, researchers, and the wider public should understand the terms used to designate and distinguish between the First Peoples found in what is now the United States. Here, *First Peoples*, just as the term implies, indicates those inhabitants of northern North America present for thousands of years before contact from Europeans and those who are their descendants. It is an all-encompassing term that includes hundreds of tribes and nations. Today's descendants in the United States include members of the 574 Federally Recognized Tribes (U.S. Department of the Interior, Indian Affairs, 2024). A synonym is the term *Indigenous,* which is used broadly and is used in this chapter when speaking about people who have been on this continent for millennia, including during the times of pre-contact and during early contact and, of course, their descendants. Other terms are *Indian*, *American Indian*, *Native American*, and *Native* as well as the hundreds of specific tribe names.

The term *Indian* is the actual legal term in the United States (U.S. Code, 2020). In modern vernacular, the term *Native* is used when it is encompassing any persons with close heritage and lineage to current or historical tribes but are not enrolled in a specific tribe. This usage is important because through the vast, purposeful interference by the U.S. federal government, many AI/AN individuals have lost any connections to their heritage groups and thus are not formally enrolled members of their tribes. In fact, they may not know their tribes or their tribes may no longer exist in the eyes of the Congress as a result of the Termination Act of 1953 (NLM, n.d.). As Pevar stated, "Nothing else that Congress can do causes tribal members to lose more of their rights than termination. Termination is the ultimate weapon of Congress and ultimate fear of tribes. Despite its drastic effect, the Supreme Court has held that Congress has the power under the Commerce Clause to terminate a tribe" (Pevar, 1992).

Importantly, the term used in this chapter is *American Indian* and, at times, *AI/AN*, both of which are being used to indicate enrolled members of one of the 574 federally recognized tribes. Notably, today many AI/AN individuals choose to directly be identified by their tribe's name rather than a blanket, "global" indication of indigeneity (National Museum of American Indians, 2024). Some examples include *Dine* as opposed to *Navajo, A:Shiwi* in lieu of *Zuni,* and *Anishinaabe* instead of *Chippewa.* Context, tribe, and individual preferences must be taken into consideration when referring to this population.

Indians are the most regulated people in the United States, with Title 25 of the U.S. Code (25 USC, Indians, 1832). In fact, no other population group in the United States is listed in the U.S. Code, making it one way that Indians are distinguished from any other race or population within the United States. Federally Recognized Tribes are solely named by the U.S. Congress (i.e., a tribe is only a tribe if Congress says it is a tribe) and "[t]he sovereignty that the Indian tribes retain is of a unique and limited character. It exists only at the sufferance of Congress and is subject to complete defeasance" (*South Dakota v. Bourland*, 1992). Tribes themselves determine who is a member. This often goes by either direct lineage or blood quantum levels or other determinative means (U.S. Department of the Interior, 2024). Consequently, in the eyes of the United States, in terms of treaties and applied case law, being eligible for Indian Health Services or Bureau of Indian Affairs–related services, one must quite literally be a card-carrying American Indian or Alaska Native.

This background is critical because the Indian Health Service (IHS) is the agency of the U.S. Department of Health and Human Services charged with providing physical and mental health care treatments and services to enrolled American Indians (IHS, n.d.). Verbal claims of being Indian alone will not hold the needed weight for these services. There is an expansive body of literature discussing the merits and pitfalls that are represented in using blood quantum to determine one's AI/AN status under current U.S. law. No other population in the United States can have their identity wiped away "by the sufferance of Congress" (as noted above), where one day you are an Indian in the eyes of the government and, by the whims of Congress, the next day you are not.

FIRST CONTACT

At initial contact, likely in the 15th century, individual Indigenous nations were acknowledged at first as sovereign nations and were formally engaged through negotiations and treaties. According to the Supremacy Clause of the U.S. Constitution, "This Constitution, and the Laws of the United States which shall be made in Pursuance thereof; and all Treaties made, or which shall be made, under the Authority of the United States, shall be the supreme Law of the Land" (U.S. Const. art. VI, cl. 2). However, looking at legal and political theories side by side with the events of American Indian issues in the United States, we can examine, "[how]...the Constitution has been applied—or not applied—to American Indians as individuals and to the lands, treaties, and rights as separate sovereign nations" (Deloria & Wilkins, 2000, p. ix). It was recognized by the early U.S. government that the Indigenous people had been here for millennia, they understood the land and context, and they held valuable knowledge and resources. However, as of 1871, the final treaty was made wherein the House of Representatives added a rider to an appropriations bill ceasing to recognize individual tribes within the United States as independent nations with whom the United States may contract by treaty. This act ended the nearly 100-year-old practice of treaty making between the federal government and Native American tribes (Indian Appropriations Act, 1871).

In the early 1800s, several Supreme Court decisions of the Marshall Court, which is the U.S. Supreme Court from 1801 to 1835, were made. Today, those decisions still guide Indian law (Library of Congress, 2024). What many do not realize is that first contact itself brought disease and premature death to Indigenous individuals and communities, and the attendant laws, policies, and court decisions that followed were the persistent, targeted, and sustained actions that forced the Indigenous population to the brink of extinction (Koch et al., 2019).

The 1900 census was the first time American Indians were enumerated in a U.S. census. At its peak, northern North American Indigenous peoples are estimated to have been in the tens of millions[2] in number (Thornton, 1987). At its lowest, roughly 230,000 Indigenous people remained, according to the 1900 U.S. census (United States Census Bureau, 2021; see **Figure 3.1**). With a population loss estimated by some to have measured as high as 90%, this population shift fits the scientific definition of "near extinction" (Kaiho, 2022). Sheehan (1973) has named Jeffersonian policy around the Removal Act, sowing the "seeds of extinction." However, Indigenous peoples are not a fauna "species," to which we usually see this term applied, but a human population. In this case then, what happened to the Indigenous people can be more appropriately termed as genocide. In simpler terms, Indigenous people indeed were 100% of the population in what is now Canada and the United States. Today, a mere 4.3% of the total U.S. population self-identifies as AI/AN only (with no other racial group selected; United States Census Bureau, 2023a; see **Figure 3.1**).

[2] Some estimates are as high as 60 million pre-contact. https://www.pri.org/stories/2019-01-31/european-colonization-americas-killed-10-percent-world-population-and-caused.

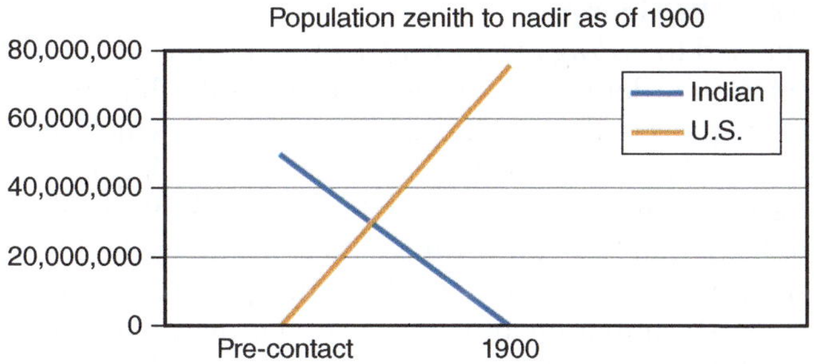

Figure 3.1 **America's Indigenous population losses from pre-contact to 1900.**

GENOCIDE

Genocide is defined by the 1948 *United Nations Convention on the Prevention and Punishment of the Crime of Genocide,* Article II as the following:

> In the present Convention, genocide means any of the following acts committed with intent to destroy, in whole or in part, a national, ethnic, racial or religious group, as such:
>
> I. Killing members of the group;
> II. Causing serious bodily or mental harm to members of the group;
> III. Deliberately inflicting on the group conditions of life calculated to bring about its physical destruction in whole or in part;
> IV. Imposing measures intended to prevent births within the group;
> V. Forcibly transferring children of the group to another group (United Nations, 1948).

Each of these elements of the definition can explicitly be shown by the laws, court cases, policies, and structures purposively put into place by the U.S. government vis-à-vis the Indigenous people found within the borders of today's America. Although few non-Indigenous Americans themselves realize this history, American Indians carry it from generation to generation. Therein lies one source of the intergenerational trauma and HT (Yellow Horse Brave Heart, 1995).

The disruption to Indigenous life in America was especially evident from the 1800s through today. The ongoing disruptions are depicted in **Figure 3.2.**

Although the federal policy periods through assimilation (see **Figure 3.2**) predate the United Nations definition of genocide, all of these named policies include and/or complement the elements of the crime of genocide, and some overlap the definitional parameters of genocide.

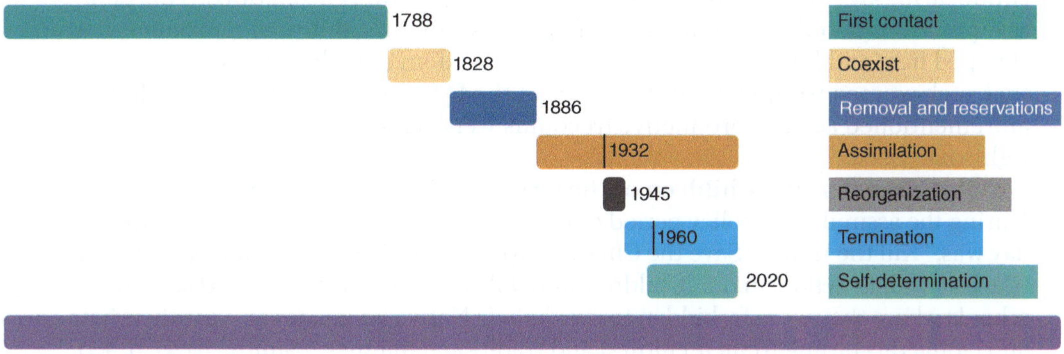

Figure 3.2 **U.S. federal policy periods, most of which caused ongoing life and death disruptions of Indigenous peoples.**

- **Killing Members of the Group**
  Several policies that led to *killing members of a group* began with certain U.S. presidents. The first extermination order was by President George Washington, when orders were given to the Iroquois to destroy Indigenous villages—which resulted in 40 villages being destroyed and the murder of the countless villagers who resided in them (Calloway, 2018). This was followed by President Thomas Jefferson, who noted on December 29, 1813, that "this unfortunate race, whom we had been taking so much pains to save and to civilize, have by their unexpected desertion and ferocious barbarities justified extermination and now await our decision on their fate" (National Archives, 2002). Jefferson then went on as architect of the Trail of Tears, which was part of the Removal Act/Era in which thousands of Indigenous people were forcibly removed from the East Coast to Oklahoma and other areas (National Park Service, 2017). Many were tortured, starved, and abused, and many even died as this unfolded.
- **Causing Serious Bodily or Mental Harm to Members of the Group**
  This element crosses several federal Indian policy periods. It often involved forcibly moving tribes to reservations, thereby completely changing the Indigenous people's way of life and religion as well as access to ceremony and history. In fact, Trennert (1975) noted that the reservation system was conceived as an "alternative to extinction." In the case of the Trail of Tears (National Park Service, 2017), people were forcibly moved and thousands died in the process. During assimilation, many children were lost, tortured, and assaulted and suffered physical, spiritual, emotional, and mental traumas. Many others were either killed or died from their injuries and/or diminished health state (Montgomery & Supernant, 2022; Williams, 2022).
- **Deliberately Inflicting on the Group Conditions of Life Calculated to Bring About Its Physical Destruction in Whole or in Part**
  This element also crosses many of the same genocidal policies. For example, once forcibly moved to "Indian Country" under the auspices of the Reservation Act, women often were abused and raped, food supplies were cut off, land was unfarmable, and weather conditions proved to be unbearable. Conditions like these are what instigated the Dakota uprising in 1862 (Martinez, 2013). As a result of that uprising—which rose from a place of protectiveness and survival—the Dakota were then banned from Minnesota. Congress passed The Dakota Removal Act on March 3, 1863, making it illegal for Dakota people to be or hold land in Minnesota. (Act of March 3, 1863). Shockingly, that law is still on the books today.
- **Imposing Measures Intended to Prevent Births Within the Group**
  It is well documented that the IHS was sterilizing women without their knowledge or consent or through coercion (Torpy, 2000). Forced sterilization of 25,000 American Indian women occurred in the 1960s and 1970s by the IHS, or one quarter of childbearing-age Native women (Dillingham, 1977; Lawerence, 2000). This policy and practice not only terminated an Indigenous woman's ability to reproduce, it also stripped her (and her family) of reproductive freedom and choice, one of the many that such women would lose at the hands of the U.S. government through all the aforementioned acts. Reproductive freedoms were removed just as so many other rights had been.
- **Forcibly Transferring Children of the Group to Another Group**
  During the assimilation policy period of federal Indian law, the saying that drove the day was, "Kill the Indian, Save the Child," adapted from "Kill the Indian, Save the Man" (Carlisle Indian School, n.d.). "Children were taken from their homes and sent to boarding schools where they were forbidden to speak their Native languages or wear their hair and clothes according to their cultural and traditional manner" (Smith, 2020, p. 45). More than 60,000 "students" were taken away to these schools by 1925, although the

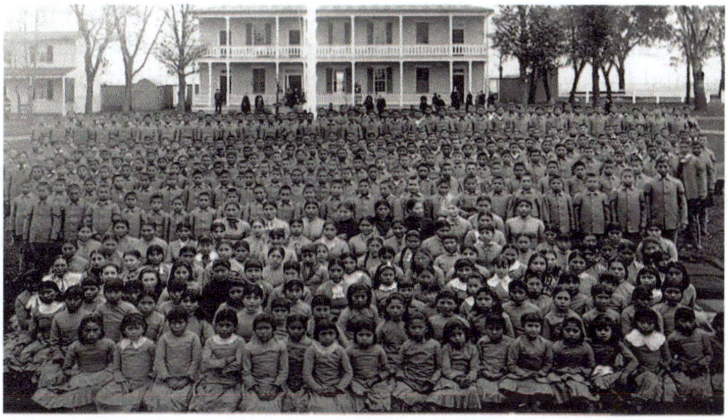

Figure 3.3 **Pupils at Carlisle Native Industrial School, Pennsylvania (c. 1900).**
Source: Manske, M. (2006). *Pupils at Carlisle Native Industrial School, Pennsylvania.* https://commons.wikimedia.org/wiki/File:Carlisle_pupils.jpg

practice and schools lasted 50 more years (National Native American Boarding School Healing Coalition, n.d.). They were not allowed to practice their ceremonies or religion and often never saw their families again. Records confirm that many were outright killed, prematurely died because of their diminished health state, or were "lost" (Little, 2017). It also is well documented that there was an abundance of physical, emotional, sexual, and mental abuse at these "schools" (Equal Justice Initiative, 2025; see **Figure 3.3**). In October 2024, President Biden offered an apology for the schools and atrocities that occurred there under the auspices of the U.S. government (Equal Justice Initiative, 2025).

The other form of removing children was in the adopting and fostering out of AI/AN children into "good" White families. Therefore, The Indian Child Welfare Act–HR12533 (S. 1214; 1977/1978) was enacted to stem the bleeding of American Indian children from their families, clans, and communities at alarming rates into non-Indian homes during the 1950s, 1960s, and 1970s (George, 1997).

MENTAL HEALTH AND AMERICAN INDIANS

Mental health in the United States is not prioritized the same as physical health. The literature shows that there are several factors driving this (e.g., stigma and lack of awareness; Pike et al., 2013). However, it is evident in terms of the resources allocated; perceived and expressed importance; equitable access to high-quality prevention, care, and treatment; and optimal outcomes for those struggling with a mental health disease or condition are not on parity with those for physical health. In fact, health professions education, including medical, nursing, dental, and social work curricula, continues to emphasize physical health over mental health (Tyerman et al., 2021). This leaves mental health a distant second in focus, importance, funding, and access, negatively affecting the pipeline of mental health care providers and educators. The unfortunate irony, however, is that we know that mental health is inextricably linked to physical health (Kwapong et al., 2023). For example, Kwapong et al. showed an association of depression and poor mental health with cardiovascular disease among young adults in the United States. Perhaps more unfortunate is that we are seeing the results of decades of actions that ignored this aspect of people's health in the high levels of those suffering from mental health disorders and illnesses in our school- and college-aged students (Harris et al., 2022), in older adults (Reynolds et al., 2022), and in incarcerated populations (Fedock et al., 2024). Fedock et al. "conceptualize prison-based mental health treatment as health harm rather than health care" (2024, p. 302). The overall lack of awareness and concern to prioritize mental health, considered in tandem with the absence of a strong, comprehensive mental health care system, only widens the gap between the great need for and the availability of adequate and appropriate mental health care services and treatments. This gap has a particularly detrimental and disproportionate impact on Indigenous individuals and communities.

AI/AN persons are often noted to be the invisible Americans (May & McDermott, 2021; Moss, 2022). Very little is understood or known about this population. *It is by design* that few Americans know much about this population, perhaps remnants of purposeful attempts to get rid of the Indian population that is prominent throughout U.S. history (May & McDermott, 2021). However, AI/AN individuals are arguably the most traumatized of any racial group in the United States, with both historical and contemporaneous traumas occurring at unprecedented levels (Moss, 2022).

As a population, it is important to note that there is a great distinguishing feature that no other racial or ethnic or otherwise minoritized group in the United States can claim. The ancestors of those now legally known as (American) Indians were the sole, original sovereigns of the land on which the United States sits today. Today, federally recognized tribes retain partial sovereignty in the eyes of the U.S. government and as such are a political body as well as a racial group. No other racial group has this designation; it is this difference that has caused the invisibility in, and the ridding of AI/AN persons from, the general U.S. population (Davis et al., 2022). Therefore, it is important to note the historical, geopolitical, and other current contexts of this Indigenous population. Once there is an understanding, only then can true planning for optimization of care and health occur. These contexts manifest in the disproportionate and persistent mental health burdens and illnesses we see in Indigenous individuals and communities today (Moss, 2022).

Mental Health Perspective

AI/AN individuals view mental health as one of the four domains of the person (Moss, 2022). The four domains are physical, mental, emotional, and spiritual and are seen as equal aspects of a person. This idea can be exemplified in the Medicine Wheel. The Medicine Wheel is understood throughout Indian country, although there are variations of labels, colors, and directions/orientation (see **Figure 3.4**).

The IHS is the federal agency charged with the provision of federal healthcare to AI/AN persons (IHS, n.d., para. 2). The IHS periodically produces a report titled *Trends in Indian Health*. In the last report (IHS, 2014), a comparison of mortality numbers for AI/

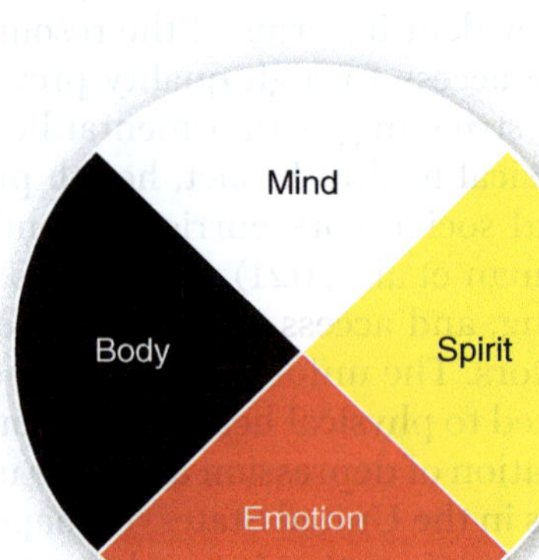

Figure 3.4 Medicine Wheel.

AN individuals and all races includes several statistics in the mental health realm versus the physical realm (see **Table 3.1**).

AI/AN populations have an array of mental health issues, running the gamut of mood and thought disorders, as in all other populations. However, there are elevations in rates of depression, anxiety, and suicide across age groups, as reported in the *IHS Trends* report. Nearly eight in 10 (87%) American Indians live off-reservation (IHS, n.d.). Little is known about the prevalence and treatment of this population. In a sample of urban AI/AN adults, primary psychiatric diagnoses in descending prevalence were found to be as follows: depressive disorders (43%), schizophrenia spectrum and other psychotic disorders (17%), bipolar and related disorders (13%), trauma and stressor-related disorders (13%), and anxiety disorders (9%; Dickerson et al., 2023). This study found that in comparison to non-AI/AN patients, AI/AN patients were diagnosed with depressive disorder, bipolar and related disorders, trauma and stressor-related disorders, or schizophrenia spectrum and other psychotic disorders at disproportionately higher rates (Dickerson et al., 2023).

Rural communities throughout the United States have unique barriers to mental health care and treatment access, exacerbated by the increased distances and lack of available mental health care providers. Recent studies show that these barriers have a disproportionate, negative impact on Indigenous individuals in rural communities. In fact, one study found that there was a higher prevalence of frequent mental distress and depression among rural AI/AN persons as compared with rural non-Hispanic Whites (Morales et al., 2020). Further, young adults aged 18 to 25 years reported the highest prevalence of mental illness within the AI/AN population in the past year (**Figure 3.5**; Substance Abuse and Mental Health Services Administration, 2023). This is due, in part, to the fact that reservation communities are especially remote and patients seeking mental health care fear the risk of explicit and implicit racism in healthcare, confidentiality issues, and racially and culturally discordant providers who are not adept at providing culturally competent mental health care (Moss, 2015).

Another study noted that among college students, AI/AN students had the largest increases in depression, anxiety, and suicidal ideation and were more likely to meet the criteria for one or more mental health problems from 2013 to 2021 (Lipson et al., 2022). There was a mental health treatment gap identified for AI/AN students in this study, and the gap was attributed to the lack of attention and resources targeted to the unique needs of this population.

Table 3.1 COMPARISON OF 2007–2009 AI/AN DEATH RATES WITH 2008 U.S. ALL-RACES DEATH RATES

MENTAL HEALTH	OVERLAPPING	PHYSICAL HEALTH
Alcohol related—520% greater	Motor vehicle crashes—207% greater	Tuberculosis—450% greater
Homicide—86% greater	Chronic liver disease and cirrhosis—368% greater	Diabetes mellitus—177% greater
Suicide—60% greater	Unintentional injuries—141% greater	Pneumonia and influenza—37% greater
Firearm injury—16% greater	Poisoning—118% greater	

Source: Indian Health Service. (2014). *Trends in Indian health: 2014 edition.* https://www.ihs.gov/sites/dps/themes/responsive2017/display_objects/documents/Trends2014Book508.pdf

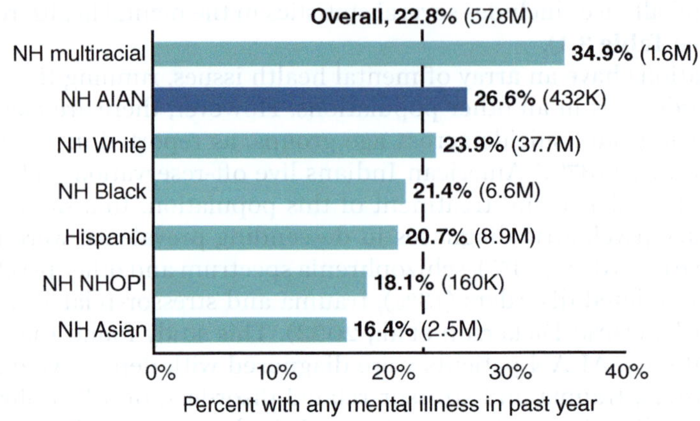

Figure 3.5 Past year mental illness, by racial and ethnic groups aged 18 years and older.

Note: AIAN adults were just as likely to have a mental illness as adults from all other racial and ethnic groups. AIAN, American Indian/Alaska Native; NH, non-Hispanic; NHOPI, Native Hawaiian or other Pacific Islander.

Source: Substance Abuse and Mental Health Services Administration. (2023). *2021 national survey on drug use and health: Among the American Indian or Alaska Native (AIAN) population aged 12 or older*. https://www.samhsa.gov/data/sites/default/files/reports/rpt41854/NSDUH%20highlighted%20population%20slides/For%20NSDUH%20highlighted%20population%20slides/2021NSDUHPopulationSlidesAIAN050323.pdf

Suicide

American Indians have the highest suicide death rates of all other racial groups in the United States (see **Figure 3.6**). Further, the 18 states that participate in the National Violent Death Reporting System (NVDRS) reported that the AI/AN population not only had the highest

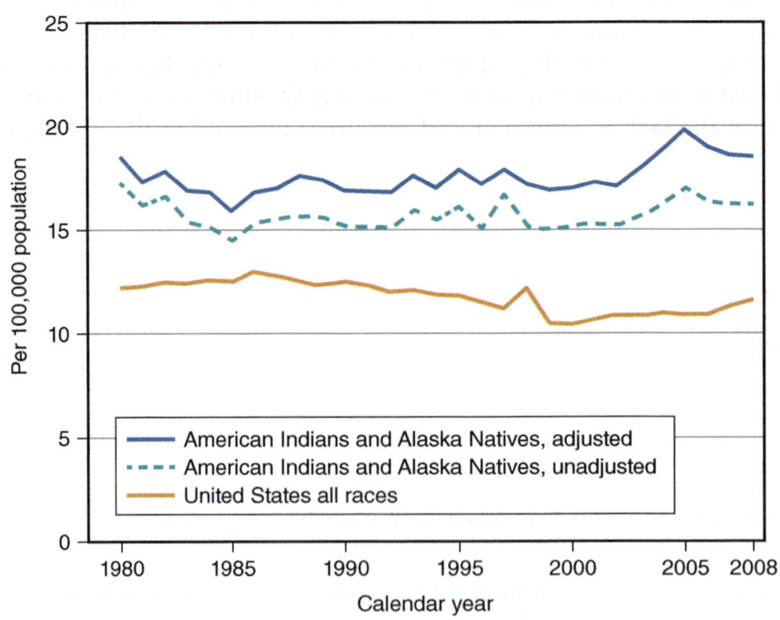

Figure 3.6 A comparison of suicide rates for AI/AN and United States all races.

AI/AN, American Indian/Alaska Native.

Source: Indian Health Service. (2014). *Trends in Indian health: 2014 edition*. https://www.ihs.gov/sites/dps/themes/responsive2017/display_objects/documents/Trends2014Book508.pdf

suicide death rates, but that these rates were up to 3.5 times higher than racial groups with the lowest rates from 2003 through 2015 (Leavitt et al., 2018).

Not only do they have the highest prevalence of mental illness across their cohort, AI/AN individuals aged 18 to 25 years reported the highest rates of suicidal thoughts, plans, and attempts in comparison with all other racial groups (Leavitt et al., 2018; see **Figure 3.7**).

Findings from the NVDRS also show that more than three in four (78%) completed suicide attempts occurred in males, with those aged 25 to 44 years having the highest rate (43%). Nearly three in four (73%) completed suicide attempts occurred at home, nearly 70% (69.4%) occurred in nonmetropolitan settings, and more than four in 10 (42%) involved the use of a firearm.

The true incidence of mental health disruptions in the AI/AN population remains largely unknown, undocumented, mis-documented, and essentially hidden. According to the IHS's last *Trends in Indian Health* report (2014), misidentification of American Indians from state data is problematic. As an example, the report "specifies a number, rate, or ratio of rates adjusted to compensate for misreporting of AI/AN race on state death certificates" (p. 64). Notations such as this appear throughout the report. Therefore, as dismal as the statistics are across all health domains, they are likely much worse across the AI/AN population (Moss, 2015).

Experiences That Contributed to Suicide Risk

Historical and contemporaneous trauma, mis- and missing treatment, and poor life conditions thrust upon the AI/AN population (as outlined earlier in the chapter) contribute to these higher suicide risk and mortality rates. One study found that suicide resulted from one or more of the following risk factors: trauma and related health problems, loss and exposure to suicide, substance misuse, lack of resources, and stigma (Shaw et al., 2019). The traumas have been well outlined, and the suicide rates and therefore exposure to suicide are higher among Indigenous individuals than any other racial group. This remains true even when issues of underreporting are taken into account.

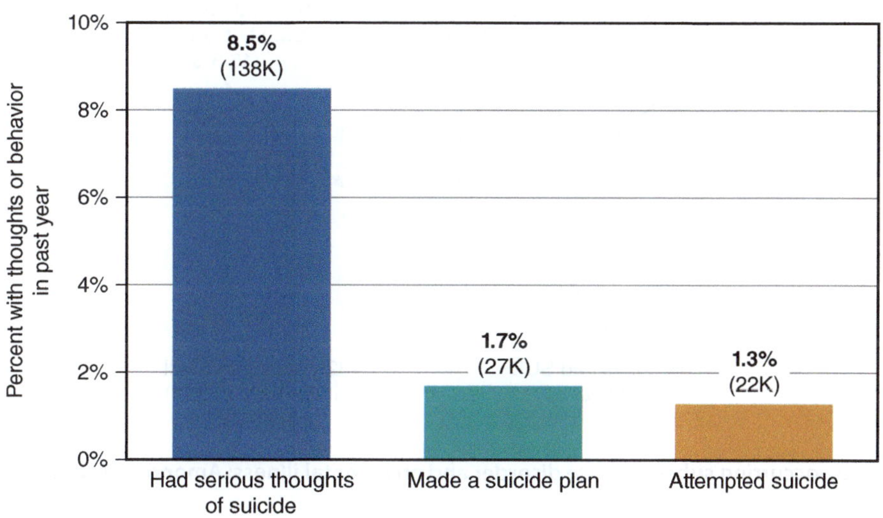

Figure 3.7 Past year serious thoughts of suicide, suicide plans, or suicide attempts among AI/AN adults aged 18 or older.

AI/AN, American Indian/Alaska Native.

Source: Substance Abuse and Mental Health Services Administration. (2023). *2021 National survey on drug use and health: Among the American Indian or Alaska Native (AIAN) population aged 12 or older*. https://www.samhsa.gov/data/sites/default/files/reports/rpt41854/NSDUH%20highlighted%20population%20slides/For%20NSDUH%20highlighted%20population%20slides/2021NSDUHPopulationSlidesAIAN050323.pdf

SUBSTANCE MISUSE

There is also a link between racial trauma and substance use among American Indians (Skewes & Blume, 2019). As seen in IHS reporting, alcohol-related deaths were 520% greater among AI/AN individuals than among all other races in the United States (IHS, 2014). Further, the Substance Abuse and Mental Health Services Administration (SAMHSA) reported substance use disorder rates without any co-occurring mental illness (AMI) as 16%, in conjunction with AMI at nearly 10% (9.7%), and AMI with no substance use disorder also at nearly 10% (9.8%; SAMHSA, 2023; see **Figure 3.8**).

According to the NVDRS, mental health and substance use challenges were present in a number of the completed suicide decedents (see **Table 3.2**). The same study found that AI/AN persons who completed suicide used alcohol hours before completion at a rate of 48.6% versus 25% for White victims, coupled with a history and current use of mental health treatment almost half that used by Whites.

CULTURAL STRATEGIES AS PROTECTIVE FACTORS

American Indians carry the burden of intergenerational trauma and grief, or *historical trauma* as coined by Maria Yellow Horse Brave Heart (1998). HT stems from the genocidal actions of the United States toward the Indigenous people of northern North America. AI/AN individuals often also suffer from posttraumatic stress disorder from contemporaneous traumas. It must be recognized, though, that HT is trauma on a group over generations, whereas posttraumatic stress disorder speaks to individualized trauma. Together, they add to the severity and rates of mental illness and the mental health disruption burden suffered by the AI/AN population (Beals et al., 2005). This burden may lead to mental illness

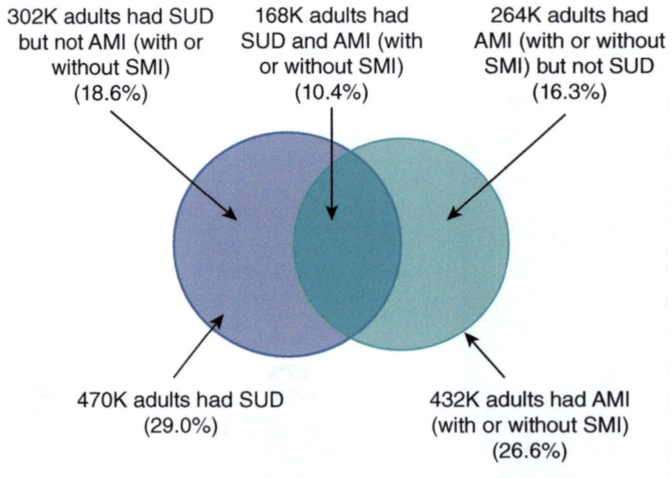

Figure 3.8 Co-occurring substance use disorder and any mental illness: Among AI/AN adults aged 18 or older.

Note: 168,000 (10.4%) AIAN adults aged 18 or older had co-occurring SUD and AMI. 734,000 AIAN adults had either SUD or AMI (with or without SMI).

AI/AN, American Indian/Alaska Native; AMI, any mental illness; SMI, serious mental illness; SUD, substance use disorder.

Source: Substance Abuse and Mental Health Services Administration. (2023). *2021 national survey on drug use and health: Among the American Indian or Alaska Native (AIAN) population aged 12 or older*. https://www.samhsa.gov/data/sites/default/files/reports/rpt41854/NSDUH%20highlighted%20population%20slides/For%20NSDUH%20highlighted%20population%20slides/2021NSDUHPopulationSlidesAIAN050323.pdf

Table 3.2 CIRCUMSTANCES PRECIPITATING SUICIDE DEATHS OF NON-HISPANIC AMERICAN INDIANS/ALASKA NATIVES COMPARED WITH NON-HISPANIC WHITES

	NO. (%)		
MENTAL HEALTH/SUBSTANCE USE	AI/AN	WHITE	AOR (95% CI)
Current mental health problem	371 (27.7)	43,614 (46.7)	0.4 (0.4–0.5)
Current depressed mood	489 (36.5)	38.940 (41.7)	0.9 (0.8–1.0)
Current mental health treatment	261 (19.5)	31,987 (34.2)	0.5 (0.4–0.5)
History of mental health treatment	311 (23.2)	37,499 (40.2)	0.4 (0.4–0.5)
Reported alcohol use in hours preceding death	651 (48.6)	23,370 (25.0)	2.7 (2.4–3.0)
Alcohol abuse problem	371 (27.7)	17,242 (18.5)	1.8 (1.6–2.1)
Substance abuse problem other than alcohol	202 (15.1)	14,365 (15.4)	—

Note: Chi-squared test result for difference between AI/AN and White significant at $p < 0.05$.

AI/AN, American Indian/Alaska Native; AOR, adjusted odds ratio; CI, confidence interval.

Source: Leavitt, R. A., Ertl, A., Sheats. K., Petrosky, E., Ivey-Stephenson, A., & Fowler, K.A. (2018). Suicides among American Indian/Alaska Natives—National violent death reporting system, 18 states, 2003–2014. *MMWR Morbidity and Mortality Weekly Report, 67*(8), 237–242. http://dx.doi.org/10.15585/mmwr.mm6708a1

and suffering as well as spiritual, emotional, and physical pain. It is a historically long and layered reality that providers must understand to offer effective, targeted, culturally relevant, and safe mental health treatment and care. Unfortunately, this type of mental health care often is unavailable to Indigenous individuals and communities (Manson, 2000).

One collaborative study on suicide protective factors in an urban setting found that intergenerational engagement and cultural connectedness were effective preventive strategies (Doria et al., 2022). Over three years, AI/AN elders, adults, and youth participated via talking circles reflecting on this issue.

Gaining a full understanding of indigeneity will not occur unless there is a purposeful and demonstrative shift in and from the Western perspective. Understanding regional as well as tribally specific cosmology, ceremony, and what is deemed sacred is necessary in understanding how “Indigenous communities relate to potent spiritual persons and powers, and express culturally specific values of divinity, community, morality and well-being (i.e., living a good life)” (Gone & Kirmayer, 2020, pp. 238). AI/AN patients understand that you may be on a learning journey, and therefore demonstrating and using the tools of cultural humility and respect to reach the goal of cultural safety for the patient will let practitioners meet the AI/AN patient where they are.

SUMMARY

AI/AN individuals have suffered huge shifts in the realities that guided their lives for millennia. With contact, they were killed, tortured, and starved over hundreds of years, all in the “get rid of the Indian problem” policies and practices of the U.S. government. This has resulted in health status and quality-of-life disruptions in which low life expectancy, high suicide rates, and other manifestations of HT are the norm in Indigenous communities today. All of these interrelated social, political, and historical forces and dynamics seem to escape the minds and practice of many of today’s practitioners on a large scale (Moss, 2015). One must understand the histories, targeted laws, and policies of the United States vis-à-vis

Indigenous people of North America to provide culturally relevant, culturally competent, and safe mental health care. This will require a monumental, coordinated effort by mental health professionals and lawmakers that is as targeted, systematic, and persistent as those efforts that disrupted Indigenous health almost since first contact generations ago. Only then would it be considered reconciliation.

DISCUSSION QUESTIONS

1. How might the Medicine Wheel's approach to health help us better understand the challenges faced by Indigenous communities today?
2. What are the major federal Indian policy periods? How do you think they have shaped the lives of Indigenous people over time?
3. What are the elements of the crime of genocide as laid out by the United Nations Genocide Convention of 1948? Why do you think the United Nations definition of genocide is important for understanding Indigenous history in the United States?
4. How have the histories and genocide of Indigenous people in the United States post contact resulted in mental health disparities today?
5. What are some cultural strategies, practices, or traditions that serve as protective factors in treating this population?

REFERENCES

25 U.S.C. § United States Code, Title 25 – Indians (1832). https://www.govinfo.gov/content/pkg/USCODE-2011-title25/html/USCODE-2011-title25.htm

Act of March 3, 1863, ch. 199, 12 Stat. 819. (1863).

Arias, E., Tejada-Vera, B., Kochanek, K., & Ahmad, F. (2022). *Provisional life expectancy estimates for 2021.* https://www.cdc.gov/nchs/data/vsrr/vsrr023.pdf. https://doi.org/10.15620/cdc:118999

Beals, J., Novins, D. K., Whitesell, N. R., Spicer, P., Mitchell, C. M., Manson, S. M., & American Indian Service Utilization, Psychiatric Epidemiology, Risk and Protective Factors Project Team. (2005). Prevalence of mental disorders and utilization of mental health services in two American Indian reservation populations: Mental health disparities in a national context. *American Journal of Psychiatry, 162*(9), 1723–1732. https://doi.org/10.1176/appi.ajp.162.9.1723

Calloway, C. G. (2018). *The Indian world of George Washington: The first president, the first Americans, and the birth of the nation.* Oxford University Press.

Carlisle Indian School. (n.d.). *Kill the Indian in him, and save the man: R. H. Pratt on the education of native Americans.* https://carlisleindian.dickinson.edu/teach/kill-indian-him-and-save-man-r-h-pratt-education-native-americans

Convention on the Prevention and Punishment of the Crime of Genocide. (1948). S. Exec. Doc.

Davis-Delano, L. R., Strother, S. L., & Gone, J. P. (2022). Perceived indicators of American Indian identity in everyday interaction: Navigating settler-colonial erasure. *Ethnic and Racial Studies, 45*(11), 2025–2048.

Deloria, V. (1969). *Custer died for your sins: An Indian manifesto.* University of Oklahoma Press.

Deloria, V., & Wilkins, D. E. (2000). *Tribes, treaties, and constitutional tribulations.* University of Texas Press.

Dickerson, D., Cain, M., & Garcia, A. (2023). Primary psychiatric diagnoses, commercialized tobacco use, and homelessness: Comparisons between urban American Indian/Alaska Native and non-American Indian/Alaska Native adult clinical samples. *American Indian and Alaska Native Mental Health Research (Online), 30*(1), 14–34. https://doi.org/10.5820/aian.3001.2023.14

Dillingham, B. (1977). Sterilization of native Americans. *American Indian Journal, 3*, 16.

Doria, C. M., Momper, S. L., & Burrage, R. L. (2022). "Togetherness:" The role of intergenerational and cultural engagement in urban American Indian and Alaskan native youth suicide prevention. *Indigenous Health Equity and Wellness* (pp. 109–126). Routledge.

Equal Justice Initiative. (2025). *President Biden apologizes to native Americans for federal Indian boarding schools.* https://eji.org/news/president-biden-apologizes-to-native-americans-for-federal-indian-boarding-schools/

Fedock, G. L., Shankar, S., Doria, C., & Malcome, M. (2024). "You have to take care of your own mental status": Incarcerated women seeking care within and beyond mental health treatment. *Affilia, 39*(2), 302–319. https://doi.org/10.1177/0886109923119622

George, L. J. (1997). Why the need for the Indian child welfare act? *Journal of Multicultural Social Work, 5*(3–4), 165–175.

Geotting, N. (2008). The Marshall trilogy and the constitutional dehumanization of American Indians. *Guild Practitioner, 65*(4), 207–226.

Gone, J. P., & Kirmayer, L. J. (2020). Advancing indigenous mental health research: Ethical, conceptual and methodological challenges. *Transcultural Psychiatry, 57*(2), 235–249. https://doi.org/10.1177/1363461520923151

Harris, B. R., Maher, B. M., & Wentworth, L. (2022). Optimizing efforts to promote mental health on college and university campuses: Recommendations to facilitate usage of services, resources, and supports. *The Journal of Behavioral Health Services & Research, 49*(2), 252–258. https://doi.org/10.1007/s11414-021-09780-2

Helgesen, E. (2011). Allotment of justice: How US policy in Indian country perpetuates the victimization of American Indians. *Journal of Law and Public Policy, 22*(3), 441.

Indian Appropriations Act. (1871). https://recordsofrights.org/records/285/indian-appropriations-act/1

The Indian Child Welfare Act HR12533, S. 1214 (1977/1978). https://www.congress.gov/95/statute/STATUTE-92/STATUTE-92-Pg3069.pdf

Indian Health Service. (n.d.). *About urban Indian organizations.* https://www.ihs.gov/Urban/aboutus/about-urban-indian

Indian Health Service. (2014). *Trends in Indian health: 2014 edition.* https://www.ihs.gov/sites/dps/themes/responsive2017/display_objects/documents/Trends2014Book508.pdf

John, R., & Baldridge, D. (1996). *The NICOA report: Health and long-term care for Indian elders.* http://moon.ouhsc.edu/rjohn/longterm.pdf

Jones, D. S. (2006). The persistence of American Indian health disparities. *American Journal of Public Health, 96*(12), 2122–2134. https://doi.org/10.2105/AJPH.2004.054262

Kaiho, K. (2022). Extinction magnitude of animals in the near future. *Scientific Reports, 12*(1), 19593. https://doi.org/10.1038/s41598-022-23369-5

Koch, A., Brierley, C., Maslin, M. M., & Lewis, S. L. (2019). Earth system impacts of the European arrival and great dying in the Americas after 1492. *Quaternary Science Reviews,* 207, 13–36. https://doi.org/10.1016/j.quascirev.2018.12.004

Kwapong, Y. A., Boakye, E., Khan, S. S., Honigberg, M. C., Martin, S. S., Oyeka, C. P., Hays, A. G., Natarajan, P., Mamas, M. A., Blumenthal, R. S., Blaha, M. J., & Sharma, G. (2023). Association of depression and poor mental health with cardiovascular disease and suboptimal cardiovascular health among young adults in the United States. *Journal of the American Heart Association, 12*(3), e028332. https://doi.org/10.1161/JAHA.122.028332

Leavitt, R. A., Ertl, A., Sheats. K., Petrosky, E., Ivey Stephenson, A., & Fowler, K.A. (2018). Suicides among American Indian/Alaska Natives—National violent death reporting system, 18 states, 2003–2014. *MMWR Morbidity and Mortality Weekly Report, 67*(8), 237–242. http://dx.doi.org/10.15585/mmwr.mm6708a1.

Library of Congress. (2024). *American Indian law: A beginner's guide. Court cases.* https://guides.loc.gov/american-indian-law/Cases

Lipson, S. K., Zhou, S., Abelson, S., Heinze, J., Jirsa, M., Morigney, J., ..., Eisenberg, D. (2022). Trends in college student mental health and help-seeking by race/ethnicity: Findings from the national healthy minds study, 2013–2021. *Journal of Affective Disorders, 306*, 138–147. https://doi.org/10.1016/j.jad.2022.03.038

Little, B. (2017). How boarding schools tried to "kill the Indian" through assimilation. https://www.history.com/articles/how-boarding-schools-tried-to-kill-the-indian-through-assimilation

Manson, S. M. (2000). Mental health services for American Indians and Alaska Natives: Need, use, and barriers to effective care. *The Canadian Journal of Psychiatry, 45*(7), 617–626. https://doi.org/10.1177/070674370004500703

Marshall, J., & Supreme Court of the United States. (1823). *U.S. reports: Johnson v. McIntosh,* 21 U.S. 8 Wheat. 543. [Periodical] Library of Congress. https://www.loc.gov/item/usrep021543/

May, A. R., & McDermott, V. (2021). Invisibility as modern racism: Redressing the experience of indigenous learners in higher education. *Journal of Communication Pedagogy, 5*, 55–61. https://doi.org/10.31446/JCP.2021.2.09

Miller, R. J. (2005). The doctrine of discovery in American Indian law. *Idaho Law Review, 42*, 1.

Montgomery, L. M., & Supernant, K. (2022). Archaeology in 2021: Repatriation, reclamation, and reckoning with historical trauma. *American Anthropologist, 124*(4), 800–812.

Morales, D. A., Barksdale, C. L., & Beckel-Mitchener, A. C. (2020). A call to action to address rural mental health disparities. *Journal of Clinical and Translational Science, 4*(5), 463–467. https://doi.org/10.1017/cts.2020.42

Moss, M. P. (Ed.). (2015). *American Indian health and nursing.* Springer Publishing Company.

Moss, M. (2022). American Indian health: The medicine wheel vs the iron triangle. In M. Halliwell (Ed.), *The Edinburgh companion to the politics of American health.* Edinburgh University Press.

National Archives. (2002). *Thomas Jefferson to David Bailie Warden, 29 December 1813.* https://founders.archives.gov/documents/Jefferson/03-07-02-0046

National Center for Health Statistics. (2016). *Health, United States, 2016.* https://www.cdc.gov/nchs/data/hus/hus16.pdf

National Library of Medicine. (n.d.). *Congress seeks to abolish tribes, relocate American Indians.* https://www.nlm.nih.gov/nativevoices/timeline/488.html

National Museum of American Indians. (2024). *Teaching & learning about Native Americans.* https://americanindian.si.edu/nk360/faq/did-you-know

National Native American Boarding School Healing Coalition. (n.d.). *US Indian boarding school history.* https://boardingschoolhealing.org/education/us-indian-boarding-school-history/

National Park Service. (2017). *Multi-state: Trail of Tears National Historic Trail.* https://www.nps.gov/articles/trailoftears.htm#:~:text=The%20Indian%20Removal%20Act%20of,occupied%20land%20for%20white%20settlers

Pevar, S. L. (1992). *The rights of Indians and tribes: The basic ACLU guide to Indian and tribal rights.* Southern Illinois University Press.

Pike, K. M., Susser, E., Galea, S., & Pincus, H. (2013). Towards a healthier 2020: Advancing mental health as a global health priority. *Public Health Reviews, 35*, 1–25. https://doi.org/10.1007/BF03391692

Reynolds C. F., III, Jeste, D. V., Sachdev, P. S., & Blazer, D. G. (2022). Mental health care for older adults: recent advances and new directions in clinical practice and research. *World Psychiatry, 21*(3), 336–363. https://doi.org/10.1002/wps.20996

Shaw, J. L., Beans, J. A., Comtois, K. A., & Hiratsuka, V. Y. (2019). Lived experiences of suicide risk and resilience among Alaska Native and American Indian people. *International Journal of Environmental Research and Public Health, 16*(20), 3953. https://doi.org/10.3390/ijerph16203953

Sheehan, B. W. (1973). *Seeds of extinction: Jeffersonian philanthropy and the American Indian* (pp. xii, 30). University of North Carolina Press.

Skewes, M. C., & Blume, A. W. (2019). Understanding the link between racial trauma and substance use among American Indians. *American Psychologist, 74*(1), 88–100. https://doi.org/10.1037/amp0000331

Smith, B. (2024). *Service delivery on Pine Ridge—Meeting the Oglala Lakota people where they are.* https://www.supremecourt.gov/DocketPDF/24/24-354/337400/20250116081739528_24-354.24-422%20AMI%20Gonzalez%20ALL%20PDFA.pdf

Smith, J. (2020). *The impact of boarding schools on Native American culture.* Native Press Publishing.

South Dakota v. Bourland, 508 U.S. 679. (1993). https://supreme.justia.com/cases/federal/us/508/679/

Steele, M. (2016). Plenary power, political questions, and sovereignty in Indian affairs. *UCLA Law Review, 63*, 666.

Substance Abuse and Mental Health Services Administration. (2023). *2021 National survey on drug use and health: Among the American Indian or Alaska Native (AIAN) population aged 12 or older.* https://www.samhsa.gov/data/sites/default/files/reports/rpt41854/NSDUH%20highlighted%20population%20slides/For%20NSDUH%20highlighted%20population%20slides/2021NSDUHPopulationSlidesAIAN050323.pdf

Thornton, R. (1987). *American Indian holocaust and survival: A population history since 1492.* University of Oklahoma Press.

Torpy, S. J. (2000). Native American women and coerced sterilization: On the Trail of Tears in the 1970s. *American Indian Culture and Research Journal, 24*(2). https://doi.org/10.17953

Trennert, R. A. (1975). Alternative to extinction: Federal Indian policy and the beginnings of the reservation system. *The Annals of the American Academy of Political and Social Science, 421*(1), 1846–1851. https://doi.org/10.1177/000271627542100144

Tyerman, J., Patovirta, A. L., & Celestini, A. (2021). How stigma and discrimination influences nursing care of persons diagnosed with mental illness: A systematic review. *Issues in Mental Health Nursing, 42*(2), 153–163. https://doi.org/10.1080/01612840.2020.1789788

United Nations. (1948). *Convention on the prevention and punishment of the crime of genocide.* https://www.un.org/en/genocideprevention/documents/atrocity-crimes/Doc.1_Convention%20on%20the%20Prevention%20and%20Punishment%20of%20the%20Crime%20of%20Genocide.pdf

United States Census Bureau. (2021). *U.S. Census Bureau history: American Indians and Alaska Natives.* https://www.census.gov/history/pdf/1890indianreport-full.pdf

United States Census Bureau. (2023a). *Detailed data for hundreds of American Indian and Alaska Native tribes.* https://www.census.gov/library/stories/2023/10/2020-census-dhc-a-aian-population.html#:~:text=The%20estimated%20American%20Indian%20and,M%20on%20July%201%2C%202022

United States Census Bureau. (2023b). *Quick facts.* https://www.census.gov/quickfacts/fact/table/US/PST045222

U.S. Code. (2020) *Title 25 Indians.* https://www.govinfo.gov/content/pkg/USCODE-2020-title25/html/USCODE-2020-title25-chap46-sec5301.htm (U.S. Const. art. VI, cl. 2).

U.S. Department of the Interior. (n.d.). *Federal law and Indian policy overview history of Indian law and policy.* https://www.bia.gov/bia/history/IndianLawPolicy.

U.S. Department of the Interior. (2024). *Tribal enrollment process.* https://www.doi.gov/tribes/enrollment#:~:text=Tribal%20enrollment%20requirements%20preserve%20the,traditions%2C%20language%20and%20tribal%20blood

U.S. Department of the Interior, Indian Affairs. (2024). *Tribal leaders directory. A resource to help connect with Indian Country.* https://www.bia.gov/service/tribal-leaders-directory

Warne, D., & Lajimodiere, D. (2015). American Indian health disparities: Psychosocial influences. *Social and Personality Psychology Compass, 9*(10), 567–579. https://doi.org/10.1111/spc3.12198

Wilkins, D. E., & Lomawaima, K. T. (2001). *Uneven ground: American Indian sovereignty and federal law.* University of Oklahoma Press.

Williams, D. R., Priest, N., & Anderson, N. B. (2016). Understanding associations among race, socioeconomic status, and health: Patterns and prospects. *Health Psychology, 35*(4), 407–411. https://doi.org/10.1037/hea0000242

Williams, S. M. (2022). *Assimilation, resilience, and survival: A history of the Stewart Indian school, 1890–2020*. University of Nebraska Press.

Wolfe, P. (1999). *Settler colonialism and the transformation of anthropology: The politics and poetics of an Ethnograph event (writing past imperialism)*. Continuum Pub.

Yellow Horse Brave Heart, M. (1995). *The return to the sacred path: Healing from historical trauma and historical unresolved grief among the Lakota* (unpublished doctoral dissertation). Smith College.

Yellow Horse Brave Heart, M. (1998). The return to the sacred path: Healing the historical trauma and historical unresolved grief response among the Lakota through a psychoeducational group intervention. *Smith College Studies in Social Work, 68*(3), 287–305. https://doi.org/10.1080/00377319809517532

4 REDLINING AND THE STRUCTURAL CONDITIONS OF MENTAL HEALTH EQUITY

OCTAVIO N. MARTINEZ, JR.

LEARNING OBJECTIVES

After reading this chapter, readers will be able to:

- Understand how redlining came to be.
- Describe the role of redlining in residential segregation.
- Explain residential segregation's effects on neighborhood characteristics.
- Discuss how redlining impacts health and mental health inequities.
- Identify the key federal policies that created redlining and its consequences.

INTRODUCTION

The term *redlining* has become a part of our vernacular. We encounter the term in the news or in print. Most individuals understand it is discriminatory and that it has to do with the process of buying real estate. However, few of us truly understand its roots and its ongoing impact beyond residential discrimination and segregation. Redlining has had a significant impact on America's culture, on the equitable distribution of resources, and on our physical and mental health. Its impact is systemic and structural. It has and continues to contribute to physical and mental health disparities through the social determinants of health and mental health; and thereby contributes to the health and mental health inequities impacting millions of Americans.

HISTORY OF REDLINING AND ASSOCIATED POLICIES AND TACTICS

To obtain a full picture of why redlining continues to be relevant to the mental health and health of communities today, it is important to have an appreciation of the historical context. After the U.S. Civil War, one of the most important demographic changes that occurred was the "Great Black Migration of the 20th Century." This was the migration of millions of Black Americans leaving the South for the northern, midwestern, and western parts of the United States for greater economic and standard-of life-opportunities (Banaji et al., 2021). Black Americans of the South lived under an oppressive caste system of racial subordination known as "Jim Crow," which lasted from approximately 1875 to 1968. Black Americans were regulated to second-class status in which the lowest status White individual was superior to the highest status Black individuals (Yearby et al., 2022). From 1876 to 1900, almost 90% of all Black Americans lived in the South, and by 1970, that percentage had declined to about 50% (Banaji et al., 2021). Over the course of these many decades, the migration was fueled by hope and the chance for a better life.

Unfortunately, discrimination and racist beliefs were not just confined to the southern states. Upon reaching their destination, the majority of Black Americans encountered laws and policies that promoted segregation, such as municipal race-based zoning ordinances; private, racially restrictive covenants and deeds; and regulations on land use (Banaji et al., 2021). Smaller towns and cities enacted “sundown laws” that required Black Americans to leave a town by sunset or face dire consequences (Banaji et al., 2021). In larger cities, municipal race-based ordinances were instituted to confine Black Americans to specific neighborhoods that often lacked the resources needed to thrive, such as well-resourced schools (Banaji et al., 2021).

In 1917, these race-based zoning ordinances were deemed unconstitutional by the U.S. Supreme Court (SCOTUS). This ruling partially led to the proliferation of racial deed restrictions and covenants to ensure racial segregation. Because racial deed restrictions and covenants are private agreements between buyers and sellers, SCOTUS ruled them, in 1926, to be constitutional. This meant it was legal to prohibit Black Americans from owning, leasing, or occupying a home in a designated White community. Given the green light, in 1927, the Chicago Real Estate Board developed a model racial covenant that would block Black Americans from living in White neighborhoods. These racial restrictions were not determined to be unconstitutional by SCOTUS until 1948 (Banaji et al., 2021; Barnett et al., 2024; Steil & Arcaya, 2023; Turner & Greene, 2024).

Violence perpetrated by Whites on Blacks also was a part of the accepted culture to keep Blacks and Whites separated. At times, it was used to destroy any measure of success by Black Americans. Numerous examples exist, including the 1906 Atlanta Race Riot; the East St. Louis, Illinois, Massacre of 1917; the Great Chicago Race Riot of 1919; and the Tulsa Massacre of 1921. In the Tulsa Massacre of 1921, the Greenwood community of Tulsa was obliterated by rioting White Tulsa residents. Up until the tragedy, the Greenwood community had developed its own Black prosperous business infrastructure, known then as the Black Wall Street (Steil & Arcaya, 2023). In addition to mass casualties, the Greenwood community suffered losses including completely destroyed homes, businesses, churches, and public buildings (Banaji et al., 2021; Steil & Arcaya, 2023).

Nationally, the real estate community was moving forward to codify racial segregation. In 1924, the National Association of Real Estate Brokers adopted a code of ethics that elevated racial discrimination. The code of ethics stated, “a realtor should never be instrumental in introducing into a neighborhood a character of property or occupancy, members of any race or nationality, or any individuals whose presence will clearly be detrimental to property values in that neighborhood” (Banaji et al., 2021).

The Great Depression that began in 1929 was a global economic phenomenon that affected everyone. It was a crisis of severe economic hardship that included the destabilization of the U.S. housing market. Home prices fell abruptly, home foreclosures rose dramatically, and the Roosevelt administration needed to stabilize the country’s financial markets. This led to a series of federal programs to address the financial crisis. Seeking to stabilize the housing market and improve financial conditions for homeowners, the Federal Home Loan Bank Board (FHLBB) was established by the Federal Home Loan Act of 1932, followed by the Home Owners’ Loan Corporation (HOLC), which was created in 1933 under the supervision of the FHLBB. With millions of middle-class White homeowners having lost their jobs and having either defaulted or being at risk of defaulting on their mortgages, the FHLBB asked HOLC to introduce a systematic appraisal process that included neighborhood-level characteristics. These appraisals would be used to refinance the mortgages of the defaulted or defaulting middle-class homeowners from short-term duration loans with balloon payments to fully amortized higher loan-to-value mortgages with 15- to 20-year durations that would be federally insured at a low interest rate (Aaronson et al., 2020; Murphy et al., 2022).

HOLC developed the "City Survey" program, which ran from 1935 through about 1940. The main purpose of the project was to provide a comprehensive assessment of mortgage lending risk. The "residential security" maps graded city neighborhoods using a standardized form. The forms included evaluation of sales, location, structural integrity, quality of the homes, access to transportation and other amenities, and proximity to industrial and commercial nuisances. Given the rampant discrimination and racist beliefs at the time, the forms also included socioeconomic, racial, ethnic, and national makeup of neighborhoods. Based on results of the surveys, urban neighborhoods were graded on a scale of A (least risky/most stable) to D (most risky/least stable; see **Table 4.1**; Aaronson et al., 2020; Murphy et al., 2022; Richardson et al., 2020).

HOLC surveyed and created residential security maps for at least 239 cities across the United States. (See **Figure 4.1** for an example of a residential security map for Austin, Texas.) HOLC officials worked with thousands of local realtors, bankers, and appraisers. Surveyors documented their observations, including quality of housing, patterns in sales

Table 4.1 HOLC GRADING SCHEMA

GRADE	COLOR	DESCRIPTORS
A	Green	Safest for investment
B	Blue	Still desirable
C	Yellow	Definitely declining
D	Red	Hazardous

HOLC, Home Owners' Loan Corporation.

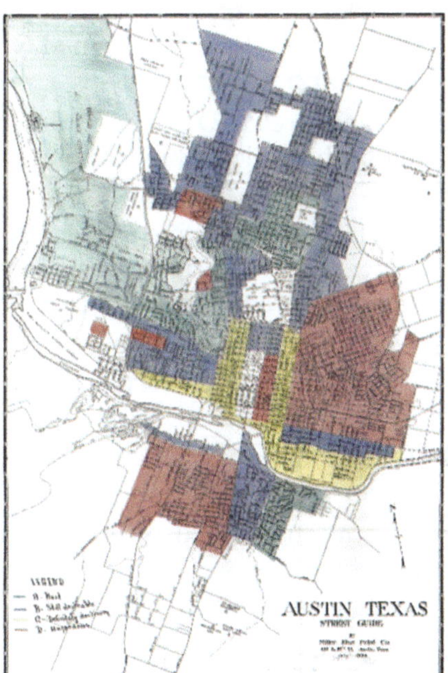

Figure 4.1 **HOLC residential security map of Austin, Texas (July 1934).**

HOLC, Home Owners' Loan Corporation.

Source: Nelson, R. K. (2023). *Mapping inequality: Redlining in New Deal America.* Digital Scholarship Lab. https://dsl.richmond.edu/panorama/redlining

and rentals, racial and ethnic composition, and socioeconomic class of residents. In total, HOLC completed more than 5 million appraisals and awarded more than one million loans to prevent foreclosures in urban areas, thereby strengthening financial markets and the banking system (Aaronson et al., 2020; Badger, 2017; Bailey et al., 2021; Banaji et al., 2021; Lynch et al., 2021; Murphy et al., 2022; Richardson et al., 2020).

It also codified, at a federal level, lawful residential segregation on the basis of race, ethnicity, and national origin (Rothstein, 2017). These residential security maps and the HOLC banking guidelines were used by both public and private banks and mortgage lenders across the country, reflecting the prejudices of the realtors and bankers who helped design the program. Redlining was a racially motivated tactic to ensure residential segregation remained in effect and explicitly refers to the red-colored parts of the residential security maps (i.e., those neighborhoods graded D). Practically all borrowers from a redlined neighborhood were denied access to credit because of the demographic composition of their neighborhood (Aaronson et al., 2020; Braveman et al., 2022; Choi, 2019; Murphy et al., 2022). Actual notations by surveyors from the Area Description Files used to create the residential security maps can be seen in **Box 4.1** (Aaronson et al., 2020).

In 1934, the Roosevelt administration created the Federal Housing Authority (FHA). The FHA was designed to offer long-term loans to prospective home buyers, not just existing homeowners. It also introduced mortgage insurance. These were positive developments in the stabilization of the housing and banking sectors. However, the FHA further solidified

Box 4.1 THE USE OF RACE IN HOME OWNERS' LOAN CORPORATION GRADING

Examples of race as a pivotal factor for Home Owners' Loan Corporation grades in area description files:

- Berkeley, Area 2, C grade: "Northeastern part of area, north of University, could be classed as High Yellow, but for infiltration of Orientals and gradual infiltration of Negroes form south to north."
- Brooklyn, Bedford-Stuyvesant, Area 8, D grade: "Colored infiltration a definitely adverse influence on neighborhood desirability although Negroes will buy properties at fair prices and usually rent rooms."
- Oakland, Piedmont, Area 14, B grade: "Some parts of this area would be considered only High Yellow but for the rigid restrictions existing in Piedmont as to type of new construction and also the fact that there are no Negroes or Asiatics allowed in the city limits."
- Richmond, VA, Area 7, C grade: "Respectable people but homes are too near negro area D2."
- Baltimore, Area 6, C grade: "No immediate danger of negro encroachment, but there is a heavy concentration of negroes in the section adjoining."
- Warren, Area 8, C grade: "Section is 'killed' by influx of negroes from D-3 to attend Francis Willard School in C-8."
- Youngstown, Area 3, D grade: "Evergrowing influx of negroes and low-class Jewish in the westerly end."

Source: Aaronson, D., Hartley, D., & Mazumder, B. (2020, August 20). *The effects of the 1930s HOLC "redlining" maps* (p. 55). Federal Reserve Bank of Chicago.

redlining by using the HOLC's Residential Security maps and creating a parallel set of maps that rated neighborhoods on a color-coded A-to-D scale, taking into consideration neighborhood demographic characteristics. In fact, the 1930s and 1940s FHA Underwriter's Manual explicitly emphasized that "if a neighborhood is to retain stability, it is necessary that properties shall continue to be occupied by the same social and racial classes." The manual additionally supported the use of racial covenants (Banaji et al., 2021). De facto, the FHA refused to insure mortgages of Black Americans. The FHA's impact was far reaching and after World War II, an aligned loan program was created in the Veterans Administration by the 1944 Servicemen's Readjustment Act, which adopted the FHA's racialized practices and procedures. Black Americans, including Black veterans, were almost completely excluded from these programs.

During the 1930s, 1940s, and 1950s, 98% of federally insured mortgages went to White households. During the postwar period, the FHA and Veterans Administration spurred suburbanization, which resulted in a mass exodus of middle- and working-class White families moving from cities to their outskirts. The "white flight" created urban cities with higher proportions of Blacks surrounded by White suburban neighborhoods. Federal transportation policies and investments further reinforced residential segregation by facilitating automobile access for the growing, mostly White suburbs and often created physical barriers that blocked Black communities by constructing inner-city highways. These policies and practices systematically denied Black Americans access to well-resourced neighborhoods and deprived racial and ethnic minority communities access to investments (Aaronson et al., 2020; Banaji et al., 2021; Richardson et al., 2020; Turner & Greene, 2024).

RESIDENTIAL SEGREGATION'S EFFECTS ON NEIGHBORHOOD CHARACTERISTICS

The combination of public and private discriminatory policies and laws created separate but not equal neighborhoods and jurisdictions. Residential segregation—the degree to which two or more groups live separately from one another, in different parts of an environment—became the norm. The lack of affordable loans and mortgages had a significant impact on every dimension of redlined neighborhoods in terms of the quality of the real estate, the willingness of investors to come in, the value of property, and the emergence of predatory financial practices (Badger, 2017). Over time, the HOLC maps impacted the degree of racial segregation. Areas graded D became more heavily Black. The lower graded side of D-to-C boundaries led to a rising share of Black households from 1930 to 1980. The same pattern occurred along the C-to-B borders, showing that yellow-lining was an important phenomenon as well. For example, before the HOLC maps, Black Americans made up about 15% of residents living in D neighborhoods and 1.5% of residents living in C neighborhoods. By 1980, the share of Black Americans living in D neighborhoods increased to 46% and almost 31% in C neighborhoods. Denial of access to capital and opportunity had the intended effect (Aaronson et al., 2020; Dinwiddie et al., 2013; Steil & Arcaya, 2023).

The lack of credit access set in motion disinvestment in redlined urban neighborhoods and in racial and ethnic minority communities. Areas that received a lower grade on the HOLC maps experienced worse housing outcomes as it related to homeownership, housing values, rents, and vacancy rates over the course of decades (Aaronson et al., 2020). Not only does racial residential segregation systematically shape the characteristics of the built environment, it also shapes the distribution of resources. This systematic disinvestment prevented these community residents from realizing the benefits of postwar economic prosperity experienced by White Americans. Existing homeowners and landlords in redlined neighborhoods struggled to obtain credit for maintenance and repairs (Aaronson et al., 2020). Business developers found redlined neighborhoods too risky to invest in grocery stores, retail establishments, and healthcare facilities. These economic dynamics worked in synergy with the discrimination and racism to devalue redlined neighborhoods. Also, because the majority of crucial local public services are based on a property tax system, property values in a neighborhood are key to how much revenue is generated to fund schools, libraries, paved streets, streetlights, sidewalks, public transit, parks, and recreation facilities. Local control over land use enables municipalities to also determine what types of dwellings (single family versus multifamily), businesses, and institutions become part of the built environment of a neighborhood through zoning regulations. All these factors work in concert to determine the physical characteristics of a neighborhood, including the quality of the air one breathes, the noise level during the day and night, who your neighbors are, and how safe the neighborhood is in general (Arcaya et al., 2024). A well-resourced, built environment increases the likelihood of access to quality food, local bank access, access to healthcare facilities and healthcare providers, adequate public transportation, safe parks, well-funded schools, and employment opportunities (Richardson et al., 2020). The socioeconomic effects of redlining resulted in racial residential segregation, neighborhood disinvestment, negative environmental impacts, lower household incomes, decreased access to quality housing, and poorer resourced schools resulting in long-term educational inequities. All of these deleterious effects are related to and increase one's health and mental health vulnerability (Aaronson et al., 2020; Arcaya et al., 2024; Clark et al., 2022; Dinwiddie et al., 2013; Kraus et al., 2023; Mentias et al., 2023; Richardson et al., 2020; Semprini et al., 2023; Steil & Arcaya, 2023).

CONTEMPORARY IMPACT ON DISPARITIES AND INEQUITIES

We currently recognize the importance of addressing the social determinants of health and mental health. What has helped to catalyze our focus on social determinants has been the identification of factors that most significantly impact quality of life, life span, health equity, and clinical outcomes. The overwhelming majority of one's health is outside the four walls of a clinic. Indeed, 80% to 90% of a person's health is the result of nonmedical factors, namely the social determinants of health and mental health: the societal conditions in which people are born, grow, live, work, play, pray, and age that impact health and well-being (Harris & Strakowski, 2024). The social–structural forces that affect health outcomes range from individual to national factors and include socioeconomic status, income inequality, racialized hierarchies, inequitable institutional policies, and geopolitical issues (Compton & Shin, 2015). Compton and Shim identified the main social determinants of mental health to include poverty, adverse life experiences, poor education, economic inequality, neighborhood deprivation, food insecurity, housing instability, poor housing, job insecurity, unemployment, underemployment, adverse features of the built environment, and poor access to healthcare (Compton & Shin, 2015).

Indeed, redlining—which has greatly contributed to racial residential segregation—is a fundamental, structural determinant of health and mental health by skewing access to education, income, employment, and housing advancements and opportunities. Consequently, it is considered an underlying cause of racial and ethnic disparities and inequities in health and mental health (Williams & Collins, 2001). Many of the same communities that were redlined more than 90 years ago today experience higher concentrations of poverty, which is highly correlated with poor physical health, especially chronic diseases such as diabetes and heart disease (Richardson et al., 2020). HOLC redlining has been associated with increased infant and maternal mortality rates, increased preterm birth rates, higher rates of childhood obesity, increased high blood pressure, and increased prevalence of cardiovascular disease and events (McCullom, 2022). It also is correlated with increased rates of stroke, diagnoses of cancer at later stages, higher risk of death from breast cancer, poorer diabetes outcomes, and increased kidney failure rates (McCullom, 2022). Additionally, it is associated with increased prevalence of visual impairment and blindness, poorer postoperative outcomes, higher COVID-19 infection and death rates, increased gunshot wound rates, increased pedestrian fatalities, and higher rates of emergency department visits for asthma as well as asthma-related deaths (McCullom, 2022). In fact, because Black Americans are 40% more likely than White Americans to experience asthma, it has led health experts to describe asthma as "the most racially and ethnically disparate health condition in the USA" (McCullom, 2022).

Black communities, in comparison with predominantly White communities, experience a 30% higher death rate from cardiovascular disease. Research has shown a direct connection between racial and ethnic disparities in housing and similar disparities in cardiovascular disease incidence and mortality. In fact, Mentias et al. (2023) observed that a greater concentration of socioeconomic distress in redlined zip codes contributed to a relationship between redlining and the incidence of heart failure. Poverty also is a major risk factor for poor mental health. It increases the likelihood of adverse childhood experiences, social isolation, loneliness, discrimination, and detachment from academic success and work opportunities and achievement, and decreases the social stigma of imprisonment. These negative experiences reflect the human experience of poverty and can diminish a person's sense of control, self-efficacy, connectedness, and hope, all of which are important factors for resilience, good mental health, and well-being (Choi, 2019).

Nardone and his fellow researchers, in 2020, studied nine U.S. cities and found associations between redlined neighborhoods and the prevalence of cancer, asthma, lack of health insurance, and poor mental health. They emphasized that "special racial segregation and poor health remain critical environmental justice issues impacting communities of color" (Nardone et al., 2020, p. 109). Further, the MITRE Corporation models indicate a significant association between HOLC grade and current poor mental health prevalence in HOLC-graded cities (Khalfani-Cox, 2023; Kraus et al., 2023; Lynch et al., 2021; Mentias et al., 2023; Murez, 2023; Murphy et al., 2022; O'Connor, 2021; Richardson et al., 2020; Steil & Arcaya, 2023; Steil & Lens, 2023; Williams & Collins, 2001).

It is clear that stable and safe housing is a critical social determinant that affects everyone's physical health and mental health. The importance of housing condition and habitability, housing stability and affordability, and neighborhood characteristics cannot be overemphasized when it comes to our collective and complete health and well-being. Like food and clothing, a home is a basic necessity of life. Having a good, stable home provides security and is crucial to well-being. It improves educational outcomes and employment opportunities and is particularly salient for early childhood development (Minott & Winkler, 2021). Green and blue spaces (e.g., vegetation and visible surface water) and walkability have been shown to have protective factors, promote physical activity, and enhance one's mood. Living in an area with abundant resources is definitely beneficial. Conversely, living in a segregated, poorly resourced area is not (Arcaya et al., 2024; Barnett et al., 2024; Khalfani-Cox, 2023; Minott & Winkler, 2021).

STRUCTURAL AND SYSTEMIC RACISM'S IMPACT

Structural racism emphasizes the role of structures. It represents the "totality of ways in which societies foster racial discrimination, through mutually reinforcing inequitable systems" of housing, education, employment, economic, finance, transportation, healthcare, justice, and politics, "that in turn reinforce discriminatory beliefs, values, and distribution of resources" (Krieger, 2014, p. 650). Structural racism functions across multiple domains that are mutually reinforcing. It simply is not the result of prejudices held by individuals, but is produced and reproduced by laws, policies, rules, and practices (Bailey et al., 2021). These structures are sanctioned and implemented by various levels of government and become embedded in cultural and societal norms. So much so, in fact, that the farther removed from its origins, racism becomes so deeply ingrained in daily life that it is no longer noticed by individuals who are not directly affected.

Systemic racism, on the other hand, emphasizes the involvement of multiple systems, if not all systems, dictating the processes and outcomes of racial inequality and inequity in life's opportunities and in health, leading to health disparities and inequities (Banaji et al., 2021). Systemic racism affects all people, but especially poor White people, disproportionately Black people, and other racial and ethnic minority individuals. It becomes so embedded in systems that it is often self-perpetuating and is assumed to reflect the natural, inevitable order of things (Braveman et al., 2022). Therein lies the unique challenge to ending structural and systemic racism, where individuals—mostly White Americans—believe, and truthfully so, that they personally did not create the rules and instead are just trying their best to succeed without awareness of its existence, without animus, and without intention to harm (Banaji et al., 2021). Simultaneously, structural and systemic racism has hindered and continues to hinder resources necessary for Black Americans and racial and ethnic minorities to achieve optimal health and well-being, thereby creating, sustaining, and exacerbating racial health disparities and inequities (Bailey et al., 2021; Banaji et al., 2021; Braveman et al., 2022; Clark et al., 2022; Dyer et al., 2023; Pearson et al., 2023; Richardson et al., 2020; Semprini et al., 2023).

Multiple research studies have investigated how and the degree to which exposure to chronic discrimination contributes to increased stress, reduces access to healthcare, and increases unhealthy behaviors (Mentias et al., 2023). Studies also have found direct relationships between childhood adversity and prevalence of poor psychosocial and behavioral outcomes later in life, including anxiety, posttraumatic stress disorder, depression, suicidal ideation, and suicide attempt (Dumornay et al., 2023). Dumornay et al. (2023) found that compared with White American children, Black American children endorsed more traumatic events and greater material hardship and lived in more disadvantaged neighborhoods. Their research showed that experiencing childhood adversity was associated with lower gray matter volumes in the amygdala, hippocampus, and prefrontal cortex of the brain. These are important brain structures that play crucial roles. The amygdala is important in the learning of a fear response and the hippocampus in memory formation, and the prefrontal cortex regulates the emotional response to fear. The mechanism appears to be toxic stress, which is defined as prolonged exposure to adverse experiences leading to excessive activation of the stress response systems. This, then, results in an accumulation of stress hormones disrupting the immune and metabolic regulatory systems. High stress also affects systemic physiology through neuroendocrine, autonomic, immune, and metabolic pathways. In the developing brain, its actual architecture is affected. The researchers included measures of neighborhood disadvantage using the Area Deprivation Index, which uses 17 socioeconomic indicators from the U.S. census (American Psychiatric Association [APA], 2023; Dumornay et al., 2023; Mentias et al., 2023).

CURRENT STATUS OF HISTORICALLY REDLINED COMMUNITIES

Lending disparities are a lasting impact of the HOLC maps, especially decreased access to credit, and mortgage lending bias not only is readily detected in contemporary data sets, but also is an active form of structural racism (see **Figure 4.2**). Despite policy changes since 1933, inequities in the number of approvals and interest rates of residential mortgage loans for Black Americans persist, and the impact on Black homeownership has been sobering. Homeownership for Black Americans is currently at about 44%, compared with about 48% for Hispanic/Latino Americans and 74% for White Americans. This reflects a percentage for

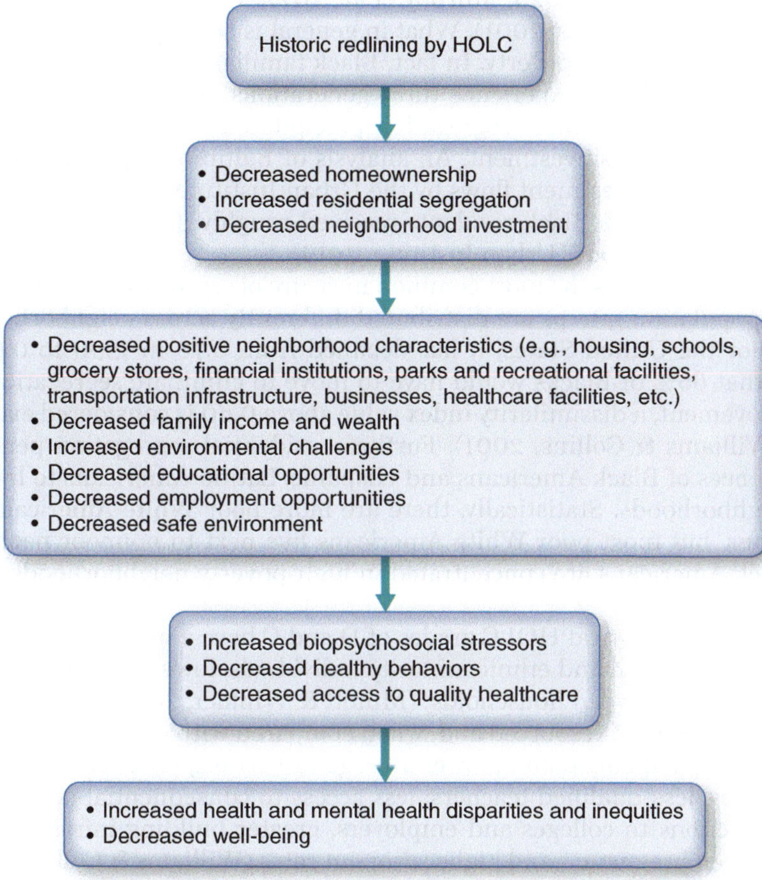

Figure 4.2 Impact of historic redlining.

Note: Postulated pathways of how historic redlining determined neighborhood characteristics and impacts health, mental health, and well-being.

HOLC, Home Owners' Loan Corporation.

Source: Adapted from Krieger, N., Van Wye, G., Huynh, M., Waterman, P. D., Maduro, G., Li, W., Gwynn, R. C., Barbot, O., & Bassett, M. T. (2020). Structural racism, historical redlining, and risk of preterm birth in New York City, 2013–2017. *American Journal of Public Health, 110*(7), 1046–1053. https://doi.org/10.2105/ajph.2020.305656

Black Americans that has not really changed in decades and is lower than when segregation was legal (Richardson et al., 2020).

The continued denial of credit reinforces preexisting patterns of economic disadvantage. Also, although redlining is no longer legal, a 2021 study by Freddie Mac, the Federal Home Loan Mortgage Corporation, found that home purchase appraisals consistently undervalue homes in predominantly Black and Hispanic/Latino neighborhoods compared with homes in White neighborhoods (Freddie Mac, 2021). Given that for most American families, housing equity is a major source of wealth, it is not surprising that given the history of HOLC and the continuing impacts of structural and systemic racism, the median Black American household wealth in 2022 was $45,000 versus $285,000 for White American households (Luhby, 2023). Little to no progress has been made in reducing wealth inequity between Black and White households, and some of the long-term effects are the decreased ability of Black households not only to build equity, but to pass equity on to the next generation

(Badger, 2017; Mentias et al., 2023; Murphy et al., 2022; Pearson et al., 2023; Richardson et al., 2020; Williams & Collins, 2001). What in general is being passed on, however, is the experience and persistence of poverty. In fact, Black families are more than 16 times more likely than White families to experience three generations of poverty (Minott & Winkler, 2021). The conditions of de facto segregation precipitated by redlining have resulted in economic exclusion and disinvestment. An analysis of Baltimore's public and private sector neighborhood-level investment flows by the Urban Institute found that neighborhoods composed of less than 50% Black residents received roughly 3.3 times the investment of majority Black neighborhoods (Urban Institute, 2019).

The dissimilarity index is the most common measure of segregation. It measures the degree to which population groups are distributed differently across neighborhoods (Arcaya et al., 2024). For the United States, it has declined from 0.70 in 1990 to 0.66 in 2000, which means that 66% of Blacks would have to move to eliminate segregation. Although this is an improvement, a dissimilarity index value above 0.60 is considered extremely high segregation (Williams & Collins, 2001). Further, residential segregation persists despite general preferences of Black Americans and Hispanic/Latino Americans to live in racially integrated neighborhoods. Statistically, there are more poor White Americans than poor Black Americans, but most poor White Americans live next to nonpoor people, whereas most poor Black Americans are concentrated in high-poverty neighborhoods (Williams & Collins, 2001).

Today, areas with historical HOLC grades of D and C have a higher percentage of Black Americans and other racial and ethnic minority individuals, lower household incomes, and a higher share of overcrowded households (Minott & Winkler, 2021). The schools in these segregated areas are poorly resourced and, when compared with schools in middle-class areas, have a more limited curriculum, lower average test scores, fewer students in advanced placement courses, less-qualified teachers, less access to consequential academic counseling, fewer connections to colleges and employers, greater building infrastructural issues, higher levels of teen pregnancy, and higher dropout rates (Williams & Collins, 2001).

There is substantial evidence that HOLC redlining has influenced the built environment. Historically redlined neighborhoods have less green space, are less likely to have access to full-service grocery stores, are more likely to have a high density of tobacco and alcohol outlets, and have a greater likelihood of toxic environmental exposures (Arcaya et al., 2024; Richardson et al., 2020). Additionally, Black Americans are more likely than White Americans to be victims of all types of crime, including homicide. Research by R.J. Sampson on the causes of urban violence determined "that the elevated homicide rate of Black Americans is a consequence of residential segregation." His research further elucidates that the "relationship between family structure and violent crime for Whites was identical in sign and magnitude to that for Blacks" (Sampson, 1987). Structurally racist redlining policies also are associated with decreased behavioral health providers, poor mental health, and delays in diagnosis and treatment of health conditions in today's historically redlined communities (Arcaya et al., 2024; Erikson et al., 2022; Minott & Winkler, 2021; Pearson et al., 2023; Richardson et al., 2020; Steil & Arcaya, 2023; Williams & Collins, 2001).

SUMMARY

According to Williams and Collins (2001), racial residential segregation "was imposed by legislation, supported by major economic institutions, enshrined in the housing policies of the federal government, enforced by the judicial system, and legitimized by the ideology of White supremacy that was advocated by churches and other cultural institutions." Racial residential segregation has and continues to impact the physical and mental health of historically redlined communities despite the enactment of federal legislation in the latter half of the 20th century (see **Table 4.2**).

Because of the complex and pervasive nature of structural and systemic racism, interventions that act at the structural and systemic levels—rather than at just the individual level—will be necessary to mitigate and eliminate physical health and mental health disparities and inequities (Clark et al., 2022). In fact, even if all conscious and subconscious racial bias and discrimination ended immediately, the structures of government, law, finance, patterns of land use, housing, and the built environment that have contributed to creating racial and ethnic health and mental health disparities and inequities would continue to generate economically segregated and inequitable neighborhoods (Arcaya et al., 2024). Therefore, ensuring optimal, equitable physical and mental health outcomes for all, and especially for Black Americans and other racial and ethnic minority individuals, will require that we intentionally and diligently address and dismantle structural and systemic racism. Going forward, we need to partner and work directly with communities. One model worth considering is by the Urban Institute, which outlines five guiding principles for "place-conscious" strategies: The first principle is to confront racism, the second principle is to empower community members, the third principle focuses on working horizontally and vertically, the fourth principle prioritizes plans for residential mobility, and the fifth principle focuses on building in accountability and continuous learning (Barnett et al., 2024). Additionally, a helpful conceptual framework comes from the Prevention Institute. The "Pillars of Well-being" framework identifies the six key elements needed for individuals and communities to not just survive, but to thrive. They include the following:

- *Pillar one*: belonging (a sense of acceptance and being part of a community)
- *Pillar two*: control of destiny (a sense of purpose, ability to influence events that shape life's circumstances)
- *Pillar three*: dignity (a sense of one's value, honor, and respect)
- *Pillar four*: hope (the belief that something better is achievable)
- *Pillar five*: safety (the experience of security)
- *Pillar six*: trust (the belief in the reliability and strength of self and others; Choi, 2019)

Table 4.2 20th CENTURY FEDERAL LEGISLATION ADDRESSING RRS

YEAR	ACTION
1962	President Kennedy banned housing discrimination by federally funded housing agencies.
1968	Fair Housing Act signed into law by President Johnson. The law made redlining in the private sector unlawful.
1974	ECOA signed into law by President Ford. Made it unlawful for any creditor to discriminate against a borrower on the basis of race, color, religion, national origin, sex, marital status, or age.
1975	The HMDA signed into law by President Ford provided additional insight into the mortgage lending process by making data on mortgage applications and decisions, along with race, ethnicity, gender, and income of borrowers and the neighborhood, publicly available.
1977	CRA signed into law by President Carter. The CRA placed an affirmative obligation for banks to provide loans and services in low- to moderate-income communities regardless of racial makeup.

CRA, Community Reinvestment Act; ECOA, Equal Credit Opportunity Act; HMDA, Home Mortgage Disclosure Act; RRS, racial residential segregation.

Source: Adapted from Richardson, J., Mitchell, B. C., Edlebi, J., Meier, H. C. S., & Lynch, E. (2020). *The lasting impact of historic "redlining" on neighborhood health: higher prevalence of COVID-19 risk factors*. National Community Reinvestment Coalition. https://ncrc.org/wp-content/uploads/dlm_uploads/2020/09/HOLC-and-public-health-affects-FINAL4.pdf

Through these types of models and frameworks, in conjunction with legislation, we can undo the harm of redlining and ensure optimal, equitable physical and mental health outcomes for all of our nation's communities.

DISCUSSION QUESTIONS

1. How is redlining from the 1930s relevant to our health and mental health today? Which communities are impacted and how?
2. Why are neighborhood characteristics important to health and mental health?
3. What is the connection between homeownership and the overall quality of life from one generation to the next? Why do you think that is an important determinant of mental health equity?
4. What are the pathways by which historic redlining affects the mental health of today's historically redlined urban neighborhoods?
5. What are potential solutions to residential segregation's impact on health and mental health? Take into consideration what can be done at the local, state, and federal levels.

ACKNOWLEDGMENT

The author acknowledges Clarissa Moreno for her review.

REFERENCES

Aaronson, D., Hartley, D., & Mazumder, B. (2020, August 20). *The effects of the 1930s HOLC "redlining" maps.* Federal Reserve Bank of Chicago. https://www.chicagofed.org/publications/working-papers/2017/wp2017-12

American Psychiatric Association. (2023, February 1). *Racial disparities in childhood adversity linked to brain structural differences in U.S. children* [Press release]. https://www.psychiatry.org/News-room/News-Releases/Racial-Disparities-in-Childhood-Adversity

Arcaya, M. C., Ellen, I. G., & Steil, J. (2024). Neighborhoods and health: Interventions at the neighborhood level could help advance health equity. *Health Affairs, 43*(2), 156–163. https://doi.org/10.1377/hltaff.2023.01037.

Badger, E. (2017, August 24). How redlining's racist effects lasted for decades. *The Upshot by The New York Times.* https://www.nytimes.com/2017/08/24/upshot/how-redlinings-racist-effects-lasted-for-decades.html

Bailey, Z. D., Feldman, J. M., & Bassett, M. T. (2021). How structural racism works—Racist policies as a root cause of U.S. racial health inequities. *The New England Journal of Medicine, 384*(8), 768–773. https://doi.org/10.1056/NEJMms2025396

Banaji, M. R., Fiske, S. T., & Massey, D. S. (2021). Systemic racism: Individuals and interactions, institutions and society. *Cognitive Research: Principles and Implications, 6,* 82. https://doi.org/10.1186/s41235-021-00349-3

Barnett, K. S., Reece, J., Mosley, B.M., Baek, M., Hyder, A., Kelleher, K., Sealy-Jefferson, S., & Chisolm, D. J. (2024). A history of the impacts of discriminatory policies on housing and maternal and infant health in an Ohio neighborhood. *Health Affairs, 43*(2), 181–189. https://doi.org/10.1377/hlthaff.2023.01045

Braveman, P. A., Arkin, E., Proctor, D., Kauh, T., & Holm, N. (2022). Systemic and structural racism: Definitions, examples, health damages, and approaches to dismantling. *Health Affairs, 41*(2), 171–178. https://doi.org/10.1377/hlthaff.2021.01394

Choi, L. (2019, July 1). Redlining and mental health: Connecting the dots across poverty, place, and exclusion. *Shelterforce.* https://shelterforce.org/2019/07/01/redlining-and-mental-health-connecting-the-dots-across-poverty-place-and-exclusion/

Clark, E. C., Cranston, E., Polin, T., Ndumbe-Eyoh, S., MacDonald, D., Betker, C., & Dobbins, M. (2022). Structural interventions that affect racial inequities and their impact on population health outcomes: A systematic review. *BMC Public Health, 22,* 2162. https://doi.org/10.1186/s12889-022-14603-w

Compton, M. T., & Shim, R. S. (Eds.). (2015). *The social determinants of mental health.* American Psychiatric Publishing.

Dinwiddie, G. Y., Gaskin, D. J., Chan, K. S., Norrington, J., & McCleary R. (2013). Residential segregation, geographic proximity and type of services used: Evidence for racial/ethnic disparities in mental health. *Social Science & Medicine, 80,* 67–75. https://doi.org/10.1016/j.socscimed.2012.11.024

Dumornay, N. M., Lebois, L. A. M., Ressler, K. J., & Harnett, N. G. (2023). Racial disparities in adversity during childhood and the false appearance of race-related differences in brain structure. *American Journal of Psychiatry, 180*(2), 127–138. https://doi.org/10.1176/appi.ajp.21090961

Dyer, Z., Alcusky, M. J., Galea, S., & Ash, A. (2023). Measuring the enduring imprint of structural racism on American neighborhoods. *Health Affairs, 42*(10), 1374–1382. https://doi.org/10.1377/hlthaff.2023.00659

Erikson, C. E., Dent, R. B., Park, Y. H., & Luo, Q. (2022). Historic redlining and contemporary behavioral health workforce disparities. *JAMA Network Open*, 5(4), e229494. https://doi.org/10.1001/jamanetworkopen.2022.9494

Freddie Mac. (2021, September). *Racial and ethnic valuation gaps in home purchase appraisals.* http://freddiemac.com/research/insight/20210920_home_appraisals.page

Harris, S. S., & Strakowski, S.M. (Eds.). (2024), *Redesigning the US mental health care system.* Oxford University Press.

Khalfani-Cox, L. (2023, December 20). For Black Americans, homeownership can mean better health: A new initiative aims to create three million new Black homeowners by 2030. *Harvard Public Health Magazine.* https://harvardpublichealth.org/equity/fighting-for-more-black-ownership-and-less-systemic-racism/

Kraus, N. T., Connors, S., Shoda, K., Moore, S. C., & Irani, E. (2023). Historic redlining and health outcomes: A systematic review. *Public Health Nursing, 41*(2), 287–296. https://doi.org/10.1111/phn.13276

Krieger N. (2014). Discrimination and health inequities. *International Journal of Health Services, 44*(4), 643–710. https://doi.org/10.2190/HS.44.4.b

Luhby, T. (2023, October 31). White Americans have far more wealth than Black Americans. Here's how big the gap is. *CNN.* https://www.cnn.com/2023/10/31/us/us-racial-wealth-gap-reaj

Lynch, E. E., Malcoe, L. H., Laurent, S. E., Richardson, J., Mitchell, B. C., & Meier, H. C. S. (2021). The legacy of structural racism: Associations between historic redlining, current mortgage lending, and health. *SSM-Population Health, 14*, 100793. https://doi.org/10.1016/j.ssmph.2021.100793

McCullom, R. (2022, October 3). What science tells us about structural racism's health impact. *Harvard Public Health.* https://harvardpublichealth.org/equity/what-science-tells-us-about-structural-racisms-health-impact/

Mentias, A., Mujahid, M. S., Sumarsono, A., Nelson, R. K., Madron, J. M., Powell-Wiley, T. M., Essien, U. R., Keshvan, N., Girotra, S., Morris, A. A., Sims, M., Capers, Q., Yancy, C., Desai, M. Y., Menon, V., Rao, S., & Pandey, A. (2023). Historical redlining, socioeconomic distress, and risk of heart failure among Medicare beneficiaries. *Circulation, 148*(3), 210–219. https://doi:10.1161/circulationaha.123.064351

Minott, O., & Winkler, A. (2021, December). *Understanding and addressing racial and ethnic disparities in housing.* Bipartisan Policy Center. bipartisanpolicy.org/download/?file = /wp-content/uploads/2021/12/BPC_Racial-Disparities-Brief_RV2-3.pdf

Murez, C. (2023, July 18). Redlining may raise heart failure risk among Black Americans. *HealthDay.* https://www.healthyday.com/health-news/cardiovascular-diseases/heart-failure-by-race-and-ethnicity-2662279067.html

Murphy, E., Bernardi, J., Bezold, C., Liberatore, A. J., Jiang, K., & De los Santos, H. (2022, August). *Exploring the association between redlining policies and poor mental health in redlined cities.* The MITRE Corporation.

Nardone, A., Chiang, J., & Corburn, J. (2020). Historic redlining and urban health today in U.S. cities. *Environmental Justice, 13*(4), 109–119. https://doi.org/10.1089/env.2020.0011

O'Connor, K. (2021, January 8). Addressing redlining, community cohesion may improve mental health. *Psychiatric News.* https://psychiatryonline.org/doi/full/10.1176/appi.pn.2021.1.16

Pearson, A. L., Zhou, Y., Buxton, R. T., Horton, T. H., Pfeiffer, K. A., & Beyer, K. M. M. (2023). The effects of contemporary redlining on the mental health of Black residents. *SSM – Population Health, 23*, 101462. https://doi.org/10.1016/j.ssmph.2023.102462

Richardson, J., Mitchell, B. C., Edlebi, J., Meier, H. C. S., & Lynch, E. (2020). *The lasting impact of historic "redlining" on neighborhood health: Higher prevalence of COVID-19 risk factors.* National Community Reinvestment Coalition. https://ncrc.org/wp-content/uploads/dlm_uploads/2020/09/HOLC-and-public-health-affects-FINAL4.pdf

Rothstein, R. (2017). *The color of law: A forgotten history of how our government segregated America* (pp. VII–XVII). Liveright Publishing Corporation.

Sampson, R. J. (1987). Urban Black violence: The effect of male joblessness and family disruption. *American Journal of Sociology, 93*(2), 348–382. https://www.jstor.org/stable/2779588

Semprini, J., Ali, A. K., & Benavidez, G. A. (2023). Medicaid expansion lowered uninsurance rates among non-elderly adults in the most heavily redlined areas. *Health Affairs, 42*(10), 1439–1447. https://doi.org/10.1377/hlthaff.2023.00400

Steil, J., & Arcaya, M. (2023. April 27). Residential segregation and health: History, harms, and next steps. *Health Affairs Health Policy Brief.* https://doi.org/10.1377/hpb20230321.580719

Steil, J., & Lens, M. (2023, April 27). Public policies to address residential segregation and improve health. *Health Affairs Health Policy Brief.* https://doi.org/10.1377/hpb20230321.466701

Turner, M. A., & Greene, S. (2024). *Causes and consequences of separate and unequal neighborhoods.* Urban Institute. https://www.urban.org/racial-equity-analytics-lab/structural-racism-explainer-collection/causes-and-consequences-separate-and-unequal-neighborhoods

Urban Institute. (2019, May). *Neighborhood disparities in investment flows in Chicago.* https://www.urban.org/sites/default/files/publication/100261/neighborhood_disparities_in_investment_flows_in_chicago_1.pdf

Williams, D. R., & Collins, C. (2001). Racial residential segregation: A fundamental cause of racial disparities in health. *Public Health Reports, 116*(5), 404–416. https://doi.org/10.1093/phr/116.5.404

Yearby, R., Clark, B., & Figueroa, J. F. (2022). Structural racism in historical and modern US health care policy. *Health Affairs, 41*(2), 187–194. https://doi.org/10.1377/hlthaff.2021.01466

5 THE LINK BETWEEN RACISM AND MENTAL HEALTH

FERNANDO DE MAIO

LEARNING OBJECTIVES

After reading this chapter, readers will be able to:

- Understand the need for empirical and theoretical research on the health effects of racism.
- Identify different levels through which racism operates in society.
- Describe key indicators of racism, including the index of concentration at the extremes.
- Explore challenges involved in moving from problem-focused to solution-focused research.
- Develop awareness of the need for antiracist research principles.

INTRODUCTION

The study of racism and its effects on health, including mental health, reveals a great deal about the limits and possibilities of scientific research and social justice activism in medicine. On one hand, scholars and activists have been writing about the effects of racism for many decades. W.E.B. Du Bois's classic (1899/1996) *The Philadelphia Negro* set the stage for this work, with detailed sociological and epidemiological analyses of Black–White inequities in mortality and a piercing analysis of what he termed the *indifference* of the White population to the unnecessary suffering of the Black population. Likewise, H.L. Harris Jr.'s (1927) study of Black–White differences in mortality rates in Chicago, published in the first ever volume of the *Social Service Review,* included a lens that we would recognize as fully compatible with contemporary notions of the political and social determinants of health.

Several decades later, the Committee to End Discrimination in Chicago Medical Institutions issued a remarkable pamphlet titled *What Color Are* Your *Germs?*, which directly challenged racial segregation—and the racism that fuels it—with data and a call to action (De Maio et al., 2019). These and many other vital works of scholarship and activism have a direct lineage to contemporary efforts to challenge racism in healthcare, including the recent statements from the American Medical Association (AMA), the American Public Health Association, and many other organizations decrying racism as a public health crisis (Benjamins et al., 2023).

Yet, on the other hand, when we review the *medical* literature for empirical studies on racism and its effects on health, we see very little, at least in terms of articles published by leading medical journals that measure racism in some form or another or even simply use racism as a concept to interpret differences between racialized groups (Krieger et al., 2021). In other words, although we know a lot about the links between racism and health, including mental health, and many people have devoted their careers to advancing this science and this activism, one might not know this if their evidence base is restricted to traditional medical journals, which for decades have restricted, censored, and even rejected knowledge about racism and health (Boyd et al., 2021; Krieger et al., 2021; Wyatt, 2021; Zambrana & Williams, 2022).

WHAT DO WE REALLY KNOW ABOUT RACISM IN THE MEDICAL LITERATURE?

To best explore and analyze the evidence linking racism and mental health, we must interrogate our own scientific discourse on racism itself, because this discourse—and the narratives that it reflects—shapes our understanding of the root problems at hand (AMA & Association of American Medical Colleges Center for Health Justice [AAMCCHJ], 2021). We now know that the scientific study of racism has been limited by the practices of medical journals (Figueroa et al., 2023; Krieger et al., 2021) and, arguably, by dominant medical culture that privileges individual-level explanations over social, structural, and historical ways of thinking. For example, consider that the first time the word *racism* was included in a paper in the *Journal of the American Medical Association* (*JAMA*) was in 1969, in a paper titled "Problems Facing the Negro in Medicine Today" (Haynes, 1969). In that paper, M. Alfred Haynes poignantly observed, "Our society tries to conceal racism by numerous devices" (Haynes, 1969, p. 1068), and presented an analysis of how racism operates in medical education, postgraduate training, and medical practice. He offered an insightful analysis, with heartbreaking contemporary relevance. With minor changes, much of the content and arguments that Haynes shared continue to apply today. What is most illuminating, however, was the response to the inclusion of the word *racism* in a medical journal. Indeed, a response was published in the very next issue of *JAMA*, critiquing Haynes's analysis and, in particular, his use of what was described as an "ugly word": *racism* (Sprunt, 1969, p. 1593).

The exchange between Drs. Haynes and Sprunt from the 1960s is relevant today. Consider a recent analysis of the use of the word *racism* in four of the leading medical journals that revealed a dire situation. Although the *British Medical Journal* (*BMJ*), *JAMA*, *The New England Journal of Medicine* (*NEJM*), and *The Lancet* dramatically increased their publication of articles that included the word *racism* in 2020 (following the public murder of George Floyd and mobilization around the Black Lives Movement), almost all of these papers were commentaries, viewpoints, or letters—undoubtedly important paradigm- and debate-setting pieces, but not formally recognized as key "science" papers by most scholars (see **Figure 5.1**).

Papers that contained data and included the word *racism* are, to this day, rare in leading medical journals. This pattern reflects real limits to knowledge about the health effects of racism. Papers that contained data and included the word *racism* are, to this day, rate in leading medical journals. This pattern reflects real limits to knowledge about the health effects of racism. As Boyd et al. (2021) observed, empirical scientific investigations have the greatest impact on medical discourse; while opinions and commentaries are valuable and often spark debates, define new terms, and challenge taken-for-granted assumptions, they are not normally regarded as definitive data. Boyd et al. concluded, "it is past time for the world's leading medical journals to name racism, publish evidence on how racism harms health, and articulate how dismantling racism can prevent racial health inequities" (Boyd et al., 2021, para. 14).

Despite the paucity of empirical studies published in leading medical journals on the health effects of racism, we do have a substantial theoretical and empirical basis from which to understand and address the links between racism and mental health, with much of it

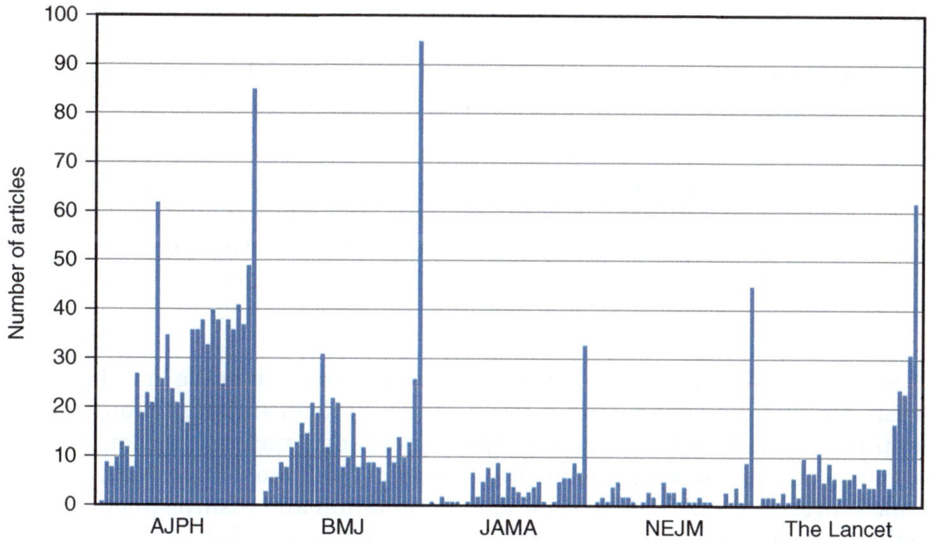

Figure 5.1 **Number of published pieces that include the word *racism*, by journal, 1990–2020.**
AJPH, *American Journal of Public Health*; BMJ, *British Medical Journal*; JAMA, *Journal of the American Medical Association*; NEJM, *The New England Journal of Medicine.*

Source: Krieger, N., Boyd, R. W., Maio, F., & Maybank, A. (2021). Medicine's privileged gatekeepers: Producing harmful ignorance about racism and health. *Health Affairs Forefront*. https://doi.org/10.1377/forefront.20210415.305480. Reprinted with permission.

published in public health and social science journals (Williams et al., 2019a; Zambrana & Williams, 2022). Many of the pathways linking racism and health mirror pathways linking income inequality and health, though these literatures have largely developed independently of one another, with little by way of citation across these seemingly connected fields (De Maio, 2010).

LINKING RACISM AND MENTAL HEALTH

Antiracist research and practice in mental health often are based on an important conceptualization of racism advanced by Camara Jones, where racism is "a system of structuring opportunity and assigning value based on phenotype ('race'), that unfairly disadvantages some individuals and communities, unfairly advantages other individuals and communities, and saps the strength of the whole society through the waste of human resources" (Jones, 2018, p. 231). Similarly, Williams and Etkins (2021) define racism as "an organized societal system in which the dominant White group categorizes individuals into 'races' and devalues, disempowers, and differentially allocates resources to ethnic groups considered to be inferior" (Williams & Etkins, 2021, p. 194). From this foundation, four levels in which racism can and does exist have been identified and defined. They include the following:

- *Structural racism* refers to "the totality of ways in which societies foster racial discrimination through mutually reinforcing systems" (Bailey et al., 2017, p. 1453; see also AMA & AAMCCHJ, 2021; Bassett, 2022; Krieger, 2014; Pallok et al., 2019).
- *Institutional racism* refers to discriminatory treatment, unfair policies and practices, and inequitable opportunities and impacts within organizations and institutions, based on race (AMA & AAMCCHJ, 2021).

- *Interpersonal racism* refers to the expression of racism between individuals (Jones, 2000, 2018).
- *Internalized racism* is acceptance by members of stigmatized races of negative messages about their own abilities and intrinsic worth (Jones, 2000, 2018).

There is a substantial body of theoretical and empirical knowledge linking racism—at each of these levels—to mental health. Some mechanisms, including *weathering* (defined by Geronimus [1992] to describe how racism wears down bodily systems), undoubtedly operate across levels of racism. There also are interactions and crossover effects among levels, all of which adversely affect mental health outcomes (Albert et al., 2021).

Structural Racism and Mental Health

Misra et al. (2022) offer a thoughtful framework for understanding the links between structural racism and mental health, with a focus on psychotic disorders. Through their work, they identified two relevant and fundamental aspects of structural racism: (a) racialized policing and incarceration (associated in the context of the United States with police brutality and mass incarceration) and (b) economic exploitation and disinvestment (particularly through the spatial concentration of poverty and disadvantage). They argue their framework might stimulate new approaches for addressing mental health inequities rooted in racism, focused on two foundational strategies: "(1) document the role of racism in the incidence, severity, and treatment of psychotic disorders; and (2) dismantle how racism operates in the United States, including defunding the police, abolishing carceral systems, and redirecting funds to invest in neighborhoods, housing, and community-based crisis response and mental health care" (Misra et al., 2022, p. 624).

Their analysis builds on earlier empirical studies that documented the foundational link between structural racism—particularly as operationalized in racialized policing—and mental health. As explained by Boyd:

> Police killing black Americans is one of the oldest forms of structural racism in the USA. The act traces its roots to slavery. Yet it remains a tool for social control that violates black bodily autonomy, engenders racial inequality in access to public services, and re-inscribes the predominant racial order any time police indiscriminately and extrajudicially take a black life. (Boyd, 2018, p. 258)

Boyd's commentary was based on a 2018 quasi-experimental study of novel data on police killings and nationally representative data from the U.S. Behavioral Risk Factor Surveillance System that demonstrated that police killings of unarmed Black people produced mental health harm at the population level. In that study, which is one of the few empirical studies of racism published in a leading medical journal, Bor et al. (2018) found that 38,993 (weighted sample share 49%) of 103,710 Black American respondents were exposed to one or more police killings of unarmed Black Americans in their state of residence in the 3 months prior to the survey. Each additional police killing of an unarmed Black American was associated with 0.14 additional poor mental health days (95% CI 0.07–0.22; $p=0.00047$) among Black American respondents (Bor et al., 2018). Notably, no effects were found for respondents interviewed before police killings, and no relationship was found between police killings of White Americans or armed Black Americans. These findings suggest that there are population-level effects of "exposure" to racialized police killing of unarmed Black people, a *spillover* or *collateral* damage felt across communities that originates in singular acts of racist violence.

There is much work to be done in this area of social epidemiology, and to be sure, there are methodological challenges and critiques that are being debated, yet the foundational point linking this particular and singular manifestation of structural racism and population-level mental health is robust (Bor et al., 2019; Lozada & Nix, 2019; Nix & Lozada, 2021). More recent studies have continued to document the mental health effects of police violence (DeVylder et al., 2022; Haile et al., 2023; Salas-Hernández et al., 2022; Williams et al., 2019a), each contributing to a nuanced model that directly connects structural racism to mental health through biopsychosocial and sociological processes. Through these modalities, the study findings show that the "public issue" of police violence and police killings has become *embodied* as a "personal trouble" in individuals.

The second component of Misra et al.'s framework for understanding the link between structural racism and mental health—economic exploitation and disinvestment—has been studied in several different ways. One of the most promising approaches involves the use of the index of concentration at the extremes as an independent variable in statistical modeling. The index of concentration at the extremes is a measure of small area inequality (i.e., it can be used at relatively small levels of geography, including cities and neighborhoods) that can be used to measure both economic polarization and racial segregation as independent and combined issues (Bishop-Royse et al., 2021; Krieger et al., 2016; Lange-Maia et al., 2018). There is a rising body of evidence linking the index of concentration at the extremes to mental health outcomes.

In a particularly important study, Acker et al. (2023) examined the link between neighborhood-level indices of concentration at the extremes and adolescent depressive symptoms and suicidality. They found that risks of depressive symptoms and suicidality increased with each level of worsening neighborhood condition. More simply, they found that as the measure of economic exploitation and disinvestment worsened in a neighborhood, so too did the mental health of the adolescents residing in the neighborhood. Acker et al. concluded that their "findings suggest that efforts to promote equity in adolescent mental health should extend beyond the clinical setting and consider the inequitable neighborhood contexts that are shaped by structural racism" (Acker et al., 2023, p. 2). Much like the Bor et al. study, Acker et al. point us toward both biopsychosocial and sociological pathways that link exposure and effect—the same pathways that have long been understood to link income inequality and adverse health outcomes, following the influential work of Richard Wilkinson (Pickett & Wilkinson, 2015; Wilkinson, 1998; Wilkinson & Pickett, 2006). Following suit, new scholarship is building on these models, adapting, extending, and enhancing new understandings of racism as a root cause of health inequities, including mental health inequities (Ribeiro et al., 2017; Tibber et al., 2022).

Institutional Racism and Mental Health

Defining characteristics of institutional racism include discriminatory treatment, unfair policies and practices, and inequitable opportunities and impacts within organizations and institutions based on race (AMA & AAMCCHJ, 2021). Although structural and institutional racism often are combined into one conceptual category, there are important differences between the two, particularly when thinking of healthcare systems and institutions that warrant their categorization as distinct levels. One might consider how the policies and systems of institutions literally *get under the skin* of individuals; how racist policies perpetuate discrimination, strain, burnout, and marginalization for racially or ethnically minoritized individuals; and how institutional racism overall advantages some while disadvantaging others. Such effects would be difficult to measure in population-level studies but come to the fore in case studies and organizational assessments (Ansell et al., 2022; Ellis, 1975; Needham et al., 2022).

There is a large body of literature that models physiological responses to chronic stress that is associated with exposure to racism (Bowen et al., 2022; Paradies et al., 2015; Shonkoff et al., 2021; Williams, 2018). Indeed, we know that the psychological experience of "othering"—describing the complex ways that society establishes and maintains some groups or individuals as different, inferior, or marginal compared with the more dominant or otherwise normative groups—has profound effects on bodily systems (Akbulut & Razum, 2022).

Complementing the literature on physiological responses to racism, there is literature that focuses on the concept of social capital to understand the links between racism and health (Gilbert et al., 2022; Husbands et al., 2022). *Social capital* is a multifaceted and contested term but in health research, has usually been defined as the strength and quality of interpersonal and community relationships (De Maio, 2010). Social capital studies point toward sociological pathways through which structural and institutional racism may—and often does—affect mental health. In particular, they highlight how the disintegration of social cohesion in communities and institutions leads to breakdowns in the quality of the social fabric, which gives rise to increased feelings of alienation and isolation in individuals. The end result is adverse mental health outcomes (Gilbert et al., 2022; Husbands et al., 2022).

Interpersonal Racism and Mental Health

Literature reviews suggest that the most studied aspect of the link between racism and mental health focuses on the effects of interpersonal racism (Paradies et al., 2015; Pieterse et al., 2012). This likely reflects the bias toward individual-level studies in many academic fields, in contrast to historical and multilevel studies that attempt to simultaneously model individual and contextual relationships (Merlo et al., 2005). Despite often lacking historical or contextual richness, individual-level studies of the relationship between interpersonal racism and mental health have demonstrated that the effects are negative and profound (Williams & Etkins, 2021). The dynamics are both nuanced and inextricably linked and incorporate psychological, biological, behavioral, healthcare utilization, and other sociological responses (Williams et al., 2019b). Further, these studies have shown that stress pathways are critical to this link, particularly when considering "fight-or-flight" responses to exposure to racist incidents wearing down bodily systems (De Maio, 2010).

Internalized Racism and Mental Health

There is an important tradition, particularly in psychology, that explores internalized racism and mental health. This is perhaps illustrated most clearly by Clark and Clark's studies in the 1940s that tested doll preferences among Black and White children, finding that by the age of 5 years, Black children had internalized racist messages and displayed preferences for White dolls (see Sims & Williams, 2024). Sims and Williams (2024) note that although internalized racism "is a well-established construct, it is a complex and multidimensional concept that has been operationalized and measured in many different ways in the literature" (Sims & Williams, 2024, p. 962). The bulk of studies that have been published in this area, however, point to an important element of the overall picture of racism and mental health, with internalized racism—commonly defined as endorsement of negative stereotypes of one's own racial group—being associated with depressive symptoms and serious psychological distress (James, 2017; Mouzon & McLean, 2017).

SHIFTING FROM PROBLEM FOCUS TO SOLUTION FOCUS

Williams and Etkins correctly observed that "research on racism and mental health, to date, has focused more on documenting that racism matters than on identifying interventions to minimize the adverse effects of exposure to racism and reduce the occurrence of racism in the first place" (2021, p. 295). This reflects a larger trend observed by many social epidemiologists who have argued that we need a subtle and important shift, from "problem-focused" to "solution-focused" research and interventions (O'Campo & Dunn, 2012). Part of this movement will necessarily involve more nuanced conceptualizations of the social construction of race as well as a greater appreciation for the heterogeneity within groups and a deeper understanding of the theoretical underpinnings of intersectionality (Ricci et al., 2023; Snyder & Mohammed, 2023). A new wave of theoretical and empirical work is needed not only to continue to monitor and document the health effects of racism (at all levels) but, more importantly, to evaluate antiracist interventions (again at all levels) using mixed-methods designs and case studies.

SUMMARY

There is a rich and rapidly growing empirical and theoretical literature on the mental health effects of racism. This literature, at its best, is deeply grounded in a history of scholarship and activism. At its best, this literature is dissatisfied with merely describing the status quo; it seeks to name and challenge racism in all manner and in all forms, moving us toward a more equitable healthcare system and a more just society. To be sure, there are real challenges; much of our research funding infrastructure incentivizes traditional research and arguably does not do enough to support novel approaches that move us from "race" to "racism" in our models, and many medical journals continue to limit the possibilities of publishing empirical, data-based papers that measure racism as a root cause of health inequity. Yet, it has become clearer to many people that truly protecting the health of all people requires an intentional and persistent effort to push through outdated and harmful mental models that have limited our collective ability to name and overcome racism.

Moving forward, we are likely to see a continued need to investigate and intervene on the links between racism (in all its form) and mental health. Such work must surely be built with multidisciplinary tools and antiracist research principles. It must challenge the *indifference* Du Bois recognized a long time ago; it must move us toward a better future and more equitable society.

DISCUSSION QUESTIONS

1. Many national organizations, including the AMA and the American Public Health Association, have recognized racism as a public health crisis. In what ways are these declarations helpful? And how might we move beyond declarations to real-world change?
2. We know that medical journals have not traditionally published many studies that measure racism in one way or another. Why do you think that is? What are some strategies we could implement to change that pattern?
3. Much of the literature on the health effects of racism has focused on anti-Black racism. How might we incorporate and collaborate with antiracist efforts focused on racism experienced by other groups as well?
4. What research strategies and approaches might be most effective for studying and supporting antiracist institutional efforts? How might quantitative and qualitative data be used to complement such work?
5. Are you optimistic or pessimistic about the potential for this area of research? What might progress look like? What needs to be done so that studies in 20 years' time show different results than studies from today?

DISCLAIMER

The ideas in this chapter are those of the author and do not necessarily represent policy of the American Medical Association.

REFERENCES

Acker, J., Aghaee, S., Mujahid, M., Deardorff, J., & Kubo, A. (2023). Structural racism and adolescent mental health disparities in northern California. *JAMA Network Open, 6*(8), e2329825. https://doi.org/10.1001/jamanetworkopen.2023.29825

Akbulut, N., & Razum, O. (2022). Why othering should be considered in research on health inequalities: Theoretical perspectives and research needs. *SSM - Population Health, 20*, 101286. https://doi.org/10.1016/j.ssmph.2022.101286

Albert, J. L., Cohen, C. M., Brockmeyer, T. F., & Malinow, A. M. (2021). Racism, chronic disease, and mental health: Time to change our racialized system of second-class care. *Healthcare (Basel, Switzerland), 9*(10), 1276. https://doi.org/10.3390/healthcare9101276

American Medical Association & Association of American Medical Colleges Center for Health Justice. (2021). *Advancing health equity: A guide to language, narrative and concepts*. https://www.ama-assn.org/about/ama-center-health-equity/advancing-health-equity-guide-language-narrative-and-concepts-0

Ansell, D. A., James, B., & De Maio, F. G. (2022). A call for antiracist action. *The New England Journal of Medicine, 387*(1), e1. https://doi.org/10.1056/NEJMp2201950

Bailey, Z. D., Krieger, N., Agénor, M., Graves, J., Linos, N., & Bassett, M. T. (2017). Structural racism and health inequities in the USA: Evidence and interventions. *The Lancet, 389*(10077), 1453–1463. https://doi.org/10.1016/S0140-6736(17)30569-X

Bassett, M. T. (2022). Tackling structural racism. *Journal of Public Health Management and Practice: JPHMP, 28*(Suppl 1), S1–S2. https://doi.org/10.1097/PHH.0000000000001457

Benjamins, M. R., Poonsapaya, J., Laflamme, E., & De Maio, F. G. (2023). Racial health equity plans in the 30 largest US cities. *Journal of Racial and Ethnic Health Disparities, 11*, 1933–1945 https://doi.org/10.1007/s40615-023-01662-x

Bishop-Royse, J., Lange-Maia, B., Murray, L., Shah, R. C., & DeMaio, F. (2021). Structural racism, socio-economic marginalization, and infant mortality. *Public Health, 190*, 55–61. https://doi.org/10.1016/j.puhe.2020.10.027

Bor, J., Venkataramani, A. S., Williams, D. R., & Tsai, A. C. (2018). Police killings and their spillover effects on the mental health of Black Americans: A population-based, quasi-experimental study. *Lancet (London, England), 392*(10144), 302–310. https://doi.org/10.1016/S0140-6736(18)31130-9

Bor, J., Venkataramani, A. S., Williams, D. R., & Tsai, A. C. (2019). Validity of details in databases logging police killings—Authors' reply. *The Lancet, 393*(10179), 1413. https://doi.org/10.1016/S0140-6736(18)33060-5

Bowen, F. R., Lewandowski, L. A., Snethen, J. A., Childs, G., Outlaw, F. H., Greenberg, C. S., Burke, P. J., Sloand, E., Gary, F., & DeSocio, J. (2022). A schema of toxic stress informed by racism, transgenerational stress, and disadvantage. *Journal of Pediatric Health Care: Official Publication of National Association of Pediatric Nurse Associates & Practitioners, 36*(2), 79–89. https://doi.org/10.1016/j.pedhc.2021.08.005

Boyd, R. W. (2018). Police violence and the built harm of structural racism. *Lancet (London, England), 392*(10144), 258–259. https://doi.org/10.1016/S0140-6736(18)31374-6

Boyd, R. W., Krieger, N., De Maio, F., & Maybank. (2021, April 21). *The world's leading medical journals don't write about racism. That's a problem*. TIME. https://time.com/5956643/medical-journals-health-racism/

De Maio, F. (2010). *Health & social theory*. Palgrave Macmillan.

De Maio, F., Shah, R. C., Mazzeo, J., & Ansell, D. A. (2019). *Community health equity: A Chicago reader*. University of Chicago Press.

DeVylder, J. E., Anglin, D. M., Bowleg, L., Fedina, L., & Link, B. G. (2022). Police violence and public health. *Annual Review of Clinical Psychology, 18*, 527–552. https://doi.org/10.1146/annurev-clinpsy-072720-020644

Du Bois, W. E. B. (1996). *The Philadelphia Negro: A social study*. University of Pennsylvania. (Original work published 1899)

Ellis, W. A. (1975). A case study of institutional racism. *Journal of the National Medical Association, 67*(2), 158–161.

Figueroa, C. A., Manalo-Pedro, E., Pola, S., Darwish, S., Sachdeva, P., Guerrero, C., von Vacano, C., Jha, M., De Maio, F., & Kennedy, C. J. (2023). The stories about racism and health: The development of a framework for racism narratives in medical literature using a computational grounded theory approach. *International Journal for Equity in Health, 22*(1), 265. https://doi.org/10.1186/s12939-023-02077-0

Geronimus, A. (1992). The weathering hypothesis and the health of African-American women and infants: Evidence and speculations. *Ethnicity & Disease, 2*(3), 207–221.

Gilbert, K. L., Ransome, Y., Dean, L. T., DeCaille, J., & Kawachi, I. (2022). Social capital, black social mobility, and health disparities. *Annual Review of Public Health, 43*, 173–191. https://doi.org/10.1146/annurev-publhealth-052020-112623

Haile, R., Rowell-Cunsolo, T., Hyacinthe, M.-F., & Alang, S. (2023). "We (still) charge genocide": A systematic review and synthesis of the direct and indirect health consequences of police violence in the United States. *Social Science & Medicine, 322*, 115784. https://doi.org/10.1016/j.socscimed.2023.115784

Harris Jr., H. L. (1927). Negro mortality rates in Chicago. *Social Service Review, 1*(1), 58–77.

Haynes, M. A. (1969). Problems facing the Negro in medicine today. *JAMA, 209*(7), 1067–1069. https://doi.org/10.1001/jama.1969.03160200031008

Husbands, W., Lawson, D. O., Etowa, E. B., Mbuagbaw, L., Baidoobonso, S., Tharao, W., Yaya, S., Nelson, L. E., Aden, M., & Etowa, J. (2022). Black Canadians' exposure to everyday racism: Implications for health system access and health promotion among urban black communities. *Journal of Urban Health: Bulletin of the New York Academy of Medicine, 99*(5), 829–841. https://doi.org/10.1007/s11524-022-00676-w

James, D. (2017). Internalized racism and past-year major depressive disorder among African-Americans: The role of ethnic identity and self-esteem. *Journal of Racial and Ethnic Health Disparities, 4*(4), 659–670. https://doi.org/10.1007/s40615-016-0269-1

Jones, C. P. (2000). Levels of racism: A theoretic framework and a gardener's tale. *American Journal of Public Health, 90*(8), 1212–1215. https://doi.org/10.2105/ajph.90.8.1212

Jones, C. P. (2018). Toward the science and practice of anti-racism: Launching a national campaign against racism. *Ethnicity & Disease, 28*(Suppl 1), 231–234. https://doi.org/10.18865/ed.28.S1.231

Krieger N. (2014). Discrimination and health inequities. *International Journal of Health Services, 44*(4), 643-710. doi:10.2190/HS.44.4.b

Krieger, N., Boyd, R. W., Maio, F., & Maybank, A. (2021). Medicine's privileged gatekeepers: Producing harmful ignorance about racism and health. *Health Affairs Forefront*. https://doi.org/10.1377/forefront.20210415.305480

Krieger, N., Waterman, P. D., Spasojevic, J., Li, W., Maduro, G., & Van Wye, G. (2016). Public health monitoring of privilege and deprivation with the index of concentration at the extremes. *American Journal of Public Health, 106*(2), 256–263. https://doi.org/10.2105/AJPH.2015.302955

Lange-Maia, B. S., De Maio, F., Avery, E. F., Lynch, E. B., Laflamme, E. M., Ansell, D. A., & Shah, R. C. (2018). Association of community-level inequities and premature mortality: Chicago, 2011–2015. *Journal of Epidemiology and Community Health, 72*(12), 1099–1103. https://doi.org/10.1136/jech-2018-210916

Lozada, M. J., & Nix, J. (2019). Validity of details in databases logging police killings. *The Lancet, 393*(10179), 1412–1413. https://doi.org/10.1016/S0140-6736(18)33043-5

Merlo, J., Chaix, B., Yang, M., Lynch, J., & Råstam, L. (2005). A brief conceptual tutorial of multilevel analysis in social epidemiology: Linking the statistical concept of clustering to the idea of contextual phenomenon. *Journal of Epidemiology and Community Health, 59*(6), 443–449. https://doi.org/10.1136/jech.2004.023473

Misra, S., Etkins, O. S., Yang, L. H., & Williams, D. R. (2022). Structural racism and inequities in incidence, course of illness, and treatment of psychotic disorders among Black Americans. *American Journal of Public Health, 112*(4), 624–632. https://doi.org/10.2105/AJPH.2021.306631

Mouzon, D. M., & McLean, J. S. (2017). Internalized racism and mental health among African-Americans, US-born Caribbean Blacks, and foreign-born Caribbean Blacks. *Ethnicity & Health, 22*(1), 36–48. https://doi.org/10.1080/13557858.2016.1196652

Needham, B. L., Ali, T., Allgood, K. L., Ro, A., Hirschtick, J. L., & Fleischer, N. L. (2022). Institutional racism and health: A framework for conceptualization, measurement, and analysis. *Journal of Racial and Ethnic Health Disparities*, 1–23. https://doi.org/10.1007/s40615-022-01381-9

Nix, J., & Lozada, M. J. (2021). Police killings of unarmed Black Americans: A reassessment of community mental health spillover effects. *Police Practice & Research, 22*(3), 1330–1339. https://doi.org/10.1080/15614263.2021.1878894

O'Campo, P., & Dunn, J. R. (Eds.). (2012). *Rethinking social epidemiology: Towards a science of change*. Springer Netherlands.

Pallok, K., De Maio, F., & Ansell, D. A. (2019). Structural racism—A 60-year-old black woman with breast cancer. *The New England Journal of Medicine, 380*(16), 1489–1493. https://doi.org/10.1056/NEJMp1811499

Paradies, Y., Ben, J., Denson, N., Elias, A., Priest, N., Pieterse, A., Gupta, A., Kelaher, M., & Gee, G. (2015). Racism as a determinant of health: A systematic review and meta-analysis. *PloS One, 10*(9), e0138511. https://doi.org/10.1371/journal.pone.0138511

Pickett, K. E., & Wilkinson, R. G. (2015). Income inequality and health: A causal review. *Social Science & Medicine, 128*, 316–326. https://doi.org/10.1016/j.socscimed.2014.12.031

Pieterse, A. L., Todd, N. R., Neville, H. A., & Carter, R. T. (2012). Perceived racism and mental health among Black American adults: A meta-analytic review. *Journal of Counseling Psychology, 59*(1), 1–9. https://doi.org/10.1037/a0026208

Ribeiro, W. S., Bauer, A., Andrade, M. C. R., York-Smith, M., Pan, P. M., Pingani, L., Knapp, M., Coutinho, E. S. F., & Evans-Lacko, S. (2017). Income inequality and mental illness-related morbidity and resilience: A systematic review and meta-analysis. *The Lancet. Psychiatry, 4*(7), 554–562. https://doi.org/10.1016/S2215-0366(17)30159-1

Ricci, F., Torales, J., Bener, A., Castaldelli-Maia, J. M., Chumakov, E., Bellomo, A., & Ventriglio, A. (2023). Mental health of ethnic minorities: The role of racism. *International Review of Psychiatry (Abingdon, England), 35*(3–4), 258–267. https://doi.org/10.1080/09540261.2023.2189951

Salas-Hernández, L., DeVylder, J. E., Cooper, H. L. F., Duarte, C. dP, Sewell, A. A., Walker, E. R., & Haardörfer, R. (2022). Latent class profiles of police violence exposure in 4 US cities and their associations with anticipation of police violence and mental health outcomes. *Journal of Urban Health: Bulletin of the New York Academy of Medicine, 99*(4), 655–668. https://doi.org/10.1007/s11524-022-00643-5

Shonkoff, J. P., Slopen, N., & Williams, D. R. (2021). Early childhood adversity, toxic stress, and the impacts of racism on the foundations of health. *Annual Review of Public Health, 42*, 115–134. https://doi.org/10.1146/annurev-publhealth-090419-101940

Sims, K., & Williams, J. C. (2024). Editorial: The relationship between internalized racism and mental health symptoms in Black adolescents. *Journal of the American Academy of Child & Adolescent Psychiatry, 63*(10), 961–963. https://doi.org/10.1016/j.jaac.2024.02.013

Snyder, C. R., & Mohammed, S. A. (2023). A critical race theory analysis of mental health disparities research. *Journal of Racial and Ethnic Health Disparities, 11*, 3900–3906. https://doi.org/10.1007/s40615-023-01840-x

Sprunt, W. H. (1969). Problems facing the Negro in medicine. *JAMA, 210*(8), 1593. https://doi.org/10.1001/jama.1969.03160340201039

Tibber, M. S., Walji, F., Kirkbride, J. B., & Huddy, V. (2022). The association between income inequality and adult mental health at the subnational level—a systematic review. *Social Psychiatry and Psychiatric Epidemiology, 57*(1), 1–24. https://doi.org/10.1007/s00127-021-02159-w

Wilkinson, R. G. (1998). Income inequality and population health. *Social Science & Medicine (1982), 47*(3), 411–412. https://doi.org/10.1016/s0277-9536(98)00101-4

Wilkinson, R. G., & Pickett, K. E. (2006). Income inequality and population health: A review and explanation of the evidence. *Social Science & Medicine, 62*(7), 1768–1784. https://doi.org/10.1016/j.socscimed.2005.08.036

Williams, D. R. (2018). Stress and the mental health of populations of color: Advancing our understanding of race-related stressors. *Journal of Health and Social Behavior, 59*(4), 466–485. https://doi.org/10.1177/0022146518814251

Williams, D. R., & Etkins, O. S. (2021). Racism and mental health. *World Psychiatry: Official Journal of the World Psychiatric Association (WPA), 20*(2), 194–195. https://doi.org/10.1002/wps.20845

Williams, D. R., Lawrence, J. A., & Davis, B. A. (2019a). Racism and health: Evidence and needed research. *Annual Review of Public Health, 40*, 105–125. https://doi.org/10.1146/annurev-publhealth-040218-043750

Williams, D. R., Lawrence, J. A., Davis, B. A., & Vu, C. (2019b). Understanding how discrimination can affect health. *Health Services Research, 54*(Suppl 2), 1374–1388. https://doi.org/10.1111/1475-6773.13222

Wyatt, R. (2021, April 5). Opinion: The health-care industry doesn't want to talk about this single word. *Washington Post*. https://www.washingtonpost.com/opinions/2021/04/05/health-care-racism-medicine/

Zambrana, R. E., & Williams, D. R. (2022). The intellectual roots of current knowledge on racism and health: Relevance to policy and the national equity discourse. *Health Affairs, 41*(2), 163–170. https://doi.org/10.1377/hlthaff.2021.01439

Part II

THE DETERMINANTS OF MENTAL HEALTH EQUITY AND INEQUITIES

6 THE ECONOMIC BURDEN OF MENTAL HEALTH INEQUITIES IN THE UNITED STATES

JOHN M. WESTFALL AND SHALE L. WONG

LEARNING OBJECTIVES

After reading this chapter, readers will be able to:

- Describe the components of the economic burden of mental health inequities.
- Explain how the political determinants of health relate to the economic burden of mental health inequities.
- Recognize the limitations of current racial and ethnic data collection practices.
- Describe the limitations in identifying the cost burden related to the underlying causes of mental health inequities.
- Identify key policy levers for mitigating mental health inequities in the United States.

INTRODUCTION

> *Investing in mental health care saves lives and dollars—we have known this for decades, but until now did not fully understand the monumental impacts of neglecting to act. For the first time, there is tangible evidence demonstrating how decades of systemic health inequities have yielded significantly worse outcomes for racial and ethnic minoritized, marginalized, and underresourced populations.*
>
> — Daniel E. Dawes, JD

In this chapter, we delve into the critical issue of mental health and its impact on overall health outcomes in the United States. Acknowledging the long-standing neglect and lack of resources dedicated to mental health, we explore the detrimental consequences it has had on the population's well-being. Moreover, we highlight how systemic health inequities have resulted in even worse outcomes for Indigenous, racial and ethnic minoritized, marginalized, and medically underresourced populations. To demonstrate the urgency of the situation, we look at the declining general health and life expectancy of the population, accompanied by the alarming deterioration of mental and behavioral health exacerbated by the COVID-19 pandemic. Particularly, we analyze the disproportionate impact on indigenous populations and racial and ethnic minoritized, marginalized, and medically underserved groups. This chapter is based on the robust report of 2022, *The Economic Burden of Mental Health Inequities in the United States*, written in collaboration with the Satcher Health Leadership Institute (Dawes et al., 2022).

Although previous studies examined the economic and life-span outcomes of health disparities, none have specifically delved into the economic burden of *mental and behavioral health* inequities. To fill the gap, we reported the consequences of an underfunded and siloed mental health care system, with a specific focus on underserved and underrepresented communities. Our investigation sought to understand the complexities and severity of the economic burden mental health concerns have among Indigenous populations and racial and ethnic minoritized groups. By analyzing public data sets, conducting case studies, and reviewing existing literature, we described a relationship between economic status, mental health status, and racial and ethnic status.

The findings, although alarming, provide clarity and define a path forward. Access to mental health services not only saves lives, but also saves dollars. Thus, we sought to answer two questions:

1. How many lives can be saved if access to mental and behavioral services becomes more equitable?
2. How many dollars can be saved if access to mental and behavioral services becomes more equitable?

Among the highlights of our findings are the staggering number of excess premature mental and behavioral health-related deaths and the associated cost burden among these vulnerable groups. However, these national estimates are likely underestimated because of the lack of accessible data for various populations living in institutional settings. A closer look reveals additional excess burden of both premature deaths and cost experienced among the unhoused and incarcerated populations.

To combat the devastating impact of mental health inequities, we offer a range of policy proposals to address systemic and structural problems. These proposals span from large-scale investments in mental and behavioral health infrastructure to immediate measures that can be implemented to address the current and future needs. Our suggestions also include adopting culturally centered mental and behavioral health care and addressing both the political and social determinants of health. By informing academic researchers, nongovernmental community organizations, and policy makers about the consequences of mental health inequities, we aim to inspire equitable policy changes to accelerate national progress. With a focus on Indigenous and racial and ethnic minoritized populations, this work seeks to enhance economic and health outcomes for all.

Background on Economic Burden of Health Inequity

Several groundbreaking reports served as the basis for our analysis and report. The study *Mental Health and the Economy* (Brenner, 1973), *Mental Health: A Report of the Surgeon General* (U.S. Department of Health and Human Services, 1999), and *The Economic Burden of Health Inequalities in the United States* (LaVeist et al., 2009) raised awareness about mental and behavioral health issues in the United States and highlighted disparities and barriers to care. However, the burden of mental health concerns has worsened since then, particularly among Indigenous populations and racial and ethnic minoritized groups, all of whom also experience disproportionate poverty rates (Around Him & Gordon, 2022; KFF, 2023). This chapter aims to provide a basic understanding of the economic burden of *mental and behavioral health* inequities and its impact on society as a whole. The COVID-19 pandemic exacerbated mental health distress and disproportionately affected marginalized communities, emphasizing the need for more equitable mental and behavioral health care policies. Definitions of significant terms, such as *health equity*, *disparities*, and *behavioral health equity*, are provided for a better understanding of this chapter.

In addition to quantitative analysis of nationally representative data, we conducted in-depth interviews with key policy makers and stakeholders in the field to gather qualitative data on the effectiveness and implementation of both existing and proposed policies. The case study methodology involved the examination of specific states or regions that have implemented policies aimed at reducing behavioral health inequities. We analyzed the impact of these policies on access to care, quality of care, and health outcomes. We also examined the barriers and challenges faced in implementing these policies, as well as the potential lessons learned for other states or regions.

Definitions

The following definitions will help the reader interpret the findings and policy recommendations:

- *Indigenous populations*: Indiginous populations are any group of people native to a specific region, who lived there before colonists or settlers arrived and began to occupy the land (World Bank Group, 2023).
- *Racial and ethnic minoritized groups*: Racial and ethnic minoritized groups are numerically smaller than the rest of the population and are not in a dominant position. These populations have culture, language, religion, or race that is distinct from that of the majority, and their members have a will to preserve those characteristics (Foa, 2015).
- *Historically marginalized*: These are groups that have been relegated to a peripheral edge of society. Many were and continue to be denied full participation in mainstream cultural, social, political, and economic activities. Marginalized communities may include racial and ethnic minority individuals, women, members of the LGBTQIA+ community, individuals with low income or education, prisoners, people with disabilities, older adults, and many more (Drake & Rose, 2018). These communities were ignored or misrepresented in traditional historical sources and may also be described as racialized, invisible, and medically underresourced.
- *Mental and behavioral health*: These include mental health and substance use concerns, life stressors and crises, stress-related physical symptoms, and health behaviors (Peek, 2013). Mental and behavioral health diagnoses and psychological distress may also be described as illness, conditions, concerns, and disorders.
- *Health equity*: Known obstacles to equity, also known as inequities, include experiences such as poverty, discrimination, power differentials, lack of access to good jobs with fair pay, quality education and housing, safe environments, and healthcare (Braveman, 2017).
- *Behavioral health equity:* Behavioral health equity includes the right to access high-quality and affordable behavioral health care services and supports for all populations (Substance Abuse and Mental Health Services Administration, 2022).
- *Equality*: As a process, equality means providing the same amounts and types of resources across populations.
- *Disparities*: Disparities are measurable differences in health outcomes.

Overall, the combination of quantitative analysis, literature review, and policy and case study analysis provides a comprehensive and multidimensional understanding of the economic burden of mental health inequities in the United States. This methodology allowed for a robust and nuanced exploration of the factors contributing to inequities, the impact of these inequities on health outcomes and healthcare costs, and potential strategies for addressing them. By framing the findings through various methodologies, this study aims to provide a holistic understanding of the economic burden of mental health inequities and inform policies and interventions that can lead to more equitable access to mental and behavioral health care for all populations.

LIVES LOST PREMATURELY DUE TO MENTAL HEALTH INEQUITIES

The quantitative findings on the impact of mental health inequities on lives lost and economic burden are stark. The data analysis focused on the period between 2016 and 2020. We found that during this period, there were a total of 116,722 excess premature mental and behavioral health–related deaths among Indigenous populations and racial and ethnic minoritized groups. These deaths are considered excess because they go beyond what would be expected for a given population. Additionally, the study estimated the total excess cost burden from these premature deaths to be $278 billion during the same period. This economic burden is attributed to mental illness, substance use, and suicide.

The excess premature deaths and economic burden were calculated following the methodology established by LaVeist et al. (2009). Our findings incorporated the prevalence of mental illness among adults, youth, and children as well as the use of mental and behavioral health care services and expenditures. The analysis focused on four categories of premature death related to mental and behavioral health: (a) death due to suicide, (b) death associated with substance use disorders, (c) death due to inadequate mental health treatment, and (d) death due to mental illness associated with comorbid illness. Mental health inequities have had a disproportionate impact on specific communities, including American Indian, Alaska Native, and Native Hawaiian populations; Asian Americans; Black/African Americans; and Hispanic/Latinx Americans.

Understanding the number of lives lost and the economic burden of mental health inequities is crucial for identifying root causes and developing prevention strategies. These deaths represent reversible inequities that persist within and beyond the healthcare and behavioral health systems in the United States.

UNDERSTANDING THE AMOUNT OF DOLLARS LOST

Although the premature loss of life is staggering, it is also important to quantify the economic burden associated with mental health inequities, specifically the excess cost burden resulting from premature deaths, the direct costs of mental health care, and the indirect costs associated with inadequate mental health care. We acknowledge that no monetary value can truly represent a human life; this study aimed to better quantify the suffering, death, and cost associated with underlying mental illness. Because direct medical costs for mental and behavioral health may be a result of overdiagnosis and overtreatment, or the downstream high cost of emergency department visits and hospitalization due to underdiagnosis and undertreatment, we were unable to adequately calculate the economic burden associated with direct medical care. Are more visits to an ambulatory care center for mental health issues the result of need or ease of access? Do fewer visits truly represent less mental illness? If patients have no access to ambulatory behavioral health, are the resulting emergency department visits for mental health exacerbations inappropriate? What is the right number of patients seeking behavioral health; being diagnosed with a mental, emotional, or behavioral health issue; or undergoing hospitalization for severe persistent mental illness or substance abuse? We do not know the answers to these questions. Because mental health has not been adequately available to nearly any population in the United States over the past 50 years, it is impossible to calculate an average or "best case" for diagnosis, treatment, and long-term outcome (Rural Health Information Hub, 2024). Future research on access, screening, diagnosis, treatment, and outcomes will improve our understanding of the costs, both human and economic, of mental, emotional, and behavioral health inequities.

Likewise, national data on the impact of mental illness on education and employment are inadequate. Some people with mental, emotional, or behavioral health issues have high rates of missed work, with resultant loss of productivity and absenteeism (de Oliveira et al., 2023). Lower educational attainment due to untreated mental health issues decreases employability or results in low-paying employment (Breslau et al., 2008; Mojtabai et al., 2015). There is wide variation in how employers support the mental, emotional, and behavioral health of their employees, ranging from no support, loss of wages, or firing, to robust health insurance, employee assistance programs, and employee wellness programs (Joseph et al., 2017; McDowell & Fossey, 2015). We found it impossible to calculate the impact of mental illness on these educational and employment outcomes. Again, future research on the impact of mental illness on education and employment will provide better opportunity to understand mental health inequities.

Therefore, the economic burden is based on the costs estimated related to premature death. Based on methodology estimates created by LaVeist, adjusted for inflation, the estimated total excess cost burden during the period under investigation was $278 billion (LaVeist et al., 2009).

The literature review highlighted that individuals affected by mental wellness concerns often face barriers to economic thriving. This is particularly true for Indigenous populations and racial and ethnic minorities, because they may already have a historically disadvantaged socioeconomic status (KFF, 2023). Mental health conditions can hinder their ability to participate fully in economic activities such as employment and workforce training. This exacerbates the economic burden of behavioral health conditions for these individuals and communities. The findings of the study also revealed inconsistencies, issues, and limitations in how the behavioral health system addresses and captures the reality of these economic burdens.

Understanding the amount of dollars lost because of mental health inequities provides insights into the economic consequences of these disparities. It highlights the real-world impact on individuals' abilities to thrive economically and calls for targeted interventions to address and reduce these burdens.

Traditional Data Collection Is Not Adequate

Approaches to studying national estimates of mental and behavioral health have traditionally collected data that exclude critical populations. Historically exclusionary data collection includes common sampling frames used by the U.S. Department of Health and Human Services and federal surveys for mental and behavioral health. Our study identified that approximately 5.8 million Americans fall into this category of exclusion, including the incarcerated, nursing home residents, residents of assisted living facilities, the unhoused, active military personnel, and individuals institutionalized in psychiatric facilities. It is important to acknowledge that the representation of these populations in existing data is insufficient. This underreporting leads to a gross underestimation of the burden of mental health inequity faced by our collective population and results in grossly underrepresenting the actual burden of mental and behavioral illness in the country.

To partially account for this underrepresentation, the study conducted an ecological analysis using published literature from multiple federal and state agencies, national advocacy organizations, and several independent local and regional studies. This analysis focused on estimating the premature deaths and excess cost burden among the unhoused and incarcerated populations. The findings were again alarming:

- The unhoused population in the United States contributes to an annual excess burden of $23 billion in terms of years of life lost.
- Among the incarcerated population in the United States, there is an excess cost of $15 billion to $44 billion among those with substance use disorders and an excess cost of $19 billion among those with mental illness. Additionally, there is a potential averted crime cost of $6 billion.

The study also highlights the overrepresentation of American Indian, Alaska Native, Native Hawaiians, Black/African Americans, and Hispanic/Latinx Americans in both the unhoused and incarcerated populations. The disproportionate burden of mental health issues among these populations leads to serious inequity in mental health outcomes and costs.

Adequate treatment for mental illness and substance use disorders could potentially save $60 billion to $90 billion each year. Policies that address mental health issues and promote improved diagnosis and treatment among historically marginalized and underresourced populations are crucial in achieving equitable strategies and better overall healthcare outcomes, ultimately benefiting the healthcare system and the country as a whole.

Understanding and addressing the exclusion of certain populations from mental and behavioral health data are essential to accurately assess the burden of mental health inequities and develop effective interventions to improve outcomes for all individuals.

ASSUMPTIONS AND LIMITATIONS

In conducting the analysis on the economic burden of mental and behavioral health inequities across Indigenous, and racial and ethnic populations, we encountered several data limitations and assumptions that must be acknowledged. These limitations and assumptions affect the reliability and representativeness of the findings and should be considered when interpreting the results. Often, limitations are reported as a tool for helping interpret the veracity of results. In the case of mental health inequities, we offer these assumptions and limitations as a contextual finding in hopes they will prompt action and policy changes. The limitations discussed are based in long-standing systemic racism and mental health stigma. They offer a first crucial step toward better understanding the economic burden of mental health inequities.

One major limitation observed throughout the literature review and the study was the lack of disaggregated data. Frequently, data were not categorized by gender, race, ethnicity, or other factors that could help identify specific populations. This inconsistency in how Indigenous, racial, and ethnic groups are classified often leads to underrepresentation or misrepresentation of certain groups in the findings. For instance, American Indian, Alaska Native, and Native Hawaiian populations are often forced to identify as "other" in survey tools. Asian Americans are grouped together yet include dozens of different languages and cultures. Such underrepresentation of these groups hampers the accuracy of the analysis, limits the ability of individuals within these communities to see themselves represented in the data, and impedes culturally specific solutions.

To address the issue of limited disaggregation, we were faced with the difficult decision of analyzing insufficient data or combining races that were not similar in language or culture. Given prior research and an effort at historical comparison, and to align with contemporary race categories, we aggregated 16 Indigenous, racial, and ethnic categories into five for analysis. However, this aggregation results in generalized findings that fail to capture the nuance and unique experiences and challenges faced by individual communities within these categories. National surveys often employ minimal standards for race and ethnicity categories, making it difficult to collect and analyze data in a more precise and comprehensive manner. Increasing efforts to disaggregate Indigenous and racial and ethnic data and improve sampling will allow for more meaningful analysis that accurately reflects the diversity of the country.

These data limitations result in the study findings not being representative of the entire U.S. population or all Indigenous, racial, and ethnic categories. The excess burden of mental and behavioral health inequities identified in this study should be understood as relative to the lowest losses among minoritized groups, with the Asian American category serving as the reference point. However, even within the Asian American category, there is evidence of underreported mental and behavioral health concerns. The limitations discussed here are further compounded by the existence of an "other" racial and ethnic category, which might include populations that do not fit conventional classification structures, including the growing number of people in the United States who have multiple races and ethnicities. As such, future research will need to disaggregate current race and ethnicity categories to capture the diversity and unique experiences of the various groups within it.

Another limitation pertains to the exclusion of behavioral health measures in many assessments of overall disease burden. State preferences regarding the interpretation of parity laws may restrict the availability of certain behavioral health data. Furthermore, inconsistency in the terminology used to describe behavioral health issues, such as variations in the terms *heavy drinking*, *alcohol use disorder*, and *alcohol misuse*, creates challenges in interpreting and comparing data across studies.

Data for youth, especially those under the age of 12, are often scarce. Disease burden is tied to diagnosable conditions rather than behavioral and emotional health that precedes a stated diagnosis. At least 50% of behavioral health conditions begin during teenage and early adult years, but are not identifiable in our data sets. Sadly, suicide is one notable distinction as a leading cause of death among teenagers.

It is crucial for the reader to be reminded that these limitations stem from systemic inequities in data collection practices, self-reporting, terminology use, and forced racial identification due to institutional policies (Dawes et al., 2022). It is essential to recognize and address these systemic inequities in order to gain a more accurate understanding of mental and behavioral health outcomes and inequities. Overall, these data limitations and assumptions underscore the need for improved data collection, disaggregation, and standardization practices. By acknowledging and addressing these limitations, future research can strive for more comprehensive and equitable analyses that provide a clearer picture of mental and behavioral health inequities across diverse populations.

A note on opioid use disorder: The opioid epidemic is strongly linked to mental health and behavioral health inequities. Communities of color, individuals with low income, and those living in rural areas have been disproportionately affected (U.S. Department of Agriculture, 2024). The opioid epidemic has also led to an increase in deaths by overdose, higher rates of substance use disorders, and an economic burden on healthcare and society as a whole. Despite national efforts to address the opioid epidemic, significant disparities remain in access to treatment, with certain communities lacking access to evidence-based opioid addiction treatment (Abraham, 2018). These disparities perpetuate existing mental and behavioral health inequities. It is crucial for healthcare systems, policy makers, and community leaders to address the drivers of mental and behavioral health inequities while tackling the opioid epidemic to ensure equitable access to effective treatments and care. Generally, over the past 20 years, the drug overdose mortality rate has increased five-fold. Rural areas experienced a dramatic rise in drug overdose mortality throughout the 2000s, with urban areas experiencing a similar rise in overdose mortalityin the 2010s (Spencer et al., 2024). In 2022 and 2023, more than 100,000 people died each year of drug overdose, with more than 80,000 deaths due to opioid overdose (National Center for Health Statistics, 2018).

DRIVERS OF INEQUITY

There are several drivers of mental health inequities. Structural barriers, biased delivery of care, social and political determinants of health, poverty, adverse childhood experiences, and historical and contemporary mistrust and misdiagnosis all contribute to inequities and subsequent health disparities. Additionally, certain populations are disproportionately affected by mental health issues, such as Native American, multiracial, and LGBTQA+ or low-income youth. Disparities are seen in how people seek and receive mental health care, including differences in access to insurance and utilization of traditional care settings. There is a disproportionate and devastating impact of suicide on certain racial groups, such as American Indian/Alaska Native and multiracial populations (KFF, 2022).

To address structural and systemic inequities, we recommend policy actions that impact policy levers at all levels: local, state, and national. Fundamental policy principles apply to all policy recommendations to ensure they effectively overcome, rather than perpetuate, inequities and prioritize the impact on marginalized communities.

FUNDAMENTAL POLICY PRINCIPLES FOR ACHIEVING EQUITY

- *Community-informed and -led research:* Community engagement and involvement are critical to understanding the unique needs and experiences of diverse populations. Policy initiatives should be initiated within the community to prioritize, inform, and lead research that actively involves the communities affected by mental and behavioral health disparities and inequities. This approach ensures that policies are developed in collaboration with those who are most affected and that interventions are culturally sensitive and relevant.
- *Truth, reconciliation, and healing:* Acknowledging historical trauma and promoting truth, reconciliation, and healing are essential components of achieving mental and behavioral health equity. This involves addressing the historical and ongoing factors that have contributed to mental health disparities and developing policies that promote healing and well-being. It may also require creating spaces for individuals and communities to share their unique stories and experiences, fostering a sense of belonging and empowerment.
- *Long-term investment with accountability:* Achieving mental and behavioral health equity requires a sustained commitment to addressing disparities. Policies should include long-term funding commitments that ensure access to quality mental health services over time. Additionally, mechanisms for accountability must be put in place to track progress, evaluate the impact of policies, and make necessary adjustments to ensure the desired outcomes are achieved and unintended outcomes are corrected.

POLICY RECOMMENDATIONS FOR IMPROVING EQUITY

To address the inequities in access to mental and behavioral health services, policy actions in three interrelated domains are recommended: (a) investment in mental health infrastructure, (b) culturally centered care, and (c) addressing the political and social determinants of mental health. *The Economic Burden of Mental Health Inequities in the United States Report* (Dawes et al., 2022) includes more than 80 specific policy recommendations based on three core rubrics:

- *Investment in mental health infrastructure:* One key policy recommendation to achieve equity in mental and behavioral health is the need for sufficient and sustainable investment in rebuilding and maintaining equitable mental health systems. This recommendation emphasizes the importance of ensuring access to the right care, in the right place, and at the right time. Adequate funding for mental health services, including workforce development and the integration of mental health into primary care, is critical for improving access and quality of care.
- *Culturally centered mental and behavioral health care:* The second policy recommendation focuses on the need for culturally centered care. Mental health services should be tailored to the unique needs and experiences of the communities they serve. This requires culturally competent providers and programs that understand and address the cultural, linguistic, and historical factors that indirectly and directly impact mental health. Collaboration with community organizations and leaders is essential to ensure that mental health services are responsive to the specific needs and preferences of diverse populations.
- *Addressing political and social determinants of mental health:* The third policy recommendation centers on addressing the political and social determinants of mental health. Mental health outcomes are influenced by a range of factors, including structural and systemic racism, poverty, discrimination, and other social inequalities. Policy action is needed to address these determinants and create environments

that promote mental and behavioral health. This includes promoting policies that address structural inequities, such as affordable housing, education, and employment opportunities, as well as addressing the social and political stigma surrounding mental health.

By implementing these policies, it is believed that mental and behavioral health equity can be achieved, benefiting all populations and leading to economic and health outcomes that have not been fully explored. The importance of research, evaluation, and tracking progress is also emphasized. Access to comprehensive and timely mental and behavioral health services is a critical component of overall healthcare. However, in the United States, there is a significant disparity in the access to these services, particularly for Indigenous populations and racial and ethnic minority groups.

SUMMARY

Improving equity in mental and behavioral health is a complex and multifaceted endeavor. It requires addressing the systemic barriers and disparities that hinder access to care and perpetuate mental health inequities. By implementing the policy recommendations outlined in this chapter—investing in mental health infrastructure, providing culturally centered care, and addressing the political and social determinants of mental health—and adhering to the fundamental policy principles of community-informed research, truth, reconciliation, healing, and long-term investment with accountability, it is possible to make significant strides toward achieving mental and behavioral health equity. Prioritizing the needs of diverse communities and ensuring access to quality care, we will move toward a future where mental and behavioral health is equitable for all.

DISCUSSION QUESTIONS

1. What impact does the economic burden of mental health inequities have on American life?
2. How do the political determinants of health shape the economic burden of mental health inequities?
3. What do you think are the root causes of mental health inequities, and when do their economic effects become visible?
4. In what ways can we better measure and understand the costs of mental health inequities?
5. What are practical local, state, and national policies that might mitigate mental health inequities?
6. What is the interplay between mental health inequities and racial inequities in the United States?
7. What challenges arise from grouping different races or ethnicities together in health and mental health data? How can we address them?
8. What are some strategies for disaggregating race data, and what are the potential risks of doing so?

REFERENCES

Abraham, A. J., Andrews, C. M., Yingling, M. E., & Shannon, J. (2018). Geographic disparities in availability of opioid use disorder treatment for Medicaid enrollees. *Health Services Research, 53*(1), 389–404. https://doi.org/10.1111/1475-6773.12686

Around Him, D., & Gordon, H. S. J. (2022). Latest census estimates show disproportionate poverty among American Indian and Alaska Native (AIAN) children and the overall AIAN population. *Child Trends*. https://

childtrends.org/blog/latest-census-estimates-show-disproportionate-poverty-among-american-indian-and-alaska-native-aian-children-and-the-overall-aian-population

Braveman, P., Arkin, E., Orleans, T., Proctor, D., & Plough, A. (2017) *What is health equity? And what difference does a definition make?* Robert Wood Johnson Foundation. https://www.rwjf.org/en/insights/our-research/2017/05/what-is-health-equity-.html

Brenner, M. H. (1973). *Mental illness and the economy.* Harvard University Press.

Breslau, J., Lane, M., Sampson, N., & Kessler, R. C. (2008). Mental disorders and subsequent educational attainment in a US national sample. *Journal of Psychiatric Research, 42*(9), 708–716. https://doi.org/10.1016/j.jpsychires.2008.01.016

de Oliveira, C., Saka, M., Bone, L., & Jacobs, R. (2023). The role of mental health on workplace productivity: A critical review of the literature. *Applied Health Economics and Health Policy, 21*(2),167–193. https://doi.org/10.1007/s40258-022-00761-w

Dawes, D., Amador, C., Jha, M., Dunlap, N., Valle, M., Lakhani, A., Konde, A., Berhanu, E., Rachel, S., Holden, K., Standifer, M., Ahmed, R., Balgobin, J., Davis, M., Wong, S. L., Gilchrist, E. C., Gold, S. B., Kenny, J., Rakeen, B., ... Jetty, A. (2022, August). *The economic burden of mental health inequities in the United States report.* Satcher Health Leadership Institute, Morehouse School of Medicine. https://satcherinstitute.org/research/ebmhi/

Drake, A., & Rose, C. (2018). Researching historically marginalized communities. *Oregon Heritage Bulletin: Tips, Ideas, Preservation Recommendations From Oregon Heritage* (p. 34). https://www.oregon.gov/oprd/OH/Documents/HB34_Researching_Historically_Marganized_Communities.pdf

Foa, R. (2015). *Creating an inclusive society: Evidence from social indicators and trends.* Expert Group on Social Development and Agenda. https://www.un.org/esa/socdev/egms/docs/2015/sd-agenda2030/RobertoFoaPaper.pdf

Joseph, B., Walker, A., & Fuller-Tyszkiewicz, M. (2017). Evaluating the effectiveness of employee assistance programmes: A systematic review. *European Journal of Work and Organizational Psychology, 27*(1), 1–15. https://doi.org/10.1080/1359432X.2017.1374245

KFF. (2022). *State health facts, suicide deaths and rates by race/ethnicity.* https://www.kff.org/other/state-indicator/suicide-rate-by-race-and-ethnicity/?dataView=1&currentTimeframe=0&sortModel=%7B%22colId%22:%22Location%22,%22sort%22:%22asc%22%7D

KFF. (2023). *State health facts, poverty rates by race/ethnicity.* https://www.kff.org/other/state-indicator/poverty-rate-by-raceethnicity/?currentTimeframe=0&sortModel=%7B%22colId%22:%22Location%22,%22sort%22:%22asc%22%7D

LaVeist, T. A., Gaskin, D. L., & Richard, P. (2009). *The economic burden of health inequalities in the United States.* Joint Center for Political and Economic Studies. Retrieved September 15, 2024 from https://hsrc.himmelfarb.gwu.edu/sphhs_policy_facpubs/225/

McDowell, C., & Fossey, E. (2015). Workplace accommodations for people with mental illness: A scoping review. *Journal of Occupational Rehabilitation, 25*(1), 197–206. https://doi.org/10.1007/s10926-014-9512-y

Mojtabai, R., Stuart, E. A., Hwang, I., Eaton, W. W., Sampson, N., & Kessler, R. C. (2015). Long-term effects of mental disorders on educational attainment in the National Comorbidity Survey ten-year follow-up. *Social Psychiatry & Psychiatric Epidemiology, 50*(10), 1577–1591. https://doi.org/10.1007/s00127-015-1083-5

National Center for Health Statistics. (2018). *U.S. overdose deaths decrease in 2023, first time since 2018.* Centers for Disease Control and Prevention, National Center for Health Statistics, Office of Communication. https://www.cdc.gov/nchs/pressroom/nchs_press_releases/2024/20240515.htm#:~:text=Provisional%20data%20from%20CDC's%20National,drug%20overdose%20deaths%20since%202018

Peek, C. (2013). *Lexicon for behavioral health and primary care integration: Concepts and definitions developed by expert consensus.* Agency for Healthcare Research and Quality , The National Integration Academy Council. https://integrationacademy.ahrq.gov/sites/default/files/2020-06/Lexicon.pdf

Rural Health Information Hub. (2024, October). *Health professional shortage areas: Mental health, by county.* https://www.ruralhealthinfo.org/charts/7

Spencer, M. R., Garnett, M. F., & Miniño, A. M. (2024). *Drug overdose deaths in the United States, 2002–2022.* NCHS Data Brief, no. 491. National Center for Health Statistics. https://dx.doi.org/10.15620/cdc:135849

Substance Abuse and Mental Health Services Administration. (2022). *Behavioral health equity.* https://www.samhsa.gov/behavioral-health-equity

U.S. Department of Agriculture. (2024). *Opioid misuse in rural America.* https://www.usda.gov/topics/opioids

U.S. Department of Health and Human Services. (1999). *Mental health: A report of the surgeon general—Executive summary.* https://www.govinfo.gov/content/pkg/GOVPUB-HE20-PURL-LPS56921/pdf/GOVPUB-HE20-PURL-LPS56921.pdf

World Bank Group. (2023). *Indigenous peoples.* World Bank. https://www.worldbank.org/en/topic/indigenouspeoples

7 SOCIAL DETERMINANTS OF MENTAL HEALTH EQUITY

RUTH S. SHIM

LEARNING OBJECTIVES

After reading this chapter, readers will be able to:

- Consider the historical context and political determinants of health leading to the development of the social determinants of mental health.
- Define several key concepts related to the social determinants of mental health.
- Review the evidence base for several important social determinants of mental health.
- Discuss how to intervene at the level of public policies and social norms to address the political and subsequent social determinants of mental health.
- Envision future directions for taking action to address the political and social determinants of mental health to achieve mental health equity.

INTRODUCTION

The principles that lay the foundation for the social determinants of mental health have been in existence for centuries, although specific terminology has only recently experienced a surge in popularity (Krieger, 2001). Modern science has come to the inescapable conclusion that societal and economic conditions are more important in shaping outcomes in health and mental health than most other factors, including genetics and biology (World Health Organization [WHO], 2008). Therefore, it is important to explore these factors, including the interventions that take action to address the social determinants of mental health, to create the greatest possibility of achieving mental health equity.

This chapter explores historical perspectives of the social determinants of mental health, because the history is critical to understanding where we need to focus interventions in the future. Additionally, this chapter provides key definitions; presents a conceptual framework for considering the social determinants of mental health and the political determinants that created, sustain, and drive them; and reviews the evidence on the association between specific social determinants of mental health and mental health inequities and poor mental health outcomes. Finally, future directions for the field are considered.

HISTORICAL CONTEXT

Although the social determinants of health have enjoyed a heightened sense of popularity within academic settings over the past few years, the concepts that have helped to shape the field of study in social determinants have existed for centuries. Rudolf Virchow, a German physician considered by many to be the father of modern pathology, was one of the first to draw a direct line between health outcomes and the sociocultural environment in the late 19th century, stating (and asking), "If medicine is to fulfill her great task, then she must enter the political and social life ... Do we not always find the diseases of the populace traceable to defects in society?" (Virchow, 1985, p. 117).

Fifty years later, with the founding of the WHO, the call to action by Virchow was enshrined in the WHO Constitution when the organization defined health as "a complete state of physical, mental, and social well-being, and not merely the absence of disease" (WHO, 1946, p.1). As time has passed, two British academics, Michael Marmot and Richard G. Wilkinson, helped to increase the recent focus on the social determinants of health with the publication of their extremely popular report, *Social Determinants of Health: The Solid Facts* in 1998 (Wilkinson & Marmot, 1998) and their textbook, *Social Determinants of Health* in 1999 (Marmot & Wilkinson, 1999), both of which have had even more successful second editions in recent years. These two publications helped to solidify the evidence that social determinants of health are deeply connected to poor health outcomes and health inequities on a global scale.

A decade later, in 2008, the WHO's Commission on Social Determinants of Health, chaired by Michael Marmot, released the report *Closing the Gap in a Generation: Health Equity Through Action on the Social Determinants of Health*, which laid out the evidence, with recommendations to take action to address social determinants on a global scale as a social justice issue (WHO, 2008). Also, in Healthy People 2020, the federal government in the United States included the social determinants of health as a leading indicator for health outcome tracking and in Healthy People 2030 demonstrated greater commitment by designating the social determinants of health as having increased and overarching focus and goals established to address them (U.S. Department of Health and Human Services [DHHS], 2023).

As the social determinants of health were becoming more mainstream, the focus on the impact of the social determinants on mental health outcomes was just coming into focus. In 2014, the WHO released a report titled *Social Determinants of Mental Health*, and a summary article based on this report was also published in the same year (Allen et al., 2014; WHO, 2014). One year later, *The Social Determinants of Mental Health* became the first U.S.-based publication to focus on the specific relevance of social determinants of health on mental health outcomes (Compton & Shim, 2015).

In recent years, several journal articles followed this publication (Shim & Compton, 2018), including the often-cited article on the topic by Alegría et al., which synthesized the literature and provided recommendations for interventions and future directions for the field to address the social determinants of mental health (Alegría et al., 2018). In December 2022, the American Psychiatric Association released its *Report of the Presidential Task Force on the Social Determinants of Mental Health*, laying out a plan for how psychiatrists should take action to address social determinants of mental health (American Psychiatric Association, 2022).

KEY DEFINITIONS

The Social Determinants of Health

The WHO defines the social determinants of health as "the conditions in which people are born, grow, work, live, and age, and the wider set of forces and systems shaping the conditions of daily life" (WHO, 2024, p. 1). Beyond this definition, the WHO highlights another important connection: that social determinants of health are the main cause of health inequities worldwide.

There is considerable debate about what constitutes the social determinants of health and mental health. For example, Healthy People 2020 (and now 2030) identified the following five social determinant areas: economic stability, education, social and community context, health and healthcare, and neighborhood and built environment (DHHS, 2023).

In considering the social determinants of mental health, Shim and Compton have described various determinants grouped into four main categories: pervasive U.S. societal problems, opportunities for accruing wealth, basic needs, and the physical environment (Compton & Shim, 2020).

Social Justice and Social Injustice

Two concepts directly relevant to the social determinants of mental health are social justice and social injustice. Social justice is a philosophical concept defined by David Miller, who was concerned with how advantages and disadvantages in society should be distributed among populations (Miller, 2001). The second concept was defined by John Rawls, who highlighted the importance of considering "the least advantaged members of society" when considering social justice (Robinson, 2010, p. 79).

In contrast, social *in*justice is the unfair and unjust distribution of advantages and disadvantages in society (Shim & Vinson, 2021). These concepts can be directly applied to the consideration of inequitable outcomes in mental health, especially when acknowledging that people with serious mental health problems are often considered to be less advantaged within our society, and so considerations of their care and treatment are issues of social justice, according to Rawls (Shim & Vinson, 2021).

Mental Health Inequities

Health inequities are defined as disparities in health that are the result of systemic, avoidable, and unjust policies and practices that create barriers to opportunity (Braveman et al., 2022). Therefore, mental health inequities are differences in mental health outcomes that result from these systemic and unjust policies and practices. The social determinants of health, which rise from political determinants of health, are implicated as the main cause of health inequities. Thus, it is important to understand how inequities are defined, how they occur, and how they apply to mental health.

Health-Related Social Needs

If social determinants of health are considered the system- and policy-level drivers of health outcomes, then health-related social needs (which are increasingly highlighted in healthcare settings) are considered the individual-level factors that occur as the result of social determinants of health (Kreuter et al., 2021). These social needs (e.g., housing and food insecurity, unemployment, lack of childcare, and utilities payment support) are commonly screened for in healthcare settings (Kreuter et al., 2021). Although the increased focus on screening for health-related social needs is occurring in Medicaid and Medicare programs, there is still further work to be done assessing for these issues in mental health care settings (Alley et al., 2016).

Additional Conceptualizations of Determinants of Mental Health

Moral Determinants of Health

The moral determinants of health are defined by Berwick as prioritizing those collective actions that could lead to greater health outcomes in society, including investing in human well-being and prioritizing solidarity and shared responsibility (Berwick, 2020). The areas of investment in moral determinants are critical to positive mental health outcomes and include ratification of human rights treaties and conventions, ensuring universal healthcare, addressing climate change, carceral system reform, reshaping immigration laws, ending food and housing insecurity in the United States, and resisting voter suppression tactics (Berwick, 2020). As with all determinants of health, successful progress in addressing the moral determinants of health will require community organizations and collaboration between people and policies.

Political Determinants of Health

According to Dawes in his landmark book *The Political Determinants of Health*, political determinants of health "involve the systematic process of structuring relationships, distributing resources, and administering power, operating simultaneously in ways that mutually reinforce or influence one another to shape opportunities that either advance health equity or exacerbate health inequities" (Dawes, 2020). Although it is an emerging concept in current health equity discourse and in the larger health equity movement, it is crucial to recognize that the political determinants of health create the social drivers—including poor environmental conditions, inadequate transportation, unsafe neighborhoods, and lack of healthy food options—that affect all other dynamics of health. In simpler terms, political determinants of health give rise to social determinants of health. Therefore, by understanding these determinants, their origins, and their impact on the equitable distribution of opportunities and resources, we can be better equipped to develop and implement actionable solutions to more meaningfully address inequities in health, including those that exist in mental health.

Calls to take action on the political determinants of health emphasize a multidisciplinary focus of politics, epidemiology, political science, and economics, centering public health to achieve health equity change at a systems level (Kickbusch, 2015).

CONCEPTUAL FRAMEWORK

Because the social determinants of mental health encompass multiple conceptual factors, it is important to consider the complexity through a framework for understanding.

At the top of the figure, which is furthest downstream, are poor mental health outcomes and mental health inequities. One level below are several risk factors for mental illness. Risk factors are characteristics that precede a disorder and are associated with the development of that disorder. In this conceptualization, relevant risk factors for the social determinants of mental health are reduced options and "poor choices," behavioral risk factors, physiologic stress responses, and psychological stress. It should be noted that poor choices are in quotations because the quality of one's choices is directly related to their environmental context. For example, a person who chooses to drink alcohol excessively may be considered as someone making a poor choice, but this decision could be a reasonable choice for someone who experiences a major trauma, develops symptoms of posttraumatic stress disorder, and/or cannot afford access to mental health services (because alcohol use/misuse represents an effective self-medication tool and thus is a reasonable choice given the limited options that this person has in their life).

Although risk factors are an important area of focus in clinical settings, including assessing for risk of self-harm or suicide and violence, the timing of this intervention, when seen through a social determinants of mental health lens, often means that clinical interventions are occurring too late to be optimally effective. Thus, when thinking about social determinants of mental health, it is important to consider intervening further upstream, to assess the "causes of the causes" (Marmot, 2007). These causes of the causes are the social determinants of mental health, in the center of the conceptualization figure. Although these social determinants do not represent every social determinant of mental health, it is helpful to consider some examples represented in this conceptualization. The social determinants of mental health highlighted in this figure consist of four categories: (a) societal problems: adverse early life experiences, discrimination and racism, exposure to violence, and interaction with the criminal justice system; (b) opportunities for wealth accrual: low education, unemployment and underemployment, poverty and income inequality, and area-level poverty; (c) basic needs: housing instability, food insecurity, transportation insecurity, and poor access to healthcare; and (d) the physical environment: adverse features of the built environment, neighborhood disorder, pollution exposure, and climate change (Compton & Shim, 2020).

Moving further upstream in the conceptualization, we encounter the drivers of the social determinants of mental health, unfair and unjust distribution of opportunity (or social injustice). Social injustice could be considered "the causes of the causes of the causes," as they set the context for the development of social determinants of mental health, which then lead to the risk factors that drive and exacerbate mental health inequities.

There are two underlying factors that create social injustice, both of which are rooted in political determinants: public policies and social norms. Public policies are the laws, policies, ordinances, and rules that regulate our institutions and governments (Shim & Compton, 2020). Social norms are the values that society places on population groups, specifically which populations society identifies as deserving of advantages and which populations society identifies as worthy of disadvantages (Shim & Compton, 2020). Social norms for people with serious mental health disorders and substance use disorders are quite negative (Shim & Compton, 2020). Because society has historically viewed this population as morally and spiritually deficient, we have passed laws that reflect our lower opinion of this population. The criminalization of people with substance use disorders and mental health problems is a clear example of how public policies have been enacted to punish and diminish opportunities for this population (Compton & Shim, 2015). This tendency has directly led to higher levels of interaction with the carceral system for this population compared with people without substance use disorders or serious mental illnesses (Dvoskin et al., 2020).

A REVIEW OF THE EVIDENCE

A review of the available evidence of specific social determinants of mental health and their impact on adverse mental health outcomes and mental health inequities is beyond the scope of this chapter. However, considering the various categories presented in the conceptualization of the social determinants of mental health, one social determinant from each of the main categories is highlighted so that the most recent evidence can be presented to illustrate how social determinants of mental health affect mental health outcomes and exacerbate mental health inequities.

Adverse Early Life Experiences

Adverse childhood experiences (ACEs) are specific adverse early life experiences that are often measured using standardized screening assessments. ACEs are considered very common, with the most recent available epidemiological data estimating that more than 6 in 10 U.S. adults (64%) have experienced one ACE (Swedo et al., 2023). More granular data from the Behavioral Risk Factor Surveillance System found a majority of people (58%) experienced one ACE, and that more than 1 in 5 people (22%) experienced three or more ACEs. Additionally, racially and sexually minoritized individuals experienced ACEs at higher rates than White individuals (Giano et al., 2020).

ACEs are closely associated with mental health problems and substance use disorders. Current research has found that there is a relationship between ACEs and suicide attempts (Thompson & Kingree, 2022), alcohol use disorder (Dube et al., 2002), substance use (Zhu et al., 2023), and borderline personality disorder (Porter et al., 2020). Further, studies confirm that among Black and Latinx adults, alcohol use disorder is a secondary driver of specific ACEs (e.g., household challenges and child abuse; Lee & Chen, 2017).

Unemployment and Underemployment

The COVID-19 pandemic helped clarify the role of employment status on mental health outcomes. Because individuals deemed "essential workers" often were exposed to greater risks in jobs with less autonomy and power, the outcomes complemented the findings of the seminal Whitehall II study (Marmot & Brunner, 2005) that occurred 35 years earlier. This study found a social gradient in health outcomes (i.e., workers with less autonomy and power in their jobs, similar to essential workers, had worse health outcomes than those with more power and control) and an association between employment rank and common mental disorders (Marmot & Brunner, 2005).

The data regarding the impacts of underemployment and unemployment on mental health are robust (Compton & Shim, 2015). For example, a 2022 systematic review of the literature found a strong association between unemployment and anxiety, mood disorders, and suicidal behavior. This same review found that men were more severely affected than women (Virgolino et al., 2022). In the United States specifically, underemployment during the COVID-19 pandemic was associated with increased rates of depression and anxiety when compared with people who had full-time jobs (Lee et al., 2021).

Food Insecurity

Food insecurity refers to the limited or uncertain availability of nutritionally adequate and safe foods due most often to a lack of financial means and/or availability of sources to acquire such food (Compton & Shim, 2015). Although rates of food security vary in the United States, the overall prevalence of households affected by food insecurity in 2022 was nearly 13% (12.8%; U.S. Department of Agriculture [USDA] Economic Research Service, 2023). Additionally, the rates of food *in*security are disproportionately higher in predominantly racial and ethnic minority, rural, and/or low-income neighborhoods (USDA Economic Research Service, 2023). Further, these rates have been trending upward from each year prior (USDA Economic Research Service, 2023).

A recent meta-analysis of studies investigating the relationship between food insecurity and mental health outcomes found an association between food insecurity and risk for depression and stress in adults (Pourmotabbed et al., 2020). Other recent studies have found that experiencing food insecurity during childhood was associated with long-standing effects on cognitive function and externalizing behaviors (Gallegos et al., 2021). Further, one study found that during the COVID-19 pandemic, food insecurity was specifically associated with high rates of anxiety and depression in adults. This same survey found that the risk for anxiety and depression associated with food insecurity was *higher* than that associated with job loss during the pandemic (Fang et al., 2021).

Climate Change

The World Meteorological Organization's 2023 *State of the Global Climate* report presented a bleak image of the climate worldwide, because 2023 was considered the warmest year on average (World Meteorological Organization, 2024). Extreme weather, including wildfires, flooding, and droughts, led to significant losses in socioeconomic measures and human lives (World Meteorological Organization, 2024). Unfortunately, as studies have shown, increased anxiety about the perception of climate change leads to poor mental health outcomes (Clayton, 2021).

One of the WHO's global research priorities for protecting human health from climate change relates to assessing the mental health risks of climate change (Charlson et al., 2021). A recent review of the existing literature found associations between negative climate exposures and poor mental health (Charlson et al., 2021). Common negative mental health outcomes from extreme weather events include depression, anxiety, and posttraumatic stress disorder. Further, children tend to be more negatively affected than adults (Palinkas & Wong, 2020). Unfortunately, long-term data regarding the mental health implications of climate change do not exist, which is a clear area for targeted research in the future.

FUTURE DIRECTIONS

An emphasis on the ever-changing conceptualization and expansion of the social determinants of health to include factors such as the political determinants of health, the moral determinants of health, and health-related social needs demonstrates the dynamic and fluid nature of the landscape and reinforces the need for flexibility in consideration. Past efforts have been preoccupied with defining and categorizing the social determinants of mental health. Future directions should focus on their root causes—the political determinants of health—as an effective strategy to design and implement impactful interventions to successfully minimize the deleterious effects of the social determinants of mental health that give rise to the persistent mental health inequities we grapple with today. Although many examples of successful interventions (often organized and implemented by community groups and organizations) exist, they have not been sufficiently evaluated and/or scaled and, thus, are not more prominent or integrated into the larger mental health care system (Alegría, 2018).

Although screening is vital during initial planning stages, successful mental health equity interventions should move beyond screening for health-related social needs and progress to interventions that address the public policies and social norms that govern unfair and unjust distribution of advantage, access, and opportunity. This work would involve shifting emphasis from clinician/provider tasks and behaviors to focus on policies and policy-driven practices, including meaningful interactions with lawmakers and policy makers. It would also include speaking up against and seeking to amend or thwart the harmful social norms that serve to divide or oppress specific populations, particularly those that are disproportionately and detrimentally affected by mental health inequities. It is the shared responsibility of all those working in healthcare fields to achieve mental health equity.

SUMMARY

Social determinants of health, which rise from political determinants of health, are the key factors that create, sustain, and exacerbate health inequities in society today. As such, social determinants of mental health serve as a foundation upon which current mental health inequities exist and persist. Although social determinants of mental health can be intervened upon at the individual level, for the greatest impact, systems-level change will have to occur by acting upon the deep-seated social norms and public policies that govern society. In simpler terms, to tackle the social determinants that drive the mental health inequities with which we currently contend downstream, it is imperative first to identify and adequately address the political determinants that gave rise to these social determinants that were created and exist upstream. Significant progress has been made toward achieving mental health equity through action on the social determinants of mental health, but there is still more work to be done.

DISCUSSION QUESTIONS

1. What role do the political and social determinants of health play in the current health inequity (and mental health inequity) crisis in the nation today?
2. Which social determinants of mental health do you identify with most based on your lived experience? Why?
3. How have health inequities personally affected you or your family members?
4. How do you personally identify with the term *social justice*? Do you consider it to be positive or negative?
5. What are some ways you can personally work to change social norms and improve public policies?
6. What commitments can you make today to work to achieve mental health equity?

REFERENCES

Alegría, M., NeMoyer, A., Falgàs Bagué, I., Wang, Y., & Alvarez, K. (2018). Social determinants of mental health: Where we are and where we need to go. *Current Psychiatry Reports, 20*(11), 95. https://doi.org/10.1007/s11920-018-0969-9

Allen, J., Balfour, R., Bell, R., & Marmot, M. (2014). Social determinants of mental health. *International Review of Psychiatry, 26*(4), 392–407. https://doi.org/10.3109/09540261.2014.928270

Alley, D. E., Asomugha, C. N., Conway, P. H., & Sanghavi, D. M. (2016). Accountable health communities—Addressing social needs through Medicare and Medicaid. *New England Journal of Medicine, 374*(1), 8–11. https://doi.org/10.1056/NEJMp1512532

American Psychiatric Association, Task Force on Social Determinants of Mental Health. (2022). *Report of the presidential task force on the social determinants of mental health.* https://www.psychiatry.org/getmedia/b73d3f7b-94dd-4a52-9267-e83328247325/2022-APA-TFSDMH-Board-of-Trustees-December-Report.pdf

Berwick, D. M. (2020). The moral determinants of health. *JAMA, 324*(3), 225. https://doi.org/10.1001/jama.2020.11129

Braveman, P. A., Arkin, E., Proctor, D., Kauh, T., & Holm, N. (2022). Systemic and structural racism: Definitions, examples, health damages, and approaches to dismantling. *Health Affairs, 41*(2), 171–178. https://doi.org/10.1377/hlthaff.2021.01394

Charlson, F., Ali, S., Benmarhnia, T., Pearl, M., Massazza, A., Augustinavicius, J., & Scott, J. G. (2021). Climate change and mental health: A scoping review. *International Journal of Environmental Research and Public Health, 18*(9), Article 9. https://doi.org/10.3390/ijerph18094486

Clayton, S. (2021). Climate change and mental health. *Current Environmental Health Reports, 8*(1), 1–6. https://doi.org/10.1007/s40572-020-00303-3

Compton, M. T., & Shim, R. S. (Ed.). (2015). *Social determinants of mental health.* American Psychiatric Publishing.

Compton, M. T., & Shim, R. S. (2020). Why employers must focus on the social determinants of mental health. *American Journal of Health Promotion, 34*(2), 215–219. https://doi.org/10.1177/0890117119896122c

Dawes, D. (2020). *The political determinants of health.* Johns Hopkins University Press.

Dube, S. R., Anda, R. F., Felitti, V. J., Edwards, V. J., & Croft, J. B. (2002). Adverse childhood experiences and personal alcohol abuse as an adult. *Addictive Behaviors, 27*(5), 713–725. https://doi.org/10.1016/s0306-4603(01)00204-0

Dvoskin, J. A., Knoll, J. L., & Silva, M. (2020). A brief history of the criminalization of mental illness. *CNS Spectrums, 25*(5), 638–650. https://doi.org/10.1017/S1092852920000103

Fang, D., Thomsen, M. R., & Nayga, R. M. (2021). The association between food insecurity and mental health during the COVID-19 pandemic. *BMC Public Health, 21*(1), 607. https://doi.org/10.1186/s12889-021-10631-0

Gallegos, D., Eivers, A., Sondergeld, P., & Pattinson, C. (2021). Food insecurity and child development: A state-of-the-art review. *International Journal of Environmental Research and Public Health, 18*(17), Article 17. https://doi.org/10.3390/ijerph18178990

Giano, Z., Wheeler, D. L., & Hubach, R. D. (2020). The frequencies and disparities of adverse childhood experiences in the U.S. *BMC Public Health, 20*(1), 1327. https://doi.org/10.1186/s12889-020-09411-z

Kickbusch, I. (2015). The political determinants of health—10 years on. *BMJ, 350*(2), h81–h81. https://doi.org/10.1136/bmj.h81

Kreuter, M. W., Thompson, T., McQueen, A., & Garg, R. (2021). Addressing social needs in health care settings: Evidence, challenges, and opportunities for public health. *Annual Review of Public Health, 42*, 329–344. https://doi.org/10.1146/annurev-publhealth-090419-102204

Krieger, N. (2001). Theories for social epidemiology in the 21st century: An ecosocial perspective. *International Journal of Epidemiology, 30*, 668–677. https://doi.org/10.1093/ije/30.4.668

Lee, J. O., Kapteyn, A., Clomax, A., & Jin, H. (2021). Estimating influences of unemployment and underemployment on mental health during the COVID-19 pandemic: Who suffers the most? *Public Health, 201*, 48–54. https://doi.org/10.1016/j.puhe.2021.09.038

Lee, R. D., & Chen, J. (2017). Adverse childhood experiences, mental health, and excessive alcohol use: Examination of race/ethnicity and sex differences. *Child Abuse & Neglect, 69*, 40-48. https://doi.org/10.1016/j.chiabu.2017.04.004

Marmot, M. (2007). Achieving health equity: From root causes to fair outcomes. *The Lancet, 370*(9593), 1153–1163. https://doi.org/10.1016/S0140-6736(07)61385-3

Marmot, M., & Brunner, E. (2005). Cohort profile: The Whitehall II study. *International Journal of Epidemiology, 34*(2), 251–256. https://doi.org/10.1093/ije/dyh372

Marmot, M., & Wilkinson, R. G. (1999). *Social determinants of health* (1st ed.). Oxford University Press.

Miller, D. (2001). *Principles of social justice.* Harvard University Press.

Palinkas, L. A., & Wong, M. (2020). Global climate change and mental health. *Current Opinion in Psychology, 32*, 12–16. https://doi.org/10.1016/j.copsyc.2019.06.023

Porter, C., Palmier-Claus, J., Branitsky, A., Mansell, W., Warwick, H., & Varese, F. (2020). Childhood adversity and borderline personality disorder: A meta-analysis. *Acta Psychiatrica Scandinavica, 141*(1), 6–20. https://doi.org/10.1111/acps.13118

Pourmotabbed, A., Moradi, S., Babaei, A., Ghavami, A., Mohammadi, H., Jalili, C., Symonds, M. E., & Miraghajani, M. (2020). Food insecurity and mental health: A systematic review and meta-analysis. *Public Health Nutrition, 23*(10), 1778–1790. https://doi.org/10.1017/S136898001900435X

Robinson, M. (2010). Assessing criminal justice practice using social justice theory. *Social Justice Research, 23*(1), 77–97. https://doi.org/10.1007/s11211-010-0108-1

Shim, R. S., & Compton, M. T. (2018). Addressing the social determinants of mental health: If not now, when? If not us, who? *Psychiatric Services, 69*(8), 844–846. https://doi.org/10.1176/appi.ps.201800060

Shim, R. S., & Compton, M. T. (2020). The social determinants of mental health: psychiatrists' roles in addressing discrimination and food insecurity. *Focus (American Psychiatric Publishing), 18*(1), 25–30. https://doi.org/10.1176/appi.focus.20190035

Shim, R. S., & Vinson S. (2021). *Social (in)justice and mental health.* American Psychiatric Publishing.

Swedo, E. A., Aslam, M. V., Dahlberg, L.L., Niolon, P. H., Guinn, A. S., Simon, T. R., & Mercy, J. A. (2023). Prevalence of adverse childhood experiences among U.S. adults—Behavioral risk factor surveillance system, 2011–2020. *MMWR, Morbidity and Mortality Weekly Report, 72*(26), 707–715. http://dx.doi.org/10.15585/mmwr.mm7226a2

Thompson, M. P., & Kingree, J. B. (2022). Adverse childhood experiences, sexual victimization, and suicide ideation and attempts: A longitudinal path analysis spanning 22 years. *American Journal of Orthopsychiatry,* 92(3), 302–309. https://doi.org/10.1037/ort0000613

U.S. Department of Agriculture Economic Research Service. (2023, October 25). *Key statistics & graphics.* https://www.ers.usda.gov/topics/food-nutrition-assistance/food-security-in-the-u-s/key-statistics-graphics/#insecure

U.S. Department of Health and Human Services, Office of the Assistant Secretary for Health, Office of the Secretary. (2023). *Healthy People 2030: Social determinants of health.* https://health.gov/healthypeople/priority-areas/social-determinants-health

Virchow, R. (1985). *Collected essays on public health and epidemiology.* Science History Publications.

Virgolino, A., Costa, J., Santos, O., Pereira, M. E., Antunes, R., Ambrósio, S., Heitor, M. J., & Vaz Carneiro, A. (2022). Lost in transition: A systematic review of the association between unemployment and mental health. *Journal of Mental Health, 31*(3), 432–444. https://doi.org/10.1080/09638237.2021.2022615

Wilkinson, R., Marmot, M. (1998). *Social determinants of health: The solid facts* (1st ed.). World Health Organization.

World Health Organization. (1946). *Constitution of the World Health Organization.* https://apps.who.int/gb/bd/pdf_files/BD_49th-en.pdf#page=6

World Health Organization. (2014). *Social determinants of mental health.* https://iris.who.int/bitstream/handle/10665/112828/9789241506809_eng.pdf?sequence=1

World Health Organization. (2024). *Social determinants of health.* https://www.who.int/health-topics/social-determinants-of-health#tab=tab_1

World Health Organization Commission on Social Determinants of Health. (2008). *Closing the gap in a generation: Health equity through action on the social determinants of health.* Commission on Social Determinants of Health Final Report. https://iris.who.int/bitstream/handle/10665/69832/WHO_IER_CSDH_08.1_eng.pdf?sequence=1

World Meteorological Organization. (2024). *State of the global climate 2023.* https://library.wmo.int/records/item/68835-state-of-the-global-climate-2023

Zhu, J., Racine, N., Devereux, C., Hodgins, D. C., & Madigan, S. (2023). Associations between adverse childhood experiences and substance use: A meta-analysis. *Child Abuse & Neglect,* 106431. https://doi.org/10.1016/j.chiabu.2023.106431

8 ENVIRONMENTAL DETERMINANTS OF MENTAL HEALTH EQUITY

BRITT WEINSTOCK, CHRISTIAN M. AMADOR, AND SHANEETA M. JOHNSON

LEARNING OBJECTIVES

After reading this chapter, readers will be able to:

- Define and discuss the importance of the major environmental determinants of mental health.
- Understand how various environmental determinants impact mental health equity.
- Discuss how politics influence environmental factors that affect mental health in minoritized communities.
- Identify effective interventions and strategies that address environmental determinants to improve mental health in minoritized communities.
- Describe how combining interventions in environmental policy and health policy may help reduce mental health disparities and inequities in minorized communities.

INTRODUCTION

Despite efforts to reduce and eliminate them, mental health inequities have affected and continue to affect individuals and communities disproportionately and detrimentally. The severity and persistence of these inequities have compelled researchers to identify and investigate the factors that led to the current mental health crisis in this nation. One key factor—the environment—has only recently gained traction among researchers as an important determinant of mental health and a driver of mental health disparities and inequities. Because the environment has a dynamic and complex impact on mental health, it is imperative to focus on *all* environmental determinants and understand how these factors often create, reinforce, sustain, and exacerbate one another. It also is important to address the political determinants that give rise to the environmental determinants of mental health as an effective strategy to design interventions and craft policies to promote and advance mental health equity.

Minoritized individuals and communities, rural communities, and lower socioeconomic communities in the United States experience disproportionately high incidence and prevalence for myriad chronic and acute conditions, as well as significant barriers in accessing affordable, high-quality healthcare when it is needed. However, one factor that has consistently plagued the health and wellness of minoritized individuals and communities is inequity. Just as physical health is not immune to inequity, neither is mental health.

Overall, mental health challenges, conditions, and diseases unfortunately tend to be an almost invisible, albeit crucial, counterpart to more widely known chronic and acute conditions and diseases that affect millions of people in the United States. However, mental health inequities have been and remain a persistent public health challenge in the United

States among minoritized individuals and communities. They were magnified over the past decade by the "dual pandemics" (or "twin pandemics") of COVID-19 and the resurgence and widespread media coverage of acts of discrimination and racism (e.g., the murders of Breonna Taylor and George Floyd; Stolberg, 2020). Although they had an effect on the mental health of all individuals, the dual pandemics had a profoundly negative impact on the mental health of African Americans and other minoritized individuals and communities. In fact, the compounded effects of the COVID-19 pandemic and heightened indirect and direct exposure to acts of racism and discrimination led to significant increases in feelings of worry and stress and in symptoms of depressive, anxiety, and trauma- and stressor-related disorders among African American, Latinx, and other population groups (Czeisler et al., 2020; Perrigo et al., 2022; Stinson et al., 2021).

Similar trends in mental health inequities in population groups and communities continue to persist today. The mental health equity crisis carries a significant human health toll, with studies finding that across nearly every age group, individuals with mental health conditions and challenges have a higher prevalence of chronic conditions (Dawes et al., 2024). Research confirms that racial and ethnic minorities with mental health conditions and disorders, when compared with their White cohort, bear a disproportionately higher burden of disability. Further, when compared with Whites, rates of suicide are rising faster among racial and ethnic minorities, especially among Black and American Indian/Alaska Native (AI/AN) populations (Panchal et al., 2022), with the latter group having disproportionately higher rates of posttraumatic stress disorder (PTSD) than any other racial and ethnic group (Budhwani et al., 2015).

The mental health equity crisis also has a devastating economic impact. According to a recent analysis by the Meharry School of Global Health, mental health inequities cost the United States more than $477 billion today. If left unaddressed, the toll could rise to $14 trillion by 2040 (Dawes et al., 2024). When the human health toll and economic impacts are considered in tandem, the urgency to address and eliminate mental health inequities comes into full focus.

As a growing body of literature emerges about the root causes of the mental health equity crisis facing population groups and communities in the United States, one important factor—environmental determinants of mental health—has received heightened attention and focus. Environmental determinants have a profound impact on all aspects of human health, including mental health and wellness. These determinants can be physical, chemical, or biological and can be man-made, natural, or caused by social conditions.

Although environmental determinants affect the health and wellness of *all* individuals, they have had and continue to have a disproportionate and often detrimental impact on the mental health and wellness of minoritized individuals and communities. Further, like other determinants of health, environmental determinants of mental health are rooted in the political determinants of health and the systematic process of structuring relationships and prioritizing and allocating resources and power that have a demonstrative impact on efforts to achieve health equity, including mental health equity (Dawes, 2020). As such, environmental determinants are among the key factors that create, sustain, and exacerbate the mental health inequities with which we contend and struggle today.

ENVIRONMENTAL DETERMINANTS OF MENTAL HEALTH AND MENTAL HEALTH EQUITY: AN OVERVIEW

Conventional thinking leads most individuals who investigate the environmental determinants of health to—with sound reason—focus on natural disasters (e.g., earthquakes, hurricanes, and floods), climate change (e.g., global warming and the recent extreme and uncharacteristically high and low temperatures experienced in communities and states throughout the country), and pollution (e.g., physical garbage that has been littered and/or improperly disposed of/recycled and harmful toxins and other chemicals in the air, water, and soil). However, there are other environmental determinants that must be considered and investigated because they also have a profound impact on mental health and wellness. They include social factors (e.g., exposure to racism and other forms of systemic and structural discrimination, and the effects of segregation through redlining) and built environments (e.g., community designs and availability of green spaces, quality of housing, sanitation practices, and public safety).

Although a more expansive body of knowledge is needed, current research has found that environmental determinants of mental health drive today's mental health equity crisis. These environmental determinants have a noted and often detrimental impact on the mental health and well-being of minoritized individuals and communities. Further, the numerous factors that fall under the umbrella of environmental determinants of mental health often have an intersectional impact on mental health and well-being and tend to recreate and/or reinforce one another. The resultant impacts and effects on mental health and well-being are enduring and profoundly negative.

As a generic example, consider the intersectional effect of built environments, climate change, pollution, and natural disasters: four factors that fall under the umbrella of environmental determinants of mental health. The direst impacts are frequently observed in individuals who live in low-income, often minoritized communities. Such individuals are more likely to live and work in communities and settings—that is, built environments—that are less healthy and less safe (i.e., substandard housing and working conditions and poor public safety). These built environments also tend to be more prone to the negative effects of social and economic inequities and the catastrophic consequences of natural disasters (e.g., hurricanes or floods). Further, they often have significantly higher rates of exposure to pollution and experience uncharacteristically extreme hot or cold temperatures that result from climate change in any given year. In tandem, all of these factors have detrimental impacts on mental health and well-being because when an individual lives and works in this type of built environment that is affected by other environmental determinants, studies confirm that they are at greater risk for experiencing symptoms of anxiety, stress, and depression. Further, when an individual suffers from poor mental health, learning, working, advancing, and thriving—particularly in subpar built environments with these compounding effects—are further compromised, thereby exacerbating the individual's already vulnerable mental state.

A growing community of researchers, particularly ecopsychologists, would refer to this dynamic as "solastalgia," a term that was introduced in 2005 to describe the anxiety and distress that individuals experience when their environments (structural, living and working, social and personal) experience negative changes and they feel powerless to do anything about it. However, the previous generic example underscores not only the intersectional impacts and consequences of environmental determinants of mental health, but also the need to address each factor's impact, both individually and in tandem, on mental health equity.

THE MENTAL HEALTH IMPACTS OF CLIMATE CHANGE

Climate change has numerous effects, including increased heat, flooding, coastal erosion, drought, air pollution, extreme weather events (e.g., wildfires), and impacts on both water and food supply and quality (Neville et al., 2023). Acute weather events pose immediate physical danger and long-term psychological trauma. Additionally, air pollution, extreme heat, and other climate-related impacts lead to an increased risk of lung and breast cancers, traumatic injuries, and cardiovascular and respiratory illnesses (Johnson et al., 2024; Nogueira et al., 2023).

The mental health consequences associated with climate change are significant and include feelings of helplessness and despair, mental stress, depression, anxiety, cognitive impairment, and increased suicidal ideation ("What Happens When," 2024). These climate-related mental health impacts are often referred to as "eco-anxiety" or "climate anxiety." The American Psychological Association has defined eco-anxiety as "a chronic fear of environmental doom" ("What Happens When," 2024). A 2021 multinational survey of 10,000 people aged 16 to 25 years found that approximately 60% were worried about climate change and nearly half (45%) reported that this worry impacted their sleep, work duties, and other aspects of their daily lives (Hickman et al., 2021).

The impacts of climate change are widespread and affect all communities and populations. However, racialized minority populations, Indigenous populations, frontline workers, fenceline populations, older adults, individuals with disabilities, and children are particularly vulnerable to these effects. The compounding effects of social and political determinants of health on environmental factors often exacerbate the overall impact. Many of these populations lack the resources for resilience, mitigation, and adaptation, the very resources that are integral to relocation following natural disasters, flooding, or coastal erosion. Research shows that this negative, intersectional impact of determinants leads to increased mental health disorders and illnesses, including heightened anxiety, mental stress, and PTSD.

For example, and perhaps without realizing it, the world witnessed the intersectional mental health impacts of environmental and political determinants when Hurricane Katrina struck New Orleans, Louisiana, in 2005. Decades before the hurricane even formed, the effects of historic redlining practices (a political determinant that led to discriminatory actions that denied access to financial and other needed services to communities on the basis of race) created mass socioeconomic insecurity and inequity in predominantly Black and other minoritized communities. By the time Hurricane Katrina struck the coast, neighborhoods in New Orleans were racially and economically segregated, with nearly every extreme-poverty neighborhood being predominantly Black. These same neighborhoods bore the brunt of the disaster. In the aftermath of Hurricane Katrina in 2005, the individuals living in these communities experienced higher levels of PTSD than their neighbors who lived in more affluent communities. Not surprisingly, Black residents, who were disproportionately more likely than White residents to live in an impoverished and marginalized community, had a twofold greater likelihood of screening positive for PTSD. They also experienced elevated rates of mental stress, anxiety, and depression (Alexander et al., 2017).

Climate change also exacerbates long-standing challenges associated with water and food insecurity, both of which disproportionately affect impoverished and marginalized communities, and both of which have a direct impact on mental health. Some of the effects of climate change (e.g., drought, flooding, and extreme temperatures) disrupt food distribution. In considering the Hurricane Katrina scenario, the disruptions in food distribution hit the poorest communities in the area the hardest, leaving millions—who already were struggling with PTSD and/or other mental health conditions in the immediate wake of the storm—now also struggling with food insecurity (Mirzabaev et al., 2023; O'Neill et al., 2022). Studies confirm that individuals who experience food and water insecurity, regardless of the cause, have higher rates of anxiety, depression, and mental stress. In fact, a 2014 World Gallup poll found that across 149 nations (including the United States), as rates of food and water insecurity rose, so too did rates of deleterious mental health conditions and disorders, including anxiety and depression (Myers, 2020).

Climate change has led to a noticeable rise in extreme heat events and wildfires, resulting in serious mental health issues among those most immediately affected (To et al., 2021). These include trauma, mental stress, mood disorders, anxiety, and PTSD. Extreme heat events and wildfires also lead to higher incidence of acute mental health crises that often require hospitalizations. Sadly, the negative mental health impacts of wildfires persist

10 to 20 years after the event occurrence, which undoubtedly poses a challenge to advancing mental health equity (Bryant et al., 2020; McFarlane & Van Hooff, 2009).

In January 2025, several wildfires raged in Los Angeles County, leading to the evacuation and displacement of hundreds of thousands of people. While this disaster caused significant loss of human life (i.e., two dozen lives lost in the first 3 days), it also caused intense mental trauma (Weber et al., 2025). Although wildfires can affect anyone, minoritized individuals and communities tend to have the greatest resultant burden, the mental health effects of which are devastating. For example, following a wildfire (or other natural disaster resulting from climate change), minoritized individuals often experience greater challenges associated with displacement, loss of livelihood, and unemployment, leading to disproportionately high levels of psychological distress. Children and adolescents who survive wildfires are also found to have higher rates of mood and anxiety disorders (To et al., 2021). Limited access to mental health services exacerbates these challenges. The psychological turmoil arising from the immediate threat to life and property is further intensified by additional social and political determinants of health, such as access to mental health care, financial insecurity, and unemployment. All of these factors, which rise from political and environmental determinants, have a compounding effect that significantly thwarts the progression of mental health equity.

THE MENTAL HEALTH IMPACTS OF AIR POLLUTION

Accounting for nearly one in eight total global deaths or 7 million premature deaths each year (Neville et al., 2023) and with 99% of the global population breathing polluted air that exceeds guidelines from the World Health Organization, air pollution has become one of the greatest environmental threats. The physical impacts of air pollution are well documented. It is linked to increased risk for and incidence and prevalence of respiratory and cardiovascular complications; exacerbation of respiratory diseases, including asthma and chronic obstructive pulmonary disease; and an increased incidence of lung, esophageal, and other cancers (Johnson et al., 2024). However, studies also indicate that air pollution exposure is a significant determinant of major depressive and anxiety disorders (Borroni et al., 2022) and schizophrenia spectrum disorder (Nobile et al., 2023). Air pollution also has a detrimental impact on cognitive impairment and learning difficulties, including impaired neurocognitive development, cognitive decline, and dementia (Chandra et al., 2022). In fact, the Lancet Commission released a report recognizing air pollution as a risk factor for dementia (Chandra et al., 2022).

Air pollution not only is a major driver of deleterious mental health conditions and disorders, it also thwarts the progress of efforts to achieve mental health equity. In 1970, the United States passed the Clean Air Act to regulate air emissions in an effort to reduce air pollution (U.S. Environmental Protection Agency [EPA], n.d.). However, in 2024, the EPA lowered air quality standards to levels that were *lower* than the *less* stringent World Health Organization's recommended guidelines (Keswani et al., 2022). Studies confirm that the highest vulnerability to the detrimental impacts of air pollution are found within the populations most exposed (Turner et al., 2020). The residual effects of redlining have left a disproportionate number of minoritized individuals living in communities with the highest vulnerabilities to air pollution exposure. For example, low-income communities and frontline communities, as well as fenceline communities (i.e., communities that directly neighbor a high-pollution facility) tend to be home for minoritized individuals. These same communities also are more likely to exist near major highways and high-polluting facilities (e.g., industrial factories and processing plants). Because most of the residents in such communities lack the resources and option to relocate, they often are left struggling with the mental health consequences of this high burden of air pollution exposure (Hajat et al., 2015).

The political determinants that were discussed earlier (e.g., redlining), when compounded with environmental determinants, leave minoritized individuals and communities at particularly high risk for the mental health disorders and conditions that are affiliated with and exacerbated by chronic exposure to air pollution. Given the ubiquitous nature of air pollution in minoritized communities, and its established deleterious impacts on mental health, interventions and strategies that centralize equity and account for the other determinants that drive these grave mental health inequities are needed.

THE MENTAL HEALTH IMPACTS OF NATURAL DISASTERS

Natural disasters—floods, hurricanes, earthquakes, and other extreme weather events—often have the most significant negative mental health impact on directly affected individuals and communities (Nogueira et al., 2023). Research has shown that exposure to natural disasters can result in myriad psychological impacts, including increased suicidal ideation and attempts, higher rates of PTSD, depression, substance use, adjustment disorder, and anxiety (Keya et al., 2023). These mental health impacts persist for significant periods, with research demonstrating that the psychological impacts of natural disasters can linger for more than 15 years (Beyeler et al., 2024).

Flooding is the most common major disaster globally and is projected to increase in frequency and severity because of increased climate-related precipitation (Stanke et al., 2012). Flooding has been linked to increased rates of anxiety, depression, PTSD, suicidal ideation, and suicide (Ahern et al., 2005). Research also demonstrates that children who experience a flooding event exhibit higher rates of aggression, bedwetting, and stress-related behaviors (Ahern et al., 2005).

Vulnerable populations, such as individuals in low-income communities, those with preexisting mental health conditions, and those with limited access to mental health care, often bear a greater mental health burden following not only flooding, but all natural disaster events (Keya et al., 2023). Research has consistently shown that in the aftermath of natural disasters, those directly affected not only exhibited increased rates of anxiety, stress, and depressive disorders, they also remained more susceptible to future psychological distress.

The intersection of environmental, social, and political determinants often exacerbates the burden on those already facing socioeconomic and other challenges and hardships. Inability or lack of resources to mitigate the effects of climate change, evacuate, or relocate, combined with policies that do not adequately provide for a population before, during, or after the occurrence of the disaster, may play a role in the increased incidence and prevalence of mental health disorders and conditions among the affected population (Keya et al., 2023). Addressing these intersecting determinants of mental health and mitigating their resultant mental health inequities, then, are essential for any effective postdisaster intervention and recovery efforts.

THE MENTAL HEALTH IMPACTS OF THE BUILT ENVIRONMENT

Built environments—the physical surroundings in which people, live, work, and play—are unequivocally important when exploring the environmental determinants of mental health and their impact on mental health equity. Extrapolating the results of the research strongly demonstrates that through their direct and indirect effects, built environments are powerful determinants of mental health. Together, these effects impact the prevalence and incidence of myriad mental health conditions and disorders, including anxiety and depression, and the progression or disruption of cognitive development, the latter of which could lead to a mental health challenge (Andrusaityte et al., 2020; Bezold et al., 2018; Evans, 2003).

Studies show that there is an intersectional relationship between built environments and other environmental determinants (e.g., natural disasters and pollution), with several factors creating, reinforcing, and exacerbating one another. There also is evidence that the mental health effects of built environments often interact with other determinants in a manner that profoundly, and often negatively, affects mental health equity. While this section highlights key aspects of built environments and their impacts on mental health and mental health equity, other factors that intersect with built environments, such as systemic discrimination, redlining, and segregation, are expanded upon in other sections throughout the chapter. However, research confirms that the negative mental health impacts of built environments, most of which have a disproportionate and often negative influence on minoritized individuals, families, and communities, are fundamental impediments to the progression of mental health equity (Halpern, 1995; Renalds et al., 2010; Wang & Li, 2023).

THE BUILT ENVIRONMENT: URBAN DESIGN

Urban designs play a fundamental role in the quality of nearly every aspect of residents' lives, including their mental health and well-being. *Urban design* is defined as the process of creating functional and aesthetically pleasing spaces that can serve as the bridge between the natural environment and the built environment (Bansal et al., 2020). However, historically in the United States, urban design has been influenced and reinforced by racist and discriminatory policies that systemically and intentionally excluded racial and ethnic minorities, low-income residents, and other minoritized individuals, creating economically and racially segregated neighborhoods. The residual impacts of this rampant segregation continue to exist today and perpetuate and exacerbate numerous pressing inequities, including those observed in mental health.

In order to explore the powerful and compounding effect that urban design has on mental health and health equity, this section discusses the factors that are considered throughout the urban design process: quality of housing, urban density and their associated environmental hazards, walkability and transit, and access to and incorporation of nature and community spaces.

Quality of Housing

There is extensive knowledge about the effects of the "outdoor" environmental determinants of mental health (e.g., pollution, natural disasters, and climate change). Although the findings are as germane as they are stark, the reality is that the majority of the U.S. population spends roughly 90% of their lives indoors (U.S. Environmental Protection Agency, 2024), making housing a vital element of built environments.

Research confirms that both quality and type of housing impact mental health and mental health inequities. Urban design plays a decisive role in housing by setting minimum space standards to prevent overcrowding and maximize exposure to natural light; determining housing design, compositions, and use; and integrating elements (e.g., appropriate infrastructure and crime- and traffic-reduction measures) to bolster both safety and property value (Mouratidis, 2021). Therefore, the resultant impact of housing on mental health and mental health equity is rooted, at least partially, in urban planning. In fact, the evidence overwhelmingly demonstrates that poor housing quality conditions often beget poor mental health outcomes (Pevalin et al., 2017).

Studies confirm that financial strain, including that related to housing, is a determinant factor of mental health and wellness. In a study of U.S. adults that investigated the relationship between financial pressures and psychological distress, Ryu and Fan (2023) found an inverse relationship between household income and psychological distress, with individuals and families with lower incomes experiencing notably higher levels of psychological distress. Further, findings from the 2024 Census Bureau's Household Pulse Survey found that nearly one in three adults report not being current on their mortgage or rent payments, with an eviction or foreclosure being "very likely" or "somewhat likely" within the next 2 months. These findings strongly imply that worsened housing instability and resultant negative mental health consequences may be on the horizon and should be central to strategies that seek to advance mental health equity through the improvement of all aspects of built environments, particularly housing.

Urban Density

Living in large cities and other densely populated areas presents a dynamic set of challenges for mental health and mental health equity that rise, in part, from urban density. With increasing global populations, migration, or desire to live within certain geographic regions, overcrowding often occurs and may result in a lack of privacy and limited access to personal space, both of which lead to increased levels of stress and anxiety (Ruiz-Tagle & Urria, 2022). Urban density also can lead to heightened exposure to environmental hazards, such as loud noise pollution, which is linked to increased levels of anxiety and impaired cognitive function (Babisch, 2002) and depressive disorders (Stansfeld & Matheson, 2003). Further, urban density often results in fewer green spaces, which is extremely detrimental to mental health and well-being. In fact, exposure to green spaces, particularly in residential environments, results in significant short- and long-term improvements in outcomes across an array of common mental health conditions and disorders (Rigolon et al., 2021).

Walkability and Transit

Environments that encourage walking, biking, and public transportation can lead to improved overall health, including mental health. Exercise is a well-known mood booster and a key factor in reducing symptoms of depression and anxiety (Tight & Baughan, 2005). Kingham and Ure (2010) highlight additional mental health benefits from the social interaction and community engagement that can rise from proper urban design promoting walkability and cycling. On the other hand, areas that leave residents heavily reliant upon cars for transportation cause, though likely unintentional, increases in rates of stress, emotional exhaustion, and burnout reactions due to traffic and long car commutes (de Reuver & Biron, 2024; Olsson et al., 2013).

Nature and Community Spaces

Exposure to nature reduces stress by lowering levels of cortisol (the stress hormone), reducing anxiety, and promoting mental relaxation. Cities, communities, and other environments with green spaces tend to have lower rates of nearly every common mental health condition and disease, including depression, anxiety, PTSD, and stress. Interestingly, there is evidence that simply having indoor plants and access to views of nature have positive mental health effects, including heightened feelings of well-being and overall life satisfaction (Chang et al., 2020; Gilchrist et al., 2015). In fact, research on "restorative environments" suggests that integrating elements of nature into physical spaces (commonly known in architecture as biophilic design) helps mitigate and reduce mental fatigue, stress, and depressive feelings (Staats, 2012), as well as enhancing mood and improving cognitive performance (Hung & Chang, 2021).

When neighborhoods create community spaces, their residents tend to experience improved mental health and well-being. These spaces—which may be parks, public squares, or community centers—often share a common purpose: to provide a safe and welcoming environment to help foster social cohesion (Chung & Kim, 2022). Studies confirm that combating social isolation and bolstering a sense of community and belonging lead to improved mental health measures across several mental wellness indicators. Further, community spaces have been found to be especially impactful in minoritized and other vulnerable populations at risk for poor mental health and wellness (Ramos-Vidal & Dominguez de la Ossa, 2023; Yan et al., 2021).

Today, one in five adults live with a mental illness and nearly half of the U.S. population will have a mental illness at some point during their lives. Additionally, research findings have shown that minoritized individuals and communities bear a greater mental health burden than other individuals and communities (National Institute for Mental Health, 2021). The documented impact of urban design on mental health, therefore, underscores the vital importance of addressing urban density in efforts seeking to mitigate the negative impacts of environmental determinants to advance mental health equity.

THE MENTAL HEALTH IMPACTS OF LEGISLATION

The law can be a powerful resource for impacting the environmental determinants of mental health. If carefully conceptualized and implemented, legislation can create new or reinforce existing protective measures by maximizing the health benefits from both the built and natural environment to those living in and around them. The evidence is in: mental health and wellness are inextricably linked to environmental determinants (Institute of Medicine Roundtable on Environmental Health Sciences et al., 2002), necessitating a holistic and inter- and transdisciplinary approach to policy making.

This increased understanding and respect for the environment as a mental health determinant has yielded a new and inclusive theoretical framework: "one health." This framework is based on the notion that human, animal, and environmental health are inextricably linked, necessitating a collaborative approach to attain optimal health for all three (One Health High-Level Expert Panel, 2022). Though still controversial, the framework is recognized for being uniquely poised to handle the increasingly complex global public health challenges of climate change, pandemics, neglected zoonotic diseases, and the collapse in biodiversity. As recent environmental incidents have shown, any one of these events singularly can have a direct or indirect effect on mental health. Collectively, the compounded impact on mental health would likely be catastrophic. The promising thrust of the one health framework, then, is that a unifying and collaborative approach can serve as a model for policy making, with room for its application within this domain to effectively mitigate the current environmental determinants and prevent the proliferation of additional ones in future.

Using the political determinants of health framework enables us to understand how voting, government, policy, advocacy, and commercial interests have been used to create and sustain or used to repeal or amend policies, regulations, practices, zoning ordinances, and resource allocations that have a direct and profound impact on mental health and well-being. For instance, the National League of Cities has highlighted an increasing trend in the use of policy—through city government—to address suboptimal housing conditions across several cities in the United States. These policies have resulted in proactive inspection programs against negligent landlords, lead hazard prevention and elimination, and rental registrations with the city to ensure compliance with housing and building codes (Ford, 2023). Indeed, there are a multitude of legislative efforts to address environmental determinants, including environmental laws, executive orders, and EPA-led initiatives to help monitor, protect, and enforce these actions. Some of these examples are intended to advance environmental justice by addressing the intersection of social, economic, and political structures that have led to disparate and inequitable outcomes for minoritized individuals and communities (Exec. Order No. 12,898, 1994; Exec. Order No. 14,096, 2023).

However, in the absence of political will, ideas and intentions to address these issues will prove futile. Collectively, the actions of the political determinants—voting, governing, and policy making—have historically been used to propagate the postcolonial legacies through seemingly race-neutral policies. For instance, residential segregation was a consequence of policies that birthed the formation of the Home Owners' Loan Corporation and whose discriminatory lending practices—redlining—were bolstered by the efforts of the Federal Housing Administration to reject mortgage insurances in and near African American and other minoritized neighborhoods (Courtemanche & Snowden, 2011). However, the Fair Housing Act of 1968 sought to dismantle the racially biased laws and policies that had created these segregated communities by outlawing the ability to (a) overtly refuse to rent or sell to racial and ethnic minority groups who had been previously discriminated against, (b) refuse to negotiate, (c) deceptively deny the availability of housing, and (d) engage in other related discriminatory practices (Franzese & Beach, 2019).

These examples demonstrate how far-reaching and impactful the actions of policy can be for a community and a nation. Policy has the power to transform well-being on a grand scale and should be carefully considered and strategically utilized to promote policies and practices that advance mental health equity. Examples of these include addressing environmental and other determinants of mental health, strengthening the resiliency of minoritized individuals and communities that are disproportionately and detrimentally affected by climate change and natural disasters, and creating solutions and interventions that are intersectional, multifactorial, and reticulated. By prioritizing mental health equity in policy agendas, governments can pave the way for healthier populations and a more just and fair society.

ACTIONABLE TOOLS AND INTERVENTIONS TO ACTUALIZE MENTAL HEALTH EQUITY

To positively influence environmental determinants and mental health outcomes, actionable steps must focus on creating supportive, sustainable, and equitable environments. Both research and history support the notion that changes that are made "upstream" can have the greatest impact on a given population "downstream" (Dawes, 2020; Ray et al., 2023). There is increasing awareness of the impact that environmental determinants, such as climate change, pollution, natural disasters, and built environments, have downstream on the health, including the mental health, of individuals. In addition to launching greater public awareness campaigns and appealing to their elected officials about the mental health impacts of green spaces, exposure to pollution, and built environments, stakeholders in communities across the nation have used ordinances and zoning laws to mitigate the negative mental health effects of environmental determinants.

Ordinances

Ordinances are powerful tools that allow for the application of laws passed by local governments (state, city, county, or town governments) to regulate issues that have an impact on public health. Communities throughout the nation have used ordinances to address pressing health issues—including mental health issues—that disproportionately and detrimentally affect their residents.

Zoning Laws

Zoning is the most prevalent land use planning tool available in the United States. Zoning laws determine what types of land uses and densities can occur in a municipality and therefore govern the range of potential environmental and health impacts resulting from the land use. As such, they have far-reaching effects on the environmental determinants that negatively affect mental health and exacerbate mental health inequities.

Case Vignette 8.1 CITY OF HOUSTON

From 2004 to 2009, the City of Houston implemented a novel, municipality-based air pollution reduction strategy to address what it considered unacceptable health risks of air pollution exposure and an insufficient regulatory response from state and federal agencies. The city's effort to exert local control over stationary sources of air pollution represents a unique opportunity to study the selection and performance of policy tools and to consider their ramifications for the design of future air pollution control strategies that could mitigate their negative mental health effects on residents. The results of this case vignette demonstrate the potential for municipal government to use a combination of cooperative and confrontational policies to stimulate responses from private industry and state and federal regulators as part of a larger strategy to address the pollution problems that exacerbate mental health inequities.

Case Vignette 8.2 COMPLETE STREETS

Complete Streets is a transportation policy and design approach that requires streets to be planned, designed, operated, and maintained to enable safe and convenient travel regardless of an individual's mode of transportation. These policies, which have been implemented in numerous cities and communities throughout the nation, have been shown to positively impact mental health by encouraging physical activity, reducing stress and depressive disorders by fostering a sense of community and connection within a neighborhood, and reducing social isolation.

Effective policies must go beyond siloed approaches, leveraging multisectoral collaboration to ensure holistic solutions—such as safe housing, accessible transportation, biophilic urban design, and thriving natural environments. Effective governance should be leveraged to ensure impactful and thoughtful interventions that engage communities throughout the process and prioritize objectives to address the environmental determinants that continue to drive the nation's mental health equity crisis. Not only would this build resilient, thriving communities equipped to weather future environmental events, but it also would address persistent mental health disparities and inequities experienced by diverse population groups.

SUMMARY

This chapter explores the profound influence of environmental determinants on mental health equity and their critical role in perpetuating mental health inequities, particularly among minoritized communities. It emphasizes that environmental determinants—encompassing natural disasters, climate change, pollution, built environments, and structural social factors such as racism and discrimination—interact and often exacerbate mental health disparities. Key themes include the disproportionate mental health burdens faced by marginalized populations due to factors such as housing, exposure to environmental hazards, and limited access to resources that mitigate these challenges.

The chapter highlights how political determinants of health underpin these environmental determinants, shaping inequities through structural and systemic discrimination and resource allocation. The mental health impacts of climate change, air pollution, and natural disasters illustrate the interconnectedness of these issues. The chapter discusses targeted interventions through policy-driven action, such as urban design and planning that promotes sustainability and equity, adoption of a more unified, comprehensive and inclusive approach to policy making, and legislative efforts to address the environmental and structural conditions impacting mental health.

Finally, the chapter underscores the importance of targeted structural-level interventions to help individuals and communities adapt to environmental challenges, emphasizing the need for comprehensive, collaborative solutions that prioritize mental health equity and sustainability.

DISCUSSION QUESTIONS

1. What are the major environmental determinants of mental health equity? Which do you think contribute the greatest impact and why?
2. What are two examples of how various environmental determinants—such as climate change, built environments, and structural factors in the environment—negatively impact mental health equity?
3. What is an example of a political determinant of health that gives rise to the environmental determinants of mental health that are associated with the mental health challenges among and within minoritized individuals and communities?
4. Consider that the built environment, one of the environmental determinants of mental health, is one entire "finished product." What multifaceted upstream approaches can be taken to address the mental health challenges facing individuals and communities?
5. How can legislation be used to mitigate (and even eliminate) the deleterious mental health impacts on minoritized individuals and communities that are created by the environmental determinants?

REFERENCES

Ahern, M., Kovats, R. S., Wilkinson, P., Few, R., & Matthies, F. (2005). Global health impacts of floods: Epidemiologic evidence. *Epidemiologic Reviews*, *27*, 36–46. https://doi.org/10.1093/epirev/mxi004

Alexander, A. C., Ali, J., McDevitt-Murphy, M. E., Forde, D. R., Stockton, M., Read, M., & Ward, K. D. (2017). Racial differences in posttraumatic stress disorder vulnerability following Hurricane Katrina among a sample of adult cigarette smokers from New Orleans. *Journal of Racial and Ethnic Health Disparities*, *4*(1), 94–103. https://doi.org/10.1007/s40615-015-0206-8

Andrusaityte, S., Grazuleviciene, R., Dedele, A., & Balseviciene, B., (2020). The effect of residential greenness and city park visiting habits on preschool children's mental and general health in Lithuania: A cross-sectional study. *International Journal of Hygiene and Environmental Health*, *223*(1), 142–150.

Babisch, W. (2002). The noise/stress concept, risk assessment and research needs. *Noise & Health*, *4*(16), 1–11.

Bansal, V., Bansal, S., & Sen, J. (2020). Assessing the role of urban design in a rapidly urbanizing historical city and its contribution in restoring its urban ecology: The case of Varanasi, India. In P. Verma, P. Singh, R. Singh, & A. S. Raghubanshi (Eds.), *Urban ecology* (pp. 413–434). Elsevier. https://doi.org/10.1016/B978-0-12-820730-7.00021-5

Beyeler, N. S., Buonocore, J., Gohlke, J., Johnson, S., Salas, R.N., & Hess, J.J. (2024). Lancet countdown on health and climate change policy brief for the United States of America. *Policy Brief* (p. 20).https://www.lancetcountdownus.org/2024-lancet-countdown-u-s-brief/

Bezold, C. P., Banay, R. F., Coull, B. A., Hart, J. E., James, P., Kubzansky, L. D., Missmer, S. A., & Laden, F. (2018). The relationship between surrounding greenness in childhood and adolescence and depressive symptoms in adolescence and early adulthood. *Annals of Epidemiology*, *28*(4), 213–219. https://doi.org/10.1016/j.annepidem.2018.01.009

Borroni, E., Pesatori, A. C., Bollati, V., Buoli, M., & Carugno, M. (2022). Air pollution exposure and depression: A comprehensive updated systematic review and meta-analysis. *Environmental Pollution*, *292*, 118245. https://doi.org/10.1016/j.envpol.2021.118245

Bryant, R. A., Gibbs, L., Colin Gallagher, H., Pattison, P., Lusher, D., MacDougall, C., Harms, L., Block, K., Ireton, G., Richardson, J., Forbes, D., Molyneaux, R., & O'Donnell, M. (2020). The dynamic course of psychological outcomes following the Victorian Black Saturday Bushfires. *The Australian and New Zealand Journal of Psychiatry, 55*(7), 666–677. https://doi.org/10.1177/0004867420969815

Budhwani, H., Herald, K., & Chavez-Yenter, D. (2015). Depression in racial and ethnic minorities: The impact of nativity and discrimination. *Journal of Racial and Ethnic Health Disparities, 2*(1), 34–42. https://doi.org/10.1007/s40615-014-0045-z

Chandra, M., Rai, C. B., Kumari, N., Sandhu, V. K., Chandra, K., Krishna, M., Kota, S. H., Anand, K. S., & Oudin, A. (2022). Air pollution and cognitive impairment across the life course in humans: A systematic review with specific focus on income level of study area. *International Journal of Environmental Research and Public Health, 19*(3), 1405. https://doi.org/10.3390/ijerph19031405

Chang, C., Oh, R., Nghiem, T., Zhang, Y., & Carrasco, L. R. (2020). Life satisfaction linked to the diversity of nature experiences and nature views from the window. *Landscape and Urban Planning, 202*, 103874. https://doi.org/10.1016/j.landurbplan.2020.103874.

Chung, S., & Kim, M. (2022). Age-friendly environment, social support, sense of community, and loneliness among middle-aged and older adults in Korea. *Aging & Mental Health, 27*, 1–8. https://doi.org/10.1080/13607863.2022.2116395

Courtemanche, C., & Snowden, K. (2011). Repairing a mortgage crisis: HOLC lending and its impact on local housing markets. *The Journal of Economic History, 71*(2), 307–337. http://www.jstor.org/stable/23018301

Czeisler, M. E., Lane, R. I., Petrosky, E., Wiley, J. F., Christensen, A., Njai, R., Weaver, M. D., Robbins, R., Facer-Childs, E. R., Barger, L. K., Czeisler, C. A., Howard, M. F., & Rajaratnam, S. M. W. (2020). Mental health, substance use, and suicidal ideation during the COVID-19 pandemic – United States, June 24–30, 2020. *MMWR Morbidity and Mortality Weekly Rep*ort, *69*(32), 1049–1057. https://doi.org/10.15585/mmwr.mm6932a1

Dawes, D. (2020). *The political determinants of health.* Johns Hopkins University Press.

Dawes, D., Bhatt, J., Dunlap, N., Amador, C., Gebreyes, K., & Rush, B. (2024). *The projected cost and economic impact of mental health inequities in the United States.* Meharry School of Global Health.

de Reuver, R., & Biron, M. (2024, January). The effect of morning commutes on emotional exhaustion and task performance: Taking mental effort and cognitive appraisal into account. *Travel Behavior and Society, 34*(100697), 1–8. https://doi.org/10.1016/j.tbs.2023.100697

Evans, G. W. (2003). The built environment and mental health. *Journal of Urban Health: Bulletin of the New York Academy of Medicine, 80*(4), 536–555. https://doi.org/10.1093/jurban/jtg063

Exec. Order No. 12,898 59 F.R. 7629. (1994). https://www.federalregister.gov/d/94-3685

Exec. Order No. 14,096 88 F.R. 25251. (2023). https://www.federalregister.gov/d/2023-08955

Ford, L. (2023, January 6). How cities are shaping policy to better ensure health housing. *National League of Cities.* https://www.nlc.org/article/2023/01/06/how-cities-are-shaping-policy-to-better-ensure-healthy-housing/

Franzese, P. A., & Beach, S. J. (2019). Promises still to keep: The fair housing act fifty years later. *Cardozo Law Review, 40*, 1207–1235.

Gilchrist, K., Brown, C., & Montarzino, A. (2015). Workplace settings and wellbeing: Greenspace use and views contribute to employee wellbeing at peri-urban business sites. *Landscape and Urban Planning, 138*, 32–40. https://doi.org/10.1016/j.landurbplan.2015.02.004

Hajat, A., Hsia, C., & O'Neill, M. S. (2015). Socioeconomic disparities and air pollution exposure: A global review. *Current Environmental Health Reports, 2*(4), 440–450. https://doi.org/10.1007/s40572-015-0069-5

Halpern, D. (1995). *Mental health and the built environment: More than bricks and mortar?* (1st ed., pp. 203–213). Routledge. https://doi.org/10.4324/9781315041131

Hickman, C., Marks, E., Pihkala, P., Clayton, S., Lewandowski, R. E., Mayall, E. E., Wray, B., Mellor, C., & van Susteren, L. (2021). Climate anxiety in children and young people and their beliefs about government responses to climate change: A global survey. *The Lancet Planetary Health, 5*(12), e863–e873. https://doi.org/10.1016/S2542-5196(21)00278-3

Hung, S., & Chang, C. (2021). Health benefits of evidence-based biophilic-designed environments: A review. *Journal of People Plants Environment, 24*(1), 1–16. https://doi.org/10.11628/ksppe.2021.24.1.1

Institute of Medicine Roundtable on Environmental Health Sciences, Research, and Medicine, Frumkin, H., Jackson, R. J., & Coussens, C. M. (Eds.). (2002). *Health and the environment in the Southeastern United States.* National Academies Press.

Johnson, S., Corbin, S., South, C., & Cawich, S. (2024). The impact of environmental health determinants in surgical oncology. *Journal of Surgical Oncology, 130*(7), 1439–1446. https://doi.org/10.1002/jso.27889

Keswani, A., Akselrod, H., & Anenberg, S. (2022). Health and clinical impacts of air pollution and linkages with climate change. *NEJM Evidence, 1*(7), EVIDra2200068. https://doi.org/10.1056/EVIDra2200068.

Keya, T. A., Leela, A., Habib, N., Rashid, M., & Bakthavatchalam, P. (2023). Mental health disorders due to disaster exposure: A systematic review and meta-analysis. *Cureus, 15*(4), e37031. https://doi.org/10.7759/cureus.37031

Kingham, S., & Ure, J. (2010). Impact of the built environment on walking and cycling. *Environment and Planning B: Planning and Design*, 37(2), 248–267.

McFarlane, A. C., & Van Hooff, M. (2009). Impact of childhood exposure to a natural disaster on adult mental health: 20-year longitudinal follow-up study. *British Journal of Psychiatry, 195*(2), 142–148. https://doi.org/10.1192/bjp.bp.108.054270

Mirzabaev, A., Kerr, R. B., Hasegawa, T., Pradhan, P., Wreford, A., Pahlen, M. C. T. V. D., & Gurney-Smith, H. (2023). Severe climate change risks to food security and nutrition. *Climate Risk Management, 39*, Article 100473. https://doi.org/10.1016/j.crm.2022.100473

Mouratidis, K. (2021). Urban planning and quality of life: A review of pathways linking the built environment to subjective well-being. *Cities, 115*, 103229.

Myers, C. A. (2020). Food insecurity and psychological distress: A review of the recent literature. *Current Nutrition Reports, 9*(2), 107–118. https://doi.org/10.1007/s13668-020-00309-1

National Institute for Mental Health.(2021). *Mental health information. Mental illness.* https://www.nimh.nih.gov/health/statistics/mental-illness

Neville, T., Schweizer, C., & Neira, M. (2023). Climate change and health: Three grand challenges. *Nature Medicine, 29*(7), 1631–1638. https://doi.org/10.1038/s41591-023-02438-w

Nobile, F., Forastiere, A., Michelozzi, P., Forastiere, F., & Stafoggia, M. (2023). Long-term exposure to air pollution and incidence of mental disorders. A large longitudinal cohort study of adults within an urban area. *Environment International, 181*, 108302. https://doi.org/10.1016/j.envint.2023.108302

Nogueira, L. M., Crane, T. E, Ortiz, A. P., D'Angelo, H., & Neta, G. (2023). Climate change and cancer. *Cancer Epidemiology, Biomarkers & Prevention, 32*(7), 869–875. https://doi.org/10.1158/1055-9965.EPI-22-1234

Olsson, L. E., Gärling, T., Ettema, D., Friman, M., & Fujii, S. (2013). Happiness and satisfaction with work commute. *Social Indicators Research, 111*(1), 255–263. https://doi.org/10.1007/s11205-012-0003-2

One Health High-Level Expert Panel, Adisasmito, W. B., Almuhairi, S., Behravesh, C. B., Bilivogui, P., Bukachi, S. A., Casas, N., Becerra, N. C., Charron, D. F., Chaudhary, A., Ciacci Zanella, J. R., Cunningham, A. A., Dar, O., Debnath, N., Dungu, B., Farag, E., Gao, G. F., Hayman, D. T. S., Khaitsa, M., ..., Zhou, L. (2022). One Health: A new definition for a sustainable and healthy future. *PLOS Pathogens, 18*(6), e1010537. https://doi.org/10.1371/journal.ppat.1010537

O'Neill, B., van Aalst, M., Zaiton Ibrahim, Z., Berrang Ford, L., Bhadwal, S., Buhaug, H., Diaz, D., Frieler, K., Garschagen, M., Magnan, A., Midgley, G., Mirzabaev, A., Thomas A., & Warren, R. (2022). Key risks across sectors and regions. In H.-O. Pörtner, D. C. Roberts, M. Tignor, E. S. Poloczanska, K. Mintenbeck, A. Alegría, M. Craig, S. Langsdorf, S. Löschke, V. Möller, A. Okem, & B. Rama (Eds.), *Climate change 2022: Impacts, adaptation, and vulnerability. Contribution of working group II to the sixth assessment report of the intergovernmental panel on climate change* (pp. 2411–2538). Cambridge University Press. https://doi.10.1017/9781009325844.025

Panchal, N., Saunders, H., & Ndugga, N. (2022, September 22). *Five key findings on mental health and substance use disorders by race/ethnicity.* KFF. https://www.kff.org/mental-health/issue-brief/five-key-findings-on-mental-health-and-substance-use-disorders-by-race-ethnicity/

Perrigo, J. L., Samek, A., & Hurlburt, M. (2022). Minority and low-SES families' experiences during the early phases of the COVID-19 pandemic crisis: A qualitative study. *Children and Youth Services Review, 140*, 106594. https://doi.org/10.1016/j.childyouth.2022.106594

Pevalin, D. J., Reeves, A., Baker, E., & Bentley, R. (2017). The impact of persistent poor housing conditions on mental health: A longitudinal population-based study. *Preventive Medicine, 105*, 304–310. https://doi.org/10.1016/j.ypmed.2017.09.020

Ramos-Vidal, I., & Dominguez de la Ossa, E. (2023). A systematic review to determine the role of public space and urban design on sense of community. *International Social Science Journal, 74*(252), 633–655. https://doi.org/10.1111/issj.12472

Ray, R., Lantz, P. M., & Williams, D. (2023). Upstream policy changes to improve population health and health equity: A priority agenda. *The Milbank Quarterly, 101*(S1), 20–35. https://doi.org/10.1111/1468-0009.12640

Renalds, A., Smith, T. H., & Hale, P. J. (2010). A systematic review of built environment and health. *Family & Community Health, 33*(1), 68–78. https://doi.org/10.1097/FCH.0b013e3181c4e2e5

Rigolon., A., Browning, M., McAnirlin, O., & Yoon, H.V. (2021). Green space and health equity: A systematic review on the potential of green space to reduce health disparities. *International Journal of Environmental Research and Public Health, 18*(5), 2563. https:/doi.org/10.3390/ijerph18052563

Ruiz-Tagle, J., & Urria, I. (2022). Household overcrowding trajectories and mental wellbeing. *Social Science and Medicine, 296*, 114051. https://doi.org/10.1016/j.socscimed.2021.114051

Ryu, S., & Fan, L. (2023). The relationship between financial worries and psychological distress among U.S. adults. *Journal of Family and Economic Issues, 44*(1), 16–33. https://doi.org/10.1007/s10834-022-09820-9

Staats, H. (2012). Restorative environments. In S. D. Clayton (Ed.), *The Oxford handbook of environmental and conservation psychology* (pp. 445–458). Oxford University Press. https://doi.org/10.1093/oxfordhb/9780199733026.013.0024

Stanke, C., Murray, V., Amlôt, R., Nurse, J., & Williams, R. (2012). The effects of flooding on mental health: Outcomes and recommendations from a review of the literature. *PLoS Currents, 4*, e4f9f1fa9c3cae. https://doi.org/10.1371/4f9f1fa9c3cae

Stansfeld, S. A., & Matheson, M. P. (2003). Noise pollution: Non-auditory effects on health. *British Medical Bulletin, 68*(1), 243–257. https://doi.org/10.1093/bmb/ldg033

Stinson, E. A., Sullivan, R. M., Peteet, B. J., Tapert, S. F., Baker, F. C., Breslin, F. J., Dick, A. S., Gonzalez, M. R., Guillaume, M., Marshall, A. T., McCabe, C. J., Pelham, W. E., III, Van Rinsveld, A., Sheth, C. S., Sowell, E. R., Wade, N. E., Wallace, A. L., & Lisdahl, K. M. (2021). Longitudinal impact of childhood adversity on early adolescent mental health during the COVID-19 pandemic in the ABCD study cohort: Does race or ethnicity moderate findings? *Biological Psychiatry Global Open Science, 1*, 324–335. https://doi.org/10.1016/j.bpsgos.2021.08.007

Stolberg, S. (2020, June 7). Pandemic within a pandemic: Coronavirus and police brutality roil Black communities. *The New York Times*. https://www.nytimes.com/2020/06/07/us/politics/blacks-coronavirus-police-brutality.html

Tight, M., & Baughan, C. (2005). The relationship between transport and mental health. *Transportation Research Part F: Traffic Psychology and Behaviour, 8*(3), 209–218.

To, P., Eboreime, E., & Agyapong, V. I. O. (2021). The impact of wildfires on mental health: A scoping review. *Behavioral Sciences, 11*(9), 126. https://doi.org/10.3390/bs11090126

Turner, M. C., Andersen, Z. J., Baccarelli, A., Diver, W. R., Gapstur, S. M, Pope, C. A, III, Prada, D., Samet, J., Thurston, G., & Cohen, A. (2020). Outdoor air pollution and cancer: An overview of the current evidence and public health recommendations. *CA: A Cancer Journal of Clinicians, 25*, 10.3322/caac.21632. doi: 10.3322/caac.21632

U.S. Census Bureau. (2024, December 19). Likelihood of eviction or foreclosure. *Household pulse survey*. https://www.census.gov/data-tools/demo/hhp/#/?measures=EVICTFOR

U.S. Environmental Protection Agency. (n.d.). *History of the clean water act*. https://www.epa.gov/laws-regulations/history-clean-water-act?

U.S. Environmental Protection Agency. (2024). What are the trends in indoor air quality and their effects on human health? *Indoor Air Quality*. https://www.epa.gov/report-environment/indoor-air-quality#:~:text=The%20potential%20impact%20of%20indoor%20air%20quality,5%20times%20higher%20than%20typical%20outdoor%20concentrations

Wang, H., & Li, D. (2023). Emergency department visits for mental disorders and the built environment: Residential greenspace and historical redlining. *Landscape and Urban Planning, 230*, 104568. https://doi.org/10.1016/j.landurbplan.2022.104568

Weber, C., Watson, J., & Seewer, J. (2025, January 13). Strong winds forecast to return and threaten Los Angeles area's fight against fires. *AP News*. https://apnews.com/article/los-angeles-wildfires-southern-california-4997fb4d4490fdaa9f2d5cf8cd5f2be7

What happens when climate change and the mental-health crisis collide? (2024). *Nature, 628*(8007), 235. https://doi.org/10.1038/d41586-024-00993-x

Yan, Y., Liu, H., & He, C. (2021). How does urban sprawl affect public health? Evidence from panel survey data in urbanizing China. *International Journal of Environmental Research and Public Health, 18*(19), 10181. https://doi.org/10.3390/ijerph181910181

9 BIOLOGICAL AND GENETIC DETERMINANTS OF MENTAL HEALTH

WALTER D. CONWELL

LEARNING OBJECTIVES

After reading this chapter, readers will be able to:

- Understand the interplay among genetics, epigenetics, and mental health disorders.
- Explain the methodologies used in psychiatric genetic epidemiology.
- Discuss the neurobiological and structural brain alterations observed in mental health disorders.
- Analyze the conceptual framework of "brain vulnerability" in the context of mental health disorders.
- Evaluate the concept of precision psychiatry and its goal of tailoring prevention, diagnosis, and treatment strategies to individual patients.

INTRODUCTION

Mental health is a multifaceted domain influenced by genetic, neurobiological, and environmental factors. This chapter explores the biological and genetic determinants of mental health, emphasizing their role in understanding, diagnosing, and treating psychiatric conditions. Through the lens of psychiatric genetics, neurobiology, and precision psychiatry, we delve into foundational and emerging insights that have shaped the field. The inclusion of real-world applications and a case vignette further bridges the gap between theory and practice, providing a comprehensive understanding of these critical determinants.

PSYCHIATRIC GENETICS

The intricate interplay between genetics and mental health has long been a subject of fascination for researchers and clinicians alike. Psychiatric genetics, a field at the intersection of genetics and psychiatry, seeks to unravel the genetic underpinnings of mental disorders. This section provides an overview of the foundations of psychiatric genetics, its methodologies, key findings, and the implications for understanding, diagnosing, and treating mental health conditions.

Psychiatric Genetic Epidemiology

Psychiatric genetic epidemiology is a field of study that investigates the genetic factors underlying psychiatric disorders and their interplay with environmental influences within populations (Kendler et al., 2011). This involves the application of epidemiological methods to understand the distribution and determinants of psychiatric disorders at the population level, with a specific focus on genetic risk factors.

Key Terms and Methods

Heritability Studies

Heritability studies aim to estimate the proportion of variance in a psychiatric disorder that can be attributed to genetic factors (heritability). Twin and family studies are commonly used to estimate heritability by comparing the rates of disorder concordance between monozygotic (MZ; identical) and dizygotic (DZ; fraternal) twins or between biological relatives.

Family Studies

Family studies examine the aggregation of psychiatric disorders within families to assess familial risk and genetic transmission patterns. They involve comparing the rates of disorder among biological relatives of affected individuals with those of relatives of unaffected individuals.

Twin Studies

Twin studies, particularly those involving MZ and DZ twins, allow researchers to disentangle genetic and environmental influences on psychiatric disorders. By comparing the concordance rates of disorders between MZ and DZ twins, genetic and environmental contributions to disorder variance can be estimated.

Adoption Studies

Adoption studies examine the risk of psychiatric disorders in adopted individuals compared with their biological and adoptive relatives. These studies help to differentiate between genetic and environmental influences by assessing whether the risk of disorder is more strongly associated with genetic relatedness or shared environment.

Molecular Genetic Studies

Molecular genetic approaches, such as genome-wide association studies (GWAS), candidate gene studies, and linkage studies, identify specific genetic variants associated with psychiatric disorders. These studies analyze the distribution of genetic variants across populations to identify susceptibility genes and genetic risk loci.

Gene–Environment Interactions

Psychiatric genetic epidemiology also investigates interactions between genetic and environmental factors in the development of psychiatric disorders. Gene–environment interaction studies examine how specific genetic variants modify the impact of environmental risk factors on disorder risk.

Polygenic Risk Scores

Polygenic risk scores (PRS) aggregate information from multiple genetic variants associated with a disorder to calculate an individual's genetic risk. Psychiatric genetic epidemiology uses PRS to assess genetic susceptibility to psychiatric disorders and to investigate relationships among genetic risk, environmental exposures, and disorder outcomes.

Population-Based Cohort Studies

Population-based cohort studies follow large cohorts of individuals over time to examine the natural history, risk factors, and outcomes of psychiatric disorders. These studies provide valuable data for understanding the complex interplay among genetic, environmental, and developmental factors in the etiology of psychiatric disorders.

Prevalence

Genetic factors contribute significantly to the vulnerability and resilience associated with mental health disorders. The prevalence of mental health disorders within the U.S. population has been found to be high, impacting approximately 23% of all adults (Kessler et al., 2005). However, the prevalence varies across sex, gender, age groups, and racial/ethnic groups. Understanding these variations is critical for tailoring interventions to specific populations (Kessler et al., 2005). Although environmental influences also play a crucial role, the heritability of conditions such as schizophrenia, bipolar disorder, and major depressive disorder has been well established through twin, family, and adoption studies. However, the degree of heritability may vary greatly (Pettersson et al., 2019; Smoller et al., 2005; Sullivan et al., 2000, 2003). Undoubtedly, environmental factors such as prenatal exposures, adverse childhood experiences (ACEs), and nutritional factors influence the trajectory of brain development, increasing the vulnerability of neurological disorders later in life (Felitti et al., 1998; Jacka et al., 2011; McEwen, 2012).

Considerations and Future Directions

As the field of psychiatric genetics progresses, ethical considerations surrounding genetic testing, privacy, and potential stigmatization become increasingly important. Balancing the benefits of genetic insights with the potential societal and individual risks necessitates ongoing dialogue and the establishment of robust ethical frameworks to guide research and clinical applications. In addition, although molecular genetics studies such as gGWAS have revolutionized our understanding of the genetic basis of various traits and diseases, beneath the promise of genomic research lies a critical issue disparities in GWAS data. Historically, GWAS have predominantly focused on populations of European descent, with individuals of African, Asian, and other non-European ancestries being underrepresented (**Figure 9.1**; MacArthur et al., 2017; Martin et al., 2019). This bias limits the generalizability of GWAS

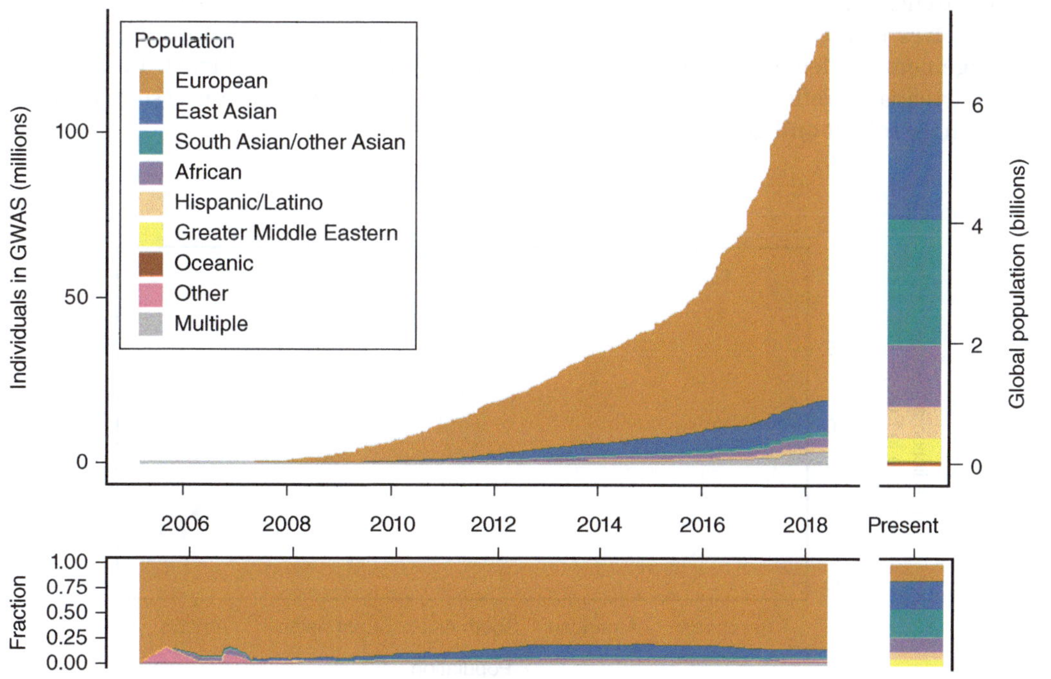

Figure 9.1 Disparities in ancestry within GWAS catalog.

Note: Ancestry of GWAS participants over time, as compared with the global population. Cumulative data, as reported by the GWAS catalog. Individuals whose ancestry is "not reported" are not shown.

GWAS, genome-wide association studies.

Source: Martin, A. R., Kanai, M., Kamatani, Y., Okada, Y., Neale, B. M., & Daly, M. J. (2019). Clinical use of current polygenic risk scores may exacerbate health disparities. *Nature Genetics, 51*(4), 584–591. https://doi.org/10.1038/s41588-019-0379-8

findings and hinders our ability to understand the full spectrum of genetic variation across diverse populations (Batai et al., 2021; Mostafavi et al., 2020; Wojcik et al., 2019).

Several factors contribute to the underrepresentation of certain populations in GWAS. Socioeconomic factors, historical injustices, and inadequate access to healthcare and research opportunities have played a role in limiting the participation of diverse populations. Additionally, ethical considerations related to informed consent, data sharing, and mistrust in medical research further complicate efforts to achieve representative and inclusive GWAS cohorts.

The implications of GWAS data disparities extend beyond the scientific realm and impact public health and healthcare equity. The lack of diversity in genetic studies perpetuates health disparities, because findings may not accurately reflect the genetic contributions to diseases in underrepresented populations. This has real-world consequences, because the prediction accuracy of polygenic risk scores in non-European populations has been found to be lower for various traits and diseases (Martin et al., 2019; Mostafavi et al., 2020; **Figure 9.2**).

Addressing GWAS data disparities requires a multifaceted and culturally humble approach. Cultural humility is a framework first described by Melanie Tervalon and Jann Murray-Garcia that has four main elements, detailed in **Box 9.1** (Tervalon & Murray-García, 1998). First and foremost, researchers themselves should represent diverse backgrounds and should engage in ongoing self-reflection to examine their own biases, assumptions, and privileges. Furthermore, researchers must seek to ethically navigate the complexities of obtaining informed consent, ensuring that participants have access to language-concordant and accessible services that allow them to become well informed about the potential uses of their genetic data and the implications of the research.

Researchers should also actively strive to increase the diversity of study populations. This involves fostering collaboration with diverse communities, incorporating community engagement strategies, and addressing historical injustices to build trust. Ensuring that study participants reflect the global diversity of the human population is essential for producing more robust and generalizable genetic data sets.

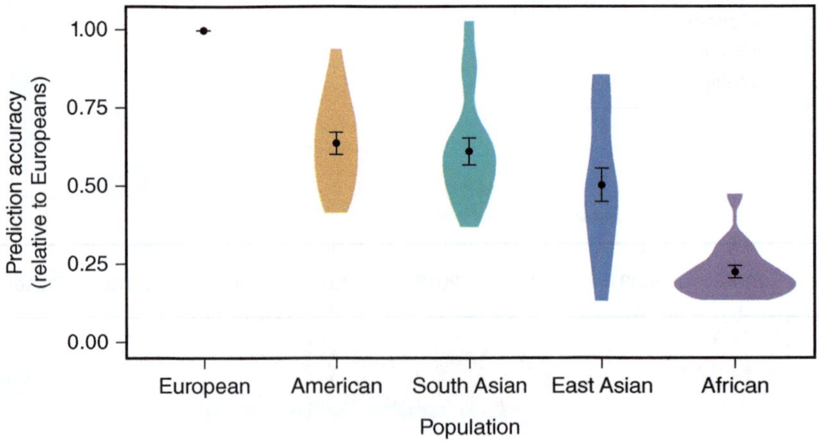

Figure 9.2 Disparities in prediction accuracy for PRS.

Note: Prediction accuracy relative to European-ancestry individuals across 17 quantitative traits and five continental populations in the UK Biobank (UKBB).

PRS, polygenic risk scores.

Source: Martin, A. R., Kanai, M., Kamatani, Y., Okada, Y., Neale, B. M., & Daly, M. J. (2019). Clinical use of current polygenic risk scores may exacerbate health disparities. *Nature Genetics, 51*(4), 584–591. https://doi.org/10.1038/s41588-019-0379-8

Box 9.1 CULTURAL HUMILITY IN GENETICS RESEARCH

- *Lifelong learning and critical self-reflection:* Researchers should engage in ongoing self-reflection to examine their own biases, assumptions, and privileges.
- *Identifying and addressing power imbalances:* Researchers should provide concordant and accessible language services, including translation and interpretation services.
- *Developing mutually beneficial dynamics:* Researchers should actively recruit participants from underrepresented populations, including individuals of different racial, ethnic, and cultural backgrounds.
- *Ensuring institutional accountability:* Researchers should maintain transparency and accountability in all aspects of the research process, including decision-making, resource allocation, and reporting of findings.

Institutional changes are also necessary to address genetic data disparities. Transparency in data-sharing practices, including clear communication regarding the handling and sharing of genetic information, is crucial for fostering trust between researchers and study participants. In addition, funding agencies and research institutions should prioritize and incentivize studies that include diverse populations. This involves allocating resources for research infrastructure in underrepresented regions, promoting diversity in research teams, and incorporating diversity and inclusion metrics into grant evaluations.

The field of psychiatric genetics continues to evolve, offering unprecedented insights into the genetic foundations of mental health disorders. As we unlock the mysteries of the genome, the integration of genetic information into clinical practice holds immense promise for revolutionizing how we diagnose, treat, and understand mental health conditions. However, to realize the promise of psychiatric genetics, collaboration and data sharing across diverse research consortia are essential. In addition, open sharing of data facilitates more robust analyses, replication studies, and the development of comprehensive PRS. However, the ethical considerations and challenges associated with disparities in data sets underscore the need for responsible and collaborative approaches to ensure the ethical and equitable application of genetic insights in psychiatry. Addressing these challenges requires a concerted effort from the scientific community, policy makers, and research institutions to ensure that genetic research is inclusive, transparent, and ethically conducted.

NEUROBIOLOGY

The neurobiology of mental illness represents a complex and dynamic intersection of genetics, neurochemistry, and structural and functional abnormalities in the brain. This section delves into the intricacies of how alterations at the molecular, cellular, and systems levels contribute to the development and manifestation of mental health disorders. Understanding the neurobiological basis of mental illness is essential for advancing therapeutic interventions and reducing the stigma surrounding these conditions.

Methodologies

Structural imaging techniques play a pivotal role in unveiling the intricacies of brain structure and vulnerability. MRI, with its high spatial resolution, allows researchers and clinicians to visualize and quantify brain anatomy. Diffusion tensor imaging (DTI) is a specialized MRI technique that provides insights into the microstructural organization of white matter tracts in the brain. Unlike traditional structural MRI, which primarily visualizes anatomical structures, DTI allows researchers to examine the diffusion of water molecules within tissues and provides insights into white matter integrity. This information is particularly valuable for mapping the orientation and integrity of white matter fibers, offering a unique perspective on the brain's connectivity and enabling the detection of subtle structural abnormalities associated with vulnerability.

PET contributes to our understanding of structural brain vulnerability by examining metabolic and molecular processes. Tracer compounds can target specific proteins, neurotransmitters, or metabolic activities associated with vulnerability and neurological disorders. Integrating PET data with structural imaging enhances our understanding of the functional consequences of structural vulnerabilities.

Neurotransmitters and Mental Health

Serotonin is a neurotransmitter known for its role in mood regulation. Dysregulation of the serotonin system is associated with several mental health disorders (Cuijpers et al., 2019; Hofmann et al., 2012). Antidepressant medications, such as selective serotonin reuptake inhibitors (SSRIs), target serotonin pathways to alleviate symptoms, emphasizing the critical role of neurotransmitter balance in mental well-being (Hofmann et al., 2012).

Dopamine is involved in various cognitive, emotional, and behavioral functions within the brain. Its role in mental health is complex, and dysregulation of dopamine levels has been implicated in several psychiatric disorders (Belujon & Grace, 2017).

Glutamate, the most abundant excitatory neurotransmitter in the brain, plays a crucial role in various aspects of mental health. Its involvement extends to learning, memory, and synaptic plasticity, making it a key player in neurological and psychiatric conditions. Dysregulation of glutamate signaling has been implicated in several mental health disorders, underscoring the importance of understanding its role in both health and pathology (Sanacora et al., 2012).

Gamma-aminobutyric acid (GABA) is the primary inhibitory neurotransmitter in the central nervous system, playing a fundamental role in modulating neural activity. GABAergic neurotransmission is crucial for maintaining a balance between excitation and inhibition in the brain. Dysregulation of GABAergic signaling has been implicated in various mental health disorders, underscoring the importance of understanding the role of GABA in mental health (Cryan & Kaupmann, 2005).

Table 9.1 briefly reviews the roles of these neurotransmitters, across several mental health disorders.

Structural and Functional Brain Factors

In the field of mental health, researchers have increasingly turned their focus to structural changes in the brain, seeking to unravel the complex interplay between neurobiology and psychiatric disorders. This section explores the structural alterations observed in mental health disorders, shedding light on how these changes contribute to the understanding and treatment of conditions such as depression, anxiety, schizophrenia, and bipolar disorder (Falkai et al., 2018).

Depression

Structural changes in the brain are notably evident in individuals with depression, particularly in the hippocampus. The hippocampus, a region crucial for memory and emotional regulation, often exhibits reduced volume in individuals experiencing depressive episodes. Chronic stress, a common precursor to depression, has been linked to the atrophy of hippocampal neurons. Understanding the structural changes in the hippocampus provides insights into the cognitive and emotional symptoms associated with depression (Lorenzetti et al., 2009).

Table 9.1 NEUROTRANSMITTER CHANGES IN COMMON MENTAL HEALTH DISORDERS

	SEROTONIN	DOPAMINE	GLUTAMATE	GABA
Major depressive disorder	Reduced serotonin activity		Changes in glutamate levels or receptor function, particularly involving the NMDA receptor, have been observed in individuals with depression.	Alterations in GABA receptor expression and function have been observed in preclinical and clinical studies.
Anxiety disorders	Reduced serotonin activity		Dysregulation of glutamate levels or altered receptor function may contribute to the development or exacerbation of anxiety disorders.	GABA receptors, particularly the GABA-A receptor, mediate inhibitory effects in the brain, helping to dampen excessive neural activity associated with anxiety. Reduced GABAergic function has been observed in individuals with anxiety disorders, contributing to heightened excitability and increased susceptibility to anxious states.
Bipolar disorder		Increased dopamine activity is thought to contribute to symptoms such as elevated mood, increased energy, and impulsivity during manic episodes.	Increased glutamatergic activity may contribute to excitability, impulsivity, and other symptoms associated with manic episodes.	
Schizophrenia		"Dopamine hypothesis" suggests that an excess of dopamine activity in certain brain regions, particularly the mesolimbic pathway, contributes to positive symptoms of schizophrenia, including hallucinations and delusions.	The glutamate hypothesis of schizophrenia posits that deficits in glutamatergic neurotransmission, especially at the NMDA receptor, contribute to cognitive impairments and positive symptoms of the disorder.	

(*continued*)

Table 9.1 NEUROTRANSMITTER CHANGES IN COMMON MENTAL HEALTH DISORDERS (*continued*)

	SEROTONIN	DOPAMINE	GLUTAMATE	GABA
Addiction		Dopamine is implicated in the reward system of the brain, and dysregulation of this system is associated with addiction. Substance use, such as drugs or alcohol, can lead to increased dopamine release in the brain's reward pathway, reinforcing addictive behaviors.		GABA is involved in the reward pathway of the brain, and alterations in GABAergic transmission are associated with substance use disorders. Chronic substance abuse can affect GABA receptor function, contributing to withdrawal symptoms and the cycle of addiction.

GABA, gamma-aminobutyric acid; NDMA, *N*-methyl-D-aspartate.

Sources: Adapted from Cuijpers, P., Karyotaki, E., Weitz, E., Andersson, G., Hollon, S. D., & van Straten, A. (2019). The effects of psychotherapies for major depression in adults on remission, recovery and improvement: A meta-analysis. *Journal of Affective Disorders, 257*, 695–704. https://doi.org/10.1016/j.jad.2019.07.074; Hofmann, S. G., Asnaani, A., Vonk, I. J., Sawyer, A. T., & Fang, A. (2012). The efficacy of cognitive behavioral therapy: A review of meta-analyses. *Cognitive Therapy and Research, 36*(5), 427–440. https://doi.org/10.1007/s10608-012-9476-1; Sanacora, G., Treccani, G., & Popoli, M. (2012). Towards a glutamate hypothesis of depression: An emerging frontier of neuropsychopharmacology for mood disorders. *Neuropharmacology, 62*(1), 63–77. https://doi.org/10.1016/j.neuropharm.2011.07.036

Anxiety

The amygdala, a key player in emotional processing and the brain's fear center, undergoes structural changes in individuals with anxiety disorders. Heightened anxiety is associated with increased amygdala volume and hyperactivity. These structural alterations contribute to exaggerated fear responses and difficulties in emotion regulation. Unraveling the structural changes in the amygdala is essential for understanding the neural basis of anxiety and developing targeted interventions (Kendler et al., 2011).

Schizophrenia

Schizophrenia, a complex and severe mental disorder, is characterized by structural changes in the brain, including ventricular enlargement. Increased ventricular size reflects a loss of brain tissue, particularly in the frontal and temporal lobes. These structural alterations are associated with cognitive deficits and the positive and negative symptoms of schizophrenia. Investigating ventricular enlargement provides valuable insights into the neuroanatomical aspects of this debilitating disorder (Shepherd et al., 2012).

Bipolar Disorder

The prefrontal cortex, responsible for executive functions and emotional regulation, is implicated in bipolar disorder. Structural abnormalities, including reduced gray matter volume and alterations in neural connectivity, are observed in the prefrontal cortex of individuals with bipolar disorder. Dysfunction in this region contributes to mood instability and impaired decision-making. Unraveling the structural changes in the prefrontal cortex enhances our understanding of the neural underpinnings of bipolar disorder (Kempton et al., 2011).

Structural Connectomes

Structural connectomes, comprehensive maps of the brain's anatomical connections, have become invaluable tools in neuroscience research (Sporns, 2011). These intricate diagrams offer a network-centric perspective on mental health disorders. Rather than focusing solely on isolated brain regions, researchers can analyze the patterns of connectivity within the entire brain network. This approach allows for a more holistic understanding of how disruptions in communication between brain regions may underlie the manifestation of various mental health conditions (Cao et al., 2015).

Major Depressive Disorder

Structural connectome studies have revealed alterations in the connectivity of brain regions involved in emotional processing, such as the amygdala and prefrontal cortex. Changes in white matter integrity and disruptions in communication pathways between mood-regulating regions contribute to the neurobiology of depression. Understanding these structural alterations provides a framework for developing targeted interventions that aim to modulate aberrant connectivity (Sullivan et al., 2003).

Anxiety Disorders

Anxiety disorders, including generalized anxiety disorder and posttraumatic stress disorder, involve disruptions in the structural connectome related to emotion regulation and fear processing. Altered connectivity patterns among the amygdala, hippocampus, and prefrontal regions contribute to heightened emotional responses and impaired regulation of anxiety (Sullivan et al., 2000).

Schizophrenia is characterized by disruptions in perception, cognition, and emotion. Structural connectome analyses have identified widespread connectivity dysregulation, including changes in the integrity of long-range connections and alterations in hub regions. These structural changes contribute to the cognitive and perceptual deficits observed in schizophrenia, offering potential targets for therapeutic interventions (Pettersson et al., 2019).

Bipolar Disorder

Structural connectome studies have revealed dysfunction in the prefrontal–subcortical circuitry, which regulates mood and emotional processing. Abnormalities in white matter connectivity within this circuitry, including the connections among the prefrontal cortex, amygdala, and striatum, have been observed in individuals with bipolar disorder. In addition, there is evidence to suggest that alterations in the structural connectome associated with bipolar disorder may have neurodevelopmental origins, with abnormalities in white matter connectivity emerging early in life. Additionally, longitudinal studies have indicated that some structural alterations may progress over time, potentially contributing to the course and progression of the disorder (Smoller et al., 2005).

BRAIN VULNERABILITY

As research advances, the challenge lies in integrating knowledge of structural changes with genetic, molecular, and environmental factors to create a comprehensive understanding of mental health disorders. The conceptual framework of "brain vulnerability" offers a potential holistic approach to addressing this interplay. This concept is particularly relevant in understanding the neurobiological basis of mental health disorders, where specific brain regions or networks may demonstrate increased vulnerability, contributing to the development, progression, or recurrence of psychiatric conditions (Taquet et al., 2021). These vulnerabilities may manifest as alterations in brain volume, changes in connectivity patterns, or disruptions in specific regions critical for cognitive and emotional processing. Brain vulnerability factors can encompass a wide range of biological and environmental influences that increase the susceptibility of the brain to dysfunction and contribute to the onset, severity, and course of mental health disorders.

Epigenetic Mechanisms

Epigenetics refers to changes in gene expression that occur without alterations to the underlying DNA sequence. These changes are mediated by various epigenetic mechanisms, such as DNA methylation, histone modifications, and noncoding RNAs, which regulate gene activity and contribute to the dynamic control of cellular processes (Kundakovic et al., 2015; Labonté et al., 2012). In the context of mental health disorders, epigenetic mechanisms play a crucial role in modulating gene expression patterns in the brain and other relevant tissues, thereby influencing susceptibility to psychiatric conditions and contributing to their etiology and pathophysiology.

Epigenetic modifications mediate interactions between genetic susceptibility and environmental factors in the development of mental health disorders. Environmental influences, such as structural and interpersonal racism, can induce epigenetic changes that alter gene expression patterns and increase susceptibility to psychiatric conditions (Simons et al., 2018).

Epigenetic mechanisms play a key role in regulating neurodevelopmental processes, including neuronal differentiation, synaptic pruning, and circuit formation. Disruptions in epigenetic regulation during critical periods of brain development may contribute to neurodevelopmental abnormalities underlying conditions such as ASD and schizophrenia (Ikegame et al., 2013).

Epigenetic modifications acquired during early development or in response to environmental exposures can also be transmitted across generations, influencing the risk of mental health disorders in offspring. Epigenetic inheritance mechanisms, such as DNA methylation and histone modifications, may contribute to the transgenerational transmission of vulnerability to psychiatric conditions (Yehuda et al., 2016).

Neuroplasticity and Adaptation

It is important to note that brain vulnerability is not static but dynamic, changing over the life span and in response to environmental factors. The brain's remarkable ability to adapt and reorganize, known as neuroplasticity, may contribute to changes in vulnerability. Chronic stress can induce changes in the brain's structure and function, affecting regions involved in stress response and emotional regulation. Neuroplasticity in these areas contributes to the adaptation to stressors or, conversely, vulnerability to stress-related disorders. Conditions such as major depressive disorder may involve maladaptive neuroplasticity in response to adverse childhood experiences and chronic stress, impacting mood-regulating circuits. Neuroplasticity is particularly relevant in neurodevelopmental disorders such as autism spectrum disorder (ASD). Altered patterns of neuroplasticity during critical periods of development may contribute to the characteristic features of these disorders (Pittenger & Duman, 2008).

Although vulnerabilities may increase the risk of mental health disorders, interventions that leverage neuroplasticity can potentially promote resilience and recovery. For instance, in the treatment of anxiety disorders, cognitive behavioral therapy (CBT) leverages neuroplasticity to help individuals relearn and adapt their responses to anxiety-provoking stimuli. In conditions in which structural vulnerabilities are identified, treatment approaches can be tailored to enhance adaptive neuroplasticity, fostering positive changes in brain structure and function.

The neurobiology of mental illness is a vast and evolving field that provides a deeper understanding of the biological underpinnings of psychiatric disorders. From neurotransmitter imbalances to structural and functional brain abnormalities, this section explores the intricate web of factors contributing to mental health conditions. The ongoing integration of genetic, molecular, and imaging technologies promises to unveil even more insights, ultimately shaping the future of mental health research and personalized treatment strategies.

PRECISION PSYCHIATRY

The integration of genetic information into psychiatric practice paves the way for precision psychiatry. Precision psychiatry aims to tailor prevention, diagnosis, and treatment strategies to individual patients based on their unique characteristics, including genetic makeup, environmental exposures, neurobiological factors, and clinical presentation. Integrating knowledge of brain vulnerability into precision psychiatry approaches allows for a more personalized understanding and management of psychiatric conditions as detailed in the following text.

Risk Stratification

Precision psychiatry uses advanced neuroimaging techniques, genetic testing, and other biomarkers to identify individuals at increased risk for mental health disorders based on their brain vulnerability profile. By assessing neurobiological markers of vulnerability, clinicians can stratify patients into different risk categories and implement targeted prevention strategies tailored to their specific needs (Baker & Holmes, 2019; Bruder et al., 2005; Dukal et al., 2020).

Early Detection and Intervention

Early identification of brain vulnerability markers associated with mental health disorders enables clinicians to intervene proactively before the onset of symptoms. Biomarker-based screening programs can identify individuals at high risk for conditions such as schizophrenia, bipolar disorder, or major depressive disorder, allowing for early intervention strategies aimed at preventing or delaying the onset of illness (Koutsouleris et al., 2018; Lui et al., 2015; Perkins et al., 2015).

Treatment Selection and Personalization

Precision psychiatry considers individual differences in brain vulnerability when selecting treatment approaches and medications for mental health disorders. Pharmacogenomic testing, which analyzes genetic variations affecting drug metabolism and response, helps guide medication selection and dosing to maximize treatment efficacy and minimize adverse effects based on an individual's genetic profile (Fabbri et al., 2018; Hall-Flavin et al., 2012; Singh, 2014; Winner et al., 2013).

Neurobiological Targets for Intervention

Understanding the neurobiological underpinnings of brain vulnerability provides insight into potential targets for novel therapeutic interventions. Precision psychiatry research focuses on developing targeted treatments that modulate specific neurobiological pathways implicated in psychiatric conditions, aiming to address underlying brain vulnerabilities and improve treatment outcomes (Duman & Aghajanian, 2012; Duman et al., 2016; Soares & Duman, 2016).

Personalized Psychotherapy Approaches

Precision psychiatry incorporates neurobiological and genetic information into the development of personalized psychotherapy approaches tailored to individual patients. By targeting neurobiological mechanisms associated with brain vulnerability, such as alterations in stress response pathways or emotion regulation circuits, psychotherapeutic interventions can be optimized to address the specific needs and challenges of each patient (Cuijpers et al., 2019; Dichter et al., 2015; Hofmann et al., 2012).

Predictive Modeling and Prognostic Assessment

Precision psychiatry uses predictive modeling techniques to integrate multiple data sources, including genetic, neuroimaging, and clinical data, to predict disease progression and treatment response in individual patients. By incorporating information about brain vulnerability into predictive models, clinicians can more accurately assess prognosis and develop personalized treatment plans that consider the unique neurobiological characteristics of each patient (Chekroud et al., 2016; Vieira et al., 2017).

Overall, precision psychiatry aims to improve patient outcomes by incorporating knowledge of brain vulnerability into personalized prevention, diagnosis, and treatment approaches for mental health disorders. By understanding the individual neurobiological factors that contribute to psychiatric conditions, clinicians can develop more targeted and effective interventions that address the specific needs and challenges of each patient, ultimately leading to better outcomes and improved quality of life. Advancements in our understanding of brain vulnerability contribute to the emergence of precision medicine. Tailoring treatments based on an individual's genetic profile, structural brain characteristics, and environmental exposures enhances therapeutic efficacy and reduces potential side effects. Precision medicine approaches represent a paradigm shift toward more targeted and personalized interventions in neurological care.

Case Vignette 9.1 GENE–ENVIRONMENT INTERACTIONS IN DEPRESSION

A 35-year-old woman presents with symptoms of major depressive disorder, including persistent low mood, anhedonia, difficulty concentrating, and fatigue. Her mother has a history of depression, and genetic testing reveals that the patient carries a short allele of the serotonin transporter gene (5-HTTLPR), which has been associated with increased sensitivity to stress. During her childhood, she experienced significant trauma, including emotional neglect and parental separation.

Treatment begins with a combination of a selective serotonin reuptake inhibitor, selected based on her genetic profile to minimize side effects, and trauma-focused cognitive behavioral therapy (TF-CBT). Over time, the patient shows improvement in mood and functional capacity. However, she experiences periodic setbacks due to situational stressors, prompting adjustments in therapy focus and medication dosage.

This case vignette illustrates the interplay between genetic vulnerability and environmental triggers in the pathogenesis of depression. It highlights the importance of a personalized treatment approach that integrates genetic insights with environmental and psychological factors.

SUMMARY

This chapter has provided an in-depth examination of the biological and genetic determinants of mental health. From psychiatric genetics to neurobiology and precision psychiatry, the discussion underscores the intricate interplay between genetic and environmental factors in shaping mental health outcomes. Real-world applications, including a case vignette and current research, illustrate the relevance of these concepts in clinical practice. By addressing disparities in genetic research and emphasizing cultural humility, the field is moving toward more inclusive and equitable approaches, ultimately enhancing mental health care for diverse populations.

DISCUSSION QUESTIONS

1. How do gene–environment interactions influence the development of psychiatric disorders, and how can psychiatric genetic epidemiology help identify specific genetic variants that modify the impact of environmental risk factors on disorder risk?
2. What are some potential implications of GWAS data disparities for public health and healthcare equity, particularly in terms of diagnostic accuracy, treatment effectiveness, and health disparities? How can addressing these disparities improve healthcare outcomes for diverse populations?
3. How do alterations in neurotransmitter systems, such as serotonin, dopamine, glutamate, and GABA, contribute to the pathophysiology of mental health disorders?
4. What role do chronic stress and other environmental factors play in inducing structural changes in the brain?
5. How does the concept of brain vulnerability broaden our understanding of the development of mental health disorders?
6. How does precision psychiatry incorporate neurobiological and genetic information into the development of personalized psychotherapy approaches?

REFERENCES

Baker, J. T., & Holmes, A. J. (2019). Can machine learning identify individuals at ultra-high risk for psychosis based on patterns of brain activity? *Journal of Personalized Medicine*, *9*(3), 32. https://doi.org/10.3390/jpm9030032

Batai, K., Hooker, S., & Kittles, R. A. (2021). Leveraging genetic ancestry to study health disparities. *American Journal of Physical Anthropology*, *175*(2), 363–375. https://doi.org/10.1002/ajpa.23972

Belujon, P., & Grace, A. A. (2017). Dopamine system dysregulation in major depressive disorders. *International Journal of Neuropsychopharmacology*, *20*(12), 1036–1046. https://doi.org/10.1093/ijnp/pyx086

Bruder, G. E., Keilp, J. G., Xu, H., Shikhman, M., Schori, E., Gorman, J. M., & Gilliam, T. C. (2005). Catechol-O-methyltransferase (COMT) genotypes and working memory: Associations with differing cognitive operations. *Biological Psychiatry*, *58*(11), 901–907. https://doi.org/10.1016/j.biopsych.2005.05.011

Cao, M., Wang, Z., & He, Y. (2015). Connectomics in psychiatric research: Advances and applications. *Neuropsychiatric Disease and Treatment*, *11*, 2801–2810. https://doi.org/10.2147/NDT.S83581

Chekroud, A. M., Zotti, R. J., Shehzad, Z., Gueorguieva, R., Johnson, M. K., Trivedi, M. H., & Corlett, P. R. (2016). Cross-trial prediction of treatment outcome in depression: A machine learning approach. *The Lancet Psychiatry*, *3*(3), 243–250. https://doi.org/10.1016/S2215-0366(15)00471-X

Cryan, J. F., & Kaupmann, K. (2005). Don't worry 'B' happy!: A role for GABA(B) receptors in anxiety and depression. *Trends in Pharmacological Sciences*, *26*(1), 36–43. https://doi.org/10.1016/j.tips.2004.11.004

Cuijpers, P., Karyotaki, E., Weitz, E., Andersson, G., Hollon, S. D., & van Straten, A. (2019). The effects of psychotherapies for major depression in adults on remission, recovery and improvement: A meta-analysis. *Journal of Affective Disorders*, *257*, 695–704. https://doi.org/10.1016/j.jad.2019.07.074

Dichter, G. S., Gibbs, D., & Smoski, M. J. (2015). A systematic review of relations between resting-state functional-MRI and treatment response in major depressive disorder. *Journal of Affective Disorders*, *172*, 8–17. https://doi.org/10.1016/j.jad.2014.09.028

Dukal, H., Gohil, D., & Henry, T. (2020). Identifying suicide risk with psychiatric diagnosis and neurocognitive profile using machine-learning algorithms. *Journal of Personalized Medicine*, *10*(4), 234. https://doi.org/10.3390/jpm10040234

Duman, R. S., & Aghajanian, G. K. (2012). Synaptic dysfunction in depression: Potential therapeutic targets. *Science*, *338*(6103), 68–72. https://doi.org/10.1126/science.1222939

Duman, R. S., Aghajanian, G. K., Sanacora, G., & Krystal, J. H. (2016). Synaptic plasticity and depression: New insights from stress and rapid-acting antidepressants. *Nature Medicine*, *22*(3), 238–249. https://doi.org/10.1038/nm.4050

Fabbri, C., Hosak, L., Mössner, R., Giegling, I., Mandelli, L., Bellivier, F., Claes, S., Collier, D. A., Corrales, A., Delisi, L. E., Gallo, C., Gill, M., Kennedy, J. L., Leboyer, M., Lisoway, A., Maier, W., Marquez, M., Massat, I., Mors, O., Muglia, P., Nöthen, M. M., O'Donovan, M. C., Ospina-Duque, J., ..., Serretti, A. (2018). Consensus paper of the WFSBP Task Force on Genetics: Genetics, epigenetics, and gene expression markers of major depressive disorder and antidepressant response. *World Journal of Biological Psychiatry*, *19*(1), 1–28. https://doi.org/10.1080/15622975.2017.1338775

Falkai P., Schmitt A., & Andreasen, N. (2018). Forty years of structural brain imaging in mental disorders: Is it clinically useful or not? *Dialogues in Clinical Neuroscience*, *20*(3), 179–186. https://doi.org/10.31887/DCNS.2018.20.3/pfalkai

Felitti, V. J., Anda, R. F., Nordenberg, D., Williamson, D. F., Spitz, A. M., Edwards, V., Koss, M. P., & Marks, J. S. (1998). Relationship of childhood abuse and household dysfunction to many of the leading causes of death in adults: The Adverse Childhood Experiences (ACE) study. *American Journal of Preventive Medicine*, *14*(4), 245–258. https://doi.org/10.1016/S0749-3797(98)00017-8

Hall-Flavin, D. K., Winner, J. G., Allen, J. D., Carhart, J. M., Proctor, B., Snyder, K. A., Drews, M. S., Eisterhold, L. L., Geske, J., & Mrazek, D. A. (2012). Utility of integrated pharmacogenomic testing to support the treatment of major depressive disorder in a psychiatric outpatient setting. *Pharmacogenetics and Genomics*, *22*(10), 762–769. https://doi.org/10.1097/FPC.0b013e3283581d3e

Hofmann, S. G., Asnaani, A., Vonk, I. J., Sawyer, A. T., & Fang, A. (2012). The efficacy of cognitive behavioral therapy: A review of meta-analyses. *Cognitive Therapy and Research*, *36*(5), 427–440. https://doi.org/10.1007/s10608-012-9476-1

Ikegame, T., Bundo, M., Murata, Y., Kasai, K., Kato, T., & Iwamoto, K. (2013). DNA methylation of the BDNF gene and its relevance to psychiatric disorders. *Journal of Human Genetics*, *58*(7), 434–438. https://doi.org/10.1038/jhg.2013.60

Jacka, F. N., Kremer, P. J., Berk, M., de Silva-Sanigorski, A. M., Moodie, M., Leslie, E. R., Pasco, J. A., & Swinburn, B. A. (2011). A prospective study of diet quality and mental health in adolescents. *PLOS ONE*, *6*(9), e24805. https://doi.org/10.1371/journal.pone.0024805

Kempton, M. J., Salvador, Z., Munafo, M. R., Geddes, J. R., Simmons, A., Frangou, S., & Williams, S. C. (2011). Structural neuroimaging studies in major depressive disorder: Meta-analysis and comparison with bipolar disorder. *Archives of General Psychiatry*, *68*(7), 675–690. https://doi.org/10.1001/archgenpsychiatry.2011.60

Kendler, K. S., Aggen, S. H., Knudsen, G. P., Røysamb, E., Neale, M. C., & Reichborn-Kjennerud, T. (2011). The structure of genetic and environmental risk factors for syndromal and subsyndromal common DSM-IV axis I and all axis II disorders. *The American Journal of Psychiatry*, *168*(1), 29–39. https://doi.org/10.1176/appi.ajp.2010.10030340

Kessler, R. C., Chiu, W. T., Demler, O., & Walters, E. E. (2005). Prevalence, severity, and comorbidity of 12-month DSM-IV disorders in the National Comorbidity Survey Replication. *Archives of General Psychiatry*, *62*(6), 617–627. https://doi.org/10.1001/archpsyc.62.6.617

Koutsouleris, N., Kambeitz-Ilankovic, L., Ruhrmann, S., Rosen, M., Ruef, A., Dwyer, D. B., Paolini, M., Chisholm, K., Kambeitz, J., Haidl, T., Schmidt, A., Gillam, J., Schultze-Lutter, F., Falkai, P., Reiser, M., Riecher-Rössler, A., Upthegrove, R., Hietala, J., Salokangas, R. K. R., Pantelis, C., Meisenzahl, E., ..., Borgwardt, S. (2018). Prediction models of functional outcomes for individuals in the clinical high-risk state for psychosis or with recent-onset depression: A multimodal, multisite machine learning analysis. *JAMA Psychiatry*, *75*(11), 1156–1172. https://doi.org/10.1001/jamapsychiatry.2018.2165

Kundakovic, M., Gudsnuk, K., Herbstman, J. B., Tang, D., Perera, F. P., & Champagne, F. A. (2015). DNA methylation of BDNF as a biomarker of early-life adversity. *Proceedings of the National Academy of Sciences*, *112*(22), 6807–6813. https://doi.org/10.1073/pnas.1408355111

Labonté, B., Suderman, M., Maussion, G., Lopez, J. P., Navaro, L., Yerko, V., Mechawar, N., Szyf, M., & Meaney, M. J. (2012). Genome-wide epigenetic regulation by early-life trauma. *Archives of General Psychiatry*, *69*(7), 722–731. https://doi.org/10.1001/archgenpsychiatry.2011.2287

Lorenzetti, V., Allen, N. B., Fornito, A., & Yücel, M. (2009). Structural brain abnormalities in major depressive disorder: A selective review of recent MRI studies. *Journal of Affective Disorders*, *117*(1–2), 1–17. https://doi.org/10.1016/j.jad.2008.11.021

Lui, S., Yao, L., Xiao, Y., Keedy, S. K., Reilly, J. L., Keefe, R. S., Tamminga, C. A., Keshavan, M. S., Pearlson, G. D., Gong, Q., & Sweeney, J. A. (2015). Resting-state brain function in schizophrenia and psychotic bipolar probands and their first-degree relatives. *Psychological Medicine*, *45*(1), 97–108. https://doi.org/10.1017/S0033291714001085

MacArthur, J., Bowler, E., Cerezo, M., Gil, L., Hall, P., Hastings, E., Junkins, H., McMahon, A., Milano, A., Morales, J., Pendlington, Z. M., Welter, D., Burdett, T., Hindorff, L., Flicek, P., Cunningham, F., & Parkinson, H. (2017). The new NHGRI-EBI Catalog of published genomewide association studies (GWAS Catalog). *Nucleic Acids Research*, *45*, D896–D901. https://doi.org/10.1093/nar/gkw1133

Martin, A. R., Kanai, M., Kamatani, Y., Okada, Y., Neale, B. M., & Daly, M. J. (2019). Clinical use of current polygenic risk scores may exacerbate health disparities. *Nature Genetics*, *51*(4), 584–591. https://doi.org/10.1038/s41588-019-0379-8

McEwen, B. S. (2012). Brain on stress: How the social environment gets under the skin. *Proceedings of the National Academy of Sciences, 109*(Suppl 2), 17180–17185. https://doi.org/10.1073/pnas.1121254109

Mostafavi, H., Harpak, A., Agarwal, I., Conley, D., Pritchard, J. K., & Przeworski, M. (2020). Variable prediction accuracy of polygenic scores within an ancestry group. *eLife, 9*, e48376. https://doi.org/10.7554/eLife.48376

Perkins, D. O., Jeffries, C. D., Addington, J., Bearden, C. E., Cadenhead, K. S., Cannon, T. D., Cornblatt, B. A., Mathalon, D. H., McGlashan, T. H., Seidman, L. J., Tsuang, M. T., Walker, E. F., Woods, S. W., & Heinssen, R. (2015). Towards a psychosis risk blood diagnostic for persons experiencing high-risk symptoms: Preliminary results from the NAPLS project. *Schizophrenia Bulletin, 41*(2), 419–428. https://doi.org/10.1093/schbul/sbu099

Pettersson, E., Lichtenstein, P., Larsson, H., Song, J., Agrawal, A., Børglum, A. D., Bulik, C. M., Daly, M. J., Davis, L. K., Demontis, D., Edenberg, H. J., Grove, J., Gelernter, J., Neale, B. M., Pardiñas, A. F., Stahl, E., Walters, J. T. R., Walters, R., Sullivan, P. F., Posthuma, D., & Polderman, T. J. C. (2019). Genetic influences on eight psychiatric disorders based on family data of 4,408,646 full and half-siblings, and genetic data of 333,748 cases and controls. *Psychological Medicine, 49*(7), 1166–1173. https://doi.org/10.1017/S0033291718002039

Pittenger, C., & Duman, R. S. (2008). Stress, depression, and neuroplasticity: A convergence of mechanisms. *Neuropsychopharmacology, 33*(1), 88–109. https://doi.org/10.1038/sj.npp.1301574

Sanacora, G., Treccani, G., & Popoli, M. (2012). Towards a glutamate hypothesis of depression: An emerging frontier of neuropsychopharmacology for mood disorders. *Neuropharmacology, 62*(1), 63–77. https://doi.org/10.1016/j.neuropharm.2011.07.036

Shepherd, A. M., Matheson, S. L., Laurens, K. R., Carr, V. J., & Green, M. J. (2012). Systematic meta-review and quality assessment of the structural brain alterations in schizophrenia. *Neuroscience & Biobehavioral Reviews, 36*(4), 1342–1356. https://doi.org/10.1016/j.neubiorev.2011.12.015

Simons, R. L., Lei, M. K., Beach, S. R., Cutrona, C. E., Philibert, R. A., & Barr, A. (2018). Economic hardship and biological weathering: The epigenetics of aging in a U.S. sample of Black women. *Social Science & Medicine, 209*, 1–10. https://doi.org/10.1016/j.socscimed.2018.04.022

Singh, A. B. (2014). Improved antidepressant remission in major depression via a pharmacokinetic pathway polygene pharmacogenetic report. *Clinical Psychopharmacology and Neuroscience, 12*(2), 150–156. https://doi.org/10.9758/cpn.2014.12.2.150

Smoller, J. W., Finn, C. T., & Family Bipolar Disorder Consortium. (2005). Family, twin, and adoption studies of bipolar disorder. *American Journal of Medical Genetics Part C: Seminars in Medical Genetics, 123C*(1), 48–58. https://doi.org/10.1002/ajmg.c.30061

Soares, J. C., & Duman, R. S. (2016). Targeting the glutamatergic system to develop novel, improved therapeutics for mood disorders. *Nature Reviews Drug Discovery, 15*(12), 865–886. https://doi.org/10.1038/nrd.2016.164

Sporns, O. (2011). The human connectome: A complex network. *Annals of the New York Academy of Sciences, 1224*(1), 109–125. https://doi.org/10.1111/j.1749-6632.2010.05888.x

Sullivan, P. F., Kendler, K. S., & Neale, M. C. (2003). Schizophrenia as a complex trait: Evidence from a meta-analysis of twin studies. *Archives of General Psychiatry, 60*(12), 1187–1192. https://doi.org/10.1001/archpsyc.60.12.1187

Sullivan, P. F., Neale, M. C., & Kendler, K. S. (2000). Genetic epidemiology of major depression: Review and meta-analysis. *The American Journal of Psychiatry, 157*(10), 1552–1562. https://doi.org/10.1176/appi.ajp.157.10.1552

Taquet, M., Smith, S. M., Prohl, A. K., Peters, J. M., Warfield, S. K., Scherrer, B., & Harrison, P. J. (2021). A structural brain network of genetic vulnerability to psychiatric illness. *Molecular Psychiatry, 26*, 2089–2100. https://doi.org/10.1038/s41380-020-0762-9

Tervalon, M., & Murray-García, J. (1998). Cultural humility versus cultural competence: A critical distinction in defining physician training outcomes in multicultural education. *Journal of Health Care for the Poor and Underserved, 9*(2), 117–125. https://doi.org/10.1353/hpu.2010.0233

Vieira, S., Pinaya, W. H., & Mechelli, A. (2017). Using deep learning to investigate the neuroimaging correlates of psychiatric and neurological disorders: Methods and applications. *Neuroscience & Biobehavioral Reviews, 74*, 58–75. https://doi.org/10.1016/j.neubiorev.2017.01.002

Winner, J. G., Carhart, J. M., Altar, C. A., Allen, J. D., & Dechairo, B. M. (2013). A prospective, randomized, double-blind study assessing the clinical impact of integrated pharmacogenomic testing for major depressive disorder. *Discovery Medicine, 16*(89), 219–227. PMID: 24229738

Wojcik, G. L., Graff, M., Nishimura, K. K., Tao, R., Haessler, J., Gignoux, C. R., Highland, H. M., Patel, Y. M., Sorokin, E. P., Avery, C. L., Belbin, G. M., Bien, S. A., Cheng, A., Cullina, S., Hodonsky, C. J., Hu, Y., Huckins, L. M., Jeff, J., Justice, A. E., Kocarnik, J. M., Lim, U., ..., Carlson, C. S. (2019). Genetic analyses of diverse populations improve discovery for complex traits. *Nature, 570*, 514–518. https://doi.org/10.1038/s41586-019-1310-4

Yehuda, R., Daskalakis, N. P., Bierer, L. M., Bader, H. N., Klengel, T., Holsboer, F., & Binder, E. B. (2016). Holocaust exposure induced intergenerational effects on FKBP5 methylation. *Biological Psychiatry, 80*(5), 372–380. https://doi.org/10.1016/j.biopsych.2015.08.005

10 POLITICAL DETERMINANTS OF HEALTH IMPACT ON ACTUALIZING MENTAL HEALTH EQUITY

DANIEL E. DAWES, J.C. GONZALEZ, ALICIA HOLLOWAY, AND NELSON J. DUNLAP

LEARNING OBJECTIVES

After reading this chapter, readers will be able to:

- Analyze the political determinants of health framework on mental health equity.
- Evaluate the role of legislation and regulation.
- Integrate public health themes with policy analysis.
- Understand the interconnection between innovation and policy on mental health equity.
- Understand public policy interventions in the context of mental health equity.

INTRODUCTION

This chapter provides a comprehensive exploration of the relationship between political determinants and mental health equity. It begins by defining mental health equity and emphasizing the profound impact of political decisions, policies, and laws on mental health outcomes and equity. By unpacking the historical context of these determinants, the chapter offers a nuanced understanding of how political structures have shaped mental health services and outcomes over time. The chapter critically analyzes how existing measures address mental health inequities and the extent to which public policy plays a pivotal role in modulating access, quality of care, and outcomes in mental health services. The text delves into a detailed assessment of the structuring of relationships, administration of power, and distribution of resources to illustrate the impacts of these actions on diverse populations. Looking to the future, the chapter explores innovative policy solutions to improve mental health equity. It engages with the challenges of political resistance, funding constraints, and the perpetuation of stigma in policy making while also underscoring the potential of policy reforms to tackle systemic inequities. The discussion culminates in emphasizing the critical role of cross-sectoral and intersectional collaborations for fostering mental health equity.

All around us exist silent or even invisible forces at play that do in fact play an outsized role in how our world is shaped. Many individuals may not be aware of their existence. These forces, or rather determinants, have a direct and tangible impact on an individual's or community's quality of life and well-being. To effect meaningful changes and advance mental health equity, it is paramount that each of us fully understands how to identify, assess, and leverage these multiple intersecting and interacting determinants of health, especially the political determinants, which have significant force over all determinants of health.

UNDERSTANDING POLITICAL DETERMINANTS

Let us begin with the bedrock principle of the social determinants of health. The World Health Organization (WHO) defines the social determinants of health as the nonmedical factors that influence health outcomes. These are the conditions in which people are born, grow, work, live, and age, and the wider set of forces and systems that shape the conditions of daily life (WHO, n.d.). In fact, you may already be familiar with the social determinants of health, even if you have not previously known what to call them. Examples of such include education, food insecurity, and housing just to name a few. Although being made aware of the social determinants of health is a good first step on your journey toward addressing mental health inequities, there's another layer of determinants that are even more determinative of your quality of life. Those would be the political determinants of health.

The political determinants of health are multidimensional and involve the systematic process of structuring relationships, distributing resources, and administering power, operating simultaneously in ways that mutually reinforce or influence one another to shape opportunities that either advance health equity, including mental health equity, or exacerbate health inequities (Dawes, 2020). Equally important to our systemic health, we must be able to address at an upstream level the political factors impacting behavioral, biological, social, economic, environmental, and spiritual determinants of health that extend far beyond the walls of a hospital or clinic. This can be achieved only by having those difficult conversations that address inequities: the allocation/reallocation of resources and prioritization and creation of policies that rectify the damage that has already been done across communities nationwide in our society. We can tackle the broad and collateral effects of the political determinants of health by targeting three major aspects that interact in various ways to advance or hinder our health equity: voting, government, and policy. In some instances, the political determinants of health have elevated efforts to advance health equity for all groups, but on more occasions, they have hindered the advancement of health equity.

Political strategies, decisions, and actions have resulted in reinforcing systems that either ensure the status quo or have dismantled systems that challenge the status quo. Overall, health inequities in the United States can be traced back to a political determinant even when the inequities are deemed to result from an environmental, social, economic, healthcare, or behavioral health determinant. The political determinants are the instigators of the causes. They are the determinants of the determinants. History is replete with examples of political systems ignoring the voice of justice. Some of these examples are embedded within policies and racist preconceptions dating back to centuries ago; some are still practiced in more recent times, such as systemic exclusion, including race norming practices in healthcare and mental health care, the practice of redlining, partisan gerrymandering, exclusion by sexism, and immigration enforcement.

Although **Figure 10.1** is informative of the entire life cycle of the political determinants of health framework, another way of thinking about these determinants can be viewed in relation to the social determinants. For every social determinant of health that you can point to, there was some preceding legal, legislative, policy, or even administrative decision that resulted in that social determinant. Think about your surroundings. Perhaps that faint buzz of the television is a local news report on the impact of social media use on the mental well-being of teenagers in high school. On the one hand, as was previously established, education is a very clear example of the social determinants of health at play. However, when you move further upstream, you begin to see the political determinants at work in the form of the school board's decision to implement policies surrounding social media use in school, a state legislature and governor passing and implementing a bill to prohibit teenagers under the age of 16 years from having a social media account, or even the Supreme Court of the United States weighing in on which social media platforms are allowed to exist at all.

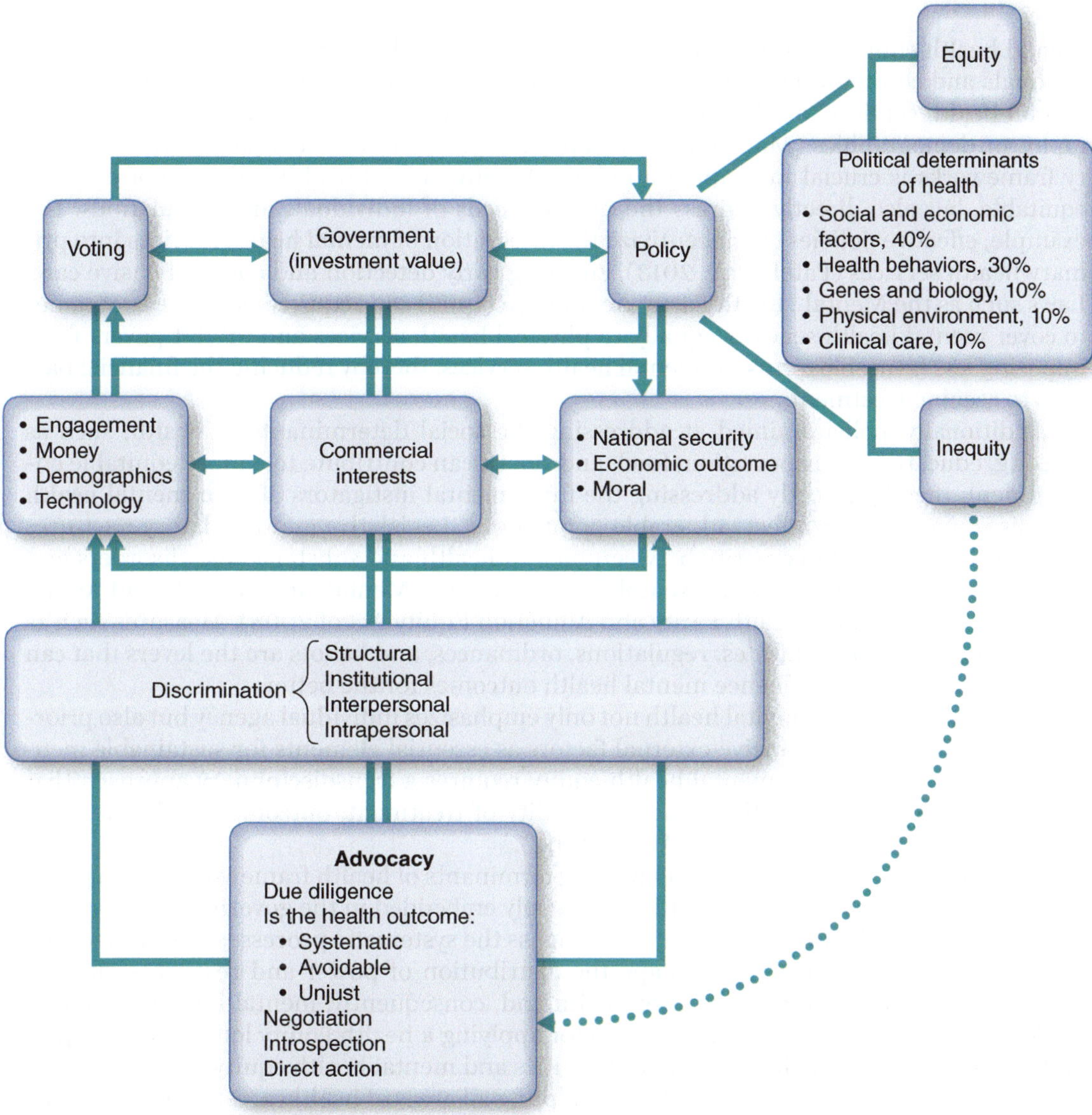

Figure 10.1 Political determinants of health framework.

Source: Dawes, D. (2020). *The political determinants of health* (p. 49). Johns Hopkins University Press. © 2020 Johns Hopkins University Press. Reprinted with permission of Johns Hopkins University Press.

Maybe those muffled sounds at the coffee shop that you have heard in the past were part of a conversation between local urban farmers excited about a new farmer's market opening. You could simply view that conversation as representative of the social determinant of food security or insecurity being addressed, or you could look upstream and consider the multitude of decisions, or political determinants, that had to be enacted for a farmer's market to seek and obtain permission to open its doors. At their most basic construction, the political determinants of health are simply a novel way for you to view the points of leverage that already exist in our society, which can help you improve outcomes and reduce inequities. This may be most potently realized in the mental health space.

THE IMPACT OF LEGISLATION AND REGULATION

Mental health equity is a fundamental aspect of public health, emphasizing the right of individuals and communities to reach their full health potential, including accessing quality mental health services for all individuals, irrespective of their socioeconomic status, geography, or demographics (Mangalore & Knapp, 2011). The role of legislation and regulatory frameworks is crucial in shaping a policy whereby mental health services not only are equitable, but also directly address the diverse needs of individuals and populations. For example, effective policies can incentivize the integration of mental health services into primary health services (Patel et al., 2013), ensuring early detection and comprehensive care. Laws such as the Mental Health Parity Act of 1996 (1996) can require insurance companies to cover mental health services equally to physical health services and inhibit payers from imposing less favorable terms for mental health services, thereby reducing the financial barriers to seeking treatment.

Additionally, policies aimed at addressing the social determinants of health, such as housing, education, transportation, food, and safety, can contribute to a more equitable environment, thereby directly addressing the fundamental instigators of poor mental health that disproportionately affect vulnerable populations. Legislative and regulatory measures have the power to enforce parity between mental health and substance use disorders and medical and surgical benefits, as exemplified by the 2008 Mental Health Parity and Addiction Equity Act (Mental Health Parity and Addiction Equity Act of 2008). Measures such as these demonstrate that statutes, regulations, ordinances, and ballots are the levers that can be pushed or pulled to influence mental health outcomes for the better.

This commitment in mental health not only emphasizes individual agency but also prioritizes investments in supportive external factors as essential elements for sustainable mental well-being. Addressing mental health equity requires a transdisciplinary approach that includes confronting inequities in access, quality of treatment, outcomes, and well-being across different population groups (WHO, 2013).

Central to this discussion is the political determinants of health framework, which posits that the root causes of health inequities are deeply embedded in the governance of societies (Dawes, 2020). Political determinants encompass the systematic processes that decide who gets what, when, and how. They shape the distribution of power and resources, directly influencing the social determinants of health and, consequently, mental health outcomes. Understanding this framework is essential for applying a health equity lens to the complex and mutually reinforcing factors between politics and mental health equity.

Legal frameworks are instrumental in sculpting all areas of healthcare, but especially the mental health sector, because policy is underdeveloped in this space. Policies that define the allocation of resources and the setting of benchmarks for care quality and availability are sorely needed. However, the impact of these legal instruments is often double edged. Legislation, though often well intentioned, can inadvertently perpetuate health inequities. When the urgent demands of mental health issues are sidelined in favor of other priorities or when budgetary allocations are not reflective of the needs of diverse populations because of unconscious bias, systemic racism, or data invisibility, the result is a healthcare chasm (Gonzalez, 2023). Laws that do not holistically address the needs of the most vulnerable—such as those suffering from mental illness, especially within marginalized communities—further entrench these inequities within our society. These populations frequently find themselves hindered by a web of inadequate services and a one-size-fits-all approach that fails to accommodate the cultural and contextual nuance needed to advance mental health equity.

Legislation, regulation, subregulation, ordinances, and ballot initiatives are some of the critical instruments of governance that hold the power to forge programs and systems that prioritize mental health resources, interventions, and equitable delivery, effectively steering the direction of funding to the most pressing needs and erecting the benchmarks for the quality and accessibility of care, treatments, and supports. Such policies can catalyze the creation of a health system that prioritizes the mental well-being of its citizens, ensuring that no individual is deprived of the care they need. Take for instance Section 2703 of the Affordable Care Act, which provided funding for states to design health homes to provide comprehensive care coordination for high-cost Medicaid beneficiaries with chronic conditions, including serious mental illnesses (Druss & Goldman, 2018). These programs have been cited as essential elements of care integration for patients with serious mental illnesses and can serve as a model of the impact of legislation to promote activities that address true needs.

Policy that is grounded in evidence-based research, compassionate understanding of mental health struggles, community-designed interventions, and a commitment to equity can transform the abstract notions of justice and fairness into concrete actions and regulations. These can pave the way for mental health services that are not just universally available but also tailored to the needs of diverse populations. The Protecting Access to Medicare Act (H.R. 4302) for instance includes behavioral health clinics, which are required to address care coordination among mental health providers and to develop partnerships for primary care. The Affordable Care Act has provided ongoing funding to these programs, which provide funding for community mental health centers to treat common medical conditions on site or via referral (Scharf et al., 2014). Increased care coordination of mental health components into primary care is an often-cited example of how impactful policy can bring these issues to the forefront of care providers' attention.

The quest for mental health equity is fundamentally a political endeavor, rooted in the administration of power, the distribution of resources, and the structuring of relationships that promote well-being for all (Dawes, 2020). By understanding and addressing the political determinants of mental health, policy makers, advocates, and public health professionals can enact meaningful changes that address these barriers and foster a more equitable society. Through the reinforcement of community-based health initiatives, we can foster a more culturally sensitive and accessible care environment. In addition, by holding systems accountable for the standards of care provided, we ensure that quality is not just a privilege but a baseline expectation for all, irrespective of socioeconomic status.

FUTURE DIRECTIONS IN POLITICAL DETERMINANTS OF MENTAL HEALTH EQUITY

The future of mental health equity demands a forward-thinking approach that anticipates the changing needs of diverse populations both domestically and globally. Prioritizing the development of policies that are not only responsive to addressing current inequities but also proactive in preventing the emergence of new ones is essential. This entails a commitment to continuous research and data analysis, ensuring that our policies are informed by the latest scientific understanding and the real-world experiences of those closest to mental health issues.

One of the most promising areas for advancing mental health equity lies in the advancement of data and technology. Emerging technologies such as telehealth applications, artificial intelligence, and mobile health platforms have the potential to revolutionize access to mental health services, treatments, and supports and improve data collection and reporting practices, breaking down traditional barriers of distance and scarcity. However, to fully harness these innovations, policy must evolve in tandem, offering support and incentive for technology-based interventions while safeguarding against new forms of bias and discrimination that such advancements might inadvertently create.

The global nature of mental health, along with increased globalization and reliance on internet-based applications, calls for international collaboration in policy making. Learning from the successes and setbacks of different nations can guide the creation of more effective mental health strategies and foster a global commitment to mental health equity. Policies that encourage cross-border sharing of resources, expertise, and best practices can serve as a catalyst for worldwide improvements in mental health and well-being.

Advocacy and public engagement must remain at the heart of political determinants. Empowering individuals with mental health experiences and expertise to have a voice in policy development is crucial. Their narratives can provide invaluable insights that shape more compassionate and practical legislation. Likewise, involving mental health professionals and community leaders and encouraging collaboration across industries to include organizations outside the traditional healthcare structures, such as data and technology companies, education, and media organizations, in the policy-making process can ensure that laws and policies are all-encompassing and strategic in their approach, development, implementation, and enforcement.

The future of mental health equity depends on our collective willingness to embrace innovation, foster international cooperation, and engage in continual advocacy. By envisioning a future where political determinants are identified and acted upon directly as tools to influence mental health outcomes, we can pave the way for a society that not only recognizes mental health as a fundamental human right but actively works to ensure that right is realized for all population groups regardless of their status.

SUMMARY

To go beyond simply naming mental health inequities to effectively addressing mental health inequities, work must be done upstream to address the root causes or origination of these inequities. The political determinants of health, which are undergirded by racism and other destructive forms of discrimination, are the creators, perpetuators, and exacerbators of structural conditions and the social drivers that affect the overall dynamics of health. The political determinants of health are multidimensional and involve the systematic process of structuring relationships, distributing resources, and administering power, operating simultaneously in ways that mutually reinforce or influence one another to shape opportunities that either advance health equity, including mental health equity, or exacerbate health inequities.

Equally important to our systemic health, we must be able to address at an upstream level the political factors impacting behavioral, biological, social, economic, environmental, and spiritual determinants of health that extend far beyond the walls of a hospital or clinic. This can be achieved only by having those difficult conversations that address inequities: the allocation/reallocation of resources and prioritization and creation of policies that rectify the damage that has already been done across communities nationwide in our society. We can tackle the broad and collateral effects of the political determinants of health by targeting three major aspects that interact in various ways to advance or hinder our health equity: voting, government, and policy. In some instances, the political determinants of health have elevated efforts to advance health equity for all groups, but on more occasions, they have hindered the advancement of health equity.

Political strategies, decisions, and actions have resulted in reinforcing systems that either ensure the status quo or have dismantled systems that challenge the status quo. Overall, health inequities in the United States can be traced back to a political determinant even when the inequities are deemed to result from an environmental, social, economic, healthcare, or behavioral health determinant. The political determinants are the instigators or fundamental causes of the causes. They are the determinants of the determinants. History is replete with a narrative filled by examples of political systems ignoring the voice of justice. Some examples of these are embedded within policies and racist preconceptions dating back to centuries ago; some are still practiced in more recent times, such as systemic exclusion, including race norming practices in healthcare and mental health care, the practice of redlining, partisan gerrymandering, exclusion by sexism, and immigration status. Yet for different reasons, people tend to shy away from the role that policy has played in creating, maintaining, and increasing the inequities we observe today as well as the impact they have on all forces that affect our health.

DISCUSSION QUESTIONS

1. Explain the differences between the social determinants of health and the political determinants of health.
2. How do political decisions influence the distribution of resources and power, ultimately impacting mental health outcomes? Provide examples that illustrate how voting, government, advocacy, commercial interests, and policy can both positively and negatively affect mental health equity.
3. Analyze the impact of specific legislative acts mentioned in the text, such as the Mental Health Parity Act of 1996 and the Mental Health Parity and Addiction Equity Act of 2008, and the Affordable Care Act on the provision and accessibility of mental health services. How do these laws contribute to or hinder the achievement of mental health equity, particularly for marginalized communities?
4. The chapter suggests that addressing social determinants of health (e.g., housing, education, transportation, food, racism, stigma, and safety) is crucial for mental health equity. How can political strategies be designed to tackle these social determinants effectively, and how can such strategies lead to improved mental health outcomes across different populations?
5. Considering the future directions outlined in the chapter, what innovative policy approaches could be developed to anticipate and respond to the evolving needs of global mental health?

REFERENCES

Dawes, D. E. (2020). *The political determinants of health*. Johns Hopkins University Press.

Druss, B., & Goldman, H. (2018). Integrating health and mental health services: A past and future history. *The American Journal of Psychiatry, 175*(12), 1199–1204. https://doi.org/10.1176/appi.ajp.2018.18020169

Gonzalez, J. (2023). There's a public health crisis lurking in our data: The census option "some other race." *STAT*. https://www.statnews.com/2023/12/19/some-other-race-census-data-disaggregation-public-health/

Mangalore, R., & Knapp, M. (2006). Equity in mental health. *Epidemiology and Psychiatric Sciences, 15*, 260–266. https://doi.org/10.1017/S1121189X00002141

Mental Health Parity Act of 1996, Pub. L. No. 104-204, 110 Stat. 2944 (1996).

Patel, V., Belkin, G., Chockalingam, A., Cooper, J., Saxena, S., & Unützer, J. (2013). Grand challenges: Integrating mental health services into priority health care platforms. *PLoS Medicine, 10*(5), e1001448. https://doi.org/10.1371/journal.pmed.1001448

Paul Wellstone and Pete Domenici Mental Health Parity and Addiction Equity Act of 2008, Pub. L. No. 110-343, 122 Stat. 3765 (2008).

Scharf, D. M., Eberhart, N. K., Hackbarth, N. S., Horvitz-Lennon, M., Beckman, R., Han, B., Lovejoy, S. L., Pincus, H. A., & Burnam, M. A. (2014). Evaluation of the SAMHSA primary and behavioral health care integration (PBHCI) grant program: Final report. *Rand Health Quarterly, 4*(3), 6.

World Health Organization. (n.d.). *Social determinants of health*. https://www.who.int/health-topics/social-determinants-of-health#tab=tab_1

World Health Organization. (2013). *Mental health action plan 2013–2020*. https://www.who.int/publications/i/item/9789241506021

11 THE ROLE OF RELIGION, SPIRITUALITY, AND FAITH COMMUNITIES IN ADDRESSING MENTAL HEALTH DISPARITIES

CARLOS FAYARD AND WONHA KIM

LEARNING OBJECTIVES

After reading this chapter, readers will be able to:

- Articulate the relevance of faith communities and religion in promoting mental well-being.
- Discuss how religion and faith communities can help reduce mental health disparities.
- Describe a model that reduces mental health inequities by taking into consideration the role of faith communities, faith leaders, religious beliefs and practices, and mental health systems of care.
- Consider ways to engage faith communities in promoting mental health equity.
- Reflect on what is needed to fully leverage the positive effects of religion and faith communities in addressing mental health disparities.

INTRODUCTION

Minoritized groups have in common the significant negative impact of health disparities and their reliance on faith-based resources to address these needs (Yamada et al., 2020). Faith communities often are the de facto frontline providers of mental health services for racialized populations, particularly for African Americans, because "spirituality is an essential component of preserving mental wellness among Black people" (Thompson Fullilove et al., 2024, p. 65). This is particularly significant in the current context of shortages of trained clinicians in general, and particularly from minoritized backgrounds (Mongelli et al., 2020). In this chapter, following a brief review on the impact of religious beliefs and practices on mental health, a case is made for the relevance of including faith communities and spiritual leaders in addressing mental health disparities. A few studies illustrate ways in which collaboration with faith-based organizations can be beneficial to communities of color. Potential obstacles to the implementation of the strategies recommended to reduce disparities are identified, followed by a description of initiatives that, when taken together, may constitute a model to support and collaborate with spiritual leaders and communities on the front lines of mental health.

RELEVANCE OF FAITH COMMUNITIES AND RELIGION IN PROMOTING POSITIVE MENTAL HEALTH

Promoting mental health equity requires a multifaceted approach that goes beyond traditional healthcare systems. Faith communities and religion, with their deep-rooted influence on individuals and societies, play a crucial role in promoting health and well-being—especially when it comes to the mental health space. Before delving deeper into the various ways in which faith communities and religion can affect mental health, however, it is important to define these terms. *Religion* is "an organized system of beliefs, practices, and symbols designed (a) to facilitate closeness to the transcendent and (b) to foster an understanding of one's relationship and responsibility to others in living together in a community" (Koenig, 2012, p. 3). A *faith community*, on the other hand, is a group of people who share a particular set of religious beliefs. Although many who espouse a particular religion or faith traditions belong to faith communities, it is possible that one could subscribe to a certain religion but not belong to a formal faith community.

Throughout history, faith communities have been at the forefront of healthcare, providing comfort, support, and healing to individuals in need. Religious institutions established the world's first hospitals and emphasized compassion and care for the sick (Koenig, 2012). Although many hospitals and healthcare systems no longer have ties to religious institutions in today's world, this historical connection remains relevant as faith communities continue to serve as pillars of strength for individuals facing health challenges, including mental health challenges.

By providing individuals with a sense of purpose, community support, coping mechanisms, and a framework for finding meaning in life, religion and faith communities can play a significant role in improving mental health. Religion can promote positive mental health outcomes, such as happiness, optimism, hope, and gratefulness, while mitigating negative outcomes such as depression, anxiety, and substance abuse (Koenig, 2012). Faith communities can also provide much-needed support not only during times of difficulties such as grief or loss, but also during everyday life. Because much research demonstrates that social isolation can lead to depression and other poor health outcomes (Brandt et al., 2022), the social support provided by faith communities can be protective. **Table 11.1** gives some detailed examples of how religion and faith communities can promote mental well-being.

THE DARK SIDE OF RELIGION AND SPIRITUALITY ON MENTAL HEALTH

Religious and spiritual coping contribute to buffering the severity of symptoms for several psychiatric conditions (e.g., depression, suicidality, substance use, posttraumatic stress disorder, anxiety, and psychosis; see Huguelet, 2020; Lopez et al., 2023; Lucchetti et al., 2021, p. 7620). However significantly positive religion and spirituality are for mental health, there is a significant body of research that shows a bidirectional relationship between religion and mental health in that negative religious coping has a deleterious impact on the severity of psychiatric symptoms such as anxiety, depression, paranoid ideation, obsessive-compulsiveness, somatization, and suicidality and may lead to an overall lower quality of life (see **Figure 11.1**). The clinical significance of what is referred to as *spiritual struggles* cannot be underestimated, particularly in populations with psychiatric disorders. Spiritual and religious struggles are defined as tensions, conflict, and strains in what individuals deem as sacred. Research has shown that spiritual struggles are ubiquitous across religious traditions and even present in individuals self-identified as agnostic but who grew up in a religious environment. Although spiritual struggles are frequent in the general population, the severity of psychiatric symptoms is worse when the tension is not resolved. In other words, someone who is clinically depressed will experience an increased severity in the symptoms of depression if struggling with spiritual issues (Pargament & Exline, 2021).

Table 11.1 WAYS IN WHICH RELIGION AND FAITH COMMUNITIES CONTRIBUTE TO MENTAL WELL-BEING

SUPPORT	EXAMPLE
Sense of purpose	Religious beliefs often provide individuals with a sense of purpose and meaning in life. The understanding that one's life is part of a larger, meaningful narrative can contribute to a positive outlook and reduce existential angst.
Values and morality	Religious teachings often emphasize ethical values and moral principles. Adhering to these values can contribute to a sense of integrity and personal fulfillment, positively impacting mental well-being.
Hope and optimism leading to resilience	Many religious traditions promote hope and optimism, encouraging individuals to face challenges with resilience and faith. Believing in a higher power or divine plan can instill a positive outlook even in difficult circumstances.
Mindfulness and meditation	Many faith traditions incorporate mindfulness and meditation practices. These techniques can promote relaxation, reduce stress, and enhance mental clarity, contributing to overall mental well-being.
Coping mechanisms	Religious practices, such as prayer, meditation, and rituals, can serve as coping mechanisms during times of stress or crisis. These practices provide a structured way to process emotions, find solace, and seek guidance.
Community support, including during times of loss	Faith communities offer a built-in support system in which individuals can find understanding, empathy, and social connections. This sense of belonging can alleviate feelings of isolation and loneliness, contributing to improved mental health. In addition, faith communities usually rally around members experiencing grief and loss, providing much-needed support during adverse moments in life.
Rituals and routines	Participating in religious rituals and routines can provide a sense of structure and predictability, promoting stability and reducing anxiety. Regular attendance at religious services or engagement in spiritual practices can establish healthy habits.
Altruism and volunteering	Many religious traditions encourage acts of kindness, charity, and volunteering. Engaging in altruistic activities can contribute to a sense of purpose, fulfillment, and improved mental well-being.

Source: Adapted from Koenig, H. G. (2012). Religion, spirituality, and health: The research and clinical implications. *International Scholarly Research Network Psychiatry, 2012*, 278730. https://doi.org/10.5402/2012/278730

Unless clinicians are attentive to their clients' worldview and explanatory model of their distress, they will not be as effective. The types of spiritual struggles are described in **Table 11.2**.

A culturally sensitive treatment of mental illness must consider positive and negative religious beliefs and practices. The next section further explores the reasons religion and faith communities should be actively considered in reducing mental health disparities.

WHY RELIGION SHOULD BE ACTIVELY CONSIDERED FOR REDUCING MENTAL HEALTH DISPARITIES

Addressing disparities requires an integrated, systemic, and clinical approach that considers the barriers that perpetuate inequity as well as the development of means to overcome them. This section explores the rationale and evidence that support the inclusion of religion and spirituality in the reduction of mental health disparities.

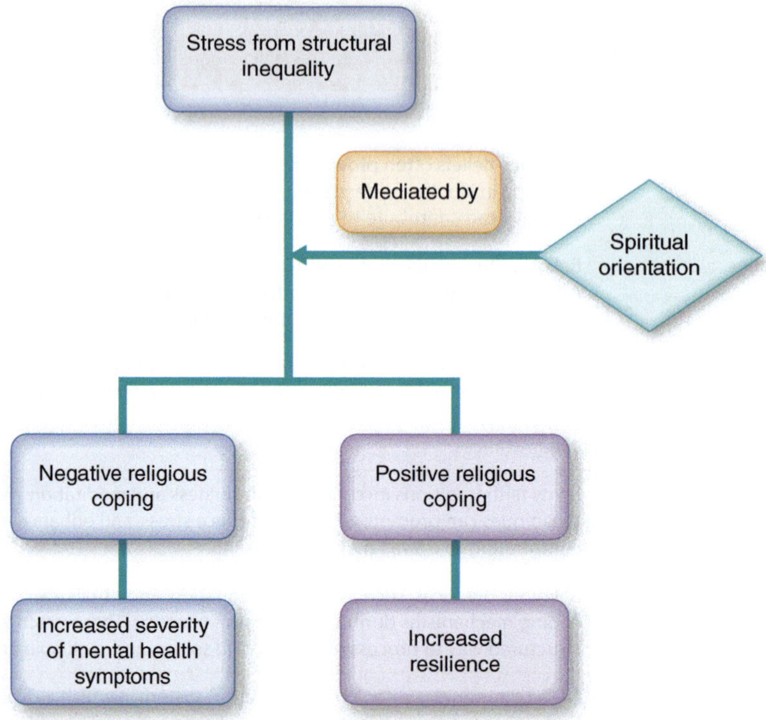

Figure 11.1 Religious coping and mental health outcomes.

Table 11.2 WAYS IN WHICH RELIGION AND SPIRITUALITY CONTRIBUTE TO PSYCHOLOGICAL DISTRESS

SPIRITUAL STRUGGLE	DESCRIPTION
Divine struggles	Anger, sadness, disappointment as one perceives to have been abandoned, punished, or no longer loved by God
Demonic struggles	Attribution that one's problems are caused or influenced by evil spiritual forces
Doubt-Related struggles	Feeling confused and troubled by one's religious beliefs and practices
Moral struggles	Tension and guilt about believing that one is failing to live up to the moral standards of the religious teachings
Struggles of ultimate meaning	Wondering whether one's life has any meaning or consequence in the world
Interpersonal sruggles	Conflict in a church, with other members, clergy, or the organized religion. Feeling isolated, criticized, mistreated or offended by fellow religionists

Source: Adapted from Exline, J. J. (2013). Religious and spiritual struggles. In K. I. Pargament (Ed.), J. Exline & J. Jones (Assoc. Eds.), *APA handbook of psychology, religion, and spirituality: Vol. 1. Context, theory, and research* (pp. 459–476). American Psychological Association.

First, there are pragmatic reasons racialized communities tend to seek mental health treatment through their faith communities (Derr, 2016; Hays & Lincoln, 2017; Maura & Weisman de Mamani, 2017; NeMoyer et al., 2019; Wang et al., 2003). Furthermore, religious people tend to cope with emotional distress by relying on spiritual strategies (Lucchetti et al., 2021; Pargament & Exline, 2021; Pomerleau et al., 2020). Failing to cooperate with spiritual leaders and faith-based organizations perpetuates a system of segregation that limits access to more complex levels of care for populations carrying the intersectional burden of the social determinants of health (Shim, 2021).

Second, research shows that religious coping is an important protective factor for racialized populations impacted by intersectional issues of racism and poverty (Ellison et al., 2008, 2012, 2017; Ellison & Flannelly, 2009; Upenieks et al., 2023). Failing to recognize the strengths and resilience embraced by minoritized groups undermines culturally relevant paths to promote and prevent mental illness in populations at risk (Ungar & Theron, 2020).

Third, there is a theoretical rationale. Most world religions provide a frame of reference for human flourishing and derailment. In other words, religious worldviews often include explanatory models of illness and healing (Dein, 2018). This is in contrast to the scientific worldview that excludes supernatural agents, activities, or events. The worldview of mental health practitioners tends to exclude or ignore religious ideas and practices (Ayvaci, 2017; Maura & Weisman de Mamani, 2017; Shafranske, 2013), which has contributed to mutual distrust with spiritual leaders (Sullivan et al., 2014). Kleinman (1980) proposed a framework that can be helpful to reduce the gap between these worldviews. He described a cultural construction of clinical reality, because the experience of illness is informed by cultural beliefs, idioms, and practices that impact help-seeking behaviors. Inequities may be reduced when providers understand the explanatory models of illness and healing and adapt their therapeutic approach to be culturally relevant (Balboni et al., 2022; Hartog & Gow, 2007), thereby reducing dropout rates and improving the quality and outcomes of the care received (Turner et al., 2019). Initial attempts to decolonize psychotherapeutic practices (Dueck, 2020) and the adaptation of psychological therapies to religious populations are showing promising results (Richards et al., 2023; Weisman de Mamani et al., 2023). Understanding the worldview of racialized communities is essential to the development of cultural competencies (Vieten & Lukoff, 2022).

Finally of note, faith communities themselves can present challenges for marginalized groups with intersectional identities that do not conform to the religious group's beliefs. For example, sexual minorities who draw on spiritual resources face unique challenges because the social context in many faith communities can be negative and potentially harmful (Lockett et al., 2023). Although spiritual struggles are present across diverse spiritual communities (Christian, Jewish, Hindu, Buddhist, and Muslim) and age, gender, and socioeconomic groups (Abu-Raiya et al., 2015; Phillips et al., 2009), they may be particularly deleterious to sexual minorities (Huffman et al., 2020). Engaging faith-based organizations to reduce stigma is crucial given their central position and influence among their members (Codjoe et al, 2021).

Taken together, all these factors make for a strong clinical rationale for paying attention to religion and including faith communities in addressing mental health inequities.

CASE VIGNETTES

As noted in the previous sections, there is significant evidence of the important role religion and faith communities can play in improving mental health and mental health disparities. In this section, we discuss some of the examples that highlight such roles. The first example demonstrates the effect of a collaboration with a faith community to provide an educational program that incorporates a faith component in preventing substance abuse among African American adolescents. The second example highlights the role that a faith community can play in providing mental health treatments in the setting familiar and comfortable to the target population (African American women, in this case). Finally, the third case vignette highlights how religion can be a protective factor in building resilience among Latinx immigrants.

Case Vignette 11.1 FAITH-BASED SUBSTANCE ABUSE AND HIV/AIDS PREVENTION PROGRAM FOR AFRICAN AMERICAN ADOLESCENTS (BRIDGE PROJECT)

The first example comes from a community-based participatory research project that designed, implemented, and evaluated a faith-based substance abuse and HIV/AIDS prevention program for African American adolescents in Houston, Texas (Marcus et al., 2004). A coalition of university-based researchers along with leaders and members of a large, 14,000-member church in Houston collaborated on a project called BRIDGE (**B**old, **R**eady, **I**ntelligent, **D**edicated, **G**uided, **E**quipped), a 3-year intervention to reduce substance abuse and HIV/AIDS in African American adolescents. Specifically, the project targeted African American middle school adolescents in grades 6 through 8 because this group was deemed vulnerable to the risks of engaging in substance abuse by virtue of their age, race, and socioeconomic status (Marcus et al., 2004).

The intervention included four components: (a) life skills training; (b) spreading the word, which is described as "Afrocentric prevention alternatives based on arts, media, communication, music and physical activity strategies" (Marcus et al., 2004, p. 350); (c) choosing the best; and (d) a faith component that incorporated scripture-based lessons to reinforce the curriculum at hand and was woven throughout the program. Project BRIDGE provided this structured curriculum on Wednesday nights during the school year. The team, consisting of African American church/community members and Anglo-American university researchers, met on a regular basis to create a common ground of understanding regarding cultural issues to ensure cultural sensitivity. Each year, a new cohort of adolescents was enrolled, and necessary modifications were made to the program based on input from students, parents, teachers, volunteers, and the research team (Marcus et al., 2004).

The result of this three-year intervention was very positive. The adolescents who participated in Project BRIDGE ($n = 34$) reported significantly less use of marijuana ($p = .024$) and other drugs ($p = .011$) in the previous 30 days than the comparison group. In addition, those who participated in the program began serving as role models for other adolescents in the church. Project BRIDGE was designated as an official ministry of the church and was extended to others in the greater metropolitan community. The church also benefited from having a well-trained volunteer staff (Marcus et al., 2004).

Case Vignette 11.2 GROUP PSYCHOTHERAPY FOR WOMEN AT CHURCH (INSIGHT THERAPY)

The second example comes from a study conducted by Mynatt et al. (2008). Because African Americans in general underutilize mental health services and, when they do seek treatment, they often seek individual counseling through their ministers (Young et al., 2003), Mynatt and colleagues decided to conduct a trial of group psychotherapy at a local church to reduce symptoms of depression, anxiety, hopelessness, and loneliness among African American women. The 12-week intervention, called INSIGHT therapy, was a cognitive behavioral therapy (CBT) approach designed specifically for women. Study participants ($n = 7$) were recruited through announcements in the church bulletin. The church was already equipped with a counseling center, and the church counselor was a faculty member at a local university. This connection facilitated the process of obtaining permission from the church pastor to conduct the study and of securing a room at the counseling center for the group to meet for therapy (Mynatt et al., 2008).

Participants' ages ranged from 24 to 53 years, with a mean of 41 years. Of the seven participants, three were single and four were married. The self-reported mean length of depressive symptoms among the participants was 10 years, with a range of 33 to 37years. Four of the participants had prior treatment for depression, and three had previous suicidal ideation without taking any further action.

To assess the effects of the INSIGHT therapy, study investigators scored the participants on the Beck Depression Inventory II (BDI-II), State and Trait Anxiety Inventory (STAI), Beck Hopelessness Scale (BHS), and UCLA Loneliness Scale. The median posttreatment scores on the BDI-II and STAI were less than pretreatment scores but not statistically significant. However, significant changes in depression were observed when analyzing data with paired *t* tests ($p = .02$; Mynatt et al., 2008).

Case Vignette 11.3 CROSS-SECTIONAL STUDY LOOKING AT THE RELATIONSHIP BETWEEN RELIGION AND MENTAL HEALTH OF LATINX IMMIGRANTS

The third example comes from a cross-sectional study using in-person survey interviews at a community center and at church during a three-month period in 2018 (Revens et al., 2021). Like the first case example, this was also a community-based participatory research (CBPR). Given that Latinx immigrants are at increased risk for mental disorders due to socioeconomic disadvantages and stressful conditions stemming from immigrating to another country and given that Latinx immigrants are also among the least likely group to seek mental health treatment, the study investigators examined the relationship between protective factors (including religion), resilience, and psychological distress in Latinx immigrants (Revens et al., 2021).

Through the in-person survey, the study investigators obtained the following data: Brief Resilience Scale, Brief Symptom Inventory, Duke University Religion Index, Multi-group Ethnic Identity measure, and the Interpersonal Support Evaluation List. A total of 128 participants completed the survey, and the results show that resilience—defined as the ability to recover from stress—was positively related to social support ($p = .001$) and religiosity ($p = .006$). The study investigators concluded that promoting social support and religion in Latinx immigrant communities can help improve well-being by increasing resilience and reducing distress (Revens et al., 2021).

FROM IDEAL TO REALITY: GAPS TO LEVERAGING FAITH-BASED ORGANIZATIONS

These examples highlight the potential benefits of collaborating with faith communities serving primarily those affected by health inequities. However, to have a meaningful impact, there should be a multilayered, systemic, and sustained process whereby spiritual leaders and their members can participate as active partners. The next section identifies the existing gaps to develop this partnership, followed by a model to redress these gaps.

Communities of faith may also address specific structural determinants of health by advocating through the political process, for instance, gaining universal health coverage, improving housing options, reducing food insecurity, denouncing racially driven policies and practices, or improving employment opportunities for persons with mental illness. Faith-based organizations assist individuals through their local agencies, such as Catholic Charities USA and others. Their activity, of necessity, is focused on individual needs rather than on the macro level.

Some of the most frequently cited strategies to reduce health disparities relevant to mental health at the meso and micro levels include developing multisector partnerships, coordinating care across community and health systems, increasing access to care, enhancing the providers' cultural competency, implementing best practices, systematically collecting data to inform clinical outcomes, and instituting policies to ensure sustainability. Each of these strategies presents both a promise and a challenge to the effective participation of faith communities in the larger mental health system. What follows is a brief discussion on the specific gaps.

Development of Multisector Partnerships

Faith-based organizations, mental health systems, and their respective practitioners have a long-standing and bidirectional measure of skepticism and mistrust (Idler et al., 2019). The mistrust may be based on the different worldviews on explanatory systems of health and healing; historical prejudice and racism in the delivery of healthcare—for instance, African Americans receiving more severe psychiatric diagnoses (van der Ven & Susser, 2023) and being more likely to be overmedicated (Smith, 2021); and one-sided benefits accrued from short-term collaboration (a pastor said, "Once you collect your data you are out of here"). The development of mutual trust over time is essential.

Coordination of Care

Spiritual leaders are perceived primarily as gatekeepers and not as partners. For instance, among the recommendations developed by a highly respected organization to reduce health disparities, it stated the following concerning the role of faith communities in the mental health among Latinx:

> Participants also described their preference for seeking support from church priests, pastors, or other nontraditional service providers in times of emotional crisis. Overall, the participants believed that churches were in a better position than agencies to effectively disseminate mental health information to the community. One strategy envisions persuading church leaders to become involved by providing them with information and training regarding mental health illness and interventions. (Aguilar-Gaxiola et al., 2012, p. 32)

In other words, even though the respondents to the survey affirmed their preference for care from spiritual leaders, the strategy recommended is to "persuade and educate." In most cases, there is no coordination of care because spiritual providers are not perceived as partners. Task sharing is emerging only recently as an accepted concept (Mongelli et al., 2020). Additionally, principles of cultural humility may facilitate the needed framework for mutual understanding and coordination (Stubbe, 2020).

Increase Access to Care

If there is no or limited trust, there are no established pathways for collaboration and coordination of care, or the preference for services provided by faith communities is ignored (Wang et al., 2003), individuals in need of higher levels of care may not have timely and seamless access to what they need. Working in a collaborative environment will enhance the competencies of both mental health clinicians and spiritual helpers for the benefit of the patient. Establishing "networks of care" (discussed in the next section) may facilitate cooperation and transition to appropriate levels of care while maintaining the support of the patient's own faith community. Increased access to care can be facilitated by cooperation in the implementation of community-based interventions to promote resilience and early identification of those in need of access to higher levels of care.

Cultural Competency

For many people, religion and spirituality provide the idioms for emotional distress, a narrative to explain mental illness, and the trusted resources to mitigate the impact of psychiatric conditions. Furthermore, racialized minorities have a distinct preference for including a spiritual perspective in their treatment (Dimmick et al., 2022). However, mental health professionals are rarely trained to address these issues in their work (Vieten & Lukoff, 2022). In fact, a study found a high frequency (39%) of religious microaggressions during treatment, resulting in a negative therapeutic alliance: the most important predictor of psychotherapeutic outcomes (Trusty et al., 2022). Although mental health professionals and the general population place a different value on religion and spirituality (Dein, 2018), there is a growing interest in gaining skills to address this dimension of diversity (Vieten et al., 2023). Training programs have been developed to enhance competencies in religion and spirituality (Pearce et al., 2019); however, a crucial missing link is the training that takes place during clinical education (Hathaway et al., 2022). What is not implemented systematically during the shaping of clinical competencies is less likely to be part of clinical practice. Furthermore, training to acquire competencies that address the intersectionality of religion and racialized groups is missing (Captari et al., 2022). Finally, although clergy often are the frontline providers, they may not have the needed skills to be as effective as they could be (Anthony et al., 2015). Mental health practitioners need to increase their literacy on religious and spiritual matters, not only conceptually but critically, in the context of their clinical education. On the other hand, spiritual leaders may also benefit from increasing their literacy and competency skills when dealing with individuals with mental health disorders.

Implementing Best Practices

Spiritually integrated psychotherapies have flourished in recent years (Richards et al., 2023). The studies consistently report greater symptom relief and spiritual well-being when compared with standard (secular) treatment (Captari et al., 2022) and highlight the importance of religion in the formation of the therapeutic alliance (Terepka & Hatfield, 2020). A strong therapeutic alliance is also important for maintaining adherence to psychotropic medication treatment (Wienke Totura et al., 2017). Paying attention to religious beliefs is an important factor because they have been identified among the contributors to nonadherence (Semahegn et al., 2020). Clinical practices that include religion and spiritual considerations need to move from academic and research environments to the real world of practice, particularly with racialized populations. Giving religion and spirituality a consideration like what is currently given (correctly) to race and identity would facilitate dissemination and implementation.

Systematic Data Collection to Inform Clinical Outcomes

Mental health treatment in general does not use systematic data collection to inform clinical practice and influence outcomes (Miller et al., 2015). Ideally, data collection would include the elements that are relevant to the reduction of health disparities, such as access to care, patient engagement, and adherence, from both the mental health system and spiritual leaders.

Institutional Policies to Support Sustainability

What an organization requires is more likely to happen. It is unclear what impact the requirement of a spiritual assessment of all hospitalized patients by the Joint Commission had, if any. The Joint Commission no longer has this requirement (Koenig et al., 2023, p. 659). It is possible that by withdrawing this standard of care, the attention of practitioners to the spirituality of their patients may be less salient and therefore less likely to be mined for patient care. On the other hand, chaplain support is an integral part of most inpatient facilities as well as in some outpatient settings. Several studies have documented the beneficial impact of chaplain care on mental health (Buelens et al., 2023; Jones et al., 2022; Macdonald, 2017; Smigelsky et al., 2022; Wortmann et al., 2023). As is the case with community clergy, chaplains often deal with individuals with serious mental disturbance. Although institutional policies to systematically include a patient-centric approach to include religion and spirituality among the interventions that can help in addressing mental health disparities at the clinical level, to be meaningful, it would need to be embedded in a robust articulation of diversity and cultural competencies.

As it is apparent, each component of these strategies could work well in isolation. However, they are best conceived as an interlocking system with the clear goal of addressing and decreasing disparities in mental health. **Table 11.3** provides a summary of each strategy and key recommendations to close the gap and support patients and their families.

The next section presents a proposal with examples based on community and international work conducted by one of us (C.F.). We highlight real-world experiences of success and unfulfilled promise. The systematic incorporation of all aspects of work with faith communities may result in a robust approach to reducing mental health disparities.

Table 11.3 STRATEGIES TO REDUCE HEALTH DISPARITIES AND KEY RECOMMENDATIONS TO CLOSE THE GAP

STRATEGY	RECOMMENDATION
Development of multisector partnerships	Convene community stakeholders to understand perceived needs and develop trust.
Coordination of care	Highlight and implement the principles of cultural humility and "task sharing" with spiritual leaders.
Increase access to care	Establish "networks of care" including spiritual leaders and mental health providers. Cooperate on community-based early intervention to promote emotional resilience, identifying those in need for higher levels of care.
Cultural competency	Increase literacy on spirituality and religion for mental health clinicians, and literacy on mental health issues for spiritual leaders. Incorporate religion and spirituality in clinical education.
Implement best practices	Disseminate spiritually integrated psychotherapies and strengthen the prescriber's therapeutic alliance to improve adherence to psychotropics by attending to the patient's religiously informed explanatory model of illness and healing.
Systematic data collection to improve clinical outcomes	Systematically track the results of collaboration efforts with faith-based organizations in facilitating access to care, and patient engagement when religion and spirituality are incorporated into treatment.
Institutional policies to support sustainability	Highlight and train clinicians on the relevance of religion and spirituality for racialized communities in a manner similar to other dimensions of culture and identity.

A WAY FORWARD: FILLING THE GAPS AND UNDERSTANDING REALITY TO REDUCE DISPARITIES

Faith-based organizations are uniquely positioned to play a substantial role in the prevention, early identification, and treatment of mental disorders. Their effectiveness can be significantly increased when embedded in a larger system that collaborates, supports, and provides a seamless path to facilitate access to appropriate levels of care and to reduce disparities. This section provides a narrative of intentional efforts to develop multisectorial cooperation with faith communities, implement strategies for early identification of individuals at risk of emotional distress, and promote resilience, leveraging the credibility and skill set of spiritual leaders, using evidence-based strategies adapted to their religious language and practices, and facilitating access to appropriate levels of care (see **Figure 11.2**). After describing an evidence-based low-intensity psychological intervention to enhance task sharing in providing mental health services in the community, a recommendation is made to support continuity in cooperation and sustainability. Finally, efforts to enhance the spiritual and religious literacy of mental health clinicians working in an integrated primary care setting are described. Throughout, challenges to implementation are highlighted. Taken together, all these components provide an actionable model to reduce mental health disparities.

The strategies for reducing health disparities rest on the assumption that community and health systems leaders and resources can seamlessly and bidirectionally connect with one another. The initial step in forging a systemic process necessitates the development of mutual trust and understanding among key stakeholders to develop a common framework for cooperation based on perceived respect and clearly identified needs, methods, and procedures. The conceptual frame of reference should be guided by the values of cultural humility and task sharing. Cultural humility in this context requires self-awareness, a keen interest in understanding what the other side brings to the table, openness to differences, and a commitment to respectfully find common ground. Task sharing is a direct implementation of cultural humility in that the practices of spiritual leaders and mental clinicians have legitimacy, although they may rest on a different worldview and use different methodologies, and yet contribute to the common goal of assisting communities in need. The following descriptions intend to convey something about the opportunities and challenges associated with this strategy.

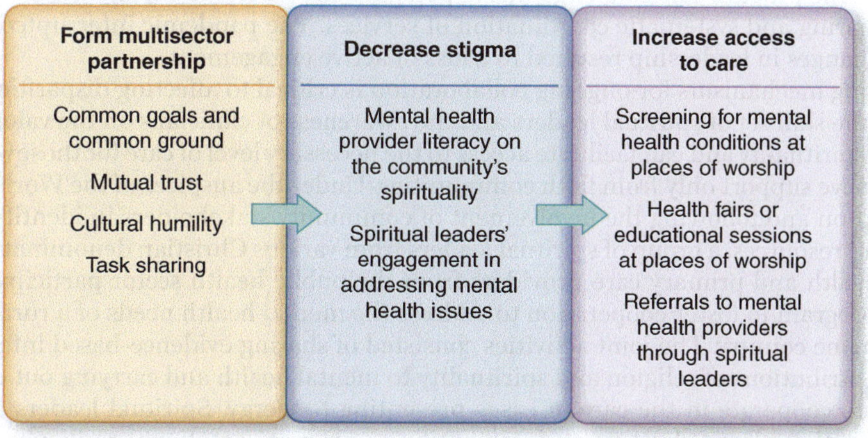

Figure 11.2 Strategy for reducing mental health disparities through partnership with faith communities.

We live and practice in a community with a large Latinx population, many of whom are recent immigrants, and a high percentage are undocumented. This is a population at risk for mental health issues given the intersectionality of poverty, racism, and exclusion from the health system. I (C.F.) have been a consultant with the largest religious body in the area, with a majority membership of Hispanics with various degrees of acculturation. After being approached by a spiritual leader asking for help to support the people in his congregation, a meeting was held including consequential community stakeholders from his faith tradition and leaders from the county health system to understand their mutual concerns and needs and to identify strategies to redress the mental health needs of this group. Both sides indicated an interest and commitment to the process. The county, being the safety net for all residents regardless of immigration status, was interested in outreach and early identification of individuals in need of services. The church was interested in supporting the work of their clergy in relieving the emotional needs of their parishioners, and in meeting the concrete needs of their community. The subsequent step involved several meetings with representatives of both parties with direct responsibilities in providing spiritual and mental health care in their region. The county identified specific geographical areas with high need, whereas the church identified the parishes in that area that could participate in planned activities. The next step consisted of meeting with the local church leaders to have a more granular understanding of needs and expectations. Following a needs assessment conducted on the day of highest church attendance, a health fair with a focus on mental health was held. On that day, the county deployed their mobile clinic, mental health clinicians, and various recourses to address substance abuse and youth behavioral health issues, on the church grounds. At the end of each church service, the pastor encouraged parishioners to take advantage of the resources, and the Patient Health Questionnaire–9 (PHQ-9) was administered to all who were willing to take it. The PHQ-9 is a short screening measure of depression, the mental health condition with the highest frequency and impact, to educate the congregants on mental health issues and invite those with scores in the clinical range to avail themselves of a consult with the county's mental health experts. Those in need of clinical services received a direct referral. Anecdotally, the wait period to see a psychiatrist went down from 2 months to 2 weeks. Access to needed care was significantly improved. Moreover, the pastor's endorsement (and the bishop's blessing through a prepared video) contributed to assuaging concerns secondary to the impact of legal status and stigma. Furthermore, particular care was given to having providers who were Latinx and Spanish speakers, because cultural affinity could ease the process. The challenge was to persuade the parties to expand the cooperation to task sharing and systematic coordination of services. The pandemic interrupted the initiative. Changes in leadership resulted in a loss of active engagement.

Creating mechanisms for ongoing collaboration is critical to affecting disparities. It can increase the skill set of spiritual leaders and the awareness of clinicians on the value of religion and spirituality and can facilitate access to the necessary level of care for thosewho need it and receive support only from faith communities. Under the auspices of the World Health Organization and following the involvement of community stakeholders in identifying priorities and resources, a group of spiritual leaders from various Christian denominations and mental health and primary care providers from the public health sector participated in a literacy program to foster cooperation to address the mental health needs of a rural area in a low-income country. The joint activities consisted of sharing evidence-based information on the contributions of religion and spirituality to mental health and carrying out exercises on ways to cooperate in the care of cases presenting to clergy. Spiritual leaders also met independently to learn skills on an intervention to promote emotional resilience through their churches. The content of the intervention consisted of learning teachable skills that although evidence based, reflected their spiritual beliefs and practices. During the intervention, the PHQ-9 was administered to identify individuals needing higher levels of care.

Coordination was facilitated through "networks of care," meaning that clinicians and clergy met regularly to continue to foster cooperation and facilitate referrals for those with a "positive" PHQ-9. After the first wave conducting the intervention, two problems were identified. One, the mental health resources were quickly overwhelmed and unable to respond to the demand. Second, transportation to the health centers made it unworkable for many. For the first concern, a local university with a psychology program was included in the program, and the advanced students were made available to help. The students, under supervision, were deployed at pastors' offices, decreasing the problem with transportation. Additionally, and in concordance with the strategies to reduce disparities, the students were also located in primary care settings to provide integrated behavioral care. The students in turn also participated in literacy efforts on the value of religion and spirituality in mental health. Sustainability became a problem. As is frequently the case, funding was not consistent, a local champion shifted direction away from this initiative, and COVID-19 happened. All of these factors conspired against maintaining and supporting the gains.

The cooperation of spiritual leaders and mental health clinicians requires the development of cultural competency. Clinicians need to become conversant on the positive and dark sides of religion and skilled in implementing best practices relevant to racialized groups. Spiritual leaders may need to become more conversant on mental health issues and enhance pastoral care skills when dealing with emotional distress. Cultural competency contributes to the implementation of best practices. Of all the strategies, this has proven to be the most challenging to implement. Having participated in the clinical education and training of psychiatrists and clinical psychologists for close to three decades and having consulted with clergy from different denominations on mental health issues for many years, the challenge essentially lies in the worldviews and education assumptions that shape the professional identity of these groups. Unless the didactic content of the training is linked to competency-based expectations, and routinely incorporated into the supervision of clinical encounters, the transfer to regular practice does not take place. In this context, clinical psychology trainees worked at outpatient medical clinics serving primarily minoritized groups. Early identification in primary care resulted in consultation and follow-up. The psychotherapeutic interventions integrated a patient-centric approach to the patients' religion and spirituality, which resulted in improved patient outcomes and engagement. The main challenge was to overcome the trainees' bias and discomfort in providing evidence-based interventions congruent with the patients' religious beliefs and practices.

Spiritual leaders' training and level of comfort in delivering mental health services vary. Frequently, those caring for racialized groups feel insufficiently prepared to respond to the demand (Bolger & Prickett, 2021). Problem Management Plus (PM+) is a low-intensity psychological intervention that has been shown to be effective in contexts of adversity (Connolly et al., 2021) and is well suited to enhance the skill set of spiritual leaders because it builds on existing competencies, teaches helpful interventions over a brief period, and targets clinical groups with mild to moderate levels of morbidity. Additionally, the pastors and lay leaders who participated in learning the PM+ were supported by mental health clinicians who planned ongoing clinical support and supervision. This initiative resulted in improving the skill set of the spiritual leaders, access to culturally sensitive care, and a systemic connection with the mental health system to facilitate access to higher levels of care when needed. Because this effort is unfolding at this time, the main challenge is sustainability. Spiritual leaders have a busy schedule that does not always allow for the ongoing consultation needed to consolidate and internalize the various elements of the training.

If all these components could be integrated into an active plan to address disparities, the way forward could look something like this:

1. Stakeholders from faith communities and mental health systems cooperate in the development of a framework based on their common ground, mutual needs, and

agreed-upon general principles of cultural humility and task sharing. The organizations involved transfer the agreement into actionable expectations for the systems they represent to facilitate implementation, dissemination, and accountability. A data collection strategy is agreed upon at this level and from the outset to inform and adapt the strategies being used.

2. Implementation champions from faith communities and mental health systems articulate processes to build community resilience, facilitate early identification of cases, and facilitate access to care.
3. Literacy efforts are conducted jointly and independently to increase cultural competencies, disseminate best practices, and highlight the role of task sharing. Particular attention should be given to the points of contact where access to care is most likely to be needed, such as integrated behavioral care in primary care and specialty clinics dealing with chronic conditions and serving racialized minorities.
4. Networks of care are implemented to facilitate ongoing cooperation and support.
5. Stakeholders meet at an established frequency to continue to cultivate trust, monitor progress, and make the necessary institutional adjustments to ensure continuity, sustainability, and integrity of the efforts.

Faith-based organizations do not initiate programs to reduce mental health disparities. Those who see the value of engaging faith communities should consider the following recommendations to facilitate engaging faith leaders.

RECOMMENDATIONS TO ENGAGE FAITH LEADERS

The principles of cultural humility and task sharing should inform how religious actors may be engaged. Cultural humility assumes a willingness to examine one's position not as dominant but open to the knowledge coming from other perspectives. Task sharing promotes the cooperation between spiritual leaders and mental health providers as equal contributors to a common goal.

Here are some recommendations primarily drawn from the work of Melissa Nozell (personal communication, May 10, 2024) at the U.S. Institute of Peace's initiative on religious communities supporting psychosocial interventions.

- *Let religious actors be religious actors.* Partner with them in ways that allow them to continue to be religious and meet them where they are, without incentivizing them to change or adapt. Recognize their work on the front lines of mental health treatment.
- *Engage religious actors early and often as partners.* If they are included from the beginning, their insights can be essential to informing effective policy and programming tailored to their context.
- *Engage inclusively.* Recognize the nuances and complexities of religion in mental health. There may be a misalignment in values. While emphasizing the common ground, it is important to recognize the boundaries that may constitute nonnegotiables for healthy cooperation.
- *Go beyond theology.* Religious actors wear many hats in their communities. They are parents, siblings, teachers, and counselors. Recognize that they bring more than only the "obviously religious" to the table.

SUMMARY

There are pragmatic, clinical, and theoretical reasons to involve religion, spirituality, and faith communities in the reduction of health disparities, because communities most affected by inequality rely on religious practices, beliefs, and their houses of worship as resources to cope with emotional distress. A comprehensive model is needed that supports the creation of sustainable "networks of care" involved in the promotion, prevention, and intervention with spiritually and culturally relevant beliefs, practices, and actors in mental health. There is a need for a sustained strategy informed by the values of cultural humility and task sharing. There is a need for "champions" who can lead with adequate institutional support and a commitment and vision that transcend the silos that keep those in need from accessing quality care. Finally, there is a need for an implementation science approach to track and adjust the interventions that can lead to a reduction in mental health disparities.

DISCUSSION QUESTIONS

1. Religion makes positive and negative contributions to mental health. How might this change the way you think about engaging faith-based organizations?
2. There are several reasons to include faith communities in the reduction of mental health disparities. Based on what you know about your local community, what rationale would you articulate to advocate cooperation?
3. One of the gaps that separate mental health systems from faith-based organizations is the worldview that informs perspectives on health and healing. Can you identify the potential points of conflict and how you might address them?
4. The implementation of best practices with minoritized people integrating religion, spirituality, and faith communities is crucial to reduce mental health disparities. Can you assess the gaps in your community and think of ways to close the gaps?
5. Consider and discuss the model that may best fit the needs of the community where you are. What makes the model you've selected effective?

REFERENCES

Abu-Raiya, H., Pargament, K. I., Krause, N., & Ironson, G. (2015). Robust links between religious/spiritual struggles, psychological distress, and well-being in a national sample of American adults. *American Journal of Orthopsychiatry*, *85*(6), 565–575. https://doi.org/10.1037/ort0000084

Aguilar-Gaxiola, S., Loera, G., Méndez, l., Sala, M., Latino Mental Health Concilio, & Nakamoto, J. (2012). *Community-defined solutions for Latino mental health care disparities: California reducing disparities project, Latino strategic planning workgroup population report.* UC Davis.

Anthony, J. S., Johnson, A., & Schafer, J. (2015). African American clergy and depression: What they know; what they want to know. *Journal of Cultural Diversity*, *22*(4), 118–126.

Ayvaci, E. (2017). Religious barriers to mental healthcare. *The American Journal of Psychiatry Resident's Journal*, *11*(7), 11–13. https://doi.org/10.1176/appi.ajp-rj.2016.110706

Balboni, A., VanderWeele, T., Doan-Soares, S., Long, K., Ferrell, B., Fitchett, G., Koenig, H., Bain, P., Puchalski, C., Steinhauser, K., Sulmasy, D., & Koh, H. (2022) Spirituality in serious illness and health. *JAMA*, *328*(2), 184. https://doi.org/10.1001/jama.2022.11086

Bolger, D., & Prickett, P. J. (2021). Where would you go? Race, religion, and the limits of pastor mental health care in Black and Latino congregations. *Religions*, *12*(12), 1062. https://doi.org/10.3390/rel12121062

Brandt, L., Liu, S., Heim, C., & Heinz, A. (2022). The effects of social isolation stress and discrimination on mental health. *Translational Psychiatry*, *12*(1), 398. https://doi.org/10.1038/s41398-022-02178-4

Buelens, E., Dewitte, L., Dezutter, J., Vandenhoeck, A., & Dillen, A. (2023). The outcomes of healthcare chaplaincy on hospitalized patients. A quasi-experimental study in Belgium. *Journal of Spirituality in Mental Health*, *25*(3), 1–24. https://doi.org/10.1080/19349637.2023.2177239

Captari, L. E., Sandage, S. J., & Vandiver, R. A. (2022). Spiritually integrated psychotherapies in real-world clinical practice: Synthesizing the literature to identify best practices and future research directions. *Psychotherapy*, *59*(3), 307–320. https://doi.org/10.1037/pst0000407

Codjoe, L., Barber, S., Ahuja, S., Thornicroft, G., Henderson, C., Lempp, H., & N'Danga-Koroma, J. (2021). Evidence for interventions to promote mental health and reduce stigma in Black faith communities: systematic review. *Social Psychiatry and Psychiatric Epidemiology*, *56*(6), 895–911. https://doi.org/10.1007/s00127-021-02068-y

Connolly, S. M., Vanchu-Orosco, M., Warner, J., Seidi, P. A., Edwards, J., Boath, E., & Irgens, A. C. (2021). Mental health interventions by lay counsellors: A systematic review and meta-analysis. *Bulletin of the World Health Organization*, *99*(8), 572–582. https://doi.org/10.2471/BLT.20.269050

Dein, S. (2018). Against the stream: Religion and mental health—The case for the inclusion of religion and spirituality into psychiatric care. *BJ Psych Bulletin, 42*(3), 127–129. https://doi.org/10.1192/bjb.2017.13

Derr, A. (2016). Mental health service use among immigrants in the United States: A systematic review. *Psychiatric Services, 67*(3), 265–273. https://doi.org/10.1176/appi.ps.201500004

Dimmick, A. A., Trusty, W. T., & Swift, J. K. (2022). Client preferences for religious/spiritual integration and matching in psychotherapy. *Spirituality in Clinical Practice, 9*(3), 202–211. https://doi.org/10.1037/scp0000269

Dueck, A. (2020). Indigenous psychologies of spirituality: Remembering, excavating, and individuating. In T. A. Sisemore & J. J. Knabb (Eds.), *The psychology of world religions and spiritualities.* Templeton Press.

Ellison, C., Bradshaw, M. Kuyel, N., & Marcum, J. (2012). Attachment to God, stressful life events, and changes in psychological distress. *Review of Religious Research, 53*, 493–511. https://doi.org/10.1007/s13644-011-0023-4

Ellison, C., & Flannelly, K. (2009). Religious involvement and risk of major depression in a prospective nationwide study of African American adults. *The Journal of Nervous and Mental Disease, 197*(8), 568-573. https://doi.org/10.1097/NMD.0b013e3181b08f45

Ellison, C. G., DeAngelis, R. T., & Güven, M. (2017). Does religious involvement mitigate the effects of major discrimination on the mental health of African Americans? Findings from the Nashville stress and health study. *Religions, 8*, 195. https://doi.org/10.3390/rel8090195

Ellison, C. G., Musick, M. A., & Henderson, A. K. (2008), Balm in Gilead: Racism, religious involvement, and psychological distress among African-American adults. *Journal for the Scientific Study of Religion, 47*(2), 291–309. https://doi.org/10.1111/j.1468-5906.2008.00408.x

Hartog, K., & Gow, K. (2007). Religious attributions pertaining to the causes and cures of mental illness. *Mental Health, Religion & Culture, 8*(4), 263–276. https://doi.org/10.1080/13674670412331304339

Hathaway, D. B., de Oliveira e Oliveira, F. H. A., Mirhom, M., Moreira-Almeida, A., Fung, W. L. A., & Peteet, J. R. (2022). Teaching spiritual and religious competencies to psychiatry residents: A scoping and systematic review. *Academic Medicine, 97*(2), 300–310. https://doi.org/10.1097/ACM.0000000000004167

Hays, K., & Lincoln, K. D. (2017). Mental health help-seeking profiles among African Americans: Exploring the influence of religion. *Race & Social Problems.* 9, 127–138. https://doi.org/10.1007/s12552-017-9193-1

Huffman, J. M., Warlick, C., Frey, B., & Kerr, B. (2020). Religiosity, spirituality, gender identity, and sexual orientation of sexual minorities. *Translational Issues in Psychological Science, 6*(4), 356–371. https://doi.org/10.1037/tps0000262

Huguelet, P. (2020). Spirituality, religion, and psychotic disorders. In D. H. Rosmarin & H. G. Koenig, (Eds.), *Handbook of spirituality, religion, and mental health. Spirituality, religion, and psychotic disorders* (2nd ed., Chapter 5, pp. 79–97). Academic Press. https://doi.org/10.1016/B978-0-12-816766-3.00005-7

Idler, E., Levin, J., VanderWeele, T. J., & Khan, A. (2019). Partnerships between public health agencies and faith communities. *American Journal of Public Health, 109*(3), 346–347. https://doi.org/10.2105/AJPH.2018.304941

Jones, K. A., Freijah, I., Carey, L., Carleton, R. N., Devenish-Meares, P., Dell, L., Rodrigues, S., Madden, K., Johnson, L., Hosseiny, F., & Phelps, A. J. (2022). Moral injury, chaplaincy and mental health provider approaches to treatment: A scoping review. *Journal of Religion and Health, 61*, 1051–1094. https://doi.org/10.1007/s10943-022-01534-4

Kleinman, A. (1980). *Patients and healers in the context of culture: An exploration of the borderland between anthropology, medicine, and psychiatry.* University of California Press.

Koenig, H. G. (2012). Religion, spirituality, and health: The research and clinical implications. *International Scholarly Research Network Psychiatry, 2012*, 278730. https://doi.org/10.5402/2012/278730

Koenig, H. G., VanderWeele, T., & Peteet, J. R. (2023). *Handbook of religion & health.* Oxford University Press.

Lockett, G. M., Brooks, J. E., Abreu, R. L., & Sostre, J. P. (2023). "I want to go to a place that's openly talking about the experiences of people of color who also identify as LGBTQ+": Cultural, religious, and spiritual experiences of LGBTQ people of color. *Spirituality in Clinical Practice, 10*(3), 261–270. https://doi.org/10.1037/scp0000288

Lopez, D., Saenz Escalante, G., & Weisman de Mamani, A. (2023). The role of religious coping on suicidality among Latinx and Black/African American individuals with schizophrenia spectrum disorders. *Spirituality in Clinical Practice, 10*(3), 219–232. https://doi.org/10.1037/scp0000317

Lucchetti, G., Koenig, H. G., & Lucchetti, A. L. G. (2021). Spirituality, religiousness, and mental health: A review of the current scientific evidence. *World Journal of Clinical Cases,* 9(26), 7620–7631. https://doi.org/10.12998/wjcc.v9.i26.7620

Macdonald, G. (2017). The efficacy of primary care chaplaincy compared with antidepressants: A retrospective study comparing chaplaincy with antidepressants. *Primary Health Care Research & Development, 18*(4), 354–365. doi:10.1017/S1463423617000159

Marcus, M., Walker. T., Swint, J. M., Smith, B. P., Brown, C., Busen, N., Edwards, T., Liehr, P., Taylor, W., Williams. D., & von Sternberg, K. (2004). Community-based participatory research to prevent substance abuse and HIV/AIDS in African-American adolescents. *Journal of Interprofessional Care, 18*(4), 347–359. https://doi.org/10.1080/13561820400011776

Maura, J., & Weisman de Mamani, A. (2017). Mental health disparities, treatment engagement, and attrition among racial/ethnic minorities with severe mental illness: A review. *Journal of Clinical Psychology in Medical Settings, 24,* 187–210. https://doi.org/10.1007/s10880-017-9510-2

Miller, S. D., Hubble, M. A., Chow, D., & Seidel, J. (2015). Beyond measures and monitoring: Realizing the potential of feedback-informed treatment. *Psychotherapy, 52*(4), 449–457. https://doi.org/10.1037/pst0000031

Mongelli, F., Georgakopoulos, G., & Pato, M. (2020). Challenges and opportunities to meet the mental health needs of underserved and disenfranchised populations in the United States. *Focus, 18*(1), 16–24. https://doi.org/10.1176/appi.focus.20190028

Mynatt, S., Wicks, M., & Bolden, L. (2008). Pilot study of INSIGHT therapy in African American women. *Archives of Psychiatric Nursing, 22*(6), 364–374. https://doi.org/10.1016/j.apnu.2007.10.007

NeMoyer, A., Alvarez, K., & Alegria, M. (2019). Understanding mental health disparities. In M. Williams, D. Rosen, & J. Kanter (Eds.), *Eliminating race-based disparities: Promoting equity and culturally responsive care across settings.* Context Press.

Pargament, K., & Exline, J. (2021). *Working with spiritual struggles in psychotherapy: From research to practice.* The Guilford Press.

Pearce, M. J., Pargament, K. I., Oxhandler, H. K., Vieten, C., & Wong, S. (2019). A novel training program for mental health providers in religious and spiritual competencies. *Spirituality in Clinical Practice, 6*(2), 73–82. https://doi.org/10.1037/scp0000195

Phillips, R. E. III, Cheng, C. M., Pargament, K. I., Oemig, C., Colvin, S. D., Abarr, A. N., Dunn, M. W., & Reed, A. S. (2009). Spiritual coping in American Buddhists: An exploratory study. *International Journal for the Psychology of Religion, 19*(4), 231–243. https://doi.org/10.1080/10508610903143263

Pomerleau, J. M., Pargament, K. I., Krause, N., Ironson, G., & Hill, P. (2020). Religious and spiritual struggles as a mediator of the link between stressful life events and psychological adjustment in a nationwide sample. *Psychology of Religion and Spirituality, 12*(4), 451–459. https://doi.org/10.1037/rel0000268

Revens, K. E., Gutierrez, D., Paul, R., Reynolds, A. D., Price, R., & DeHaven, M. J. (2021). Social support and religiosity as contributing factors to resilience and mental wellbeing in Latino immigrants: A community-based participatory research study. *Journal of Immigrant Minority Health, 23*(5), 904–916. https://doi.org/10.1007/s10903-021-01179-7

Richards, P., Allen, G., & Judd, D. (2023). *Handbook of spiritually integrated psychotherapies.* American Psychological Association Publishing.

Richards, P., Pargament, K., Exline, J., & Allen, G. (2023). Introduction: Bringing spiritually integrated psychotherapies into the health care mainstream. In P. Richards, G. Allen, & D. Judd (Eds.), *Handbook of spiritually integrated psychotherapies.* American Psychological Association.

Semahegn, A., Torpey, K., Manu, A., Assefa, N., Tesfaye, G., & Ankomah, A. (2020). Psychotropic medication non-adherence and its associated factors among patients with major psychiatric disorders: A systematic review and meta-analysis. *Systematic Reviews, 9*(1), 17. https://doi.org/10.1186/s13643-020-1274-3

Shafranske, E. (2013). Religious involvement and professional practices of psychiatrists and other mental health professionals. *Psychiatric Annals, 30*(8), 525–532. https://doi.org/10.3928/0048-5713-20000801-07

Shim, R. (2021). Dismantling structural racism in psychiatry: A path to mental health equity. *American Journal of Psychiatry, 178*(7), 592–598. https://doi.org/10.1176/appi.ajp.2021.21060558

Smigelsky, M. A., Trimm, V., Meador, K. G., Jackson, G. L., Wortmann, J. H., & Nieuwsma, J. A. (2022). Core components of moral injury groups co-facilitated by mental health providers and chaplains. *Spirituality in Clinical Practice, 9*(3), 159–174. https://doi.org/10.1037/scp0000297

Smith, J. R. (2021). Diagnosis issues with African Americans. In: M. O. Adekson (Eds.), *African Americans and mental health.* Springer. https://doi.org/10.1007/978-3-030-77131-7_6

Stubbe, D. (2020). Practicing cultural competence and cultural humility in the care of diverse patients. *Focus, 18*(1), 49–51. https://doi.org/10.1176/appi.focus.20190041

Sullivan, S., Pyne, J. M., Cheney, A. M., Hunt, J., Haynes, T. F., & Sullivan, G. (2014). The pew versus the couch: Relationship between mental health and faith communities and lessons learned from a VA/clergy partnership project. *Journal of Religion & Health, 53*(4), 1267–1282. https://doi.org/10.1007/s10943-013-9731-0

Terepka, A., & Hatfield, D. R. (2020). Effects of assessing religious beliefs in initial sessions on aspects of the therapeutic alliance. *Spirituality in Clinical Practice, 7*(1), 3–17. https://doi.org/10.1037/scp0000213

Thompson Fullilove, M., Dix, E., Hankerson, S., Lassiter, J., & Jordan, A. (2024). Systems that promote mental health in the teeth of oppression. *The Lancet Psychiatry, 11*(1), 65–74. https://doi.org/10.1016/S2215-0366(23)00344-9

Trusty, W. T., Swift, J. K., Black, S. W., Dimmick, A. A., & Penix, E. A. (2022). Religious microaggressions in psychotherapy: A mixed methods examination of client perspectives. *Psychotherapy, 59*(3), 351–362. https://doi.org/10.1037/pst0000408

Turner, E. A., Malone, C. M., & Douglas, C. (2019). Barriers to mental health treatment for African Americans: Applying a model of treatment initiation to reduce disparities. In M. T. Williams, D. C. Rosen, & J. W. Kanter (Eds.), *Eliminating race-based mental health disparities: Promoting equity and culturally responsive care across settings* (pp. 27–42). Context Press/New Harbinger Publications.

Ungar, M., & Theron, L. (2020). Resilience and mental health: how multisystemic processes contribute to positive outcomes. *The Lancet Psychiatry, 7*(5), 441–448. https://doi.org/10.1016/S2215-0366(19)30434-1

Upenieks, L., Louie, P., & Hill, T. D. (2023). Welcome to the dark side: The role of religious/spiritual struggles in the Black-White mental health paradox. *Society and Mental Health, 13*(2), 151–168. https://doi.org/10.1177/21568693221119786

van der Ven, E., & Susser, E. (2023). Structural racism and risk of schizophrenia. *The American Journal of Psychiatry, 180*(11), 782–784. https://doi.org/10.1176/appi.ajp.20230733

Vieten, C., & Lukoff, D. (2022). Spiritual and religious competencies in psychology. *American Psychologist, 77*(1), 26–38. https://doi.org/10.1037/amp0000821

Vieten, C., Oxhandler, H. K., Pearce, M., Fry, N., Tanega, C., & Pargament, K. (2023). Mental health professionals' perspectives on the relevance of religion and spirituality to mental health care. *BMC Psychology, 11*, 4. https://doi.org/10.1186/s40359-023-01466-y

Wang, P. S., Berglund, P. A., & Kessler, R. C. (2003). Patterns and correlates of contacting clergy for mental disorders in the United States. *Health Service Research, 38*(2), 647–673. https://doi.org/10.1111/1475-6773.00138

Weisman de Mamani, A., Lopez, D., McLaughlin, M. M., Ahmad, S. S., & Altamirano, O. (2023). A pilot study to assess the feasibility and efficacy of a transdiagnostic, religiously/spiritually-integrated, culturally informed therapy. *Spirituality in Clinical Practice, 10*(3), 233–244. https://doi.org/10.1037/scp0000308

Wienke Totura, C. M., Fields, S. C., & Karver, M. (2017). The role of the therapeutic relationship in psychopharmacological treatment outcomes: A meta-analytic review. *Psychiatric Services, 69*(1), 41–47. https://doi.org/10.1176/appi.ps.201700114

Wortmann, J. H., Nieuwsma, J. A., Cantrell, W., Fernandez, P., Smigelsky, M., & Meador, K. (2023). Chaplain training in evidence-based practices to promote mental health and improve care for suicidality in veterans and service members, *Archives of Suicide Research, 27*(1), 122–134. https://doi.org/10.1080/13811118.2021.1972884

Yamada, A.-M., Lukoff, D., Lim, C. S. F., & Mancuso, L. L. (2019). Survey of individuals receiving mental health services & their families. *Psychology of Religion and Spirituality, 12*(3), 276-287. https://doi.org/10.1037/t71832-000

Young, J. L., Griffith, E. E., Williams, D. R., Young, J. L., Griffith, E. E. H., & Williams, D. R. (2003). The integral role of pastoral counseling by African-American clergy in community mental health. *Psychiatric Services, 54*(5), 688–692. https://doi.org/10.1176/appi.ps.54.5.688

Part III

KEY INTERSECTIONAL ISSUES IMPACTING MENTAL HEALTH EQUITY

12 INTERSECTIONAL DRIVERS OF MENTAL HEALTH INEQUITIES

KAREN A. SCOTT AND SUNG-JAE LEE

LEARNING OBJECTIVES

After reading this chapter, readers will be able to:

- Define intersectionality and explain the utility of intersectionality in healthcare, research, public health, and policy.
- Explain the difference between mental health equity and mental health inequity.
- Explain how intersectionality shapes mental health inequities and impacts access to care for minoritized communities.
- Describe the impact of at least three intersectional drivers of mental health on the patient experience by focusing on patient dignity, safety, and autonomy.
- List intersectional approaches in policy, public health, healthcare, and research to reduce or eliminate the harm caused by intersectional drivers of mental health inequity.

INTRODUCTION

The term *intersectionality* was first coined by Kimberlé Crenshaw (Crenshaw, 1989). Intersectionality encompasses the idea that we have more than one identity, with a combination of various identity markers, such as gender, race, religion, and sexuality. These identity markers intersect with one another and shape our unique experiences and challenges. The concept of intersectionality pertains to mental health because our mental health oftentimes does not exist separately from our identity markers. For example, mental health can be affected by gender. There may be unique sexuality, age, religion, and more life stressors that accompany these identity markers.

INTERSECTIONALITY AND MENTAL HEALTH

Mental health inequities are disparities in mental health outcomes and access to mental health care that disproportionately affect certain groups of people. Many mental health disparities exist among minoritized populations. For those belonging to multiple disadvantaged or minoritized groups, these disparities are often even more prevalent and pervasive. Some inequities in the mental health care field include lack of access to care, lack of resources, discrimination, underdiagnosis, overdiagnosis, and stigma such as disproportionate overdiagnosis of psychotic disorders (e.g., schizophrenia) and underdiagnosis of mood disorders (e.g., depression). These inequities may be explained by a lack of representation, awareness, and education or institutional and systemic racism, homophobia, or transphobia, among other drivers.

For minoritized groups, recognizing, treating, and recovering from mental illness might be difficult. Depending on one's identity, mental illness may be a result of the stigma surrounding mental health care that can occur in specific communities. For example, Black,

Indigenous, and people of color (BIPOC) communities are less likely to seek support or receive quality mental health care because of cultural stigmas, internalized shame, and poverty. Those living in poverty often face difficulty seeking proper care for their mental health, and individuals in LGBTQ+ community may face discrimination at a higher rate by being exposed to homophobia or transphobia. Finally, older populations may not have the resources to reach out for support.

In the aforementioned examples, each of these communities faces challenges because of a singular identity marker. However, someone who faces more than one of these identities might be at a more significant disparity. For example, a gay Black man in his 80s who lives below the poverty line may face more challenges than a straight Black man who is in his 20s and has a high-paying job. Without an intersectional lens to look through, it might be harder to spot all the potential disadvantages each person faces.

TERMINOLOGY AND DEFINITIONS OF KEY TERMS

Throughout this chapter, we use key terms to address intersectional drivers of mental health inequities. In **Table 12.1**, we start by providing terminology and definitions of specific terms mentioned throughout this chapter.

Table 12.1 CHAPTER TERMINOLOGY AND DEFINITIONS

TERM	DEFINITION
Intersectionality	Encompasses the idea that we have more than one identity, with a combination of various identity markers, such as gender, race, and sexuality (Crenshaw, 1989). These identity markers intersect with one another and shape and influence our experience. Intersectionality is intimately tied to mental health because our mental health oftentimes does not exist separately from our identity markers. Mental health can be affected by gender, sexuality, age, and other intersectional drivers of health.
Intersectionality paradox	The phenomenon of adverse health outcomes and experiences at the intersection of high-status identity (i.e., middle-class SES) with race and gender for Black middle-class women and men. Despite an abundance of empirical data that outline the association between higher SES and better health outcomes, we observe the inverse relationship between higher SES and the disproportionate rates of homicide among Black middle-class men and infant mortality among Black middle-class women (when compared with White women with less education; Bowleg, 2012; Jackson & Williams, 2006)
Health equality	The same healthcare treatment and availability of healthcare services for all people. The goal of equality is to promote fairness, but it can work only if everyone starts from the same place and needs the same things. Realistically, people with diseases such as diabetes or physical disabilities, and people who live in communities where healthcare services are limited, will need different things to achieve and maintain their overall level of wellness.
Health inequality	Differences in the determinants, distribution, and burden of disease, injury, violence, or opportunities to achieve optimal health between one or more groups.
Health equity	Providing communities with opportunities, options, and resources to achieve the highest level of health for all people based on individual and community-level needs, independent of their social, economic, demographic or geographic circumstances. In 2019, Dr. Camara Phyliss Jones defined *health equity* as the assurance of optimal conditions for all people, a perpetual process whereby systems and structures are required to value everyone equally, rectify historic inequities, and distribute resources according to need (National Academies of Sciences, Engineering, and Medicine, 2019).

(continued)

Table 12.1 CHAPTER TERMINOLOGY AND DEFINITIONS (*continued*)

TERM	DEFINITION
Health inequity	Preventable, predictable, unfair differences in health status, disease distribution, determinants, and burden, or in the distribution of health resources among different population groups, arising from the social conditions in which people are born, grow, live, work, and age. Health inequities could be reduced and/or eliminated by the right mix of government policies. Health injustice leads to health inequity.
Health justice	A series of intentional actions designed to facilitate pathways and processes toward achieving, sustaining, or advancing health equity, through the deliberate removal of structural, systemic, and discriminatory risks, barriers, and burdens at the level of individual, interpersonal, community, and policy and politics, to actualize equal access to healthcare and health education and optimal healthy living and well-being. It rights the injustices, inequalities, and inequities that affect healthcare access, education, and outcomes.
Health injustice	A policy, practice, procedure, program, or process at the system/institutional or structural level that creates, promotes, and/or worsens a preventable, predictable, unfair health difference that disproportionately, simultaneously favors one group and harms another group; that policy, practice, procedure, program, or process is an example of a health injustice that then creates, promotes, or worsens health inequity.
Intersectional health equity	Influenced by the scholarship of Jones (2014) about health equity and Collins and Bilge (2016) about intersectionality, Lopez and Gadsden (2016) define an intersectionality health equity lens as ongoing critical knowledge theory, projects, inquiry, and praxis that can include research, teaching, and practice approaches that are attentive to the ways in which systems and structures (a) offer the assurance of optimal conditions for all people, a perpetual process whereby systems and structures are required to value everyone equally, rectifying historic inequities and (re)distributing resources according to need; (b) design and provide opportunities, options, and resources for communities to achieve their highest level of health, independent of their social, economic, demographic, or geographic circumstances; and (c) consider *how* the multiplicity of identities and systems of historical and contemporary oppressions, and age, race, sexual orientation, gender identity, national origin, immigration status, religion, ability, body size/shape, hair texture, and language shape our complex and dynamic relationships, connectedness, power, and social positioning as well as our individual and community-level social, political, cultural, legal, financial, and health capital to achieve the highest level of health free of racism, gender oppression, sexism, gendered racism, trans/queer/homophobia, xenophobia, ageism, body terrorism, and linguistic injustice (Lopez & Gadsden, 2016). In activating, affirming, amplifying, and advancing intersectional health equity, one must avoid single-issue problem identification, characterization, analysis, or solutions. According to Audre Lorde, "There is no such thing as a single-issue struggle, because we do not live single-issue lives" (Lorde, 2012, p. 138).
Mental health	Mental health includes our emotional, psychological, and social well-being. It affects how we think, feel, and act. It also helps determine how we handle stress, relate to others, and make healthy choices. Mental health is important at every stage of life, from childhood and adolescence through adulthood (WHO, 2022).
Mental health equity	Mental health equity is the state in which everyone has a fair and just opportunity to reach their highest level of mental health and emotional well-being (Stewart & Shim, 2020).
Mental health inequity	Mental health inequities are disparities in mental health outcomes and access to mental health care that disproportionately affect certain groups of people.
Equitable care	Equity is the process of ensuring that practices and programs are impartial and fair and provide optimal outcomes for all. Equitable care is when every person has the options, opportunities, and resources to attain their full and optimal potential of health with the assurance of optimal condition, where systems and structures amplify patient dignity, rectify historic inequities, and (re)distribute resources based on need, without patient disadvantage from attaining their optimal potential needs due to demographics or geographical background.

SES, socioeconomic status; WHO, World Health Organization.

Intersectional Drivers of Mental Health Inequities

When identifying factors associated with mental health inequities, we offer a list of intersectional drivers that could facilitate and/or exacerbate mental health inequities. These intersectional drivers represent analytic frameworks, phenomena, medical conditions, systems, or structures that interact in interlocking simultaneous and overlapping ways to create burdens for and/or barriers to community access to and/or utilization of opportunities, options, and resources to achieve the highest level of mental health for all people based on individual and community-level needs, independent of their social, economic, demographic, or geographic circumstances. According to Camara Phyliss Jones, MD, PhD, MPH, U.S. physician scientist, epidemiologist, and antiracist scholar activist, health equity is the assurance of optimal conditions for all people, a perpetual process whereby systems and structures are required to value everyone equally, rectify historic inequities, and distribute resources according to need (Jones, 2014).

Therefore, we offer a curated "living list" of intersectional determinants and drivers of mental health inequities that disrupt, delay, deny, and/or diminish the process of care access at the patient and community levels (e.g., ability to perceive, seek, reach, pay, and engage) and the system level (e.g., approachability, acceptability, availability and accommodation, affordability, and appropriateness; Levesque et al., 2013). Specifically, the living list of intersectional determinants and drivers of mental health inequities defines, values, and shapes options, opportunities, and optimal conditions by which individuals and communities choose to protect, secure, and actualize mental health equally and equitably, independent of individual and community demographics. Additionally, intersectional determinants and drivers of mental health inequities worsen historic oppressions and inequities and further deter the redistribution of resources according to need, favoring historically and structurally centered, protected, and privileged communities. The intentional use of language such as a curated *living list* invites the reader to consider intersectional drivers of mental health inequities not recognized or reported in our book chapter or section. **Box 12.1** outlines the curated living list of intersectional drivers of mental health inequities. The authors invite the readers to consider the historical context and contemporary implications of ecological influences within their communities, such as relational, structural, and/or political inequities, on the manifestations, measurements, and monitoring and mitigation strategies in addressing mental health inequities.

METHODS

Case Vignettes Highlighting Intersectional Drivers of Mental Health Inequities

When examining the presence and impact of intersectional drivers of mental health inequities, including a wide range of narratives on health inequality and injustice, the discrimination, erasure, and violence that structurally minoritized and marginalized communities experience are important because they impact mental health experiences and outcomes. Individual identity markers are not the issue; the problem lies within power systems and structure that cause and/or exacerbate stigma, discrimination, and oppression, including risks, barriers, and burdens to institutional care provision and community care utilization. To illustrate the impact and implications of intersectional drivers of mental health inequities, we offer two case vignettes along with the application of key strategies to consider in your intersectional analysis of harms and synthesis of solutions and recommendations.

Box 12.1 CURATED LIVING LIST OF INTERSECTIONAL DRIVERS OF MENTAL HEALTH INEQUITIES

- Racial capitalism
- Gentrification and sociocultural isolation
- Medical misogynoir (racism + sexism)
- Obstetric racism (medical racism + obstetric violence)
- Structural and systemic barriers to life and thriving (e.g., maternity care desert, housing desert, medication access)
- ACEs, chronic medical conditions, and adverse sexual and reproductive health outcomes (e.g., HIV, sexually transmitted infections, preterm birth)
- Historical and generational trauma
- SGBV
- Shame, stigma, and stigmatization
- Chronic pain syndrome, chronic medical conditions, and other comorbidities (e.g., hypertension, cardiovascular disease, diabetes, cancer)
- Co-occurring disorders (e.g., coexisting mental illness, neurodiversity, substance use disorder)
- SAVA syndemic
- Chronic pain syndrome, ACEs, and SGBV
- Intersectional violence: workplace violence (e.g., bullying, harassment, gaslighting, misogyny, and misogynoir from peers, supervisors, department chair, university deans and presidents), community violence (e.g., sexual abuse by faith-based leaders and teachers), and family/home (e.g., trans/homo/queerphobia, intimate partner violence)
- Police brutality and violence
- Mass incarceration
- Flawed carceral system and criminal justice system
- Patient-centered access to healthcare at the interface of health systems and populations: five institutional dimensions of accessibility (approachability, acceptability, availability and accommodation, affordability, and appropriateness) and five corresponding dimensions of patient abilities (to perceive, to seek, to reach, to pay, and to engage; Levesque et al., 2013)
- Restrictive reproductive health laws and financing mechanisms
- Structural competency and incompetency in health professional education

ACE, adverse childhood experience; SAVA, substance abuse, violence, and AIDS; SGBV, sexual and gender-based violence and victimization.

Case Vignette 12.1 BRE'S EXPERIENCE

A Black transgender woman, aged 19, named Bre (pronounced with a long-sounding *e*, rhymes with *bee*), with undiagnosed autism shares her lived experience managing her depression through navigating systems and structures such as healthcare, pharmacy, housing, and food insecurities. One significant contributing factor to her relapse in depression is because the pharmacy cannot find her prescription under her chosen name. Her story also includes significant intersectional determinants and drivers of mental health inequities, including undiagnosed neurodivergent condition, social isolation, stigma, abandonment, adverse childhood experiences (ACEs), and past history of sex- and gender-based violence. In order to secure food and housing, Bre must also rely on informal economies such as survival sex. In spite of these intersectional barriers, she embodies resilience and strives to continue her education and training to become a community health worker at a local community college.

In Bre's own words:

> In the labyrinth of the healthcare system, I found myself lost, my chosen name seemingly erased at the pharmacy counter. The dissonance between my identity and the prescription label triggered a relapse, a cascade of memories echoing isolation, stigma, family abandonment, and past trauma of sexual abuse. My plea for recognition echoed in empty spaces, and the pharmacist's confusion mirrored society's struggle to acknowledge my existence. The weight of family abandonment compounded with the solitude imposed by the healthcare system left me adrift. Struggling to survive, I reluctantly turned to sex work, an informal economy, to secure the basic necessities of food and shelter, caught in a web of systemic neglect that perpetuates mental health inequities.

Case Vignette Analysis

Bre's case exemplifies how intersecting identity markers and systemic barriers exacerbate mental health inequities. As a 19-year-old Black transgender woman with undiagnosed autism, her story highlights the compounded challenges of navigating healthcare, social services, and personal safety while managing depression. Her inability to access her prescription under her chosen name underscores systemic neglect and the discrimination faced by transgender individuals in healthcare settings. This experience triggers a cascade of psychological distress and reaffirms societal neglect, amplifying the stigma and isolation she endures. Family abandonment and societal marginalization further exacerbate her mental health challenges, leaving her with limited social support.

To support Bre, addressing her legal and systemic challenges is essential. Facilitating her name change and providing advocacy for inclusive healthcare practices can mitigate barriers and create a more affirming experience in healthcare interactions. Partnering with LGBTQ+ advocacy organizations can help ensure healthcare providers are educated about transgender health needs, fostering a more inclusive and respectful system. Mental health support tailored to Bre's unique needs, including trauma- and resilience-informed care for neurodivergent individuals, is also critical. Connecting her to peer support groups for transgender women offers her a sense of belonging and understanding, countering the profound isolation she faces.

Bre's reliance on survival sex to meet basic needs highlights the importance of addressing her economic and safety concerns. Connecting her to social services that provide stable housing and food security can alleviate the financial pressures that compel her to engage in high-risk activities. Concurrently, developing a safety plan with Bre, including harm-reduction strategies, offers a pragmatic approach to enhancing her immediate safety while working toward long-term solutions. These measures can provide her with the stability necessary to focus on her well-being and future aspirations.

Supporting Bre's educational and career goals can serve as a pathway to empowerment and financial independence. Assisting her in accessing financial aid and connecting her with resources at her community college, such as disability services and LGBTQ+ organizations, can help her achieve her goal of becoming a community health worker. This, in turn, positions her to advocate for herself and others in her community. Additionally, fostering connections to supportive communities can offer her the emotional reinforcement needed to navigate her challenges with resilience.

The support strategies outlined here align closely with the recommendations in **Table 12.2**, emphasizing a holistic approach to addressing Bre's intersecting challenges. By integrating

Table 12.2 TYPES OF SUPPORT AND RECOMMENDATIONS TO ADDRESS INTERSECTIONAL DRIVERS OF MENTAL HEALTH INEQUITIES

TYPE OF SUPPORT	RECOMMENDATION
Legal support	Assist Bre in accessing legal aid services to facilitate her name change and address any current and predictable legal challenges.
Advocacy for inclusive healthcare and clinical encounter	Connect Bre with LGBTQ+ organizations and healthcare advocacy groups that can provide support in advocating for inclusive healthcare practices and guidance on navigating legal and policy frameworks, barriers, and burdens. Identify healthcare allies and collaborate with local pharmacies to provide education and training on transgender health, ensuring that staff can better assist individuals with chosen names.
Mental health support	Help Bre find mental health professionals who specialize in supporting transgender women with neurodivergent conditions; offer trauma- and resilience-informed care that activates individual and community resistance. Encourage Bre to join peer support groups and identify peer mentors for transgender women, creating a space where she can share experiences and receive understanding and encouragement. Connect Bre to trauma- and resilience-informed and resource-activating therapy to address ACEs, SGBV, and generational and intersectional violence.
Housing and food insecurities	Connect Bre with local social services agencies that can provide housing, food, financial, and work assistance programs designed for transgender women, preventing and mitigating survival sex.
Safety planning and education	Provide Bre with resources and education on harm reduction practices to minimize risks associated with survival sex, including codevelopment of a safety plan that includes resources and strategies to enhance her safety while engaging in survival sex.
Education and training	Celebrate her resilience and acts of refusal and resistance. Assist Bre in exploring financial aid options and scholarships that can support her education and training as a community health worker. Connect Bre with support services at her community college, including mental health counseling, disability services, and LGBTQ+ student organizations.
Community engagement	Help Bre to connect with supportive communities that celebrate her identity and her softness, resilience, refusal, and resistance. These communities can provide emotional support and a sense of belonging. Explore mentorship opportunities at the community college to connect Bre with experienced individuals who can offer guidance and encouragement.

ACE, adverse childhood experience; SGBV, sexual and gender-based violence and victimization.

legal, social, economic, and psychological interventions, these measures uphold patient-centered care principles, focusing on dignity, safety, and autonomy. They not only address Bre's immediate needs but also empower her to overcome systemic barriers and build a foundation for long-term mental health equity and justice.

Case Vignette 12.2 BIANCA'S EXPERIENCE

A highly educated and affluent Black cisgender woman aged 42 years, named Bianca, is a first-time single mother by design, who shares her story of bullying, harassment, isolation, and stigma while navigating intersectional oppressions within and across systems of healthcare, family, and work. After battling infertility treatments, miscarriages, and broken romantic partnerships, she designed her first-time motherhood experience through donor sperm and surrogacy. Despite achieving success in family building through pregnancy, birth, and postpartum by design, severe and frequent bouts of postpartum stress and anxiety overwhelm her. She feels like she is in a war to be seen, heard, and believed in while navigating the ongoing denials and dismissals of the existence, value, and validity of her unique parenting journey by so many she trusted, starting with her team of physicians and nurses. In her extended family of Christian married heteronormative families, where wives stay home, birth large families, and care for everyone but themselves, her family members undermine her parenting lifestyle and choices. She cannot convince her postpartum medical team that she needs to start medications and see a trauma-informed, Black woman–focused therapist, (not the same as a Black woman therapist) because they fail to believe her daily episodes of anxiety and stress because publicly, "we see you on the news, on social media, and in magazines winning lots of awards and grants at work." At work, she can't convince her CEO and board of directors that she needs to extend her parental leave beyond 12 weeks, even taking unpaid leave for at least an additional 12 weeks, because "the company can't function without her unique areas of expertise and portfolio of clients." Currently, she is having suicidal ideations and fears losing her baby and her job, which adds to the fear of losing her baby and being labeled as an unfit mother.

In Bianca's own words:

> In the intricate dance of my life, I grapple with the silent storm of postpartum stress and anxiety, a tempest intensified by the relentless waves of misogynoir. Despite my public achievements, I find myself caught in a paradox where accolades at work belie the internal battles I face. The medical team, blind to my struggles, refuses the lifeline of medication and mental health therapy because I don't perform or test as "depressed," dismissing my pleas and my symptoms. My cries for help are met with disbelief from a medical team blind to intersectional struggles of affluent, highly educated, high-performing Black women.
>
> At work, the rigid and unrealistic trope of the Black superwoman schema denies me the space I need to be vulnerable and gently cared for and supported, forcing me to confront the harsh dual reality of being indispensable yet invisible. Obstetric racism, mother blame, and workplace violence weave a tapestry of isolation, stigmatization, and degradation, pushing me toward the precipice of despair, where thoughts of losing my child and job become haunting echoes in my daily existence. And then I become the thing I feared the most when growing up, an emotionally unavailable and broken mother.

Case Vignette Analysis

Immediately, one may think that Bianca's healthcare team missed an opportunity to diagnose and treat her for postpartum depression. She screened negative for postpartum depression based on the misalignment between common symptom presentation as detected by dominant instruments and actual dominant symptomatology of depression among Black women, particularly Black mothers. Among Black women, depression can manifest as emotional exhaustion, irritability and anger, heightened awareness of stress and danger, and "superwoman syndrome" (the pressure to meet heightened expectations of others while simultaneously neglecting and dismissing one's needs and self-care; Anderson & Robinson, 2023). Based on data analysis of variations in and predictors of depressive symptoms among 227 Black mothers, the authors found that Black mothers with greater depressive symptoms reported somatic symptoms (e.g., fatigue, insomnia, decreased libido) and self-critical symptoms (e.g., self-hate, self-blame, feeling unattractive) at higher rates than stereotypical depression symptoms, such as feelings of hopelessness or depressed mood. Black women also reported experiences of anhedonia (an inability to experience pleasure) and irritability. These data from 227 Black mothers also showed an association between high stress overload and greater depressive symptoms (Perez et al., 2023). In the United States, one in five pregnant or postpartum women are diagnosed with a mood or anxiety disorder during the perinatal period. *Perinatal mood and anxiety disorder* (PMAD) is a commonly used term to describe a mental health disorder occurring during pregnancy, after having a new baby, adopting, or experiencing pregnancy/infant loss. Although *postpartum depression* is often used as the umbrella term, PMAD is a more accurate and precise yet inclusive term. Any expectant or new parent can experience PMAD, particularly if navigating any of the following risk factors: stressful life evets, previous history of depression or anxiety, difficulty getting pregnant, pregnancy with twins or multiple babies, adolescent-aged parent, preterm labor or birth (prior to pregnancy age of 37 weeks), and pregnancy and birth complications (Minnesota Department of Health, 2023).

We identified and used data sources and descriptions that highlighted structural incompetency in health professional education and epistemic redlining in the dominant knowledge and narrative of depression, specifically PMAD among Black mothers and parents. Unfortunately, the systems of health, workplace, and home fail to prepare and respond to predictable adverse health experiences and outcomes among high socioeconomic status Black women, as explained by the intersectionality paradox. Bianca's fear of failing at work, with family, and at home is a manifestation of the superwoman/strong Black Woman trope that determines the cognitive and behavioral norms and narratives of Black womanhood, including a perpetual display of strength, service to others, suppression of emotions, and succeeding despite limited resources. The symptomatology was indirectly associated with depression through social isolation. Yet, Black women's moral imperative to exhibit a posture of power and an extreme motivation to succeed was associated with resilience and gendered racial centrality. Thus, the investigators determined that Black women's perpetuation of he superwoman schema may be adaptive in navigating both intersectional oppressions and psychological distress (Nelson et al., 2024). When Bianca asked for additional leave but without pay, sacrificing her own needs in service to protecting the company's finances, she embodied the strong black woman trope. *Misogynoir*, defined as anti-Black and misogynistic representation about Black women manifesting as hatred, vitriol, and violence, particularly in visual culture and digital spaces (Bailey & Trudy, 2018), fuels the denial, dismissal, and diminishing of Bianca's humanity, autonomy, and psychological distress by family, health, and work systems.

Likewise, obstetric racism serves as an analytic and a phenomenon that describes the mechanisms of subordination to which Black birthing people are subjected that track along histories of anti-Black racism and eugenics. Obstetric racism comprises attitudes and behaviors leveled against the reproducing Black body during service provision by any healthcare professional, independent of race, that sit at the intersection of obstetric violence and medical racism (Davis, 2019, 2020, 2022). During Bianca's attempts to secure medication treatment and a referral to a mental health therapist, we immediately recognize two of six dimensions of obstetric racism: (a) neglect, dismissiveness, and disrespect as a result of the health team ignoring Bianca's worsening symptoms and desperate cries for help and treating her with disdain and (b) diagnostic lapses as a result of a clinician's uninterrogated belief that Blackness is pathological, leading them to diminish, ignore, or exaggerate a patient's symptoms, resulting in an inappropriate or lapsed diagnosis. We also see reproduction of two additional dimensions of obstetric racism dominating Bianca's care experiences: (a) a health system's acts of intentionally causing pain, as manifested by the absence of empathy for Black people's physical suffering, leading to a lack of internal motivation to alleviate or reduce Black suffering, and (b) coercion, as manifested by intimidating patients to make decisions such as working longer than one's desire and/or capacity.

Bianca's fears and frustrations highlight the complex intersectional challenges faced by the professional Black mother that go unnamed, ignored, and/or diminished, emphasizing the hierarchy of priority and power in healthcare that cultivates a vicious cycle of harm, as demonstrated by repeated provider and system failures (**Figure 12.1**).

For more holistic and humane approaches to advancing mental health equity and mental health justice in healthcare systems, we invite providers and systems to elicit patient desires (see **Figure 12.2**) and identify areas of alignment and misalignment between patient expectations and patient experiences.

The areas and actions of misalignment can then be translated into provider and systems levers for policy and practice changes.

DISCUSSION

Addressing mental health inequities and improving patient/family/community-centered access to care demand a comprehensive and transformative intersectional approach—one that moves beyond the current standards of fragmented, negligent, and dehumanizing care. An intersectional approach must embody curiosity, creativity, critical thinking, compassion, and

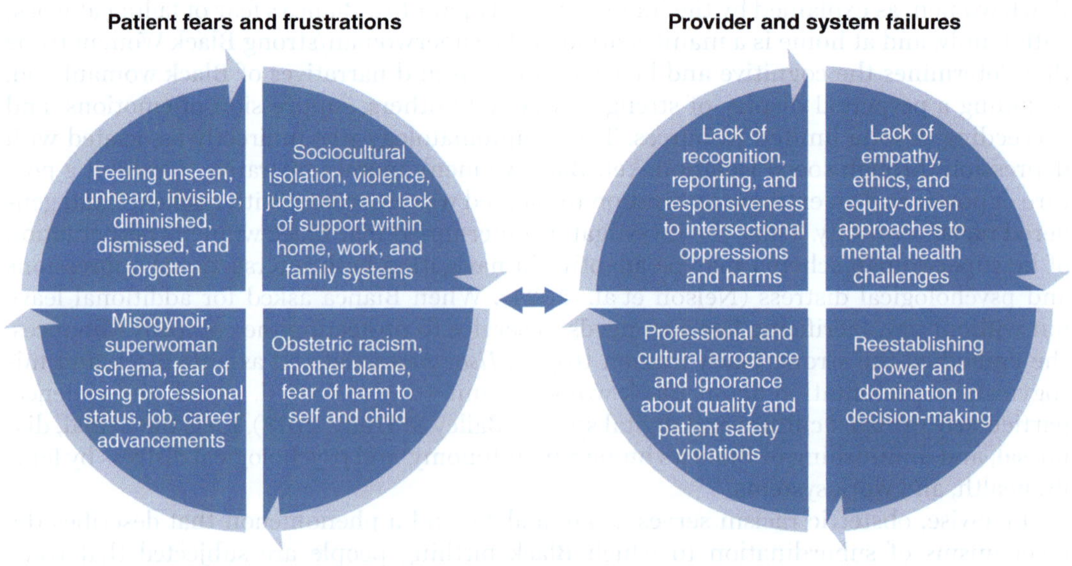

Figure 12.1 Comparison of multilevel intersectional fears, frustrations, and failures.

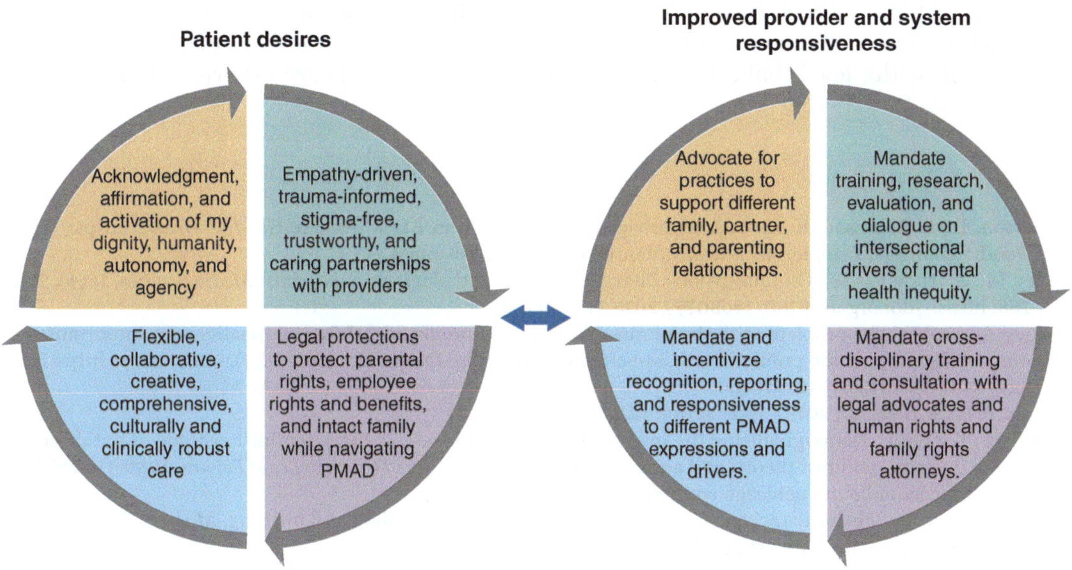

Figure 12.2 Comparison of multilevel intersectional desires and improved responsiveness.
PMAD, perinatal mood and anxiety disorder.

active community participation to identify and dismantle the systemic inequities and injustices entrenched in the design, delivery, funding, evaluation, and training within healthcare, especially in mental health. Bre's and Bianca's narratives highlight the long-standing, predictable, preventable, and unjust disparities that arise from navigating multiple interlocking systems of harm, while simultaneously contending with the intersectional forces driving mental health inequities. Through patient-centered stories, case study analyses, and visual aids, along with discussion questions, we invite readers to reimagine the overwhelming burden of navigating these powerful intersecting inequities—without the safety, security, or protection that healthcare professionals and systems are supposed to provide.

SUMMARY

Through Bre's and Bianca's narratives, we shed light on two distinct yet interconnected experiences that reveal the risks, facilitators, barriers, burdens, and rewards involved in both providing and receiving care. By centering the voices and experiences of those from structurally marginalized and minoritized communities, we invite providers, policy makers, payers, researchers, and educators to rethink and transform mental health care. This approach offers an opportunity to gain deeper insights into improving care for everyone. We present these tools, techniques, and discussion prompts as a call to action for all to envision a more compassionate and equitable health system—one that better supports individuals and communities as they navigate mental health challenges and conditions.

DISCUSSION QUESTIONS

1. What do the data reveal about mental health disparities and their causes in your work?
2. How might the way we collect and describe mental health data worsen stigma or limit healthcare training?
3. What intersectional drivers contribute most to mental health inequities in the community under consideration in your work? How does each of the intersectional drivers affect patients and providers?

4. What do patients seek in achieving mental health equity and mental health justice?
5. What are policy changes to address intersectional drivers of mental health inequities at the provider level that align patient desires for improved care experiences and outcomes?

REFERENCES

Anderson, B., & Robinson, K. (2023). Eight signs of depression in Black women. *GoodRx Health*. https://www.goodrx.com/health-topic/black-health/depression-in-black-women.

Bailey, M., & Trudy. (2018). On misogynoir: Citation, erasure, and plagiarism. *Feminist Media Studies, 18*(4), 762–768. https://doi.org/10.1080/14680777.2018.1447395

Bowleg, L. (2012). The problem with the phrase "women and minorities": Intersectionality—An important theoretical framework for public health. *American Journal of Public Health, 102*(7), 1267–1273. https://doi.org/10.2105/AJPH.2012.300750

Collins, P. H., & Bilge, S. (2016). *Intersectionality*. Polity Press.

Crenshaw, K. (1989). Demarginalizing the intersection of race and sex: A Black feminist critique of antidiscrimination doctrine, feminist theory, and antiracist politics. *University of Chicago Legal Forum, 1989*(1), Article 8. http://chicagounbound.uchicago.edu/uclf/vol1989/iss1/8

Davis, D.-A. (2019). Obstetric racism: The racial politics of pregnancy, labor, and birthing. *Medical Anthropology, 38*(7), 560–573. https://doi.org/10.1080/01459740.2018.1549389

Davis, D.-A. (2020). Reproducing while Black: The crisis of Black maternal health, obstetric racism, and assisted reproductive technology. *Reproductive Biomedicine and Society Online, 11*, 56–64. https://doi.org/10.1016/j.rbms.2020.10.001

Davis, D.-A. (2022, May 13). *A grammar of obstetric racism*. Paper presented at the Sarah Parker Redmond Center for the Study of Race and Racialisation, University College of London (Live).

Jackson, P. B., & Williams, D. R. (2006). The intersection of race, gender, and SES: Health paradoxes. In A. J. Schulz & L. Mullings (Eds.), *Gender, race, class, & health: Intersectional approaches* (pp. 131–162). Jossey-Bass.

Jones, C. P. (2014). Systems of power, axes of inequity: Parallels, intersections, braiding the strands. *Medical Care, 52*(10 Suppl 3), S71–S75. https://doi.org/10.1097/MLR.0000000000000216

Levesque, J. F., Harris, M. F., & Russell, G. (2013). Patient-centered access to healthcare: Conceptualising access at the interface of health systems and populations. *International Journal for Equity in Health, 12*, 18. https://doi.org/10.1186/1475-9276-12-18

Lopez, N., & Gadsden, V. L. (2016). *Health inequities, social determinants, and intersectionality. NAM Perspectives* (Discussion paper). National Academy of Medicine. https://doi.org/10.31478/201612a

Lorde, A. (2012). *Sister outsider: Essays and speeches*. Crossing Press.

Minnesota Department of Health. (2023). *Perinatal mood and anxiety disorders*. https://www.health.state.mn.us/people/womeninfants/pmad/index.html

National Academies of Sciences, Engineering, and Medicine; Health and Medicine Division; Division of Behavioral and Social Sciences and Education; Board on Children, Youth, and Families; Roundtable on the Promotion of Health Equity; Forum for Children's Well-Being: Promoting Cognitive, Affective, and Behavioral Health for Children and Youth; Keenan, W., Sanchez, C. E., Kellogg, E., & Tracey, S. M. (Eds.). (2019). *Achieving behavioral health equity for children, families, and communities: Proceedings of a workshop*. National Academies Press. https://www.ncbi.nlm.nih.gov/books/NBK540766/

Nelson, T., Cardemil, E. V., Overstreet, N. M., Hunter, C. D., & Woods-Giscombé, C. L. (2024). Association between superwoman schema, depression, and resilience: The mediating role of social isolation and gendered racial centrality. *Cultural Diversity and Ethnic Minority Psychology, 30*(1), 95–106. https://doi.org/10.1037/cdp0000533

Perez, N.B., D'Eramo Melkus, G., Wright, F., Yu, G., Vorderstrasse, A.A., Sun, Y.V., Crusto, C.A., & Taylor, J.Y. (2023). Latent class analysis of depressive symptom phenotypes among Black/African American mothers. *Nursing Research, 72*(2), 93–102. https://doi.org/10.1097/NNR.0000000000000635

Stewart, A.J., & Shim, R.S. (2020). Achieving mental health equity. *The Psychiatric Clinics of North America, 43*(3), xiii–xiv. https://doi.org/10.1016/j.psc.2020.06.004

World Health Organization. (2022). *World mental health report: Transforming mental health for all*. https://www.who.int/publications/i/item/9789240049338

13 GENDER BIAS, MENTAL HEALTH INEQUITIES, AND HEALTH JUSTICE

RUQAIIJAH YEARBY, PRASHASTI BHATNAGAR, CASEY GLASSER, AND DAYNA BOWEN MATTHEW

LEARNING OBJECTIVES

After reading this chapter, readers will be able to:

- Define the two levels of gender bias and how they are different.
- Identify gender bias in social systems, such as employment and medicine.
- Explain the connection of gender bias in employment and medicine to mental health inequities.
- Explain the impact of gender bias on immigrant women and their mental health.
- Describe the health justice framework and how it can be used to address gender bias and mental health inequities.

INTRODUCTION

Women have made significant gains in obtaining employment and accessing medical care after the passage of laws that prohibit sex discrimination, such as Title VII of the Civil Rights Act of 1964 (Title VII), the Equal Pay Act of 1963, and Section 1557 of the Patient Protection and Affordable Care Act of 2010 (ACA). However, research and data show that women continue to experience gender bias in employment and medicine, which has been associated with poor mental health outcomes (Khattar & Estep, 2024; Shuffrey et al., 2022; Yearby, 2019).

Also referred to as sex or gender discrimination, gender bias includes a complex array of social systems, institutional practices, norms, and interpersonal interactions used to limit women's equal access to resources and opportunities (Mullings & Schulz, 2006; Williams et al., 2019). This chapter focuses on two different levels of gender bias: structural and interpersonal. Structural gender bias is the way that individuals and organizations use institutional practices and norms to organize social systems in a manner that advantages men's access to resources and opportunities and disadvantages women's access to resources and opportunities (Mullings & Schulz, 2006; Yearby, 2018). This chapter uses the social systems of employment and medicine to illustrate gender bias experienced by cisgender women.

In employment, structural gender bias is evidenced by the practice of using prior salary history to pay women less than men even when they have the same skill, effort, and job responsibility. In 2023, 75% of women between the ages of 25 and 54 were employed; however, the women's median (middle value of) weekly earnings were $1,005, whereas men's median weekly earnings were $1,202 (Institute for Women's Policy Research, 2024). For some racial and ethnic minority women, the difference was even greater. Black women's median weekly earnings were $889 and Latinas' median weekly earnings were $800, whereas White men's median weekly earnings were $1,352 (Institute for Women's Policy Research, 2024). Structural gender bias in medicine is evidenced by medical gaslighting, where medical professionals use institutional practices and norms to dismiss women's health problems or label them as psychological in nature. Immigrant women also experience structural gender bias as a result of U.S. immigration laws that restrict opportunities for safe (im)migration and employment.

Gender bias on the interpersonal level operates through individual interactions, where an individual's conscious and/or unconscious prejudice limits women's access to resources and opportunities (Yearby, 2019). Interpersonal gender bias in employment is shown by an individual's decision to deny qualified women an interview or job because of the individual's conscious and/or unconscious prejudice against women. In medicine, interpersonal gender bias is evidenced by differences in treatment by healthcare providers. For example, Black expecting mothers frequently report experiencing mistreatment and neglect by medical providers (Markin & Coleman, 2023). Healthcare providers' conscious and unconscious biases shape the quality of the treatment Black women receive and contribute to their disproportionately high rates of maternal mortality (Kennedy-Moulton et al., 2022; Njoku et al., 2023; Owens & Fett, 2019). Immigrant women also experience interpersonal gender bias whereby they are steered to jobs that align with traditional gendered expectations, such as domestic jobs, because of an individual's conscious and/or unconscious prejudice (Menjívar & Salcido, 2013; Varela, 2023).

Experiencing gender bias has been associated with increased rates of psychological distress and depression in women, especially racial and ethnic minority women. Research shows that there is a positive correlation between anticipation of prejudice and increased psychological and cardiovascular stress among Latinas (Sawyer et al., 2012). Additionally, research shows that U.S. women are twice as likely to suffer from depression than men, which has been associated with gender inequalities (Gueltzow et al., 2023). Compared with men, women have a greater prevalence of depressive symptoms in all age groups (Gueltzow et al., 2023). Employment and educational attainment have been shown to decrease these mental health inequities for some women (Gueltzow et al., 2023). **Figure 13.1** shows the connection between gender bias, social systems, and health outcomes.

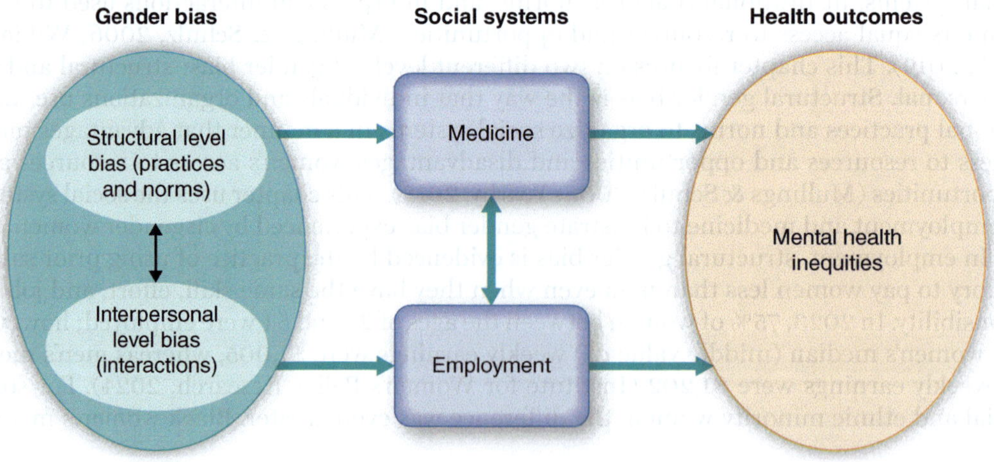

Figure 13.1 The connection between gender bias, social structures, and health outcomes.

To address gender bias and eliminate mental health inequities, individuals and organizations need to take affirmative steps to eliminate structural and interpersonal gender bias, such as using the Health Justice Framework. Based in part on principles from the reproductive justice, environmental justice, food justice, and civil rights movements, the Health Justice Framework includes three guiding principles: (a) truth and reconciliation, (b) community-driven structural change, and (c) financial supports (Yearby, 2022). By using these principles, individuals and organizations can improve their efforts to eliminate gender bias and mental health inequities by acknowledging the problem of gender bias, implementing interventions for structural change created by women, and providing support to redress the harm women have suffered. **Figure 13.2** shows the application of the three guiding principles of the Health Justice Framework to gender bias, social systems, and health outcomes.

The chapter proceeds by first examining gender bias in employment, highlighting inequities in hiring, compensation, and benefits. It then reviews gender bias in medicine, followed by a discussion on how gender bias in employment and medicine is associated with mental health inequities. The experiences of immigrant women and the resulting mental health inequities are also explored. Finally, the chapter discusses how the Health Justice Framework should be used to guide efforts for eliminating gender bias and addressing mental health inequities among cisgender women (**Table 13.1**).

GENDER BIAS IN EMPLOYMENT

In a 2019 study that surveyed 1,596 U.S. women about their experiences of gender bias, 31% reported bias in applying for jobs, whereas 41% of the women reported bias in pay and being considered for promotions (SteelFisher et al., 2019). Among those participating in the study, Asian women were less likely to report experiencing bias in employment, whereas American Indian and Black women were more likely to report experiencing bias in employment. For

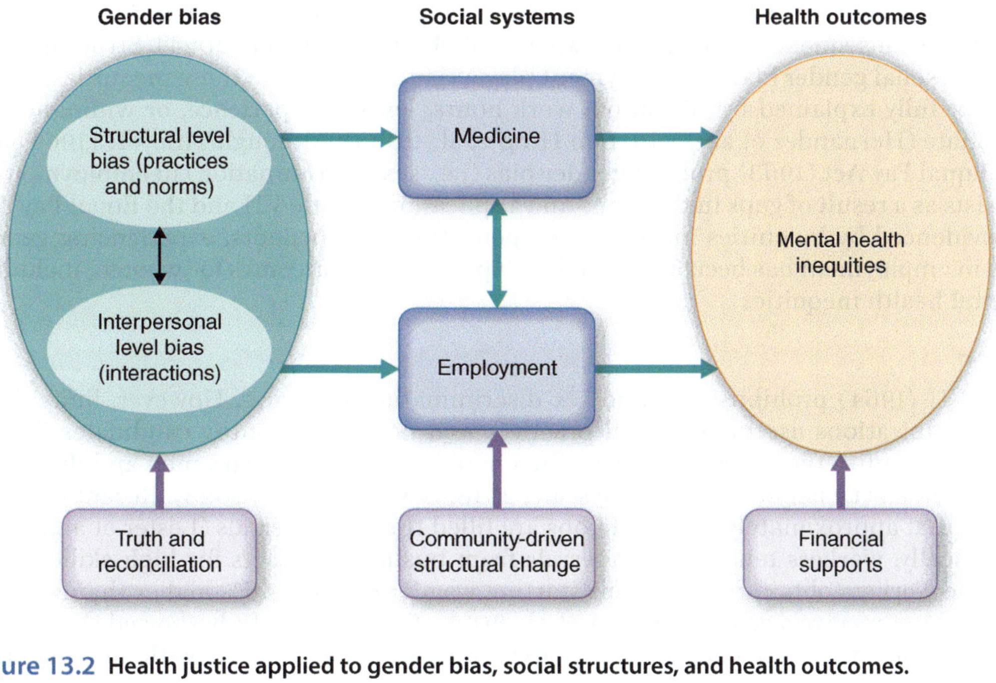

Figure 13.2 Health justice applied to gender bias, social structures, and health outcomes.

Table 13.1 DEFINITIONS OF KEY CONCEPTS

CONCEPT	DEFINITION
Gender bias	Also referred to as sex or gender discrimination, gender bias includes a complex array of social systems, institutional practices, norms, and interpersonal interactions used to limit women's equal access to resources and opportunities. There are two different levels of gender bias: structural gender bias and interpersonal gender bias.
Structural gender bias	Structural gender bias is the way that individuals and organizations use institutional practices and norms to organize social systems in a manner that advantages men's access to resources and opportunities and disadvantages women's access to resources and opportunities.
Interpersonal gender bias	Gender bias on the interpersonal level operates through individual interactions, whereby an individual's conscious and/or unconscious prejudice limits women's access to resources and opportunities.
Health justice	Health justice is achieved when gender bias is eliminated and women have the power to develop solutions to achieve health equity for their communities. The Health Justice Framework includes three guiding principles: (a) truth and reconciliation, (b) community-driven structural change, and (c) financial supports.

example, 57% of American Indian women and 50% of Black women reported experiencing gender bias in pay or being considered for a promotion, compared with 34% of Asian women (SteelFisher et al., 2019). Additionally, 49% of American Indian women and 40% of Black women reported experiencing gender bias in applying for jobs, compared with 27% of Asian women (SteelFisher et al., 2019). Despite the differences in numbers, all women reported experiencing bias in hiring, compensation, and benefits, which is further supported by the data.

Data show that between 1967 and 2021, U.S. women "experienced a cumulative loss of $61 trillion in wages due to the gender wage gap," and "lost more than $1.6 trillion in 2022 as a consequence of the gender wage gap" (Khattar & Estep, 2024). Structural and interpersonal gender bias in employment play a significant role in these inequities, which are not fully explained by education, work hours, level of experience, or willingness to negotiate (Hernandez et al., 2019; Son Hing et al., 2023). Although Title VII (1964) and the Equal Pay Act (1963) prohibit gender bias (i.e., sex discrimination) in employment, it persists as a result of gaps in the scope and application of Title VII and the Equal Pay Act. As evidenced by inequities in hiring, compensation, and benefits, experiencing gender bias in employment has been associated with poor health outcomes for women, including mental health inequities.

Hiring

Title VII (1964) prohibits race and sex discrimination in hiring. However, individuals and organizations use institutional practices and norms to identify candidates for the job and organize the interview process in a manner that advantages men and disadvantages women (Lester et al., 2021; Payscale, 2018; Son Hing et al., 2023). Recent research shows that approximately half of all jobs are filled through referrals (Lester et al., 2021). Specifically, workers tend to use referrals from business contacts for high-skilled jobs. If these workers obtain the job, their starting wages are about 16% higher than workers who did not receive a referral (Lester et al., 2021). Overall, the study showed that "referrals from business contacts primarily help high productivity workers with high incomes, particularly in high skill occupations, and thus exacerbate earnings inequality" (Lester et al., 2021). This practice disadvantages women, particularly racial and ethnic minority women.

Regardless of the job title, industry, or location, women job applicants were much less likely than men to report receiving an employee referral. More specifically, White women were 12% less likely and racial and ethnic minority women were 35% less likely to receive a job referral compared with White men, who received the most referrals for jobs (Payscale, 2018). Studies show that nearly 33% of all interviews are the result of referrals, which increases the likelihood of a job offer and a higher starting salary (Lester et al., 2021; Payscale, 2018). Structural gender bias also negatively impacts the interviewing process. When the interviewing process does not include a fixed set of questions, individual and organizational norms can influence the ratings of women candidates. Data show that women are rated lower than men during the interview process when it does not include fixed questions (Son Hing et al., 2023).

These institutional practices and gender norms used to identify candidates and organize the interview process structure the employment system in a biased manner (Lester et al., 2021; Payscale, 2018; Son Hing et al., 2023). Using referrals to create a pool of job applicants limits the pool to those with social contacts and networks rather than creating a pool of all qualified applicants. Because men tend to have greater social contacts and networks than women, the use of referrals provides more employment opportunities for men and fewer opportunities for women (Son Hing et al., 2023). The use of unstructured interviews also disproportionately benefits men and harms women because it allows interviewers to ask men and women different questions and rate them differently based on their biases. Both of these practices are examples of structural gender bias.

Interpersonal gender bias in employment also prevents qualified women from being hired. For example, research has shown that résumés with women's names submitted for high-skill jobs received half the number of callbacks as résumés with men's names, even though the résumés showed the same qualifications (Son Hing et al., 2023). When interviewers exhibit strong unconscious gender bias, they give women lower ratings than men during the interview process (Son Hing et al., 2023). Interpersonal gender bias also disadvantages women in the final hiring decision. Decision-makers favor men over women in male-dominated occupations, such as construction or engineering, because there is a presumption that women are not qualified for the job (Son Hing et al., 2023). However, even when women are clearly competent for the job, these women "are seen as having weaker social skills, and therefore are less liked and less likely to be recommended for hire, compared with a matched male candidate" (Son Hing et al., 2023, p. 4). Overall, structural and interpersonal gender biases are present in the recruitment, interview, and hiring decision-making process, which advantages men and disadvantages women. These biases are also present in compensation.

Compensation and Benefits

Title VII (1964) prohibits race and sex discrimination in compensation, whereas the Equal Pay Act (1963) prohibits differential pay between women and men working in the same establishment who perform jobs that require substantially the same skill, effort, and responsibility. Notwithstanding these laws, women continue to be paid less than men. Recent data collected by the U.S. government from 70,000 private employers and some federal contractors with 100 or more employees showed the median pay for men was higher than the median pay for women in all industries except accommodation and food services (U.S. Equal Employment Opportunity Commission, 2024). Overall, Black and American Indian women had the lowest median pay of all women and men (U.S. Equal Employment Opportunity Commission, 2024).

This difference in pay is partly the result of structural gender bias. For instance, the federal government and many states allow employers to use prior salary history to pay women less than men even when women are performing the same jobs that require substantially the same skill, effort, and job responsibility (*Rizo v. Yovino*, 2019). Women entering the workforce are often paid less than men doing the same job, which locks women into a lower prior salary throughout their entire careers (Bleiweis, 2021). By structuring the employment system in a manner that uses prior salary, which is not tied to skill, effort, or responsibility, organizations and employers are limiting women's access to equal compensation, which is evidence of structural level gender bias.

Interpersonal gender bias also limits women's compensation. Studies have shown that individuals recommend lower initial salaries for women compared with men (Son Hing et al., 2023). When women try to negotiate salaries, they are often penalized for violating gender norms (Son Hing et al., 2023). Male and female evaluators were also less inclined to work with female candidates who initiated salary negotiations compared with female candidates who did not initiate negotiations (Son Hing et al., 2023). After controlling for performance, occupation, tenure level, and business unit, men are still paid more than women regardless of whether they work in male-dominated or female-dominated occupations (Son Hing et al., 2023).

Illustrative of this point, only 32% of chief executives are women; it is a male-dominated occupation (Institute for Women's Policy Research, 2024). Although women chief executives have more elite education than men chief executives, women chief executives' median weekly earnings are $2,520 and men chief executives' median weekly earnings are $2,983 (Institute for Women's Policy Research, 2024; Son Hing et al., 2023). Even in female-dominated occupations, women still earn less than their male counterparts. About 85% of bookkeepers, accountants, and auditing clerks are women; they are female-dominated occupations (Institute for Women's Policy Research, 2024). Women bookkeepers, accountants, and auditing clerks' median weekly earnings are $922, whereas men bookkeepers, accountants, and auditing clerks' median weekly earnings are $1,100 (Institute for Women's Policy Research, 2024).

Gender differences in compensation are also associated with job segregation and promotions. Evidence shows that "[w]ithin organizations, women tend to be shuffled into different jobs than men, and these differences account for 55% of the gender wage gap" (Son Hing et al., 2023, p. 9). A 2020 study showed that even when women become well represented in an occupation, gender bias remains. For example, in the study, managers evaluating an employee based on materials randomly assigned a male name versus a female name rated "the male as more competent and advis[ed] a $3,475 higher salary, equating to an 8% pay gap" (Begeny et al., 2020). These discrepancies were partly the result of gender bias perpetuated by individuals who believe that gender bias is not happening (Begeny et al., 2020). Moreover, well-educated women receive fewer promotions than men, but if they do get promoted, the salary increase is less than men's (Son Hing et al., 2023). Research has found that these differences are tied to individuals' prejudice against women (Son Hing et al., 2023). These biases are also present in the distribution of employment benefits.

Women workers in the United States have "approximately $266 more out-of-pocket spending [for healthcare] per year than male employees (just over 18% more than men's out-of-pocket costs), which excludes pregnancy-related services" (Gebreyes et al., 2023). This results in women paying $15.4 billion more than men in annual out-of-pocket costs for healthcare, which excludes premium costs (Gebreyes et al., 2023). In all, under employer-sponsored health insurance plans, "women pay more dollars out-of-pocket than men and tend to get less coverage for every premium dollar spent" (Gebreyes et al., 2023). This is an example of structural gender bias. Employers have used institutional practices in a manner that disadvantages women by making them pay more for health benefits. Women also experience gender bias in medicine (**Table 13.2**).

Table 13.2 SUMMARY OF HOW STRUCTURAL GENDER BIAS AND INTERPERSONAL GENDER BIAS MANIFEST IN EMPLOYMENT

LEVELS OF GENDER BIAS	HOW GENDER BIAS MANIFESTS IN EMPLOYMENT
Structural gender bias	• Hiring through referrals and unstructured interviews to advantage men over women • Use of prior salary history to pay women less • Requiring women to pay more for health benefits
Interpersonal gender bias	• Fewer callbacks for résumés with female names • Employers giving women lower ratings during interviews • Recommending lower initial salaries for women compared with men • Penalizing women for negotiating salary increases

GENDER BIAS IN MEDICINE

A recent study that surveyed U.S. women showed that 18% reported experiencing gender bias when going to the doctor or health clinic and 10% reported avoiding care because they were concerned about gender bias and poor treatment (SteelFisher et al., 2019). For those participating in the study, Asian women were less likely to report experiencing bias in medicine, whereas American Indian women, Black women, and Latinas were more likely to report experiencing bias in medicine. For example, 29% of American Indian women and 22% of Black women reported experiencing gender bias in going to the doctor or a health clinic compared with 12% of Asian women (SteelFisher et al., 2019). Additionally, 27% of American Indian women and 19% of Latinas reported avoiding care because they were concerned about gender bias and poor treatment, compared with 6% of Asian women (SteelFisher et al., 2019).

Data show that although women are more likely than men to use preventive care services, there are gender inequities between men and women in the diagnosis and treatment of medical conditions (Kent et al., 2012). Structural and interpersonal gender bias in medicine—as evidenced by gender inequities in access to healthcare, medical gaslighting, and maternal mortality—play a significant role in these inequities. Although Section 1557 of the ACA (2010) prohibits gender bias (i.e., sex discrimination) in medicine, it persists as a result of gaps in the scope and application of the ACA. Experiencing gender bias in medicine has been associated with poor health outcomes for women, including mental health inequities.

Gender Inequities in Access to Healthcare

Few studies have discussed gender inequities in access to healthcare and their impact on U.S. women. The most informative study was published in 2012 (Kent et al., 2012). The study found that gender bias persists in access to healthcare in surgery, peripheral artery disease, cardiovascular disease, critical care, and cardiovascular risk factors and optimization of medical management, which was associated with health inequities for women (Kent et al., 2012). For instance, although "osteoarthritis is the leading cause of long-term disability [for women]," research indicates that women are less likely than men to be offered and receive the prescribed treatment for osteoarthritis, which improves a patient's quality of life (Kent et al., 2012).

Moreover, women are less likely than men to be admitted to the ICU, less likely than men to receive life-supporting treatments, and more likely than men to die after a critical illness, "despite similar severity of illness at the time of admission to the ICU" (Kent et al.,

2012). These inequities in access to healthcare have been associated with healthcare providers' failure to offer women the same level of care as men. This is an example of interpersonal gender bias, whereby some healthcare providers' conscious and/or unconscious prejudice against women prevents them from offering women the medically recommended care. The medical gaslighting phenomenon, on the other hand, contains aspects of both structural and interpersonal gender bias.

Medical Gaslighting

In 2022, *The New York Times* published an article on the phenomenon of medical gaslighting (Moyer, 2022). The term *medical gaslighting* was popularized by patients to describe experiences where they felt "their symptoms were inappropriately dismissed as minor or primarily psychological by doctors" (Moyer, 2022). Women report experiencing medical gaslighting at disproportionately high rates compared with men, which has been associated with health inequities (Moyer, 2022). For women in particular, physical ailments are often attributed to psychological disorders. For example, a study by Chiaramonte and Friend (2006) found that when female patients expressed experiencing coronary heart disease symptoms as well as stress, they were less likely than men to be diagnosed with coronary heart disease (Chiaramonte & Friend, 2006). Instead, their symptoms were said to have psychological origins (Chiaramonte & Friend, 2006). More specifically, doctors attributed all of the women's symptoms to mental health issues, rather than physical problems. Comparatively, the presence of stress in male patients made the same doctors more confident in diagnosing the patient with coronary heart disease, rather than attributing their heart disease symptoms entirely to the stress they reported, as they did their female patients (Chiaramonte & Friend, 2006). These results were supported by another study on gender and heart disease that found "psychological symptoms may take a central role in the assessment of female, but not male, patients" (Maserejian et al., 2009).

Medical gaslighting in this manner is an example of both interpersonal and structural gender bias in medicine. The biases of healthcare professionals are expressed in their interactions with patients and shape the diagnostic and treatment processes. Physicians use institutional practices to organize treatment in a manner that advantages men's access to healthcare resources, while disadvantaging women's access to healthcare resources (Mullings & Schulz, 2006; Yearby, 2018). Evidence shows that this can have a myriad of harmful impacts on women, including delaying treatment for women, diminishing women's trust in their ability to evaluate their own physical experiences, deteriorating women's doctor–patient relationship, and decreasing women's faith in medical professionals (Markovic et al., 2004). Illustrative of this point is a study on gynecological cancer diagnoses. In the study, women whose doctors "minimized or ignored symptoms and discomforts ... were forced to question whether their concerns were genuine ... Once their underlying illness was discovered, they questioned the competency of the health professionals who contributed to delays in the diagnosis" (Markovic et al., 2004).

Gaslighting, however, can go far beyond the exploitation of individuals. In *The Sociology of Gaslighting,* Dr. Paige L. Sweet argued that the true power of gaslighting is fundamentally a social phenomenon that involves powerful groups leveraging social narratives to manipulate the lived reality of vulnerable groups to strengthen and legitimize structural inequality (Sweet, 2019). In a variety of social contexts, politicians, psychoanalysts, academics, and journalists have appropriated the term *gaslight* to describe macro-level behavior intended to mislead a person or group of people who stand in inequitable relationship to another person or group until they lose their "sense of reality, autonomy, mobility, identity, and social supports" (Sweet, 2019). Gaslighting is an example of structural gender bias. Medical institutions and healthcare providers have used institutional practices to recreate reality, to create norms and practices that defy women's reality. These practices and recreated norms have disproportionately harmed women not only by failing to provide the medical care that they need, but also by pathologizing women as mentally unstable.

Although medical gaslighting has been used against several groups, historical and medical records indicate that this phenomenon has disproportionately harmed women. Although women of all races face challenges in receiving the same quality of care as male patients, racial and ethnic minority women disproportionately experience gender bias in medicine. The high rates of maternal mortality in Black women from preventable causes are one striking example.

Maternal Mortality

Gender bias is also racialized, as evident in the maternal health crisis disproportionately impacting Black women in the United States. Black women in the United States are at least 3 times more likely to die as a result of pregnancy-related causes than White women (Njoku et al., 2023). This gap has only widened over the past two decades (Hoyert, 2022; Huang et al., 2024). Black mothers and infants experience significantly worse health outcomes than White mothers and infants, regardless of their socioeconomic status (Kennedy-Moulton et al., 2022). A 2022 study by the National Bureau of Economic Research found that the "maternal mortality rate for Black mothers in the top quintile of the income distribution is ... about 60 percent higher than the rate among white mothers in the bottom quintile of the income distribution" (Kennedy-Moulton et al., 2022).

Since the 1990s, research has consistently shown that these inequities are in large part a result of healthcare providers' gender and racial bias (Kennedy-Moulton et al., 2022; Owens & Fett, 2019). Yet, Black mothers report being blamed by their doctors for illnesses during pregnancy and having their complaints of painful symptoms ignored (Owens & Fett, 2019). Additionally, Black mothers are more likely to experience birth trauma and posttraumatic stress disorder as a result of having higher rates of trauma exposure during their lifetime (Policy Center for Maternal Mental Health, 2023). Black women are also 3 to 4 times more likely to have a dangerous complication during labor (Policy Center for Maternal Mental Health, 2023).

Furthermore, Black women are more likely to report experiencing mistreatment, neglect, disrespect, gender bias, and racism from healthcare professionals during childbirth, which "affects their health and that of their infants" (Markin & Coleman, 2023; McLemore et al., 2018). This is an example of interpersonal gender bias, whereby some healthcare providers' conscious and/or unconscious prejudice against Black pregnant women prevents them from providing these women with medically necessary care. Gender bias in medicine, as well as in employment, has been associated with gender mental health inequities (**Table 13.3**).

Table 13.3 SUMMARY OF HOW STRUCTURAL GENDER BIAS AND INTERPERSONAL GENDER BIAS MANIFEST IN MEDICINE

LEVELS OF GENDER BIAS	HOW GENDER BIAS MANIFESTS IN MEDICINE
Structural gender bias	• Reduced access to care for women in comparison with men • Medical gaslighting, which includes failing to provide women with the medical care that they need and pathologizing women as mentally unstable
Interpersonal gender bias	• Differential and poor treatment of women compared with men with respect to receiving medically recommended care • Medical gaslighting, that is, dismissal of women's symptoms as minor or psychological

GENDER BIAS AND MENTAL HEALTH INEQUITIES

A recent study observed that there was a gender disparity in depression and anxiety disorders when women earned less than their male counterparts, which was substantially reduced when women earned more than their male counterparts (Platt et al., 2016). Thus, the researchers noted that bias embeds inequality in pay policies, which impacts the health of women. Furthermore, experiencing bias has been associated with increased depression symptoms and decreased well-being during pregnancy for Black women (Curry Owens & Jackson, 2015). Research suggests that pregnant Black women experiencing higher levels of racial bias have higher rates of depression and depressive symptoms (Curry Owens & Jackson, 2015; Ertel et al., 2012). More specifically, "well-educated Black women reported having financial pressures and fewer opportunities than White women," and this income inequity was a significant stressor for Black women throughout their life, including during pregnancy (Curry Owens & Jackson, 2015).

Moreover, experiencing gender and racial bias at work has been associated with poor mental health for women, especially racial and ethnic minority women (Harnois & Bastos, 2018). Specifically, research shows that experiencing bias is associated with higher psychological stress for racial and ethnic minority women and with self-reported poor mental health (Harnois & Bastos, 2018; Velez et al., 2018). Experiencing gender and racial bias at work has also been linked to lower psychological well-being for Black women, including "higher job stress and posttraumatic stress symptoms" (Velez et al., 2018).

Furthermore, a 2023 study showed a connection between gender bias in employment and older women's depressive risk (Gueltzow et al., 2023). Compared with men, women have a greater prevalence of depressive symptoms in all employment categories, including employment status, occupation group, and income (Gueltzow et al., 2023). These mental health inequities are greatest for Latina and Black women. Overall, the gender depression gap for all women is reduced when employment status, occupation, and prior income are equalized (Gueltzow et al., 2023). Latinas experience the greatest reduction in the gender depression gap when employment status, occupation, and prior income are equalized (Gueltzow et al., 2023). "Hence, on average, 32% of the gender depression gap can be explained by unequal opportunities in the labor market" (Gueltzow et al., 2023). Mental health inequities have also been associated with experiencing gender bias in medicine.

In addition to contributing to an increased risk of maternal mortality, Black women's experiences of gender and racial bias significantly harm their mental and physical health in numerous other ways. Historically, Black women's mental health challenges have been underdiagnosed, misdiagnosed, and undertreated (Nelson et al., 2022). Black women are also less likely to seek or obtain treatment for mental health conditions (Nelson et al., 2022). This has been attributed to factors such as the inaccessibility of mental health care, poor quality of care, and difficulties associated with cultural matching, meaning insufficient access to culturally competent mental health care professionals (Ward & Heidrich, 2009). Additionally, prior negative experiences with healthcare professionals and a "sociopolitical history involving trauma and victimization of African Americans [which has] foster[ed] cultural mistrust toward the U.S. health care system" negatively influence Black women's help-seeking behaviors (Ward & Heidrich, 2009).

In addition, sometimes healthcare providers have misdiagnosed women in the United States with mental illness for a myriad of reasons: to exercise social control, to discredit them, and as a result of internalized biases. Utilizing a misrepresentation of a woman's mental health status to restrict her freedom gained prominence as a tool of gender oppression during the 19th century. This practice is exemplified by the case of *Packard v. Packard* (Wheeler, n.d.). In 1864, Elizabeth Packard was committed to an "insane asylum" by her husband, who claimed that she was "insane" because of her views on abolitionism and women's rights (Wheeler, n.d.). Her confinement was made possible by a law passed in her home state of Illinois in 1851, which deprived married women accused of "insanity" of the right to a jury trial (Wheeler, n.d.). Packard was placed in an asylum for more than 3 years before a doctor declared her "incurably insane" and recommended her discharge (Wheeler, n.d.). Her husband prepared to have her admitted to another asylum out of state and kept her prisoner in their house in the meantime (Wheeler, n.d.). She managed to get a note to a friend who facilitated her writ of habeas corpus (Himelhoch & Shaffer, 2009). Her husband was ordered to appear before the Fifth Circuit (Himelhoch & Shaffer, 2009). The issue brought by Packard's friends was that of false imprisonment, but the judge declared it an "insanity trial" (Himelhoch & Shaffer, 2009). Packard was ultimately found "sane"; however, her husband took their children away and left her homeless (Himelhoch & Shaffer, 2009). Although Packard's husband and the asylum doctor were ultimately unsuccessful in their attempts to gaslight Packard and the court into believing she was "insane," Packard was subjected to tremendous suffering by their efforts to do so.

In the 20th century, the practice of using the diagnosis and treatment of mental illness to gaslight women evolved beyond forced institutionalization to less obvious but just as insidious manifestations. For example, the tranquilizer diazepam was marketed in the late 1960s as a treatment for "socially dysfunctional women" (Tone & Koziol, 2018). This definition included "excessively ambitious" women, "the visually unkempt, the unmarried[,] and the menopausal misfits" (Tone & Koziol, 2018). In the 1970s, clinicians believed psychologically "healthy" women were "more submissive, less independent, less adventurous, more easily influenced, less aggressive, less competitive, more excitable in minor crises, more easily hurt, more emotional, vainer, and less objective" (Roth & Lerner, 1974). Traits and behaviors that fell outside of accepted norms, such as being ambitious, adventurous, or unmarried, were deemed "unhealthy" and therefore in need of correction. Today, the treatment of women's mental health challenges continues to be riddled with inequities. At present, women are more likely to be diagnosed with depression and anxiety and to consume prescription psychotropic drugs (Bacigalupe & Martín, 2021). These differences are not explained by the prevalence of their visits or differences in their mental health, but rather by structural and interpersonal gender bias in medicine, where biased healthcare providers use institutional practices to overmedicate women for mental health issues (Bacigalupe & Martín, 2021). Immigrant women in the United States also experience gender bias, which has been associated with mental health inequities.

IMMIGRANT WOMEN AND MENTAL HEALTH INEQUITIES

There are an estimated 23 million immigrant women in the United States (American Immigration Council, 2023), nearly 5 million of whom are undocumented (Millet, 2022). Although largely overlooked in research, the mental health of immigrant women is significantly shaped by structural and interpersonal gender bias at various stages of their migration journeys to the United States (Ellman, 2019; Olukotun et al., 2019). This section focuses on gender bias in employment and detention, and the resulting mental health inequities.

Employment and Mental Health Inequities

According to the latest data released by the American Immigration Council (2023), 12.7 million immigrant women are active in the labor force; however, immigrant women earn less than any other demographic in the labor force. For example, the median household income of immigrant women is estimated to be $59.9K, whereas U.S.-born women have a median household income of $64.3K and immigrant men have a median household income of $79.0K (American Immigration Council, 2023). Undocumented women are especially overrepresented in occupations that are devalued as low wage—such as housekeeping, cooking, janitorial, and agricultural work—as a result of structural gender bias (Bhatnagar, 2022; Millet, 2022; Yearby et al., 2023).

Structural gender bias is evident in immigration law whereby governmental practices are used to limit some immigrant women's scope of employment to the domestic sphere (Legal Momentum, n.d.; Menjívar & Salcido, 2013; Varela, 2023). Specifically, a majority of immigrant women are treated as "dependents" in the U.S. immigration process; they are expected to rely on male spouses or relatives to apply for family-based or employment-based immigration status (Legal Momentum, n.d.; Menjívar & Salcido, 2013). Even after entering the legalization process, women experience long delays in receiving work permits that would allow them to enter the formal labor sector (Legal Momentum, n.d.; Menjívar & Salcido, 2013). As a result, immigrant women have no other choice than to "conform to the image of the 'non-working' or 'stay-at-home' woman" (Menjívar and Salcido, 2013) or work "underground" without legal authorization (Legal Momentum, n.d.). Immigrant women, especially those working without legal authorization, also experience interpersonal gender bias.

By working underground, immigrant women are limited to jobs that align with traditional gendered expectations and are exposed to exploitation in the form of pay gaps. For example, undocumented women are rarely hired in transportation and construction, which are relatively well paying compared with jobs associated with the domestic sphere (Varela, 2023). Additionally, undocumented women are paid "52 cents for every dollar paid to White men" and "83 cents for every dollar paid to undocumented men" (Varela, 2023). Thus, as a result of structural gender bias, immigrant women, especially undocumented women, experience "double punishment" for their gender and legal status.

Immigrant women's precarious position of working low-wage jobs has significant health implications. Women farmworkers are routinely tasked with the lowest paying jobs on the field and experience sexual abuse from employers due to structural gender bias (Goldman et al., 2021). After completing a day of work, women farmworkers are expected to provide caregiving and childcare responsibilities (Goldman et al., 2021). Women farmworkers characterize the increased labor of maintaining precarious employment while fulfilling childcare responsibilities at home as "double work days" (Goldman et al., 2021). Together, the cumulative stress of enduring gender bias and double work days contributes to women farmworkers reporting high levels of physical and psychological stress, fatigue, family conflict, marital strain, and depression (Goldman et al., 2021). The ever-expanding U.S. immigration enforcement apparatus, which includes detention, is also an example of structural gender bias, which endangers the mental health and well-being of immigrant women.

Detention and Mental Health Inequities

Most recently, the U.S. House of Representatives approved a $1.2 trillion package that heavily invests in expanding detention, specifically, "funding the detention of 41,500 people at a time, which is 7,500 above the [Fiscal Year] 2023 level and nearly three times the number of people detained when Biden took office" (Garsd, 2024; Zamore, 2024). The continued investments into the immigration enforcement apparatus keep the legacy and implementation of the 1996 Illegal Immigration Reform and Immigrant Responsibility Act (IIRIRA) ongoing. IIRIRA is a "set of laws that criminalized immigrants and centered imprisonment and punishment as core components of the nation's immigration system" (Matos & Bryant, 2022). Notably, IIRIRA, which is still in effect today, granted U.S. immigration authorities broad discretion to detain migrants, expanded the category of immigrants subject to mandatory detention, and allowed state and local law enforcement agencies to enforce immigration law (Kerwin, 2018; Matos & Bryant, 2022).

As of June 2025, 51,302 people are being held by the U.S. Immigration and Customs Enforcement (ICE) in detention facilities (Transactional Records Access Clearinghouse, 2025). There is a lack of comprehensive data on who is detained, where, and for how long by ICE due to a lack of transparency from and oversight of these detention facilities (Ellman, 2019). Detention of immigrant women, especially those who are pregnant, has been on the rise (U.S. Government Accountability Office, 2020; Ellman, 2019). Between 2016 and 2018, the number of pregnant immigrant women increased by more than 50%: from 1,380 pregnant immigrants in 2016 to 2,098 pregnant immigrants in 2018 (U.S. Government Accountability Office, 2020). Between these years, ICE detained more than 4,600 pregnant immigrant women for about 50,300 days (U.S. Government Accountability Office, 2020).

The continued expansion of detention through government-level funding while targeting immigrant women can be understood as a feature of structural gender bias. As discussed previously, immigrant women already have limited pathways to formal legal status, often having to depend on male spouses or relatives to enter the legalization process (Legal Momentum, n.d.; Menjívar & Salcido, 2013). At the same time, women and girls disproportionately experience gender-based violence across the world and, as a result, attempt to leave their home countries where they experience violence (Ellman, 2019; Kerf et al., 2023). Accordingly, more and more family units and women, who serve as the head of household, have no choice but to migrate to the United States without legal status, thus coming into increased contact with the U.S. immigration enforcement and detention systems (Kerf et al., 2023). Increasing detention of immigrant women in a gendered and racialized immigration system not only reduces their access to critical resources, but also exposes immigrant women to unsafe and health-harming conditions (Ellman, 2019; Warsi, 2023).

Detention is associated with mental health inequities because it separates immigrants from their families, children, communities, and critical services while also exposing immigrants to hazardous environments in detention (Bhatnagar, 2022; Diaz et al., 2023; Ellman, 2019). There is mounting evidence demonstrating the negative physical and mental health impacts of detention (Diaz et al., 2023; Forrest & Steel, 2023; Minero et al., 2022; von Werthern et al., 2018). Women and LGBTQIA+ immigrants, especially, face rampant gendered and sexual violence and medical neglect in detention facilities (Ellman, 2019; Gruberg, 2018; Minero et al., 2022; Pepe et al., 2023). Consequently, detention further creates and exacerbates negative mental health outcomes for women and LGBTQIA+ immigrants, who already struggle with histories of abuse and trauma (Ellman, 2019; Minero et al., 2022).

In the United States, immigrant women are exposed to structural and interpersonal gender bias through the employment and detention systems, which have severe negative implications for their mental health. The Health Justice Framework provides principles that can be used to guide governmental, organizational, and individual efforts to address gender bias and eliminate mental health inequities for all women.

ACHIEVING HEALTH JUSTICE

The Health Justice Framework includes three guiding principles: (a) truth and reconciliation, (b) community-driven structural change, and (c) financial supports (Yearby, 2022). By using these principles, employers, healthcare providers, organizations, and governments can improve their efforts to eliminate gender bias and address mental health inequities by acknowledging the problem of gender bias, implementing interventions for structural change created by women, and providing support to redress harm. Health Justice is achieved when gender bias is eliminated, and women have the power to develop solutions to achieve health equity for their communities (Yearby, 2022).

Truth and Reconciliation

To address structural and interpersonal gender bias, organizations should implement a *truth and reconciliation* process that acknowledges the existence of gender bias and offers women a mechanism to recover from the trauma of experiencing bias in the employment and medical systems. Truth and reconciliation processes provide an opportunity for women to heal and build trusting and respectful relationships with employers, healthcare providers, organizations, and governments, which are necessary for meaningful community-driven change. Some governments have already adopted this process to address racial inequities.

For instance, in 2016, Battle Creek, Michigan, adopted a truth and reconciliation process to address the historical and modern-day impacts of racism (Battle Creek Truth, Radical Healing, & Transformation, n.d.). Led by community members, the truth and reconciliation process seeks to achieve sustainable and transformative change in Battle Creek by taking the Truth, Racial Healing, and Transformation (TRHT) principles and "weaving them into the fabric of the community; embedding TRHT in all aspects of the work completed independently and in collaboration with one another" (Battle Creek Truth, Radical Healing, & Transformation, n.d.). The TRHT principles include authentic relationships; compassion, empathy, and healing; respect; historical context matters; truth; antiracism; courage; justice; lived experience; and curiosity, learning, and growth. The Battle Creek truth and reconciliation process has resulted in an anthology about racial healing in Battle Creek, and focused on transformational change in the cultural, economic, and legal systems in Battle Creek. This process should be used as a model (Battle Creek Truth, Radical Healing, & Transformation, n.d.).

In the case of gender bias in employment, employers need to admit that their practices and norms to identify candidates for the job, organize the interview process practices, decide compensation, and determine employee health insurance rates and coverage are examples of gender bias that harm women. Employers then need to provide women with an opportunity to share their experiences and stories. In the case of gender bias in medicine, healthcare providers need to admit how gender bias in medicine limits women's access to healthcare, which has resulted in harm. The healthcare system has tried to address medical malpractice by having providers apologize for their mistakes, building on the restorative justice movement "as a way for an offender to accept responsibility for hurting a victim" who did not deserve the harm (Curtis, 2010). The process should be adopted to address gender bias in medicine. Healthcare providers and institutions would have to apologize and listen to women discuss the impact that gender bias has had on them. To address mental health inequities, the truth and reconciliation processes for gender bias in employment and medicine must also include therapy and restorative services for the women who have been harmed. Women, including immigrant women, who have suffered from gender bias in employment and medicine should have the power to design the truth and reconciliation processes.

For immigrant women, governments must acknowledge that immigration laws and systems are neither gender neutral nor race neutral (Ellman, 2019; Menjívar & Salcido, 2013; Varela, 2023). More specifically, governments must admit that gendered and racialized pathways to formal legalization limit safe migration and employment opportunities for immigrant women. Furthermore, governments should provide opportunities for immigrant women to discuss how these practices have pushed immigrant women to work underground with low pay and under precarious environments, exposing them to increased contact with immigration enforcement systems. As one example of a truth and reconciliation model, immigrant women have organized several public "people's tribunals" to hold ICE accountable for its structural abuse and violence, especially toward women (Bernd, 2018). The purpose of these survivor-centered tribunals conducted with "survivors' truth commission–style testimonies" and judges who have lived experiences with detention/deportation systems is "to air the stories of survivors and others affected by the abuses there, and center them in a national discourse increasingly focused on abolition as a solution to the agency's impunity for its state-sanctioned, racist violence" (Bernd, 2018). Using such survivor-centered models offers "a space for the community to start having those conversations about what a world without ICE, without detention centers, without prisons looks like" (Bernd, 2018). Similar models can be used not only to imagine and implement community-focused solutions related to the U.S. immigration system, but also to spark community-driven change for the employment and medical systems for all women.

Community-Driven Structural Change

Employers, healthcare providers, organizations, and governments need to change their practices, norms, and behaviors that structure the employment and medical systems in a gender-biased way. These changes must be done in partnership with women to ensure that the changes address their needs. As discussed previously, eliminating the gender pay gap and equalizing employment status, occupation, income, and prior income decreases women's depression risk. Some states have already begun to adopt practices that would eliminate the gender pay gap.

For instance, California, Hawaii, and Oregon have passed equal pay laws banning employers from the use of pay history to determine salary. On July 5, 2018, Hawaii Governor David Y. Ige signed Senate Bill 2351, which prohibits prospective employers in the state from requesting or considering the wage or salary history of job applicants as part of an employment application process or compensation offer. Additionally, it prohibits enforced wage secrecy and retaliation or discrimination against employees who disclose, discuss, or inquire about their own wages or the wages of a coworker (Senate Bill 2351, 2018). On July 18, 2018, California Governor Jerry Brown signed Assembly Bill 2282, which clarified the state's existing law prohibiting salary history inquiries by employers. The law also made clear that under the California Equal Pay Act (2018), employers cannot pay employees at wage rates less than the rates paid to employees of the opposite sex for substantially similar work, except where the employer demonstrates the wage differential is based on one or more listed factors. Finally, Oregon's Equal Pay Initiative (2017), first passed in 2017 and fully implemented in 2019, prohibits employers from screening applicants or setting starting pay for new hires based on salary history. Oregon employers are also banned from seeking an applicant's salary history, either from the applicant or from other employers.

Data also show that other structural changes, including ones that are led by women, have reduced gender bias in employment. Hiring practices that remove names from résumés and blind interviewing (where the candidate's gender cannot be ascertained) have been shown to decrease gender bias in hiring (Son Hing et al., 2023). Furthermore, creating hiring decision criteria before interviewing candidates, providing only job-relevant information to the decision-makers, and having more women on the hiring committee result in more women being hired (Son Hing et al., 2023). Publicly publishing all salaries as well as increasing the pay for women (without decreasing the pay for men) has been shown to decrease the gender pay gap (Son Hing et al., 2023). In addition, there has been a reduction in gender inequities in pay and benefits when "more women are in authority positions responsible for allocating those rewards" (Son Hing et al., 2023, p. 10). Thus, as evidenced by research studies, women need to play a role in creating and implementing the structural changes necessary to eliminate gender bias in employment.

In medicine, healthcare institutions and providers need to adopt patient-centered approaches whereby patients have an equal role in determining their care. For example, research conducted by McLemore et al. (2018) showed that racial and ethnic minority pregnant women wanted more input in their care, including being able to develop birthing plans with providers. In fact, "[p]articipants saw birth plans as a way to use their voice during their birthing experiences particularly when they perceived that the staff would control when and how their social support could be present during birth. Half of the participants felt that the birth plan would protect them from stressful interactions with staff" (McLemore et al., 2018). Furthermore, racial and ethnic minority pregnant women wanted their care team to include "people who looked like them" to improve communication and lessen the stressful interactions.

Additionally, state legislatures can implement measures to address implicit bias. The California Dignity in Pregnancy and Childbirth Act provides a model. This bill requires hospitals to implement an "evidence-based implicit bias program for all healthcare providers involved in the perinatal care of patients" to combat pregnancy-related deaths among Black women caused by implicit bias among providers (California Dignity in Pregnancy and Childbirth Act, 2023). Implicit bias programs used in California and other states should be drafted in partnership with the members of the communities they are intended to serve.

Immigrant women continue to lead the way in demanding their protection and safety, including expositions of sexual violence and medical neglect they face in detention facilities (Bernd, 2018; Hodges, 2022; Warsi, 2023) and policy-level changes that expand worker protections against pesticides and heat in the workplace (Bhatnagar, 2024; Goldman et al., 2021). For example, immigrants in detention have successfully inspired and pursued state-level policy changes across the nation that prohibit public/private contracts with ICE (e.g., California, Washington, Illinois, New Jersey, Maryland, and Oregon), cut numerous contracts with ICE (e.g., Alabama, California, Georgia, Maryland, Massachusetts, Oregon, and New Jersey), and limit immigration detention (e.g., Florida, Louisiana, and North Carolina; Hodges, 2022). Such structural change should be pursued across more states and on the federal level as well.

In partnership with immigrant women, governments must build pathways to inclusion and citizenship that are "open, affordable, and accessible to all immigrant women, including those whose work is unpaid (e.g., those in the care economy), and those employed in the informal economy" (Menjívar & Salcido, 2013). For starters, governments need to put an end to the ever-expanding immigration enforcement system, including detention systems, and instead build safe pathways to (im)migration for all (im)migrants (Achiume, 2019; Walia, 2022). These examples should serve as a model for community-driven structural change in the immigration system.

Financial Supports

Employers, healthcare providers, organizations, and governments must provide financial supports to redress the harm caused by structural and interpersonal gender bias. Some governments have tried to provide financial support for individuals who have experienced bias. For example, California is working to provide reparations to Black individuals. This financial relief should be provided to women to offset the decades of unequal social and economic conditions they have experienced. For employment and healthcare inequities, this could be achieved by providing women, including immigrant women, with additional compensation and health benefits as well as discounts for employer-sponsored health insurance coverage.

In addition, many immigrant women who work in low-wage jobs do not have access to basic health and public benefits, including health insurance and paid leave (Goldman et al., 2021; National Latina Institute for Reproductive Justice & National Asian Pacific American Women's Forum [NAPAWF], 2023). The Personal Responsibility and Work Opportunity Reconciliation Act, in particular, excludes a majority of immigrants from accessing public benefits such as Medicaid, disproportionately reducing immigrant women's access to healthcare (Yearby et al., 2023). Thus, it is critical for governments and employers to provide financial support to immigrant women in the form of health and public benefits by passing, for example, the Health Equity and Access under the Law (HEAL) for Immigrant Families that "removes the five-year bar in Medicaid/CHIP [Children's Health Insurance Program], opens up the ACA marketplace, and expands access to Medicare, so that immigrants can access the affordable health care they need" (National Latina Institute for Reproductive Justice and NAPAWF, 2023). Additionally, federal and state governments should pass robust paid-leave laws that offer paid leave to *all* workers for *any* reason, including immigrant women who are often excluded from such protections.

SUMMARY

Structural and interpersonal gender biases have resulted in centuries of unequal social and economic conditions for women, which have exacerbated mental health inequities among women and will take generations to fix. A 2024 report found that "if the gender wage gap continues on its path from 2000 to 2002, it would take until 2067 for it to close for women working full time, year round" (Khattar & Estep, 2024). Thus, it is going to take a long time, even generations, of intentional work to eradicate gender bias and eliminate mental health disparities. During this time, employers, healthcare providers, organizations, and governments must acknowledge the problem of structural and interpersonal gender bias, implement interventions for structural change created by women, and provide support to redress harm women have suffered.

DISCUSSION QUESTIONS

1. How does gender bias limit women's access to medicine and employment?
2. How is gender bias connected to mental health inequities?
3. What are some ways the medical system can use the truth and reconciliation process to eliminate gender bias and mental health inequities?
4. What are some ways that employers can work with women to eliminate gender bias and mental health inequities?
5. What are two ways that immigrant women are disproportionately harmed by gender bias?
6. Why is it necessary to adopt measures to redress harm for gender bias?

REFERENCES

Achiume, E. T. (2019). The postcolonial case for rethinking borders. *Dissent*, *66*(3), 27–32. https://doi.org/10.1353/dss.2019.0043

American Immigration Council. (2023). *A snapshot of immigrant women in the United States*. https://www.americanimmigrationcouncil.org/research/snapshot-immigrant-women-united-states

Assembly Bill 2282, Reg. Sess. § 432.3 (Cal 2018).

Bacigalupe, A., & Martín, U. (2021). Gender inequalities in depression/anxiety and the consumption of psychotropic drugs: Are we medicalising women's mental health? *Scandinavian Journal of Public Health*, *49*(3), 317–324. https://doi.org/10.1177/1403494820944736

Battle Creek Truth, Radical Healing, & Transformation. (n.d.). *About Battle Creek coalition for TRHT.* https://www.bctrht.org/about

Begeny, C. T., Ryan, M. K., Moss-Racusin, C. A., & Ravetz, G. (2020). In some professions, women have become well represented, yet gender bias persists—Perpetuated by those who think it is not happening. *Science Advances*, *6*(26), eaba7814. https://doi.org/10.1126/sciadv.aba7814

Bernd, C. (2018, May 8). Survivor-centered tribunals find ICE guilty of abuses, push for agency's abolition. *Truthout*. https://truthout.org/articles/survivor-centered-tribunals-find-ice-guilty-of-abuses-push-for-agency-s-abolition/

Bhatnagar, P. (2022). Deportable until essential: How the neoliberal U.S. immigration system furthers racial capitalism and operates as a negative social determinant of health. *Georgetown Immigration Law Journal*, *36*(3), 1017–1040.

Bhatnagar, P. (2024). The pregnant workers fairness act leaves agricultural workers behind. *Journal of Law, Medicine & Ethics*, *52*(S1), 12–15. https://doi.org/10.1017/jme.2024.34

Bleiweis, R. (2021). *Why salary history bans matter to securing equal pay*. Center for American Progress. https://www.americanprogress.org/article/salary-history-bans-matter-securing-equal-pay/

California Dignity in Pregnancy and Childbirth Act, A.B. 2319, Cal. Leg. (2023).

California Equal Pay Act, Cal. Lab. Code § 432.3 (2018).

Chiaramonte, G., & Friend, R. (2006). Medical students' and residents' gender bias in the diagnosis, treatment, and interpretation of coronary heart disease symptoms. *Health Psychology, 25*(3), 255–266. https://doi.org/10.1037/0278-6133.25.3.255

Curry Owens, T., & Jackson, F. M. (2015). Examining life-course socioeconomic position, contextualized stress, and depression among well-educated african-american pregnant women. *Women's Health Issues: Official Publication of the Jacobs Institute of Women's Health, 25*(4), 382–389. https://doi.org/10.1016/j.whi.2015.05.001

Curtis, D. (2010, July). Sometimes, an apology can deter a lawsuit. *California Bar Journal.* https://www.calbarjournal.com/July2010/TopHeadlines/TH1.aspx

Diaz, C., Ortiz, V., Sanchez, L., Fernandez, J., Andrade, E. A., Akiyama, M. J., & Ross, J. (2023). Harmful by design—A qualitative study of the health impacts of immigration detention. *Journal of General Internal Medicine, 38*(9), 2030–2037. https://doi.org/10.1007/s11606-022-07914-6

Ellman, N. (2019). *Immigration detention is dangerous for women's health and rights.* Center for American Progress. https://www.americanprogress.org/article/immigration-detention-dangerous-womens-health-rights/

The Equal Pay Act of 1963, 29 U.S.C. § 206 (1963).

Ertel, K. A., James-Todd, T., Kleinman, K., Krieger, N., Gillman, M. W., Wright, R., & Rich-Edwards, J. (2012). Racial discrimination, response to unfair treatment, and depressive symptoms among pregnant black and African American women in the United States. *Annals of Epidemiology, 22*(12), 840–846. https://doi.org/10.1016/j.annepidem.2012.10.001

Forrest, W., & Steel, Z. (2023). The impact of immigration detention on the mental health of refugees and asylum seekers. *Journal of Traumatic Stress, 36*(3), 642–653. https://doi.org/10.1002/jts.22944

Garsd, J. (2024, March 22). House appropriations bill would increase border enforcement capacity. *NPR.* https://www.npr.org/2024/03/22/1240273427/immigration-migrants-house-budget-border-patrol-ice-enforcement

Gebreyes, K., Davis, A., Farina, M., Broaden, T., & Smilanich, S. (Klapperich). (2023). *Hiding in plain sight: The health care gender toll* (pp. 1–12). Deloitte. https://www2.deloitte.com/content/dam/Deloitte/us/Documents/life-sciences-health-care/us-lshc-health-gender-gap.pdf

Goldman, S., Aspenson, A., Bhatnagar, P., & Martin, R. (2021). *Essential and in crisis: A review of the public threats facing farmworkers in the US.* Johns Hopkins Center for a Livable Future. https://clf.jhsph.edu/sites/default/files/2021-05/essential-and-in-_crisis-a-review-of-the-public-health-threats-facing-farmworkers-in-the-us.pdf

Gruberg, S. (2018, May 30). *ICE's rejection of its own rules is placing LGBT immigrants at severe risk of sexual abuse.* Center for American Progress. https://www.americanprogress.org/article/ices-rejection-rules-placing-lgbt-immigrants-severe-risk-sexual-abuse/

Gueltzow, M., Bijlsma, M. J., van Lenthe, F. J., & Myrskylä, M. (2023). The role of labor market inequalities in explaining the gender gap in depression risk among older US adults. *Social Science & Medicine, 332,* 116100. https://doi.org/10.1016/j.socscimed.2023.116100

Harnois, C. E., & Bastos, J. L. (2018). Discrimination, harassment, and gendered health inequalities: Do perceptions of workplace mistreatment contribute to the gender gap in self-reported health? *Journal of Health and Social Behavior, 59*(2), 283–299. https://doi.org/10.1177/0022146518767407

Hernandez, M., Avery, D. R., Volpone, S. D., & Kaiser, C. R. (2019). Bargaining while Black: The role of race in salary negotiations. *The Journal of Applied Psychology, 104*(4), 581–592. https://doi.org/10.1037/apl0000363

Himelhoch, M. S., & Shaffer, A. H. (1979). Elizabeth Packard: Nineteenth-century crusader for the rights of mental patients. *Journal of American Studies, 13*(3), 343–375. https://doi.org/10.1017/S0021875800007404

Hodges, E. (2022). *Building power: Charting recent victories in the movement to end immigration detention in the United States* (pp. 1–111). NY Dignity Not Detention. https://nydignitynotdetention.org/wp-content/uploads/2022/06/Building-Power_Charting-Recent-Victories-Report.pdf

Hoyert, D. L. (2022). *Maternal mortality rates in the United States, 2020* (pp. 1–5). Centers for Disease Control and Prevention, National Center for Health Statistics, Division of Vital Statistics. https://www.cdc.gov/nchs/data/hestat/maternal-mortality/2020/E-stat-Maternal-Mortality-Rates-2022.pdf

Huang, R. S., Spence, A. R., & Abenhaim, H. A. (2024). Racial disparities in national maternal mortality trends in the United States from 2000 to 2019: A population-based study on 80 million live births. *Archives of Gynecology and Obstetrics, 309*(4), 1315–1322. https://doi.org/10.1007/s00404-023-06999-6

Institute for Women's Policy Research. (2024, March). *Women earn less than men whether they work in same or different occupations.* https://iwpr.org/wp-content/uploads/2024/03/Occupational-Wage-Gap-2024-Fact-Sheet-1.pdf

Kennedy-Moulton, K., Miller, S., Persson, P., Rossin-Slater, M., Wherry, L., & Aldana, G. (2022). *Maternal and infant health inequality: New evidence from linked administrative data* (Working paper 30693). National Bureau of Economic Research. https://doi.org/10.3386/w30693

Kent, J. A., Patel, V., & Varela, N. A. (2012). Gender disparities in health care. *The Mount Sinai Journal of Medicine, New York, 79*(5), 555–559. https://doi.org/10.1002/msj.21336

Kerf, M., Contreras-Urbina, M., Aguilera, A. I., Padron, E., & Burgos, C. X. M. (2023, June 6). *Migrant women and girls in Central America risk their lives in search of a better future.* World Bank Blogs. https://blogs.worldbank.org/en/latinamerica/migrant-women-girls-search-better-future-central-america

Kerwin, D. (2018). From IIRIRA to trump: Connecting the dots to the current US immigration policy crisis. *Journal on Migration and Human Security, 6*(3), 192–204. https://doi.org/10.1177/2331502418786718

Khattar, R., & Estep, S. (2024, March 14). *Playbook for the advancement of women in the economy.* https://www.americanprogress.org/article/playbook-for-the-advancement-of-women-in-the-economy/

Legal Momentum. (n.d.). *Gender bias and immigration policy.* The Women's Legal Defense and Education Fund. Retrieved March 24, 2024, from https://www.legalmomentum.org/gender-bias-and-immigration-policy

Lester, B., Rivers, D. A., & Topa, G. (2021). *The heterogeneous impact of referrals on labor market outcomes* (No. 987, pp. 1–52). Federal Reserve Bank of New York. https://www.newyorkfed.org/medialibrary/media/research/staff_reports/sr987.pdf?sc_lang=en

Markin, R. D., & Coleman, M. N. (2023). Intersections of gendered racial trauma and childbirth trauma: Clinical interventions for Black women. *Psychotherapy (Chicago, Ill.), 60*(1), 27–38. https://doi.org/10.1037/pst0000403

Markovic, M., Manderson, L., & Quinn, M. (2004). Embodied changes and the search for gynecological cancer diagnosis. *Medical Anthropology Quarterly, 18*(3), 376–396. https://doi.org/10.1525/maq.2004.18.3.376

Maserejian, N. N., Link, C. L., Lutfey, K. L., Marceau, L. D., & McKinlay, J. B. (2009). Disparities in physicians' interpretations of heart disease symptoms by patient gender: Results of a video vignette factorial experiment. *Journal of Women's Health, 18*(10), 1661–1667. https://doi.org/10.1089/jwh.2008.1007

Matos, K., & Bryant, E. (2022, June 28). *25 Years of IIRIRA shows immigration law gone wrong.* Vera Institute of Justice. https://www.vera.org/news/25-years-of-iirira-shows-immigration-law-gone-wrong

McLemore, M. R., Altman, M. R., Cooper, N., Williams, S., & Rand, L. (2018). Health care experiences of pregnant, birthing, and postnatal women of color at risk for preterm birth. *Social Science & Medicine, 201*, 127–135. https://doi.org/10.1016/j.socscimed.2018.02.013

Menjívar, C., & Salcido, O. (2013). *Gendered paths to legal status: The case of Latin American immigrants in Phoenix, Arizona* (pp. 1–11). American Immigration Council. https://www.americanimmigrationcouncil.org/sites/default/files/research/genderedpaths052813.pdf

Millet, E. (2022, March 23). *A demographic profile of undocumented immigrant women and estimates of those potentially eligible for permanent residence under pending bills.* The Center for Migration Studies of New York (CMS). https://cmsny.org/undocumented-women-032322/

Minero, L. P., Domínguez, S., Budge, S. L., & Salcedo, B. (2022). Latinx trans immigrants' survival of torture in U.S. detention: A qualitative investigation of the psychological impact of abuse and mistreatment. *International Journal of Transgender Health, 23*(1–2), 36–59. https://doi.org/10.1080/26895269.2021.1938779

Moyer, M. W. (2022, March 28). Women are calling out 'medical gaslighting.' *The New York Times.* https://www.nytimes.com/2022/03/28/well/live/gaslighting-doctors-patients-health.html

Mullings, L., & Schulz, A. J. (2006). Intersectionality and health: An introduction. In A. J. Schulz & L. Mullings (Eds.), *Gender, race, class, & health: Intersectional approaches* (pp. 3–17). Jossey-Bass/Wiley.

National Latina Institute for Reproductive Justice & National Asian Pacific American Women's Forum. (2023). *The Health Equity and Access Under the Law (HEAL) for Immigrant Families Act of 2023: Talking points.* https://napawf.org/wp-content/uploads/2023/08/July-2023-HEAL-Talking-Points.pdf

Nelson, T., Ernst, S. C., Tirado, C., Fisse, J. L., & Moreno, O. (2022). Psychological distress and attitudes toward seeking professional psychological services among Black women: The role of past mental health treatment. *Journal of Racial and Ethnic Health Disparities, 9*(2), 527–537. https://doi.org/10.1007/s40615-021-00983-z

Njoku, A., Evans, M., Nimo-Sefah, L., & Bailey, J. (2023). Listen to the whispers before they become screams: Addressing black maternal morbidity and mortality in the United States. *Healthcare, 11*(3), Article 3. https://doi.org/10.3390/healthcare11030438

Olukotun, O., Gondwe, K., & Mkandawire-Valhmu, L. (2019). The mental health implications of living in the shadows: The lived experience and coping strategies of undocumented African migrant women. *Behavioral Sciences, 9*(12), 127. https://doi.org/10.3390/bs9120127

Oregon Equal Pay Initiative, ORS § 659A.357 (2017).

Owens, D. C., & Fett, S. M. (2019). Black maternal and infant health: Historical legacies of slavery. *American Journal of Public Health, 109*(10), 1342–1345. https://doi.org/10.2105/AJPH.2019.305243

Payscale. (2018). *The impact of job referrals: Effects on pay, engagement, diversity.* https://www.payscale.com/research-and-insights/impact-of-job-referrals/

Pepe, C. S., Saadi, A., & Molina, R. L. (2023). Reproductive justice in the U.S. immigration detention system. *Obstetrics and Gynecology, 142*(4), 804–808. https://doi.org/10.1097/AOG.0000000000005335

Platt, J., Prins, S., Bates, L., & Keyes, K. (2016). Unequal depression for equal work? How the wage gap explains gendered disparities in mood disorders. *Social Science & Medicine, 149*, 1–8. https://doi.org/10.1016/j.socscimed.2015.11.056

Policy Center for Maternal Mental Health. (2023, December 11). *Issue brief: Black maternal mental health.* Policy Center for Maternal Mental Health—Formerly 2020 Mom. https://www.2020mom.org/blog/issue-brief-black-maternal-mental-health

Rizo v. Yovino, 887 F.3d 453 (9th Cir. 2018), vacated, 139 S. Ct. 706, 710 (2019).

Roth, R. T., & Lerner, J. (1974). Sex-based discrimination in the mental institutionalization of women. *California Law Review, 62*(3), 789–815.

Sawyer, P. J., Major, B., Casad, B. J., Townsend, S. S. M., & Mendes, W. B. (2012). Discrimination and the stress response: Psychological and physiological consequences of anticipating prejudice in interethnic interactions. *American Journal of Public Health, 102*(5), 1020–1026. https://doi.org/10.2105/AJPH.2011.300620

Section 1557 of the Patient Protection and Affordable Care Act, 42 U.S.C. § 18116(a) (2010).

Senate Bill 2351, 30th Leg., Reg. Sess. § 1, § 378-2.4 (Haw. 2018).

Shuffrey, L. C., Thomason, M. E., & Brito, N. H. (2022). Improving perinatal maternal mental health starts with addressing structural inequities. *JAMA Psychiatry, 79*(5), 387–388. https://doi.org/10.1001/jamapsychiatry.2022.0097

Son Hing, L. S., Sakr, N., Sorenson, J. B., Stamarski, C. S., Caniera, K., & Colaco, C. (2023). Gender inequities in the workplace: A holistic review of organizational processes and practices. *Human Resource Management Review, 33*(3), 100968. https://doi.org/10.1016/j.hrmr.2023.100968

SteelFisher, G. K., Findling, M. G., Bleich, S. N., Casey, L. S., Blendon, R. J., Benson, J. M., Sayde, J. M., & Miller, C. (2019). Gender discrimination in the United States: Experiences of women. *Health Services Research, 54*(S2), 1442–1453. https://doi.org/10.1111/1475-6773.13217

Sweet, P. L. (2019). The sociology of gaslighting. *American Sociological Review, 84*(5), 851–875. https://doi.org/10.1177/0003122419874843

Title VII of the Civil Rights Act of 1964, 42 U.S.C. § 2000e-2(a)(1) (1964).

Tone, A., & Koziol, M. (2018). (F)ailing women in psychiatry: Lessons from a painful past. *CMAJ: Canadian Medical Association Journal, 190*(20), E624–E625. https://doi.org/10.1503/cmaj.171277

Transactional Records Access Clearinghouse. (2025). Immigration detention quick facts. *TRAC Immigration.* https://tracreports.org/immigration/quickfacts/detention.html#detention_held

U.S. Equal Employment Opportunity Commission. (2024, March 12). *EEOC releases data dashboard for 2017 & 2018 pay data collection.* https://www.eeoc.gov/newsroom/eeoc-releases-data-dashboard-2017-2018-pay-data-collection

U. S. Government Accountability Office. (2021, February 25). *Immigration detention: Care of pregnant women in DHS facilities.* U.S. GAO. https://www.gao.gov/products/gao-20-330

Varela, N. V. (2023). *Double disadvantage: A profile of undocumented women in the United States* (pp. 1–20). Gender Equity Policy Institute. https://thegepi.org/wp-content/uploads/2023/06/GEPI-Double-Disadvantage.pdf

Velez, B. L., Cox, R., Polihronakis, C. J., & Moradi, B. (2018). Discrimination, work outcomes, and mental health among women of color: The protective role of womanist attitudes. *Journal of Counseling Psychology, 65*(2), 178–193. https://doi.org/10.1037/cou0000274

von Werthern, M., Robjant, K., Chui, Z., Schon, R., Ottisova, L., Mason, C., & Katona, C. (2018). The impact of immigration detention on mental health: A systematic review. *BMC Psychiatry, 18*(1), 382. https://doi.org/10.1186/s12888-018-1945-y

Walia, H. (2022, November 16). There is no "migrant crisis." *Boston Review.* https://www.bostonreview.net/articles/there-is-no-migrant-crisis/

Ward, E. C., & Heidrich, S. M. (2009). African American women's beliefs about mental illness, stigma, and preferred coping behaviors. *Research in Nursing & Health, 32*(5), 480–492. https://doi.org/10.1002/nur.20344

Warsi, Z. (2023, July 21). "Immensely invisible": Women fighting ICE's inaction on sexual abuses. *Futuro Investigates.* https://futuroinvestigates.org/investigative-stories/immensely-invisible/immensely-invisible-women-fighting-ices-inaction-on-sexual-abuses/

Wheeler, S. (n.d.). *Illinois Supreme Court history: Elizabeth Packard and mental health laws.* Administrative Office of the Illinois Courts. https://www.illinoiscourts.gov/News/1037/Illinois-Supreme-Court-history-Elizabeth-Packard-and-mental-health-laws/news-detail/

Williams, D. R., Lawrence, J. A., & Davis, B. A. (2019). Racism and health: Evidence and needed research. *Annual Review of Public Health, 40,* 105–125. https://doi.org/10.1146/annurev-publhealth-040218-043750

Yearby, R. (2018). The impact of structural racism in employment and wages on minority women's health. *Human Rights Magazine, 43*(3), 21–25. https://www.americanbar.org/groups/crsj/publications/human_rights_magazine_home/the-state-of-healthcare-in-the-united-states/minority-womens-health/

Yearby, R. (2019). Internalized oppression: The impact of gender and racial bias in employment on the health status of women of color. *Seton Hall Law Review, 49*(5), 1037–1066. https://scholarship.shu.edu/cgi/viewcontent.cgi?article=1700&context=shlr

Yearby, R. (2022). The social determinants of health, health disparities, and health justice. *The Journal of Law, Medicine & Ethics, 50*(4), 641–649. https://doi.org/10.1017/jme.2023.3

Yearby, R., Lewis, C., & Gibson, C. (2023). Incorporating structural racism, employment discrimination, and economic inequities in the social determinants of health framework to understand agricultural worker health inequities. *American Journal of Public Health, 113*(S1), S65–S71. https://doi.org/10.2105/AJPH.2022.307166

Zamore, M. (2024, March 21). *ACLU statement on FY24 appropriations bill funding immigrant detention, anti-immigrant policies.* American Civil Liberties Union. https://www.aclu.org/press-releases/aclu-statement-on-fy24-appropriations-bill-funding-immigrant-detention-anti-immigrant-policies

14 THE RELATIONSHIP BETWEEN MENTAL HEALTH AND VIOLENCE: UNMASKING THE MYTHS

JOSEPH V. SAKRAN, IFE SHOYOMBO, AND DEBRA M. FURR-HOLDEN

LEARNING OBJECTIVES

After reading this chapter, readers will be able to:

- Describe temporal trends and the public health burden of violence in the United States.
- Explicate how mental health and violence are correlated at the individual and community levels.
- Identify strategies to address community violence and mental health through evidence-based interventions, programs, and policies.
- Describe research gaps at the nexus of mental health and violence and evidence-based interventions to reduce disparities and inequities.
- Discuss opportunities for effective communication of data and science to improve community violence and mental health.

INTRODUCTION

The Epidemiology of Violence

The epidemiology of violence in the United States is complex and includes the study of the distribution and determinants of violence at both a personal and a community level. Violence often affects geographic and demographic subgroups at different rates, in a variety of ways, and has different underlying risk factors that contribute to violence perpetration and victimization. Important factors, such as the prevalence, incidence, and patterns of violent behaviors, are assessed to identify interventions to prevent and reduce various forms of violence.

Violence presents in multiple forms, including intimate partner violence (IPV), domestic violence (DV), homicide, and suicide. National estimates of IPV confirm that at least one in four women and one in seven men aged 18 and older in the United States have been the victim of severe physical violence by an intimate partner in their lifetime, and approximately one in four women and one in 10 men report experiencing some form of IPV annually (Smith et al., 2018). Despite these alarming statistics, the rates of IPV have been decreasing over time (Catalano, 2012). According to the U.S. Department of Justice, from 1994 to 2010, the overall rate of IPV in the United States declined by 64%, from 9.8 victimizations per 1,000 to 3.6 per 1,000 among those aged 12 or older. In the same period, 80% of IPV victims were female, with females aged 18 to 34 experiencing the highest rates of IPV. The rate of IPV decreased the most for Hispanic females, declining 78%, compared with nearly 61% for White women, 62% for Black women, and 40% for women of other races.

Whereas the term *intimate partner violence* references abuse or aggression within a romantic relationship, including the behavior of current and former spouses or dating partners, domestic violence includes violence against children, older adults, and other familial members. Data collection for elder abuse is difficult to quantify because of underreporting, and elder abuse represents a significant public health problem on a global scale (Pillemer et al., 2016). Child abuse also varies by age, socioeconomic status, geography, race, and ethnicity, and according to the National Children's Alliance, impacts more than 600,000 children in the United States annually (National Children's Alliance, 2024).

In the United States, homicide continues to disproportionately affect young Black males aged 15 to 24 at almost 17 times the rate of other demographic groups, and continues to increase even as homicide rates for older Black men have fallen over the past half-century (Evans & Kotowski, 2024; Jones-Eversley et al., 2020). Suicide rates, on the other hand, have reached an all-time high in the United States, with the highest rates found among men, Native Americans, and non-Hispanic Whites. In 2020, more than half of all homicides and all suicides in the United States involved firearms (Centers for Disease Control and Prevention [CDC], 2022). The number of firearm-related injuries and deaths has fluctuated over the past several decades and significantly increased during the COVID-19 pandemic.

The Impact of the COVID Pandemic on Violence

Globally, the COVID-19 pandemic was associated with increased rates of DV (Wake & Kandula, 2022). A review of DV in the United States included local police departments reporting as much as a 27% increase in reported rates of DV in 2020 compared with 2019 (Boserup et al., 2020). The mental health impacts generated by the pandemic's effects on economic uncertainty, isolation, depression, and substance use that contribute to increased rates of DV were widely expected to also affect suicide rates (Wasserman et al., 2020). However, other forms of violence also saw significant rises during the pandemic. In Connecticut, for example, there was a 55% increase in violence-related trauma in 2020 and 2021 compared with the prior 2 years (O'Neill et al., 2023). Nationally, research found that the average number of weekly emergency department visits for firearm injury was 20% to 37% higher in the years immediately following the outbreak of the pandemic compared with 2019 (Zwald et al., 2023). Data from the CDC show a 23% increase in total firearm deaths since the pandemic began, attributable to both suicides and homicides (Gramlich, 2023). According to the Pew Research Center, firearm-related homicides increased 45% during the pandemic between 2019 and 2021, whereas the number of gun suicides rose 10% during that span. Pew also notes that the overall increase in U.S. firearm deaths since the beginning of the pandemic includes a sharp increase in firearm fatalities among children and adolescents, which rose 50% from 1,732 in 2019 to 2,590 in 2021 (Gramlich, 2023). In 2020, firearms became the number one cause of death in young people, a trend that has persisted in the 3 years since (Villarreal et al., 2024).

THE RELATIONSHIP BETWEEN MENTAL HEALTH AND VIOLENCE

The relationship between violence and mental health is complex and often marred by misconceptions. Although there is some scientific support for the claim that persons with mental illness are more likely to be violent, a systematic review and meta-analysis of research on schizophrenia, other psychoses, and violence found that there is substantial heterogeneity between studies reporting risk of violence and uncertainty over the causes of this heterogeneity. This systematic review also noted that the increased risk of violent acts among persons with mental illness is often mediated by substance use comorbidity, because the risk of violence among patients with comorbid conditions is comparable with the risk among patients with only substance use (Fazel et al., 2009). One limitation of the extant literature on mental illness and violence is the selection of study samples, which are often inpatient populations, who are also at higher risk of having severe mental illness (Crump et al., 2013). Violence perpetration and victimization are more common among people with severe mental illness than in the general population (Choe et al., 2008; Marr et al., 2024).

From a public perception, schizophrenia is often highlighted as a mental illness that increases the chances of an individual being at high risk for violence. However, this has not been verified in literature reviews. A variety of features may characterize schizophrenia. What are often termed *negative symptoms* tend to include a lack of social connectedness, lack of energy, and dullness. Negative symptoms are rarely associated with acts of violence, whereas positive features of the disorder, including hallucinations, command delusions, and audiovisual illusions, have a more direct relationship with violence. Nonetheless, several studies demonstrate that the vast majority of individuals with schizophrenia never perpetrate acts of violence. In a 6-month study that clinically assessed 1,410 patients with schizophrenia, the prevalence of any violence was 19.1%, with 3.6% of participants reporting serious violent behavior (Swanson et al., 2006).

Although psychotic symptoms may present in schizophrenia and other related serious mental disorders, they can also be a representation of certain types of depression and even bipolar disorder (Witt et al., 2013). Depression is one of the most common diagnoses in the United States, and it is not usually associated with violent behavior. In rare circumstances, violent behavior may be seen in cases of depressive psychosis, which is seen in about 10% to 20% of patients with depressive disorders (Elkington et al., 2015). Patients with mania are among the most likely types of patients to commit violent acts or display aggression in an inpatient unit. Their victims are usually random bystanders rather than predetermined targets (Rueve & Welton, 2008).

Often discussed is the association between substance use disorders and violence. Substance use and personality disorders are the two most common mental illnesses that are seen in the population of violent offenders with mental illnesses. Alcohol and drug use can trigger impulsive acts, enhance an already dysfunctional emotion regulation, and add excessive stress to cognitive load. Furthermore, illicit drug markets introduce an environment for sellers, buyers, and users to be exposed to risks of violence. This is also why IPV increases with substance use disorder, with a four-fold increase in risk with alcohol use disorder and cocaine use disorder (Crane et al., 2014). Research in Baltimore suggests that the density of liquor stores in a neighborhood is associated with higher rates of violence and lower life expectancy, and that illegally operating alcohol outlets were concentrated in predominately low-income and African American communities, illustrating the need to examine the racial and economic disparities that inform a community's vulnerability to mental illness and violence (Furr-Holden et al., 2018, 2020).

Regardless, it is important to note that patients with stable mental illness generally have the same risk of perpetuating violence as the general population (Rueve & Welton, 2008; Skeem & Mulvey, 2020). Although most people with mental illness, in the absence of other factors, are not violent and mental illness alone does not appear to be a direct cause of violence, people with mental illness, regardless of the severity of the mental illness, are more likely than the general population to be victims of violence (Bhavsar et al., 2019; Dean et al., 2018; Latalova et al., 2014). Victimization, in turn, can exacerbate mental health struggles; an abundance of literature has shown a correlation between exposure to or victimization of violence with subsequent incidence of posttraumatic stress disorder (PTSD), depression, and substance use disorder (Alloush & Bloem, 2022; Nathanson et al., 2012; Ziaei & Hammarström, 2023).

It is also important to identify historical violence perpetration or victimization among those with mental illness, because a history of violence is a salient predictor of future violence perpetration and victimization, despite mental health status. This includes childhood trauma and abuse (Jung et al., 2018; Wilkins et al., 2014). Notably, persons with mental illness are more vulnerable than the general population to recurrent victimization and perpetration, in the absence of intervention (Marr et al., 2024).

Early identification of unmet mental health needs and risks, as well as access to quality, affordable healthcare and treatment, can mitigate the risk of future violence. Research in the past decade has tied the expansion of Medicaid, and ensuing access to healthcare and substance use treatment by low-income adults, to a decrease in both violent and property crime rates (Vogler, 2017; Wen et al., 2017). In addition, other individual and social drivers to consider that may increase the risk of violence among persons with mental illness include living in poverty, educational and socioeconomic disadvantage, housing and food insecurity, social isolation, and societal stigma around mental illness (Murray et al., 2024; Niño et al., 2017). Among the general population, those with a lack of economic opportunity and lack of social integration are more likely to be both victims and perpetrators of child maltreatment, IPV, self-directed violence, and suicide (Wilkins et al., 2014). Remedying these factors can positively impact both mental health and violence exposure (Sadowski & Casteel, 2010).

Gun Violence and Mental Health

Gun violence is a pressing public health crisis that intersects significantly with mental health challenges. The relationship is multifaceted, requiring careful consideration of data to foster informed discourse and evidence-based action. Understanding this intersection involves recognizing distinct patterns across various forms of gun violence, including suicide, victimization, and trauma.

Firearm-related deaths account for a significant portion of suicides, with clear links to mental health conditions such as major depression, bipolar disorder, and schizophrenia. Individuals experiencing these conditions often face heightened risks of suicidal ideation and attempts. Firearms exacerbate this risk because of their lethality, making access to mental health care, safe storage practices, and preventive policies such as red flag laws critical components of intervention. These measures not only reduce access to lethal means but also provide an opportunity to engage individuals in mental health care at critical junctures.

Contrary to pervasive stigmatization, individuals with mental illness are significantly more likely to be victims of violence rather than perpetrators (Swanson et al., 2015; Teplin et al., 2005). This reality underscores the importance of protecting vulnerable populations through community-based interventions and supportive services. Data-driven initiatives must highlight these patterns to dismantle harmful stereotypes and prioritize victim support programs. Expanding trauma recovery centers and other community resources tailored to the needs of gun violence victims can improve outcomes and foster resilience.

Exposure to gun violence—whether as a survivor, witness, or family member—has profound psychological effects. Communities plagued by gun violence often experience higher rates of anxiety, depression, and PTSD (Abba-Aji et al., 2024; Buggs et al., 2022). Addressing these outcomes requires trauma-informed care frameworks that integrate mental health support with broader community safety strategies. Incorporating culturally competent mental health interventions and ensuring accessibility for underserved communities are critical to mitigating the long-term impacts of exposure to violence.

Although public narratives often conflate gun violence with mental illness, most violent acts are not committed by individuals with severe mental health conditions. Communication efforts must emphasize this distinction to prevent further stigmatization and to refocus attention on broader systemic drivers of violence, such as poverty, inequality, and access to firearms. Framing gun violence as a multifaceted issue that includes structural inequities and public health solutions can help shift public understanding and inspire comprehensive, evidence-based approaches to prevention.

VIOLENCE PREVENTION AND INTERVENTION STRATEGIES/PROGRAMS AND POLICIES

Research on the epidemiology of violence informs the development of prevention and intervention strategies aimed at reducing the burden of violence and promoting public health and safety. This research includes efforts to identify and address risk factors, strengthen protective factors, improve surveillance and data collection, and implement evidence-based programs and policies. Contemporary violence prevention programs have a heightened focus on laws, policies, and interventions to reduce the excess burden of firearm injury, including homicide, suicide, and nonfatal firearm injury (City of Baltimore, 2021; Los Angeles County Office of Violence Prevention, 2021; NYC Health, 2023; Oakland Department of Violence Prevention, 2024a, 2024b).

Individual-Level Interventions (Domestic Violence, Interpersonal Violence, Suicide Prevention Programs)

City-led violence prevention plans predominantly focus on reducing gun and group violence community-wide, but given the interlinked nature of forms of violence as well as cycles of victimization and perpetration, many devote a smaller percentage of resources to DV and IPV prevention efforts. The City of Baltimore's Comprehensive Violence Prevention Plan notes that "children who experience domestic violence are 9 times more likely to become involved in criminal activity" (City of Baltimore, 2021). Although this acknowledgment is significant, limited resource allocation often leaves prevention efforts underfunded and underexplored. Many plans begin by calling for collecting data to better understand the landscape of IPV and identifying opportunities to incorporate IPV/DV prevention, and there can be a variation of thought around what solutions are actually effective IPV/DV prevention strategies that are ready to implement. Plans were more likely to include funding to victim support services, including emergency housing, hotlines, and legal support. Although investments into immediate crisis support and response are necessary, expanding funding and research specific to DV and IPV *prevention* within broader violence prevention frameworks could strengthen these plans.

The City of Oakland funds an intervention program in city schools intended to address multiple forms of violence affecting youth, including gender-based violence, by placing service teams in high schools (Oakland Department of Violence Prevention, 2024b). Universal, school-based IPV education programs are a popular model of IPV prevention, especially targeted toward young people who are entering the dating stage of their lives. Students may undergo training in communication and conflict resolution, healthy relationship skills, bystander intervention tactics, and recognition of abusive relationships. Yet although there is some evidence that these programs improve adolescents' knowledge and attitudes toward DV, meta-analyses of studies have not found significant reductions in the DV perpetration or victimization rates of participants (Arrojo et al., 2024).

Additionally, it is important to note that not all young people are equally at risk for IPV/DV victimization and perpetration. Adolescents who live in economically disadvantaged neighborhoods, as well as adolescents who are ethnic minorities, are more likely to be affected by DV than those who do not belong to these groups (Arrojo et al., 2024). Yet, there is little research focusing specifically on the effectiveness of prevention and education programs on these at-risk subgroups, highlighting a need for further attention and consideration of how preventive programs can serve those most likely to encounter DV (An et al., 2024). Expanding these programs to include culturally tailored curricula and targeted outreach efforts for these populations could yield more effective outcomes.

Another gap in many violence prevention strategies concerns interventions targeted toward perpetrators of IPV. Intervention programs for perpetrators have traditionally been recommended through the legal system and have commonly taken the form of psychoeducation programs paired with cognitive behavioral programming—a two-pronged approach intended to dismantle individual-level beliefs about "power and control" and improve communication and emotional control skills (Campbell et al., 2024). However, in addition to limited evidence of these programs' efficacy, these models also face criticism for failing to adequately address the mental health and trauma histories of offenders, who, according to research, are more likely to have experienced adverse childhood experiences (ACEs) and associated trauma than the general population (Campbell et al., 2024). Expanding these programs to incorporate trauma-informed care and mental health support tailored for perpetrators could address underlying issues that contribute to IPV behaviors.

Research has found that primary care doctors and nonpsychiatric practitioners are more likely to interact with future suicide decedents in the period immediately preceding a suicide, as opposed to psychiatrists or consulting mental health professionals (Luoma et al., 2002). Indeed, improved training on screening and treating depression that targets primary care doctors and nurses at the state and local levels, with support from psychiatrists, was associated with lower rates of suicide, nonfatal suicide attempts, and suicide ideation (Mann et al., 2021). In addressing youth suicide, direct education of students in mental health and suicide prevention has been found to be more effective in reducing suicide attempts than education efforts targeted to "gatekeepers" such as parents or teachers (Mann et al., 2022). Expanding this model to include adults, particularly those presenting at hospitals for IPV-related injuries, could fill a significant gap in suicide prevention efforts.

Community-Level Interventions

Violence Interrupter Programs

Violence interrupter programs, such as Safe Streets, based in Baltimore (Mayor's Office of Neighborhood Safety and Engagement, 2024a), or Cure Violence (formerly known as CeaseFire), based in Chicago (Cure Violence Global, 2024), are evidence-based public health interventions that train outreach workers to form relationships with youth at high risk for involvement in gun violence. These programs aim to reduce beliefs that lead to aggressive behaviors, teach techniques for emotional regulation and coping strategies for trauma, and intervene in conflicts to find nonviolent resolutions. The outreach programs primarily target youth, because homicide and unintentional injury—including with a firearm—are leading causes of mortality for ages 15to 24 (CDC, 2023). The program's mission is to reduce shootings and violence in the target community.

Outreach workers, often called violence interrupters, typically come from high-violence communities and may have previously been involved in violent crimes. Their connections and trust within the community are essential for being aware of existing conflicts that could escalate into violence and for being respected enough to intervene effectively. In addition to preventing violence, violence interrupters aim to change individual attitudes and community norms regarding gun violence and retaliation. Research has shown that attitudes toward gun violence in high-violence communities are predictive of having been arrested or shot at in the past, highlighting the importance of such attitudinal shifts (Milam et al., 2018).

Violence interrupter programs also create metrics to evaluate community attitudes toward violence before and after program implementation, enabling data collection to measure their success. These metrics help refine interventions and guide replication or scaling efforts in other high-violence communities. For example, in one Baltimore community where Safe Streets was implemented, 43% of assessed attitudes improved post intervention, compared with 13% in the control community (Milam et al., 2016). Another study found that Safe Streets was associated with a 23% reduction in nonfatal shootings across implementation sites, and in five sites where the program had been running for at least 4 years, it was linked to an average 32% reduction in homicides (Webster et al., 2023). Similarly, an evaluation of Chicago's CeaseFire program reported significant declines in shooting rates in four of seven neighborhoods, with reductions of up to 24% (Skogan et al., 2008).

Hospital-Based Interventions

Hospital-based violence intervention programs (HVIPs) work directly with inpatients recovering from penetrating trauma, typically caused by assaults involving guns or knives. The goal is to address the psychological trauma of being violently victimized, discourage retaliatory violence, and connect patients to resources that enhance their resilience and support networks. These interventions often include a comprehensive assessment of the patient's needs, such as evaluating the safety of their home environment, screening for mental health and substance use issues, and determining access to social support systems. Referrals to community-based services, counseling, or other support programs are provided as needed (Zufer et al., 2024).

Clinicians involved in HVIPs may include social workers, occupational or physical therapists, physicians, hospital chaplains, or case managers specifically trained in violence intervention. Beyond the immediate patient, HVIPs also aim to provide support to hospital staff exposed to repeated trauma cases. A survey of emergency medics and surgeons who have responded to mass shooting incidents recommended implementing standardized grieving and debriefing processes and active outreach mental health programs for clinicians at trauma centers who respond to such incidents (Goolsby et al., 2023).

HVIPs also represent an underutilized opportunity to prevent IPV and DV, particularly for adults. Emergency departments and primary care settings can serve as critical touchpoints for screening for IPV risk among trauma victims. For example, follow-up programs for patients who present with injuries or mental health symptoms associated with IPV could include partnerships with community advocates, access to counseling, and safety planning services. Integrating these interventions into hospital workflows can ensure that victims receive support before returning to potentially dangerous environments. Further research into hospital-based follow-up care for trauma victims at high risk of IPV or DV could also identify effective strategies for intervention and long-term support.

Although HVIPs show promise, significant research gaps remain regarding their efficacy in reducing rates of reinjury and future violence. There is a need for robust, longitudinal data on trauma survivors involved in HVIPs to develop evidence-based best practices. Additionally, integrating HVIPs into broader community-level interventions, such as violence interrupter programs, may enhance their overall impact by creating a continuum of care that extends beyond the hospital setting (Zwaiman et al., 2022).

Expanding funding for HVIPs and promoting cross-sector collaboration among hospitals, community organizations, and policy makers could address existing gaps and improve program effectiveness. For example, coordinated efforts to track patients after discharge and provide long-term support can help reduce recidivism and foster safer communities. Ensuring that HVIPs are part of broader public health strategies will be critical to their success in addressing violence and its systemic causes.

Policies (e.g., Violence as a Public Health Crisis, Laws, Policies)

In 2024, the U.S. Surgeon General released an advisory declaring firearm violence a public health crisis, citing not only rising rates of firearm-related injuries and suicides, but also the traumatic mental health impacts that shootings cause community members, including children, first responders and health workers, and family members of survivors or victims of gun violence. The advisory explicitly calls for a public health approach to violence prevention. Federal recognition of violence as a public health issue dates to the 1980s, as the risk of suicide and homicide rose sharply in the leading causes of death for Americans (Dahlberg & Mercy, 2009). Yet, years of federal policy have also contributed to concentrated disadvantage among communities of color, where violence now bears a disproportionate burden. Just one example may be found beginning in the New Deal era and continuing for decades, where the Federal Housing Administration refused to insure mortgages in and around African American neighborhoods, a practice known as "redlining" that not only racially segregated cities and towns but also contributed to "locking in" economic deprivation in areas populated by Black Americans. Recent research has found that contemporary residents of historically redlined communities on average face a 4.8% higher probability of violent victimization and increased rates of firearms violence, as compared with those who live in nonredlined areas, illustrating the lingering effects of decades-old discriminatory policy on modern public health and safety (Poulson et al., 2021; Testa et al., 2024). Advocates have also argued that "tough on crime" legislation in the 1980s and 1990s spurred mass incarceration and juvenile imprisonment, again predominantly affecting Black communities and creating a cycle of trauma and economic deprivation that feeds into community violence.

After years of decline, rates of homicides, suicides, and DV rose across the nation during the outbreak of the pandemic. The American Rescue Plan Act (ARPA) delivered $350 billion in aid to localities around the United States; the federal government created a Community Violence Intervention (CVI) collaborative to support 15 cities that used part of these funds to invest in evidence-informed CVI programs that aim to disrupt cycles of violence. The Bipartisan Safer Communities Act, passed in 2022, added $1.4 billion in funding for violence prevention and intervention programs, as well as enhancing background checks for gun purchasers under 21 years old and closing the purchasing "boyfriend loophole" for those convicted of domestic violence in a romantic relationship. In 2023, the first-ever White House Office of Gun Violence Prevention was created to expedite implementation of the Bipartisan Safer Communities Act and identify further executive actions to reduce firearm-related harm to communities.

Although federal sources offer funding and technical assistance, much of the innovative work of violence prevention happens at the state and local levels, where local authorities oversee implementation of strategies and play an instrumental role in marshaling additional funding, coordinating partnerships across sectors, and tailoring approaches to fit the unique background and challenges of their locality. In 2014, Oakland voters approved the Safety & Services Act, known as Measure Z, which allocated $30 million of tax revenue to fund violence prevention efforts that included community investments such as life coaching for at-risk youth and adults, adult employment and education programs, and work opportunities for youth (Open Budget Oakland, 2024). Preliminary findings from Urban Institute's evaluation of Measure Z suggest improvements in community cohesion and reductions in arrest rates for those engaged in life coaching, with a comprehensive review expected in mid-2025 (Jannetta et al., 2024).

In 2021, the Baltimore Mayor's Office of Neighborhood Safety and Engagement released a comprehensive Violence Prevention Plan, formulated with the input of residents, youth, immigrant voices, and local and state partner agencies. The plan's first pillar was a "public health approach to violence" that called for increased investment in both the response to violence—expanding victim services and training in trauma-informed approaches—and active violence prevention strategies, including investing in the community violence intervention ecosystem, funding prevention and education efforts in schools, and accelerating behavioral health intervention options. A key component of the plan, the Group Violence Reduction Strategy, launched in 2022, leveraged collaboration among law enforcement, social service providers, and community members to engage with residents at high risk of gun violence. Preliminary research indicates that the strategy's pilot has resulted in the reduction of homicides and shootings by a quarter, without moving crimes to other parts of the city (Crime and Justice Lab, 2024).

State-level innovations also merit attention. California's Office of Gun Violence Prevention, established in 2021, has worked to fund targeted interventions such as HVIPs. These programs provide wraparound services to gun violence survivors, addressing trauma while connecting them to employment opportunities and community resources, reducing the likelihood of reinjury or retaliation. Similarly, New Jersey's violence intervention program initiative integrates community-based organizations with law enforcement to build trust and implement tailored solutions in high-risk neighborhoods. Evaluations of these programs highlight reductions in recidivism rates and increased community trust (New Jersey Office of the Attorney General, 2024).

Policies that recognize the structural contributors to violence, such as concentrated poverty and systemic inequities, remain essential. Local governments, such as in Minneapolis, have experimented with participatory budgeting initiatives that allow communities most affected by violence to allocate funding toward neighborhood improvement projects and youth engagement programs. These models, alongside federal and state efforts, reflect the multilevel strategies needed to address violence as a complex public health crisis.

EFFECTIVE COMMUNICATION OF DATA AND SCIENCE TO IMPROVE COMMUNITY VIOLENCE AND MENTAL HEALTH

Effective communication of data and science plays a pivotal role in addressing the intertwined challenges of community violence and mental health. By ensuring that evidence-based information is accessible, engaging, and actionable, stakeholders can foster understanding, drive interventions, and inspire systemic change. In this section, we explore key opportunities for optimizing the communication of data and science in this context.

Translating complex data into accessible formats is crucial, because data on violence and mental health may be intricate and overwhelming for nonexpert audiences. Strategies such as using graphs, infographics, and dashboards help convey trends and disparities in violence and mental health outcomes, making the information more relatable. Avoiding jargon and using clear, concise language ensure that scientific findings are understandable, whereas combining quantitative data with compelling narratives highlights the human impacts of violence and fosters emotional connections (Milam et al., 2018).

Engaging diverse stakeholders is another essential component of effective communication. To create community-wide impact, messages must resonate with audiences such as policy makers, community leaders, healthcare providers, educators, and the general public. Cultural competence—understanding and respecting cultural contexts—plays a vital role in framing these messages. Collaborative partnerships with local organizations can enhance the codevelopment and dissemination of content while leveraging audience-specific channels, such as social media, town halls, or academic journals, ensuring that messages reach their intended recipients effectively (Mayor's Office of Neighborhood Safety and Engagement, 2024b).

Digital platforms and technology offer unprecedented opportunities to educate communities about violence and mental health. Social media campaigns can raise awareness with shareable content that highlights actionable solutions, whereas web-based dashboards provide publicly accessible platforms for exploring data on violence trends and mental health resources. Additionally, apps and tools offering real-time information, such as crisis hotline access or violence prevention resources, can directly support those in need (Zufer et al., 2024).

Promoting data-driven policy advocacy is critical for enacting evidence-based solutions. Concise policy briefs summarizing research findings and their implications can influence policy makers effectively. Legislative testimony by experts presenting compelling data narratives further bridges the gap between research and action. Visual storytelling through infographic-driven reports highlights key data points, emphasizing the urgency and feasibility of policy changes (Webster et al., 2023).

Building trust and transparency is essential to fostering community engagement with data and science. Clearly explaining methodologies, limitations, and potential biases in data ensures transparency. Inclusive communication actively involves affected communities in the research process, providing them with findings and ensuring that their voices are heard. Consistency in providing updates and maintaining open channels for dialogue strengthens trust and encourages ongoing collaboration (Goolsby et al., 2023).

Empowering communities through education equips individuals to interpret and use data, fostering grassroots advocacy. Workshops and training programs can teach basic data literacy and demonstrate its relevance to violence prevention and mental health. Citizen science initiatives, which involve community members in data collection and analysis, build ownership and engagement. Resource guides that connect data to real-world challenges and solutions can further empower individuals and communities (Zwaiman et al., 2022).

Leveraging media partnerships is another vital strategy. The media shape public perceptions of violence and mental health, offering opportunities for impactful communication. Training scientists to communicate their findings effectively to journalists ensures accurate reporting. Collaborative storytelling with media outlets can create in-depth reports blending data with personal stories, whereas public service announcements deliver targeted campaigns to raise awareness about available resources and interventions (Gramlich, 2023).

Effective communication of data and science is foundational to improving community violence and mental health outcomes. By translating complex information into accessible formats, engaging diverse stakeholders, and leveraging digital and media platforms, we can bridge the gap between research and action. Building trust, empowering communities, and driving policy advocacy ensure that data not only inform but also transform, fostering safer and healthier communities for all.

FUTURE DIRECTIONS FOR RESEARCH, POLICY AND PRACTICE

There remain significant research gaps on the complex and interconnected nature of violence, mental illness, and firearm use. Despite the issue's urgency and increasingly recognized relevance to public health, the politically charged nature of the gun violence debate has chilled research to the extent that funding and publication rates of gun violence research are significantly lower than that of research dedicated to other leading causes of death in the United States (Stark & Shah, 2017). As a result, more research, including longitudinal studies, are necessary to unpack causal relationships among firearms access, mental health, and violence, and better understand how these factors intersect to influence violent behavior and victimization.

As cities and states continue to pilot a range of interventions, from education to violence interruption to reforming perpetrators of IPV, thorough research will be needed to determine the efficacy, long-term impacts, and scalability of program models. Evaluations of hospital-based interventions, such as violence interruption programs, and trauma-informed care initiatives are particularly vital to understanding how healthcare systems can better support both victims and perpetrators. Additionally, more comprehensive studies on how interventions at the individual, community, hospital, and policy levels interact and compound to effectively reduce violence are critical. For example, understanding how hospital-based interventions link with community violence interruption programs or how policy-level reforms influence individual and group behaviors could enhance integrated approaches to violence prevention.

In the meantime, there are strategies that can be implemented in the short-, medium-, and long-term to address violence and minimize its harms to communities. Increasing training in trauma-informed care for community members, including hospital workers, first responders, teachers, law enforcement, and primary care practitioners, is necessary because rising incidences of violence result in collective community mental health impacts beyond the incident's immediate victims. Expanding access to mental health resources and implementing simple follow-up contact interventions with survivors of violence or suicide as well as the frontline workers who witness and respond to incidents of violence could help improve community resilience to violence (Mann et al., 2021).

Restricting access to the lethal means to commit suicide has been shown to reduce associated suicide rates; in the United States, where firearms are used in half of all suicides, this would entail meaningful gun safety reform (Mann et al., 2021). Strategies such as safe firearm storage campaigns, red flag laws, and waiting periods for firearm purchases can serve as effective measures to limit impulsive acts of violence, including suicides. These interventions require broader public support, which can be fostered through educational campaigns highlighting their evidence-based effectiveness.

Long term, there is a need to mimic the work of local violence interrupter programs in their efforts to change social norms around violence, not just at an individual level but on a large scale. Changing cultural attitudes toward violence and reducing stigma around mental illness and IPV/DV will require working across sectors of society, including the government, health, education, and entertainment. Partnerships and knowledge sharing across industries can translate to shifts in public attitudes and behavior, as seen in successful public health campaigns to reduce smoking and tobacco use among Americans (Jamieson & Romer, 2015). Media partnerships and social media platforms can amplify these efforts by delivering targeted messaging to diverse audiences, especially those in high-risk environments.

SUMMARY

This chapter illustrates that there is no one single determining factor for violence. Mental illness, geography, poverty, social norms, and access to firearms are not individually responsible for incidences of community violence but instead interact with one another and a range of other environmental factors to perpetuate violence. Therefore, any solution that addresses just one factor is unlikely to effectively reduce rates of violence long term. However, evidence-based programs have shown that identifying risks and protective factors of violence and creating models that address multiple factors through specific interventions are possible and can result in the prevention of violence. For instance, integrating mental health services into schools, primary care settings, and community centers could address upstream risk factors while simultaneously increasing access to care.

To expand our understanding of what works in violence prevention models, more funding is necessary to adapt and implement evidence-based programs across communities. Public health strategies can dig deeper into risk factors impacting mental health and violence, including exploring primary and secondary prevention of substance abuse (Fazel, 2009). It is critical that approaches engage the perspective and insight of those who are especially at risk or vulnerable to violence. Past policies have shown the detrimental and long-term impacts of solutions that do not sufficiently address root causes of violence and instead feed into patterns of disadvantage, trauma, and retribution (Sakran et al., 2021). Comprehensive community engagement—including listening to those directly impacted by violence—is essential for designing interventions that address inequities and improve health outcomes sustainably.

The racial and economic disparities that characterize the epidemiology of violence in the United States demonstrate the critical importance of designing solutions with equity at the forefront. Interventions must consider structural contributors such as systemic racism, concentrated poverty, and historical disinvestment in communities. Policies that prioritize equitable resource allocation, community empowerment, and sustained investment in marginalized neighborhoods are vital to achieving lasting change. The increasing adoption of a public health lens by governments and policy makers to address violence is a positive development. It will require extensive collaboration across fields and professions, and its foundations in the scientific method and evidence provide a major opportunity for clinicians and medical practitioners to contribute their knowledge and expertise to impact health outcomes at scale. Addressing violence effectively will ultimately demand coordinated efforts that blend rigorous research, thoughtful policy, and community-centered practice.

DISCUSSION QUESTIONS

1. How does access to weapons affect the propagation of violence?
2. What are some public health interventions that can address the prevalence of violence?
3. How does structural systemic bias perpetuate violence and mental illnesses, and how do you think these effects vary across different communities and identities?
4. How does adopting a public health perspective shape your policy solutions to violence? What are the impacts of nonpublic health perspectives on policy solutions related to violence?
5. How can policy decrease violence that is attributable to mental health?

REFERENCES

Abba-Aji, M., Koya, S. F., Abdalla, S. M., Ettman, C. K., Cohen, G. H., & Galea, S. (2024). The mental health consequences of interpersonal gun violence: A systematic review. *SSM - Mental Health*, *5*, 100302. https://doi.org/10.1016/j.ssmmh.2024.100302

Alloush, M., & Bloem, J. R. (2022). Neighborhood violence, poverty, and psychological well-being. *Journal of Development Economics*, *154*, 102756. https://doi.org/10.1016/j.jdeveco.2021.102756

An, S., Welch-Brewer, C., & Tadese, H. (2024). Scoping review of intimate partner violence prevention programs for undergraduate college students. *Trauma, Violence, & Abuse*, *25*(4), 3099–3114. https://doi.org/10.1177/15248380241237201

Arrojo, S., Santirso, F.A., Lila, M., Gracia, E., & Conchell, R. (2024). Dating violence prevention programs for at-risk adolescents: A systematic review and meta-analysis. *Aggression and Violent Behavior*, *74*, 101893. https://doi.org/10.1016/j.avb.2023.101893

Bhavsar, V., Dean, K., Hatch, S. L., MacCabe, J. H., & Hotopf, M. (2019). Psychiatric symptoms and risk of victimisation: A population-based study from Southeast London. *Epidemiology and Psychiatric Sciences*, *28*(2), 168–178. https://doi.org/10.1017/S2045796018000537

Boserup, B., McKenney, M., & Elkbuli, A. (2020). Alarming trends in US domestic violence during the COVID-19 pandemic. *The American Journal of Emergency Medicine*, *38*(12), 2753–2755. https://doi.org/10.1016/j.ajem.2020.04.077

Buggs, S. A. L., Zhang, X., Aubel, A., Bruns, A., & Kravitz-Wirtz, N. (2022). Heterogeneous effects of spatially proximate firearm homicide exposure on anxiety and depression symptoms among U.S. youth. *Preventative Medicine*, *165*(Pt A), 107224. https://doi.org/10.1016/j.ypmed.2022.107224

Campbell, J. K., Nicolla, S., Weissman, D. M., & Moracco, K. E. (2024). The uptake and measurement of alternative approaches to domestic violence intervention programs: A scoping review. *Trauma, Violence, & Abuse*, *25*(4), 3269–3284. https://doi.org/10.1177/15248380241244398

Catalano, S. (2012). *Intimate partner violence, 1993–2010*. U.S. Department of Justice Office of Justice Programs Bureau of Justice Statistics Special Report. https://bjs.ojp.gov/content/pub/pdf/ipv9310.pdf

Centers for Disease Control and Prevention. (2022). *Firearm deaths grow, disparities widen*. https://www.cdc.gov/vitalsigns/firearm-deaths/index.html

Centers for Disease Control and Prevention, National Center for Injury Prevention and Control. (2023). *Leading causes of death and injury*. http://www.cdc.gov/injury/wisqars/leadingcauses.html

Choe, J. Y., Teplin, L.A., & Abram, K. M. (2008). Perpetration of violence, violent victimization, and severe mental illness: Balancing public health concerns. *Psychiatric Services*, *59*(2), 153–164. https://doi.org/10.1176/ps.2008.59.2.153

City of Baltimore. (2021). *Violence prevention framework and plan, February 2021*. https://monse.baltimorecity.gov/sites/default/files/MayorBMS__Draft_ViolenceReductionFrameworkPlan.pdf

Crane, C.A., Oberleitner, L. M. S., Devine, S., & Easton, C. J. (2014). Substance use disorders and intimate partner violence perpetration among male and female offenders. *Psychology of Violence, 4*(3), 322–333. https://doi.org/10.1037/a0034338.

Crime and Justice Policy Lab at the University of Pennsylvania. (2024). *Analyzing the impact of Baltimore's group violence reduction strategy in the Western District.* https://crimejusticelab.org/wp-content/uploads/2024/01/GVRS-Baltimore-Evaluation-Public-Summary-vFINAL.pdf

Crump, C., Ioannidis, J. P., Sundquist, K., Winkleby, M. A., & Sundquist, J. (2013). Mortality in persons with mental disorders is substantially overestimated using inpatient psychiatric diagnoses. *Journal of Psychiatric Research, 47*(10),1298–303. https://doi.org/10.1016/j.jpsychires.2013.05.034

Cure Violence Global. (2024). *About Cure Violence Global.* https://cvg.org/about/

Dahlberg, L. L., & Mercy, J. A. (2009). *The history of violence as a public health issue.* https://www.cdc.gov/violenceprevention/pdf/history_violence-a.pdf

Dean, K., Laursen, T. M., Pedersen, C. B., Webb, R. T., Mortensen, P. B., & Agerbo, E. (2018). Risk of being subjected to crime, including violent crime, after onset of mental illness: A Danish National Registry study using police data. *JAMA Psychiatry, 75*(7), 689–696. https://doi.org/10.1001/jamapsychiatry.2018.0534

Elkington, K. S., Teplin, L. A., Abram K. M., Jakubowski J. A., Dulcan M. K., & Welty L. J. (2015). Psychiatric disorders and violence: A study of delinquent youth after detention. *Journal of the American Academy of Child & Adolescent Psychiatry, 54*(4), 302–312.e5. https://doi.org/10.1016/j.jaac.2015.01.002

Evans, W. N., & Kotowski, M. H. (2024). The demand for protection and the persistently high rates of gun violence among young black males. *Journal of Public Economics, 234*, 105114. https://doi.org/10.1016/j.jpubeco.2024.105114

Fazel, S., Gulati, G., Linsell, L., Geddes, J. R., & Grann, M. (2009). Schizophrenia and violence: Systematic review and meta-analysis. *PLoS Medicine, 6*(8), e1000120. https://doi.org/10.1371/journal.pmed.1000120

Furr-Holden, C. D. M., Milam, A. J., Nesoff, E. D., Linton, S., Reboussin, B., Sadler, R. C., & Leaf, P. J. (2020). Using zoning as a public health tool to reduce alcohol outlet oversaturation, promote compliance, and guide future enforcement: A preliminary analysis of transform baltimore. *Journal of Urban Health: Bulletin of the New York Academy of Medicine, 97*(4), 568–582. https://doi.org/10.1007/s11524-020-00453-7

Furr-Holden, C. D., Nesoff, E. D., Nelson, V., Milam, A. J., Smart, M., Lacey, K., Thorpe, R. J., & Leaf, P. J. (2018). Understanding the relationship between alcohol outlet density and life expectancy in Baltimore city: The role of community violence and community disadvantage. *Journal of Community Psychology, 47*(1), 63–75. https://doi.org/10.1002/jcop.22099

Goolsby, C., Schuler, K., Krohmer, J., Gerstner, D. N., Weber, N. W., Slattery, D. E., Kuhls, D. A., & Kirsch, T. D. (2023). Mass shootings in America: Consensus recommendations for healthcare response. *Journal of the American College of Surgeons, 236*(1), 168–175. https://doi.org/10.1097/XCS.0000000000000312

Gramlich, J. (2023). *What the data says about gun deaths in the U.S.* Pew Research Center. https://www.pewresearch.org/short-reads/2023/04/26/what-the-data-says-about-gun-deaths-in-the-u-s/

Jamieson, P. E., & Romer, D. (2015). Portrayal of tobacco use in prime-time TV dramas: Trends and associations with adult cigarette consumption—USA, 1955–2010. *Tobacco Control, 24*(3), 243–248. https://doi.org/10.1136/tobaccocontrol-2012-050896

Jannetta, J., Oglesby-Neal, A., Kim, K., DeLouya, L., Thompson, P. S., Ahmed, R., Salcido White, M., & Cajina, A. (2024). An interim process and outcome evaluation of Oakland's Measure Z-funded services: The Department of Violence Prevention's Group Violence Response Strategy, July 2022 to June 2024. *The Urban Institute.* https://www.urban.org/sites/default/files/2024-12/Interim_Evaluation_of_Oakland%E2%80%99s_Measure_Z_Funded_Services_Department_of_Violence_Prevention%E2%80%99s_Group_Violence_Response_Strategy.pdf

Jones-Eversley, S. D., Rice, J., Adedoyin, A. C., & James-Townes, L. (2020). Premature deaths of young black males in the United States. *Journal of Black Studies, 51*(3), 251–272. https://doi.org/10.1177/0021934719895999

Jung, H., Herrenkohl, T. I., Skinner, M. L., Lee, J. O., Klika, J. B., & Rousson, A. N. (2018). Gender differences in intimate partner violence: A predictive analysis of IPV by child abuse and domestic violence exposure during early childhood. *Violence Against Women, 25*(8), 903–924. https://doi.org/10.1177/1077801218796329

Latalova, K., Kamaradova, D., & Prasko, J. (2014). Violent victimization of adult patients with severe mental illness: A systematic review. *Neuropsychiatric Disease and Treatment, 10*, 1925–1939. https://doi.org/10.2147/NDT.S68321

Los Angeles County Office of Violence Prevention. (2021). *OVP strategic plan goals 2020–2024.* http://www.publichealth.lacounty.gov/ovp/docs/2021_OVP%20Overview.pdf

Luoma, J. B., Martin, C. E., & Pearson, J. L. (2002). Contact with mental health and primary care providers before suicide: A review of the evidence. *American Journal of Psychiatry, 159*(6), 909–916.

Mann, J. J., Michel, C. A., & Auerbach, R. P. (2021). Improving suicide prevention through evidence-based strategies: A systematic review. *American Journal of Psychiatry, 178*(7), 611–624. https://doi.org/10.1176/appi.ajp.2020.20060864

Marr, C., Webb, R. T., Yee, N., & Dean, K. (2024). A systematic review of interpersonal violence perpetration and victimization risk examined within single study cohorts, including in relation to mental illness. *Trauma, Violence & Abuse, 25*(1), 130–149. https://doi.org/10.1177/15248380221145732

Mayor's Office of Neighborhood Safety and Engagement. (2024a). Safe streets. *City of Baltimore.* https://monse.baltimorecity.gov/safe-streets-new

Mayor's Office of Neighborhood Safety and Engagement. (2024b). *Baltimore city comprehensive violence prevention plan.* https://mayor.baltimorecity.gov/sites/default/files/MayorScott-ComprehensiveViolencePreventionPlan-1.pdf

Milam, A. J., Buggs, S. A., Furr-Holden, C. D., Leaf, P. J., Bradshaw, C. P., & Webster, D. (2016). Changes in attitudes toward guns and shootings following implementation of the Baltimore Safe Streets intervention. *Journal of Urban Health, 93*(4), 609–626. https://doi.org/10.1007/s11524-016-0060-y

Milam, A. J., Furr-Holden, C. D., Leaf, P., & Webster, D. (2018). Managing conflicts in urban communities: Youth attitudes regarding gun violence. *Journal Of Interpersonal Violence, 33*(24), 3815–3828. https://doi.org/10.1177/0886260516639584

Murray, J., Degli Esposti, M., Loret de Mola, C., Martins, R., Smith, A. D. A. C., Moffitt, T. E., Heron, J., Miranda, V. I., Lima, N., & Horta, B. L. (2024). Life-course influences of poverty on violence and homicide: 30-year Brazilian birth cohort study. *International Journal of Epidemiology, 53*(4), dyae103. https://doi.org/10.1093/ije/dyae103

Nathanson, A. M., Shorey, R. C., Tirone, V., & Rhatigan, D. L. (2012). The prevalence of mental health disorders in a community sample of female victims of intimate partner violence. *Partner Abuse, 3*(1), 59–75. https://doi.org/10.1891/1946-6560.3.1.59

National Children's Alliance. (2024). *National statistics on child abuse.* https://www.nationalchildrensalliance.org/media-room/national-statistics-on-child-abuse/

New Jersey Office of the Attorney General. (2024). *Governor Murphy, Attorney General Platkin announce $14.5 million in violence intervention and prevention grants available for community organizations.* https://www.njoag.gov/governor-murphy-attorney-general-platkin-announce-14-5-million-in-violence-intervention-and-prevention-grants-available-for-community-organizations/

Niño, M., Ignatow, G., & Cai, T. (2017). Social isolation, strain, and youth violence. *Youth Violence and Juvenile Justice, 15*(3), 299–313. https://doi.org/10.1177/1541204016636435

NYC Health. (2023). *The violence prevention initiative.* https://www.nyc.gov/assets/doh/downloads/pdf/vio/violence-prevention-initiative.pdf

Oakland Department of Violence Prevention. (2024a). *Department of Violence Prevention service strategy: Gender-based violence.* https://cao-94612.s3.us-west-2.amazonaws.com/documents/DVP-funded-services-brochure_GBV_06.22.24.pdf

Oakland Department of Violence Prevention. (2024b). *Department of Violence Prevention service strategy: School Violence Intervention and Prevention (VIP) program.* https://cao-94612.s3.us-west-2.amazonaws.com/documents/DVP-funded-services-brochure_School-VIP-Program_06.22.24.pdf

O'Neill, K. M., Dodington, J., Gawel, M., Borrup, K., Shapiro, D. S., Gates, J., Gregg, S., & Becher, R. D. (2023). The effect of the COVID-19 pandemic on community violence in Connecticut. *American Journal of Surgery, 225*(4), 775–780. https://doi.org/10.1016/j.amjsurg.2022.10.004

Open Budget Oakland. (2024). *How does Oakland fund violence prevention? A summary of Measure Z funding.* https://openbudgetoakland.org/measure-z/

Pillemer, K., Burnes, D., Riffin, C., & Lachs, M. S. (2016). Elder abuse: Global situation, risk factors, and prevention strategies. *The Gerontologist, 56*(Suppl 2), S194–S205. https://doi.org/10.1093/geront/gnw004

Poulson, M., Neufeld, M. Y., Dechert, T., Allee, L., & Kenzik, K. M. (2021). Historic redlining, structural racism, and firearm violence: A structural equation modeling approach. *The Lancet Regional Health Americas, 3*, 100052. https://doi.org/10.1016/j.lana.2021.100052

Rueve, M. E., & Welton, R. S. (2008). Violence and mental illness. *Psychiatry, 5*(5), 34–48.

Sadowski, L., & Casteel, C. (2010). Intimate partner violence towards women. *BMJ Clinical Evidence, 24*, 1013.

Sakran, J. V., Lunardi, N., & Dawes, D. (2021, October). Confronting the political determinants of gun violence. *Scientific American.* https://www.scientificamerican.com/article/confronting-the-political-determinants-of-gun-violence/

Skeem, J., & Mulvey, E. (2020). What role does serious mental illness play in mass shootings, and how should we address it? *Criminal Public Policy, 19*(1), 85–108. https://doi.org/10.1111/1745-9133.12473

Skogan, W. G., Hartnett, S. M., Bump, N., & Dubois, J. (2008). *Evaluation of CeaseFire-Chicago.* https://www.ojp.gov/pdffiles1/nij/grants/227181.pdf

Smith, S. G., Zhang, X., Basile, K. C., Merrick, M. T., Wang, J., Kresnow, M., & Chen, J. (2018). *The National Intimate Partner and Sexual Violence Survey: 2015 data brief—Updated release.* National Center for Injury Prevention and Control, Centers for Disease Control and Prevention. file:///C:/Users/jsakran1/Downloads/cdc_60893_DS1.pdf

Stark, D. E., & Shah, N. H. (2017). Funding and publication of research on gun violence and other leading causes of death. *JAMA, 317*(1), 84–85. https://doi.org/10.1001/jama.2016.16215

Swanson, J. W., McGinty, E. E., Fazel, S., & Mays, V. M. (2015). Mental illness and reduction of gun violence and suicide: Bringing epidemiologic research to policy. *Annals of Epidemiology*, *25*(5), 366–376. https://doi.org/10.1016/j.annepidem.2014.03.004

Swanson, J. W., Swartz, M. S., Van Dorn, R. A., Elbogen, E. B., Wagner, H. R., Rosenheck, R. A., Stroup, T. S., McEvoy, J.P., & Lieberman, J. A. (2006). A national study of violent behavior in persons with schizophrenia. *Archives of General Psychiatry*, *63*(5), 490. https://doi.org/10.1001/archpsyc.63.5.490

Teplin, L. A., McClelland, G. M., Abram, K. M., & Weiner, D. A. (2005). Crime victimization in adults with severe mental illness. *Archives of General Psychiatry*, *62*(8), 911–921. https://doi.org/10.1001/archpsyc.62.8.911

Testa, A., Jackson, D. B., DeAngelis, R., Heard-Garris, N., Semenza, D. C., & Johnson, O. (2024). Historical redlining and contemporary violent victimization over the life course. *American Journal of Preventative Medicine*, *67*(4), 477–484. https://doi.org/10.1016/j.amepre.2024.06.013

Villarreal, S., Kim, R., Wagner, E., Somayaji, N., Davis, A., & Crifasi, C. (2024). *Gun violence in the United States 2022: Examining the burden among children and teens.* Johns Hopkins Center for Gun Violence Studies. https://publichealth.jhu.edu/sites/default/files/2024-09/2022-cgvs-gun-violence-in-the-united-states.pdf

Vogler, J. (2017). *Access to health care and criminal behavior: Short-run evidence from the ACA Medicaid expansions.* http://dx.doi.org/10.2139/ssrn.3042267

Wake, A. D., & Kandula, U. R. (2022). The global prevalence and its associated factors toward domestic violence against women and children during COVID-19 pandemic—"The shadow pandemic": A review of cross-sectional studies. *Women's Health*, *18*, 17455057221095536. https://doi.org/10.1177/17455057221095536

Wasserman, D., Iosue, M., Wuestefeld, A., & Carli, V. (2020). Adaptation of evidence-based suicide prevention strategies during and after the COVID-19 pandemic. *World Psychiatry*, *19*(3), 294–306. https://doi.org/10.1002/wps.20801.

Webster, D. W., Tilchin C. G., & Mitchell L. D. (2023). *Estimating the effects of Safe Streets Baltimore on gun violence.* Johns Hopkins Bloomberg School of Public Health Center for Gun Violence Studies. https://publichealth.jhu.edu/sites/default/files/2023-10/estimating-the-effects-of-safe-streets-baltimore-on-gun-violence-july-2023.pdf

Wen, H., Hockenberry, J. M., & Cummings, J. R. (2017). The effect of Medicaid expansion on crime reduction: Evidence from HIFA-waiver expansions. *Journal of Public Economics*, *154*, 67–94. https://doi.org/10.1016/j.jpubeco.2017.09.001

Wilkins, N., Tsao, B., Hertz, M. F., Davis, R., & Klevens, J. (2014). *Connecting the dots: An overview of the links among multiple forms of violence.* National Center for Injury Prevention and Control (U.S.). Division of Violence Prevention Institute. https://stacks.cdc.gov/view/cdc/31552

Witt, K., Van Dorn, R., & Fazel, S. (2013). Risk factors for violence in psychosis: Systematic review and meta-regression analysis of 110 studies. *PLoS ONE*, *8*(2), e55942. https://doi.org/10.1371/journal.pone.0055942

Ziaei, S., & Hammarström, A. (2023). The relationship between interpersonal violence in adulthood and mental health: A longitudinal study based on the Northern Swedish Cohort. *BMC Public Health*, *23*(1), 637. https://doi.org/10.1186/s12889-023-15525-x

Zufer, I., Fix, R. L., Stone, E., Cane, R., Sakran, J. V., Nasr, I., & Hoops, K. (2024). Documentation of trauma-informed care elements for young people hospitalized after assault trauma. *The Journal of Surgical Research*, *296*, 665–673. https://doi.org/10.1016/j.jss.2024.01.030

Zwaiman, A., da Luz, L. T., Perrier, L., Hacker Teper, M., Strauss, R., Harth, T., Haas, B., Nathens, A. B., & Gotlib Conn, L. (2022). The involvement of trauma survivors in hospital-based injury prevention, violence intervention and peer support programs: A scoping review. *Injury*, *53*(8), 2704–2716. https://doi.org/10.1016/j.injury.2022.06.032

Zwald, M. L., Van Dyke, M. E., Chen, M. S., Radhakrishnan, L., Holland, K. M., Simon, T. R., Dahlberg, L. L., Friar, N. W., Sheppard, M., Kite-Powell, A., & Mercy J. A. (2023). Emergency department visits for firearm injuries before and during the COVID-19 pandemic—United States, January 2019–December 2022. *Morbidity and Mortality Weekly Report*, *72*(13), 333–337. https://doi.org/10.15585/mmwr.mm7213a2

15 MEN'S MENTAL HEALTH AND AGING: UTILIZING A HEALTH EQUITY LENS

LESLIE ADAMS, DARRELL HUDSON, AND ROLAND J. THORPE, JR.

LEARNING OBJECTIVES

After reading this chapter, readers will be able to:

- Explain the role of structural and psychosocial barriers in men's mental health outcomes, particularly during aging.
- Describe the intersection between masculinity norms, help-seeking behavior, and emotional vulnerability in older men.
- Analyze the impact of social isolation and loneliness on the mental health of aging men.
- Evaluate the significance of applying a health equity lens to address disparities in mental health care for older men.
- Propose strategies for inclusive recruitment and interventions tailored to the mental health needs of diverse aging populations.

INTRODUCTION

Background on Men's Mental Health

For many years, mental health researchers have recognized discrepancies in how frequently men and women seek assistance for emotional issues (Kessler et al., 1981; Liddon et al., 2018; Möller-Leimkühler, 2002; Wendt & Shafer, 2016). Despite men facing comparable, or sometimes heightened, risk of psychiatric disorders compared with women (Kessler et al., 2005), they are also less likely to seek help from a mental health professional. According to the 2022 National Survey on Drug Use and Health (NSDUH), 16% of adults aged 60 or older received mental health treatment in the past year. This includes 11.9% of men and 19.6% of women, indicating a statistically significant difference in treatment rates between genders (**Figure 15.1**; Substance Abuse and Mental Health Services Administration, 2024).

Furthermore, men are less likely to use informal support networks, such as family, friends, or religious clergy, to address emotional concerns (Berger et al., 2013; Mahalik & Di Bianca, 2021; Wendt & Shafer, 2016). As global epidemiologic trends suggest that people are living longer and healthier lives (Robine, 2021; Robine et al., 2020; Salomon et al., 2012), scholars who study aging are grappling with the challenge of maintaining quality of life. Americans are living longer lives and quality of life. Despite advancements in aging, men consistently live shorter lives than women (Rochelle et al., 2015). Moreover, men encounter different challenges in maintaining their mental well-being as they age, experiencing a growing crisis of loneliness, depression, and less robust social support networks compared with women to combat these challenges (Barreto et al., 2021; Nummela et al., 2011). Indeed, scholars assert that the intersection of men's mental health and aging is complex and multifaceted.

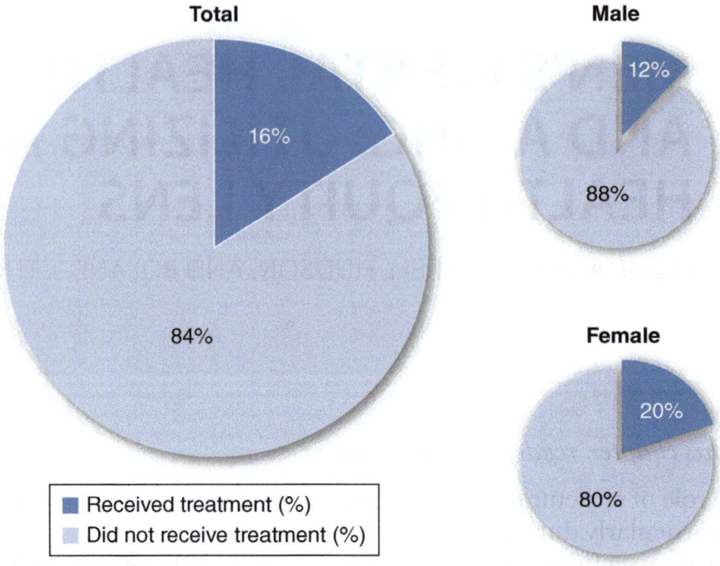

Figure 15.1 Percentage of mental health treatment among adults aged 60 or older (2021–2022).
Source: Substance Abuse and Mental Health Services Administration. (2024). *Behavioral health among older adults: Results from the 2021 and 2022 National Surveys on Drug Use and Health* (SAMHSA Publication No. PEP24-07-018). https://www.samhsa.gov/data/report/older-adult-behavioral-health-report-2021-2022

However, many key factors that link mental health and poor aging outcomes among men are socially constructed and intrinsically linked to structural factors (Addis & Mahalik, 2003; Courtenay, 2000). These influences constrain men's willingness to disclose, access, and seek adequate treatment for mental health challenges. In this chapter, we present a guiding framework, derived from a review of both seminal and recent literature, to explore the state of the field on men's mental well-being throughout the aging process.

Men's vulnerability to mental health challenges are, in some cases, dependent on their stage in the life course. For instance, scholars have demonstrated an alarming increase in rates of suicide among males during vulnerable periods of early adolescence to emerging adulthood (Bachmann, 2018; Gordon et al., 2020). During this critical stage of identity development and life transition, factors such as societal norms and expectations around gender, peer influences, and academic pressures can significantly influence mental well-being (Brausch & Gutierrez, 2010; Feigelman & Gorman, 2008; Fried et al., 2013). Similarly, as men progress through other stages of life, they encounter distinct stressors that influence their mental well-being or may exacerbate existing mental health concerns (Elder et al., 1994; Thorpe & Whitfield, 2021). Understanding men's mental health from a life course perspective is critical for developing adequate strategies tailored to the dynamic needs of aging men.

Overview of Challenges for Men's Mental Health

Scholars assert that addressing men's mental health from an aging perspective presents its own set of challenges (Elder & Johnson, 2018). Research in the field of men's health have identified key psychosocial and structural barriers that influence the access of adequate mental health care in the United States. Overall, researchers have determined that both attitudinal and socioeconomic barriers, such as help-seeking preferences, emotional disclosure, expressions of vulnerability, and structural barriers to mental health services, present distinct challenges among men seeking care for mental health needs as they grow older

(Addis & Mahalik, 2003; Thorpe & Whitfield, 2021; Williams, 2008). These barriers often contribute to delayed or inadequate access to mental health services, exacerbating the risk of undetected and untreated mental health conditions, including depression, anxiety, and suicidal ideation and behavior (Ahmedani et al., 2014; Berger et al., 2013; Powell et al., 2019). Gendered and cultural norms and stigmas surrounding mental health further compound these challenges, underscoring the urgent need for targeted interventions and culturally sensitive approaches to improve mental health outcomes among men.

Help-Seeking Behavior

Mental health help-seeking behavior, characterized as the act of searching for and receiving help for emotional and behavioral issues, has been well studied in men's mental health research. Early pioneers in this field, such as Addis and Mahalik (2003), offered theoretical foundations to clarify the ways and reasons why men do or do not seek help. Although this formative work outlines help-seeking as a core tenant of observed gender differences between men and women, the authors did not exclusively focus on mental health help-seeking.

Understanding psychosocial factors related to help-seeking will also highlight motivational influences on healthcare use that are driven by race- and gender-related factors. Mental health help-seeking barriers among men may also be further exacerbated by male gender norms (Berger et al., 2013; Coleman, 2015). These traditionally held norms associate emotional challenges with weakness and vulnerability and may ultimately discourage help-seeking behavior in professional or peer settings (Connell & Messerschmidt, 2005; Courtenay, 2000).

Extant studies examining help-seeking by race and gender cite emotion restriction, described as limited disclosure of emotional issues, as a unique psychosocial factor driving men's greater reluctance to seek professional help compared with women (Leaf et al., 1985; Möller-Leimkühler, 2002; Vogel et al., 2011). These barriers to help-seeking among men, compared with women, may be a result of the incongruence between masculine norms of strength and the vulnerable state of seeking clinical services (Idris et al., 2017; Sileo & Kershaw, 2020). Masculine role norm salience, defined as the shared cultural expectation of the male gender role, is one socialized aspect of identity that has been linked to health-promoting behaviors (Levant et al., 1992). Masculine role norm salience is viewed as socially constructed and often positions male help-seeking as a form of weakness (Vogel & Heath, 2016).

Scholars suggest that while men's healthcare engagement is shaped by gender norms, the influence of these norms largely depends on the salience or level of importance assigned to them (Addis & Mahalik, 2003). Researchers also posit that prevailing masculine role norm salience sanctions the appropriateness of disclosing issues to others and, thus, inhibits help-seeking for mental health concerns. Restrictive emotionality is one dimension of masculine role norm salience that limits disclosure of problems in order to preserve one's masculine self-concept (Levant et al., 2007) and negatively influences attitudes toward help-seeking (Berger et al., 2013; Mansfield et al., 2005). Among men, studies also show that depressive symptoms may be further exacerbated by masculine role norm salience such as restrictive emotionality, which censures crying, sadness, and vulnerability (Hammond & Mattis, 2005; Vogel et al., 2011).

Emphasizing the Need for a Health Equity Approach

Research applying a health equity lens to clarify the interplay of multiple systems and help-seeking attitudes for men's mental health remains scarce. Yet, such an approach is pivotal in unraveling the interconnected influences of race- and gender-related factors that serve as significant barriers within the mental health care system. The disparities in risk factors related to mental health conditions become starkly evident when considering the alarming relationships among major depressive disorder and suicide, posttraumatic stress, and physical health comorbidities that impact historically marginalized men as they age (Kessler et al., 2005). These realities highlight the pressing imperative to examine men's aging from a health equity lens and the unique inequities that inform barriers to effective mental health care.

GUIDING DEFINITIONS

Equity

According to the World Health Organization (WHO), "equity is the absence of unfair, avoidable or remediable differences among groups of people, whether those groups are defined socially, economically, demographically, or geographically or by other dimensions of inequality (e.g., sex, gender, ethnicity, disability, or sexual orientation)" (WHO, 2010). Further, WHO describes health equity as the absence of unfair disparities in health outcomes among various groups of people, regardless of social, economic, demographic, or other defining characteristics, such as sex, gender, ethnicity, disability, or sexual orientation. It asserts that everyone should have the opportunity to achieve their fullest potential for health and well-being. Achieving health equity involves addressing the social determinants of health, including the conditions in which individuals are born, grow, live, work, play, and age, along with structural determinants such as political, legal, and economic factors that shape access to resources and power within society.

Structural determinants, alongside social norms and institutional processes, play a pivotal role in shaping health equity in the United States by influencing the distribution of resources and opportunities among different populations (Bailey et al., 2017; Gómez et al., 2021). Discriminatory practices rooted in biases and prejudices exacerbate disparities in living conditions and access to healthcare, perpetuating inequities among marginalized groups (Bailey et al., 2020; Swope & Hernández, 2019). Thus, advancing health equity for aging men necessitates not only addressing health disparities but also dismantling systemic barriers embedded in institutional and systemic processes that influence the aging process. It entails recognizing and rectifying injustices stemming from differences in health and overall living conditions, thereby moving toward a society where everyone can enjoy equal opportunities for optimal health and well-being. Bravemen (2022) has argued that health inequities are not a result of immutable differences across race/ethnicity, social class, gender, or other identity-related factors. Rather, health inequities are driven by social stratification factors such as racism and sexism in addition to policies and practices that shape social and physical environments.

Racism

Racism is considered a multilevel factor that, while fueled by societal norms and stereotypes, impacts society in multiple ways, ranging from the individual level (e.g., racial discrimination) to the societal level (e.g., institutional racism). David Williams et al. define *racism* as "an organized societal system in which the dominant White group categorizes individuals into 'races' and devalues, disempowers, and differentially allocates resources to ethnic groups considered to be inferior" (Williams et al., 2019, as cited in Williams & Etkins, 2021, p. 194). It is important to note that in contemporary times, it is largely no longer considered polite or socially acceptable to overtly use racial epithets or explicitly promulgate stereotypes (Bonilla-Silva, 2006; Bonilla-Silva & Baiocchi, 2001). However, racism is often manifest in the structure of society, such as racial residential segregation and health inequities, which go beyond the interpersonal level.

Aging men who have experienced racism across their life course often carry the cumulative burden of these traumatic experiences (Chatters et al., 2021; Glymour & Manly, 2008).

These men carry the pain not only of interpersonal racism (e.g., microaggressions, everyday racial discrimination), but also of the enduring legacy of systemic racism. For these individuals, the impact extends beyond personal experiences to encompass historical and institutional injustices that are embedded in the fabric of society (Williams & Mohammed, 2013). Living through these tumultuous periods, which includes periods of legalized segregation, criminalization, and racial oppression, leaves a profound impact on the health and well-being of men who have navigated these experiences across the life course. As such, it is critical to understand the complex influence of health disparities and systemic inequities that may influence aging.

Life Course Perspective

Health does not occur in a vacuum. People are embedded in contexts, and exposure to physical and social stressors can negatively affect people across the life course. There are many different conceptual frameworks to understand the life course perspective. Some scholars have argued that there are critical periods of development that could negatively affect health trajectories (Halfon et al., 2014). Others, such as Krieger and Davey Smith (2004), argue that the physical and social world around us is "embodied" such that key exposure and experiences affect our health trajectories. Another life course framework, weathering, was proposed by Geronimus (1992). This framework asserts that inequities in exposure to chronic stress over the life course contribute to racial/ethnic health inequities.

CURRENT EVIDENCE ON MEN'S MENTAL HEALTH AND AGING

Growing Trends (Prevalence and Incidence) of Social Isolation and Loneliness Among Men

Social isolation, defined as the objective lack of contact with others, is a prevalent issue among older adults, particularly in the context of aging populations. The University of Michigan's National Poll on Healthy Aging (NPHA) assessed feelings of social isolation among adults aged 50 to 80 from 2018 to 2023 (**Figure 15.2**). In October 2018, 27% of respondents reported feeling isolated from others some of the time or often. This percentage increased to 56% in June 2020, coinciding with the COVID-19 pandemic, and then gradually declined to 34% by January 2023 (Kullgren et al., 2023). As men age, they may face various challenges that contribute to social isolation, such as retirement, loss of friends or family members, mobility limitations, and changes in social roles. Moreover, men have 4 times greater odds of experiencing social isolation compared with women (Cudjoe et al., 2020), which demonstrates the importance of positioning social isolation prevention strategies to support aging men. Social isolation has significant implications for the health and well-being of men as they progress across the life course, because it is associated with an increased risk of morbidity and mortality (Steptoe et al., 2013), including mental health disorders, cognitive decline, cardiovascular diseases, and decreased immune function.

Moreover, the impact of social isolation on men's aging is a topic of growing concern (Holt-Lunstad et al., 2015). Research suggests that older men may be particularly vulnerable to social isolation due to factors such as traditional gender norms that discourage emotional expression and seeking social support (Robbins et al., 2016; Willis et al., 2022; Willis & Vickery, 2022). Addressing social isolation among older men is essential for promoting healthy aging and preventing adverse health outcomes. Understanding the relationship between social isolation, men's health, and aging is crucial for developing effective interventions and policies to support the well-being of older adults.

A recent study, based on a representative sample of 7,788 Medicare beneficiaries aged 65 and older, assessed the relationship between social isolation and homebound status by race over 9 years (Cudjoe et al., 2020). The authors found that both Black and White older adults

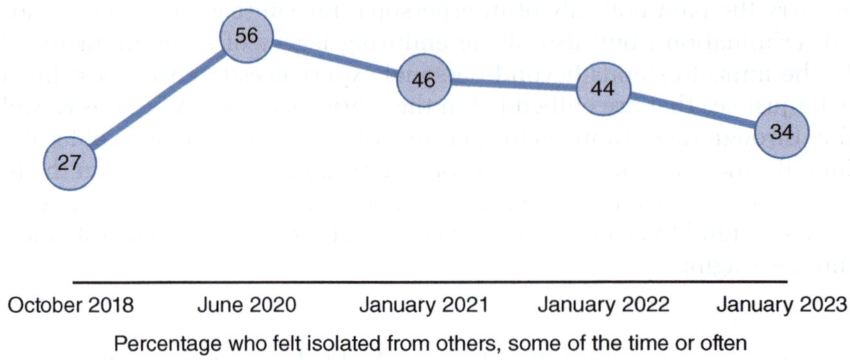

Figure 15.2 Changes in feeling of social isolation (2018–2023) among adults aged 50 to 80.
Source: Malani, P., Singer, D., Kirch, M., Solway, E., Roberts, S., Smith, E., Hutchens, L., & Kullgren, J. (2023). *National poll on healthy aging: Trends in loneliness among older adults from 2018–2023*. https://www.healthyagingpoll.org/reports-more/report/trends-loneliness-among-older-adults-2018-2023

were more likely to be homebound at baseline and also to become homebound over the 9-year study period, emphasizing the profound consequences of social isolation on mobility and independence in later life. This research highlights the urgency of addressing social isolation as a key determinant of men's health and aging and the need for community-based strategies and policies that identify and mitigate social isolation to enhance the quality of life and promote healthy aging among older adults. A follow-up study using National Health and Aging Trends Study data found that social isolation among older adults is significantly associated with a higher risk of incident dementia over a 9-year period, after adjusting for demographic and health factors (Huang et al., 2023). These studies underscore the critical importance of addressing social isolation as a potential area of intervention for men's aging research and highlight the need for targeted interventions aimed at promoting social connectedness among older adults to mitigate future cognition-related conditions. The consistency of these findings across race and ethnicity also highlights the universal relevance of addressing social isolation in dementia prevention efforts. Overall, this research illuminates the imperative of fostering social connections to safeguard the mental health and emotional well-being of men as they age.

Contemporary Challenges

The last comprehensive national psychiatric epidemiological studies were conducted more than 20 years ago. The world has changed quite a bit since then. Unfortunately, this means that national surveillance estimates of mental health are not up to date and do not capture current demographic or technological shifts. For example, although scholars have inquired about the effects of social media on overall population mental health, little is known about how social media and other technologies are affecting the mental health of men. As with most things, there are potential benefits and challenges that have emerged with greater social media. Isolation, which is strongly associated with poorer mental health outcomes and is more common among men, is reduced with greater connectivity through social media platforms (e.g., Facebook; Primack et al., 2019). However, greater social media consumption is often linked to poorer mental health, particularly among youth (Rice et al., 2013). For instance, popular images promoting muscular builds or the depiction of luxurious lifestyles may fuel feelings of inadequacy among men, negatively affecting self-esteem and increasing the likelihood of mental health concerns. Another concern with social media is negative interaction, including but not limited to online bullying, harassment, and "doxing" (i.e., the act of gathering and publicly sharing private or personally identifiable information about an individual online, often with harmful intent). As ubiquitous as social media use is in the United States, there is much to be learned about the connection between mental health and social media use among men.

LIFE COURSE EXPOSURES AND CHRONIC STRESS

Cumulative Impact of Stressors for Aging Men

There are clear connections between stress and poor mental health. Additionally, there is a growing body of evidence that indicates that stress accumulates over the life course, which can increase vulnerability to poor health outcomes through a myriad of ways. Chronic stress is especially damaging because some stressors do not have resolutions. According to social stress theory, stressors arise and individuals appraise the stressor, determining how much control they have over the situation and what resources they have to address or cope with the stressor. Depending on individuals' control (or perceptions of control) along with their resources, stressors often reach a resolution. However, there are many stressors that become chronic insofar as they have no natural resolution. For example, poverty is a significant stressor, impacting people and communities on a day-to-day basis. Each day brings additional stressors, ranging from housing insecurity to swings in work schedules to unreliable transportation. Chronic stressors are particularly deleterious to health in general, as our stress response systems are primed to activate (i.e., fight or flight), but too much activation of this response system can overwhelm our bodies. Chronic stress is linked to poor mental health in addition to physical health outcomes such as cardiovascular disease. As mentioned previously, integrated health is incredibly important here as scholars continue to investigate how stress gets under the skin, damaging our mental health while simultaneously affecting our physical health.

Inequality

Related to the need to understand the life course perspective is also the need to examine how inequality affects the mental health of men as they age. Researchers have consistently demonstrated that lower socioeconomic status is associated with poor mental health (Dohrenwend et al., 1992; Marbin et al., 2022). For example, men who experience poverty are more likely to have depression and anxiety. In many ways, inequality becomes an unrelenting vicious cycle. Living in impoverished communities affects individuals' ability to obtain educational credentials that can lead to better paying jobs, which contributes to financial insecurity. Financial insecurity is stressful, especially when individuals are not able to control when or how long bouts of poverty occur or develop savings in case of unemployment or other financial downturns. This also contributes to housing insecurity, as scholars have documented that mental health is strongly associated with homelessness (Padgett, 2020).

It is important to note that stratification policies and practices undergird the patterning of inequality in the United States. As mentioned in the previous section on racism, inequities across race and ethnicity have been largely fueled by racist policies and practices, which contribute to growing inequities across a broad range of outcomes. For example, there are significant wealth inequities across race/ethnicity in the United States that have been fueled by discriminatory practices such as redlining (Rothstein, 2017). Nonetheless, rising levels of inequality affect men across race and ethnicity. For example, data from multiple studies indicate that poorer White men are disproportionately impacted by substance use, particularly the sharp rise in opioid use during the past 30 years (Lim et al., 2022). In areas that have been disproportionately affected by deindustrialization and where there are fewer opportunities for stable employment and pathways for men to care for their family, there have been increases in suicide and substance abuse risk.

RECOMMENDATIONS AND CALL TO ACTION

Inclusive Recruitment of Diverse Samples in Aging Studies

As we identify a forward path in aging research, it is crucial to prioritize inclusive recruitment strategies that ensure the representation of diverse aging populations. This approach includes but is not limited to individuals from various racial, ethnic, socioeconomic, and cultural backgrounds. Currently, there is a lack of data focused on American Indian/Alaska Native (AI/AN) men's mental health. Indigenous communities often face systemic barriers to healthcare access and quality, leading to disparities in health outcomes. Without accurate surveillance data specific to AI/AN men's mental health, it becomes challenging to develop targeted approaches to engage this population, allocate resources effectively, and address the underlying social determinants that perpetuate mental health disparities within these communities. Immigrant men represent another demographic group that is often overlooked in aging research and prevention efforts. Immigrant and undocumented men may encounter various barriers to healthcare access, including language barriers, lack of insurance coverage, and fear of immigration enforcement. Finally, the carceral system, including prisons and detention centers, can exacerbate existing mental health conditions and increase the risk of premature mortality among aging men in these systems. Ultimately, prioritizing inclusive recruitment of these groups, and many other underrepresented communities, not only enhances the validity and relevance of aging research but also fosters a more comprehensive understanding of the multifaceted challenges faced by marginalized men, paving the way for more targeted and equitable healthcare interventions and policies. Inclusive recruitment also fosters equity in research participation and contributes to the development of interventions and services that are relevant and accessible to all aging individuals. By embracing this approach in our samples, researchers who study aging can enhance the generalizability of findings and gain a more comprehensive understanding of these processes across vulnerable groups. Such approaches may include:

- *Enhancing community partnerships to include activity spaces where aging men dwell*: By leveraging community partnerships to include activity spaces where aging men reside, such as senior living centers, retirement communities, and veterans' associations, scholars can greatly enhance their understanding of men's health. Additionally, incorporating community centers, local libraries, religious institutions, and recreational facilities into such partnerships can provide aging men with diverse opportunities for social engagement, physical activity, and mental stimulation. By expanding access to inclusive activity spaces within their immediate environments, aging men can foster meaningful connections, combat social isolation, and promote overall health and quality of life as they age.
- *Enhance language access in aging research*: Expanding the linguistic diversity of services, programs, and research available is an important consideration to ensure inclusivity and equitable participation among diverse populations. This can be achieved by providing educational materials and adapting evidence-based interventions to be accessible across multiple languages. Moreover, the intentional inclusion of multilingual research staff and interpreters can facilitate effective communication and mitigate language barriers.
- *Tailored outreach strategies*: To ensure equitable representation in aging research, developing tailored outreach strategies targeting underrepresented aging men is critical. These strategies could involve utilizing a variety of communication channels, such as community spaces, local radio stations, and online platforms frequented by men, across the life course. Additionally, leveraging social media platforms and organizing community events can serve as effective means to encourage diverse participation among aging men.

- *Inclusive study designs*: Designing research studies with flexibility to accommodate the needs and preferences of diverse aging populations will foster more inclusive and equitable focus in aging research and practice efforts. Factors such as transportation barriers, compensation of caregiver responsibilities, and mobility limitations must be carefully considered when designing programs for aging men.
- *Inclusive recruitment*: Inclusive recruitment for aging research among men is paramount because it ensures representation from diverse backgrounds, including those who experience intersecting and systemic challenges such as racism, involvement with the criminal justice system, or immigration status. By including these individuals, researchers can gain nuanced insights into the complex interactions between social determinants of health and aging, fostering more equitable and effective interventions to support the well-being of all men as they age. The absence of comprehensive data on underrepresented groups contributes to their underrepresentation in mental health research, advocacy efforts, and policy making, thus perpetuating a cycle of neglect and invisibility.

Mixed-Methods Approaches to Research

Adopting mixed-methods approaches can enrich our understanding of aging phenomena among men by combining quantitative and qualitative data collection techniques. This approach allows researchers to triangulate findings, validate results, and explore complex relationships that may not be fully captured by quantitative measures alone. Furthermore, mixed-methods research enables us to address issues such as recall bias, which may disproportionately affect older adults because of cognitive decline or memory impairments. By integrating qualitative insights with quantitative data, we can generate more nuanced and contextually grounded interpretations of aging experiences and inform the development of tailored interventions and support services.

Addressing Recall Bias

Recognizing the potential impact of recall bias on aging research, it is essential to employ strategies that mitigate its effects. This may involve using innovative data collection methods, such as mobile health or smartphone-based approaches, to capture real-time experiences and minimize reliance on retrospective memory (Burke et al., 2017). Integrating objective measures such as biomarkers, cognitive assessments, and physical performance tests can ensure a more nuanced understanding of the biological, cognitive, and functional changes that occur with aging. This approach not only enhances the rigor and validity of research findings but also allows for the identification of early indicators of mental health issues and potential preventive interventions. Additionally, leveraging observational techniques, such as longitudinal studies and community-based participatory research, can capture the dynamic interactions among individual, social, and environmental factors that influence mental health outcomes in aging men.

Extending and Integrating Services to Serve Aging Men

Given the unique challenges and needs faced by aging men described in this chapter, it is crucial to extend and integrate services that specifically target this expanding population. Historically, aging men have been underserved in healthcare settings, with limited access to preventive care, mental health services, and social support networks. To address this gap, we must prioritize the development of gender-sensitive programs and interventions that acknowledge and respond to the diverse needs and preferences of aging men. Selected approaches may include promoting men's health screenings, fostering peer support groups, and integrating and co-locating mental health services into primary care settings. In implementing such practices, it is essential for researchers, healthcare providers, policy makers, and community stakeholders to collaborate effectively and advocate for inclusive and equitable approaches to aging research and service delivery.

SUMMARY

Examining men's mental health and aging research through a health equity lens highlights the critical need to address multilevel inequities that shape the experiences of aging men. This chapter offers additional insights into how the marginalization of race, gender, and cultural background has a profound influence on mental health outcomes among older adults. By recognizing and addressing disparities in healthcare access, social support systems, and opportunities for healthy aging, we can strive toward a future where all men, irrespective of their circumstances, have equal opportunities to achieve optimal mental well-being as they grow older. As the field advances, it is imperative to continue applying a health equity perspective in research, policy, and practice to ensure that aging men receive the necessary support and resources to thrive in their later years.

DISCUSSION QUESTIONS

1. How do cultural and gendered norms influence the reluctance of aging men to seek mental health care? Do you see this reluctance in your own community or network? In your opinion, how can health professionals and practitioners better reach aging men?
2. In what ways does social isolation uniquely impact the mental health outcomes of aging men compared with women?
3. How can a health equity lens be applied to dismantle systemic barriers and improve access to mental health care for marginalized groups of aging men?
4. What are the challenges associated with studying men's mental health and aging using traditional research methodologies?
5. Discuss the role of inclusive recruitment and mixed-methods approaches in creating more equitable mental health interventions for diverse populations of aging men.

REFERENCES

Addis, M. E., & Mahalik, J. R. (2003). Men, masculinity, and the contexts of help seeking. *American Psychologist, 58*(1), 5–14. https://doi.org/10.1037/0003-066x.58.1.5

Ahmedani, B. K., Simon, G. E., Stewart, C., Beck, A., Waitzfelder, B. E., Rossom, R., Lynch, F., Owen-Smith, A., Hunkeler, E. M., Whiteside, U., Operskalski, B. H., Coffey, M. J., & Solberg, L. I. (2014). Health care contacts in the year before suicide death. *Journal of General Internal Medicine, 29*(6), 870–877. https://doi.org/10.1007/s11606-014-2767-3

Bachmann, S. (2018). Epidemiology of suicide and the psychiatric perspective. *International Journal of Environmental Research and Public Health, 15*(7), 1425. https://doi.org/10.3390/ijerph15071425

Bailey, Z. D., Feldman, J. M., & Bassett, M. T. (2020). How structural racism works—Racist policies as a root cause of U.S. racial health inequities. *New England Journal of Medicine, 384*(8), 768–773. https://doi.org/10.1056/NEJMms2025396

Bailey, Z. D., Krieger, N., Agénor, M., Graves, J., Linos, N., & Bassett, M. T. (2017). Structural racism and health inequities in the USA: Evidence and interventions. *The Lancet, 389*(10077), 1453–1463. https://doi.org/10.1016/S0140-6736(17)30569-X

Barreto, M., Victor, C., Hammond, C., Eccles, A., Richins, M. T., & Qualter, P. (2021). Loneliness around the world: Age, gender, and cultural differences in loneliness. *Personality and Individual Differences, 169*, 110066. https://doi.org/10.1016/j.paid.2020.110066

Berger, J. L., Addis, M. E., Green, J. D., Mackowiak, C., & Goldberg, V. (2013). Men's reactions to mental health labels, forms of help-seeking, and sources of help-seeking advice. *Psychology of Men & Masculinity, 14*(4), 433. https://doi.org/10.1037/a0030175

Bonilla-Silva, E. (2006). *Racism without racists: Color-blind racism and the persistence of racial inequality in the United States*. Rowman & Littlefield Publishers.

Bonilla-Silva, E., & Baiocchi, G. (2001). Anything but racism: How sociologists limit the significance of racism. *Race and Society*, *4*(2), 117–131.

Brausch, A. M., & Gutierrez, P. M. (2010). Differences in non-suicidal self-injury and suicide attempts in adolescents. *Journal of Youth and Adolescence*, *39*(3), 233–242. https://doi.org/10.1007/s10964-009-9482-0

Burke, L. E., Shiffman, S., Music, E., Styn, M. A., Kriska, A., Smailagic, A., Siewiorek, D., Ewing, L. J., Chasens, E., French, B., Mancino, J., Mendez, D., Strollo, P., & Rathbun, S. L. (2017). Ecological momentary assessment in behavioral research: Addressing technological and human participant challenges. *Journal of Medical Internet Research*, *19*(3), e77. https://doi.org/10.2196/jmir.7138

Chatters, L. M., Taylor, H. O., & Taylor, R. J. (2021). Racism and the life course: Social and health equity for Black American older adults. *Public Policy & Aging Report*, *31*(4), 113–118. https://doi.org/10.1093/ppar/prab018

Coleman, D. (2015). Traditional masculinity as a risk factor for suicidal ideation: Cross-sectional and prospective evidence from a study of young adults. *Archives of Suicide Research: Official Journal of the International Academy for Suicide Research*, *19*(3), 366–384. https://doi.org/10.1080/13811118.2014.957453

Connell, R. W., & Messerschmidt, J. W. (2005). Hegemonic masculinity: Rethinking the concept. *Gender & Society*, *19*(6), 829–859. https://doi.org/10.1177/0891243205278639

Courtenay, W. H. (2000). Constructions of masculinity and their influence on men's well-being: A theory of gender and health. *Social Science & Medicine*, *50*(10), 1385–1401. https://doi.org/10.1016/s0277-9536(99)00390-1

Cudjoe, T. K., Roth, D. L., Szanton, S. L., Wolff, J. L., Boyd, C. M., & Thorpe Jr, R. J. (2020). The epidemiology of social isolation: National health and aging trends study. *The Journals of Gerontology: Series B*, *75*(1), 107–113. https://doi.org/10.1093/geronb/gby037

Dohrenwend, B. P., Levav, I., Shrout, P. E., Schwartz, S., Naveh, G., Link, B. G., Skodol, A. E., & Stueve, A. (1992). Socioeconomic status and psychiatric disorders: The causation-selection issue. *Science*, *255*(5047), 946–952. https://doi.org/10.1126/science.1546291

Elder, G. H., & Johnson, M. K. (2018). The life course and aging: Challenges, lessons, and new directions. In *Invitation to the life course* (pp. 49–81). Routledge.

Elder, G. H., Shanahan, M. J., & Clipp, E. C. (1994). When war comes to men's lives: Life-course patterns in family, work, and health. *Psychology and Aging*, *9*(1), 5–16. https://doi.org/10.1037//0882-7974.9.1.5

Feigelman, W., & Gorman, B. S. (2008). Assessing the effects of peer suicide on youth suicide. *Suicide & Life-Threatening Behavior*, *38*(2), 181–194. https://doi.org/10.1521/suli.2008.38.2.181

Fried, L. E., Williams, S., Cabral, H., & Hacker, K. (2013). Differences in risk factors for suicide attempts among 9th and 11th grade youth: A longitudinal perspective. *The Journal of School Nursing*, *29*(2), 113–122. https://doi.org/10.1177/1059840512461010

Geronimus, A. T. (1992). The weathering hypothesis and the health of African-American women and infants: Evidence and speculations. *Ethnicity & Disease*, *2*(3), 207–221.

Glymour, M. M., & Manly, J. J. (2008). Lifecourse social conditions and racial and ethnic patterns of cognitive aging. *Neuropsychology Review*, *18*(3), 223–254. https://doi.org/10.1007/s11065-008-9064-z

Gómez, C. A., Kleinman, D. V., Pronk, N., Gordon, G. L. W., Ochiai, E., Blakey, C., Johnson, A., & Brewer, K. H. (2021). Addressing health equity and social determinants of health through healthy people 2030. *Journal of Public Health Management and Practice*, *27*(Suppl 6), S249–S257. https://doi.org/10.1097/PHH.0000000000000129

Gordon, J. A., Avenevoli, S., & Pearson, J. L. (2020). Suicide prevention research priorities in health care. *JAMA Psychiatry*, *77*(9), 885–886. https://doi.org/10.1001/jamapsychiatry.2020.1042

Halfon, N., Larson, K., Lu, M., Tullis, E., & Russ, S. (2014). Lifecourse health development: Past, present and future. *Maternal and Child Health Journal*, *18*(2), 344–365. https://doi.org/10.1007/s10995-013-1346-2

Hammond, W. P., & Mattis, J. S. (2005). Being a man about it: Manhood meaning among African American men. *Psychology of Men & Masculinity*, *6*(2), 114–126. https://doi.org/10.1037/1524-9220.6.2.114

Holt-Lunstad, J., Smith, T. B., Baker, M., Harris, T., & Stephenson, D. (2015). Loneliness and social isolation as risk factors for mortality: A meta-analytic review. *Perspectives on Psychological Science*, *10*(2), 227–237. https://doi.org/10.1177/1745691614568352

Huang, A. R., Roth, D. L., Cidav, T., Chung, S.-E., Amjad, H., Thorpe R. J., Jr., Boyd, C. M., & Cudjoe, T. K. (2023). Social isolation and 9-year dementia risk in community-dwelling Medicare beneficiaries in the United States. *Journal of the American Geriatrics Society*, *71*(3), 765–773. https://doi.org/10.1111/jgs.18140

Idris, D. R., Forrest, S., & Brown, S. (2017). Integrative review of literature on masculinity, health service utilization and health outcomes. *Brunei Darussalem Journal of Health*, *7*(1), 26–42.

Kessler, R. C., Berglund, P., Demler, O., Jin, R., Merikangas, K. R., & Walters, E. E. (2005). Lifetime prevalence and age-of-onset distributions of DSM-IV disorders in the National Comorbidity Survey Replication. *Archives of General Psychiatry*, *62*(6), 593–602. https://doi.org/10.1001/archpsyc.62.6.593

Kessler, R. C., Brown, R. L., & Broman, C. L. (1981). Sex differences in psychiatric help-seeking: Evidence from four large-scale surveys. *Journal of Health and Social Behavior*, *22*(1), 49–64.

Krieger, N., & Davey Smith, G. (2004). "Bodies count," and body counts: Social epidemiology and embodying inequality. *Epidemiologic Reviews*, *26*(1), 92–103. https://doi.org/10.1093/epirev/mxh009

Kullgren, J., Solway, E., Roberts, S., Singer, D., Kirch, M., Malani, P., Smith, E., & Hutchens, L. (2023). *Trends in loneliness among older adults from 2018-2023.* https://dx.doi.org/10.7302/7011

Leaf, P. J., Livingston, M. M., Tischler, G. L., Weissman, M. M., Holzer, C. E., III, & Myers, J. K. (1985). Contact with health professionals for the treatment of psychiatric and emotional problems. *Medical Care, 23*(12), 1322–1337. https://doi.org/10.1097/00005650-198512000-00002

Levant, R. F., Hirsch, L. S., Celentano, E., & Cozza, T. M. (1992). The male role: An investigation of contemporary norms. *Journal of Mental Health Counseling, 14*(3), 325–337.

Levant, R. F., Smalley, K. B., Aupont, M., House, A. T., Richmond, K., & Noronha, D. (2007). Initial validation of the male role norms inventory-revised (MRNI-R). *The Journal of Men's Studies, 15*(1), 83-100. https://doi.org/10.3149/jms.1501.83

Liddon, L., Kingerlee, R., & Barry, J. A. (2018). Gender differences in preferences for psychological treatment, coping strategies, and triggers to help-seeking. *British Journal of Clinical Psychology, 57*(1), 42–58. https://doi.org/10.1111/bjc.12147

Lim, T. Y., Stringfellow, E. J., Stafford, C. A., DiGennaro, C., Homer, J. B., Wakeland, W., Eggers, S. L., Kazemi, R., Glos, L., & Ewing, E. G. (2022). Modeling the evolution of the US opioid crisis for national policy development. *Proceedings of the National Academy of Sciences of the United States of America, 119*(23), e2115714119. https://doi.org/10.1073/pnas.2115714119

Mahalik, J. R., & Di Bianca, M. (2021). Help-seeking for depression as a stigmatized threat to masculinity. *Professional Psychology: Research and Practice, 52*(2), 146–155. https://doi.org/10.1037/pro0000365

Mansfield, A. K., Addis, M. E., & Courtenay, W. (2005). Measurement of men's help seeking: Development and evaluation of the barriers to help seeking scale. *Psychology of Men & Masculinity, 6*(2), 95–108. https://doi.org/10.1037/1524-9220.6.2.95

Marbin, D., Gutwinski, S., Schreiter, S., & Heinz, A. (2022). Perspectives in poverty and mental health. *Frontiers in Public Health, 10,* 975482. https://doi.org/10.3389/fpubh.2022.975482

Möller-Leimkühler, A. M. (2002). Barriers to help-seeking by men: A review of sociocultural and clinical literature with particular reference to depression. *Journal of Affective Disorders, 71*(1–3), 1–9. https://doi.org/10.1016/s0165-0327(01)00379-2

Nummela, O., Seppänen, M., & Uutela, A. (2011). The effect of loneliness and change in loneliness on self-rated health (SRH): A longitudinal study among aging people. *Archives of Gerontology and Geriatrics, 53*(2), 163–167. https://doi.org/10.1016/j.archger.2010.10.023

Padgett, D. K. (2020). Homelessness, housing instability and mental health: Making the connections. *BJPsych Bulletin, 44*(5), 197–201. https://doi.org/10.1192/bjb.2020.49

Powell, W., Richmond, J., Mohottige, D., Yen, I., Joslyn, A., & Corbie-Smith, G. (2019). Medical mistrust, racism, and delays in preventive health screening among African-American men. *Behavioral Medicine (Washington, D.C.), 45*(2), 102–117. https://doi.org/10.1080/08964289.2019.1585327

Primack, B. A., Karim, S. A., Shensa, A., Bowman, N., Knight, J., & Sidani, J. E. (2019). Positive and negative experiences on social media and perceived social isolation. *American Journal of Health Promotion, 33*(6), 859–868. https://doi.org/10.1177/0890117118824196

Rice, S. M., Fallon, B. J., Aucote, H. M., & Möller-Leimkühler, A. M. (2013). Development and preliminary validation of the male depression risk scale: Furthering the assessment of depression in men. *Journal of Affective Disorders, 151*(3), 950–958. https://doi.org/10.1016/j.jad.2013.08.013

Robbins, M. J., Wester, S. R., & McKean, N. B. (2016). *Masculinity across the life span: Implications for older men* (pp. 389–409). American Psychological Association.

Robine, J.-M. (2021). Ageing populations: We are living longer lives, but are we healthier. *United Nations, 2,* 1–24. https://desapublications.un.org/file/653/download

Robine, J.-M., Jagger, C., Crimmins, E. M., Saito, Y., & Van Oyen, H. (2020). Trends in health expectancies. *International handbook of health expectancies* (pp. 19–34). Springer.

Rochelle, T. L., Yeung, D. K., Bond, M. H., & Li, L. M. W. (2015). Predictors of the gender gap in life expectancy across 54 nations. *Psychology, Health & Medicine, 20*(2), 129–138. https://doi.org/10.1080/13548506.2014.936884

Rothstein, R. (2017). *The color of law: A forgotten history of how our government segregated America.* Liveright Publishing.

Salomon, J. A., Wang, H., Freeman, M. K., Vos, T., Flaxman, A. D., Lopez, A. D., & Murray, C. J. (2012). Healthy life expectancy for 187 countries, 1990–2010: A systematic analysis for the Global Burden Disease Study 2010. *The Lancet, 380*(9859), 2144–2162. https://doi.org/10.1016/S0140-6736(12)61690-0

Sileo, K. M., & Kershaw, T. S. (2020). Dimensions of masculine norms, depression, and mental health service utilization: Results from a prospective cohort study among emerging adult men in the United States. *American Journal of Men's Health, 14*(1), 1557988320906980. https://doi.org/10.1177/1557988320906980

Steptoe, A., Shankar, A., Demakakos, P., & Wardle, J. (2013). Social isolation, loneliness, and all-cause mortality in older men and women. *Proceedings of the National Academy of Sciences of the United States of America, 110*(15), 5797–5801. https://doi.org/10.1073/pnas.1219686110

Substance Abuse and Mental Health Services Administration. (2024). *Behavioral health among older adults: Results from the 2021 and 2022 National Surveys on Drug Use and Health* (SAMHSA Publication No. PEP24-07-018). https://www.samhsa.gov/data/report/older-adult-behavioral-health-report-2021-2022

Swope, C. B., & Hernández, D. (2019). Housing as a determinant of health equity: A conceptual model. *Social Science & Medicine, 243*, 112571. https://doi.org/10.1016/j.socscimed.2019.112571

Thorpe, R., Jr., & Whitfield, K. (2021). Social determinants of men's health across the life course. *Innovation in Aging, 5*(Suppl_1), 420. https://doi.org/10.1093/geroni/igab046.1629

Vogel, D. L., & Heath, P. J. (2016). *Men, masculinities, and help-seeking patterns.* American Psychological Association. https://doi.org/10.1037/14594-031

Vogel, D. L., Heimerdinger-Edwards, S. R., Hammer, J. H., & Hubbard, A. (2011). "Boys don't cry": Examination of the links between endorsement of masculine norms, self-stigma, and help-seeking attitudes for men from diverse backgrounds. *Journal of Counseling Psychology, 58*(3), 368. https://doi.org/10.1037/a0023688

Wendt, D., & Shafer, K. (2016). Gender and attitudes about mental health help seeking: Results from national data. *Health & Social Work, 41*(1), e20–e28. https://doi.org/10.1093/hsw/hlv089

Williams, D. R. (2008). The health of men: Structured inequalities and opportunities. *American Journal of Public Health, 98*(Suppl_1), S150–S157. https://doi.org/10.2105/ajph.98.supplement_1.s150

Williams, D. R., & Etkins, O. S. (2021). Racism and mental health. *World Psychiatry, 20*(2), 194–195.

Williams, D. R., Lawrence, J. A., & Davis, B. A. (2019). Racism and health: Evidence and needed research. *Annual Review of Public Health, 40*, 105–125. https://doi.org/10.1146/annurev-publhealth-040218-043750

Williams, D. R., & Mohammed, S. A. (2013). Racism and health. I. Pathways and scientific evidence. *American Behavioral Scientist, 57*(8), 1152–1173. https://doi.org/10.1177/0002764213487340

Willis, P., & Vickery, A. (2022). Loneliness, coping practices and masculinities in later life: Findings from a study of older men living alone in England. *Health & Social Care in the Community, 30*(5), e2874–e2883. https://doi.org/10.1111/hsc.13732

Willis, P., Vickery, A., & Symonds, J. (2022). Caring, old age, and masculinities: Men's experiences of caring and maintaining social connections in later life. In A. Tarrant, L. Ladlow, & L. Way (Eds.), *Men and welfare* (pp. 242–254). Routledge.

World Health Organization. (2010). *Health equity.* https://www.who.int/health-topics/health-equity#tab=tab_1

Part IV

FROM THEORY TO POLICY

16 SHAPING STATE POLICY TO ADDRESS MENTAL HEALTH INEQUITIES

SIDNEY D. WATSON

LEARNING OBJECTIVES

After reading this chapter, readers will be able to:

- Identify how federalism can help and hinder state efforts to address mental health inequities.
- Describe how state policy has contributed to mental health inequities.
- Explain how Medicaid expansion has reduced historic mental health inequities.
- Understand how states can regulate commercial insurance and the limits of state authority.
- Discuss how Medicaid provides opportunities to states to address mental health inequities.

INTRODUCTION

This chapter discusses how state law and policy can address and reduce mental health inequities. Historically, state coercion, incarceration, and warehousing have contributed to mental health inequities. Going forward, two principles should guide states in shaping policies to address mental health inequities. First, state policies should reduce reliance on law enforcement, involuntary interventions, and forced treatment as a response to mental health and substance use crises.[1] Second, state commercial health insurance and Medicaid policies should promote preventive, early, and long-term community-based recovery-oriented mental health treatment over acute or long-term inpatient care.

States operate within a federal system in which federal law authorizes, influences, funds, and constrains state lawmaking. For example, states have significant authority to enact laws to protect the health and safety of their citizens, but states are also constrained by the U.S. Constitution, which protects people's rights to liberty, autonomy, and due process. **Table 16.1** offers a typology of the types of federalism that frequently impact state lawmaking related to mental health inequities. As you read this chapter, consider which kinds of federalism interact with state lawmaking to address mental health inequities.

[1] This chapter often uses *mental health* to include behavioral health and substance use disorder.

Table 16.1 TYPES OF FEDERALISM

FEDERALISM TYPE	DESCRIPTION	EXAMPLE
State police power	The Constitution gives states inherent "police power" to protect public health and safety.	Civil commitment laws
Constitutional rights	States must respect U.S. Constitutional rights to liberty, autonomy, and due process.	The Supreme Court has held that states can involuntarily commit people for treatment only if they present a danger to themselves or others.
Spending clause federalism	The federal government offers funding to the states for a specific purpose. States are not required to accept the federal money, but if they do, they must comply with federal rules for using the funds.	Medicaid
Fallback federalism	The federal government offers states the opportunity to establish, enforce, or administer a program authorized by federal law. If a state declines the offer, the federal government will take up the role.	The Affordable Care Act's health insurance exchanges
Federal preemption	Federal law prohibits states from enforcing specific laws.	ERISA prohibits states from regulating employee benefit plans.

ERISA, Employee Retirement Income Security Act.

ROLE OF STATE LAW AND POLICY IN CREATING MENTAL HEALTH INEQUITIES

Historically, state policies have contributed mightily to mental health inequities. For most of the 20th century, state laws confined and segregated people identified as "mentally ill" or "mentally retarded" in massive state institutions, typically hidden in faraway rural areas. State criminal laws imprisoned those found "criminally insane." State civil commitment laws locked away others using labels like *imbecile*, *mentally defective*, and *abnormal* (Burt, 2001). Public health and criminal laws locked away Black men, grossly mislabeling them as "drug fiends" and "schizophrenics" (Hylton, 2024).

Beginning in the late 1960s, state mental health policies began to change. State and federal courts declared punitive involuntary commitment laws and the terrible conditions under which people were confined to be unconstitutional. New federal and state laws called for people with mental illness to be released from institutions and provided treatment in the community (Burt, 2001). Medicaid and Medicare, passed in 1965, severely restricted payment for "institutions for mental illness," incentivizing states to quickly reduce their state mental hospital populations, which were not eligible for payment, and move people into Medicaid and Medicare–funded nursing homes or general hospitals with psychiatric beds or send them back into the community (Davoli, 2003, p. 170).

Sadly, commercial health insurance resisted paying for mental health and substance use treatment. State and federal governments were slow to fund community-based services adequately. The stigma surrounding mental health and substance use, fueled by a century of punitive laws and policies, made people reluctant to talk about mental health and substance use problems or to seek what little community-based treatment was available. People with mental illness and substance use often went untreated until they went into an acute crisis, which was often hastily brought under control in a prison, jail, or inpatient bed. Only rarely could people access recovery-oriented community-based services.

As we entered the 21st century, the state and local policy response was to police people with mental illness and substance abuse, arresting and locking them up for minor infractions or unusual behavior. Our jails and prisons filled as people with mental illness and substance abuse rotated in and out. Many received treatment and became stabilized while incarcerated, only to crash when released back into communities that offered insufficient mental health and substance abuse treatment and other supportive services, such as housing.

Looking forward, states need to reform their policies to replace old patterns of state coercion, incarceration, and warehousing that have contributed to mental health inequities. Two principles should guide states in shaping policies addressing mental health inequities. First, state policies should reduce reliance on law enforcement, involuntary interventions, and forced treatment as a response to mental health and substance use crises. Second, state insurance policies and Medicaid should promote preventive, early, and long-term community-based, recovery-oriented mental health treatment over acute or long-term inpatient care (Swadley, 2023).

SHAPING STATE POLICY TO REDUCE RELIANCE ON LAW ENFORCEMENT AND FORCED TREATMENT

Historically, police have played a central role in triaging and transporting people in mental health crises to jails and involuntary psychiatric treatment, particularly low-income people and people of color. Police get involved with people having a mental health crisis in several ways:

- Police respond to calls related to suspected criminal behavior related to symptoms of mental illness.
- Bystanders, neighbors, and families call the police, asking them to remove a person experiencing symptoms of psychosis and behaving in ways that alarm them.
- Family members and clinicians may call the police specifically to assist with emergency detention for acute psychiatric treatment.
- People experiencing mental health crises may call the police themselves seeking help (Watson & El-Sabawi, 2023).

Using police as first responders for people experiencing mental health crises puts people at risk.

Involving police increases the risk that people in mental health crises will be involuntarily hospitalized or incarcerated (Swadley, 2023). It also puts people with mental illness at increased risk of police use of force, injury, and death. One of four people killed in interactions with the police show signs of mental illness (see Watson & El-Sabawi, 2023), and people with mental illness are at a sevenfold increased risk of death when police intervene (Swadley, 2023).

It should not be the job of police to respond to healthcare crises. People in mental health crisis, just as people with physical health emergencies, need quick access to effective mental health care. The federal Substance Abuse and Mental Health Services Administration (SAMSHA, 2020) has developed best practice guidelines for a behavioral health crisis continuum of care that contains the following three core mental health services to which every person having a mental health crisis should have access:

- *Someone to call*: local crisis call centers answering 24/7
- *Someone to respond:* mobile crisis teams staffed by behavioral health professionals who provide face-to-face stabilization services quickly in a person's home, workplace, or other community-based location
- *Somewhere to go*: crisis stabilization facilities that offer short-term (under 24 hours) observation and stabilization services in a home-like, nonhospital environment (**Figure 16.1**)

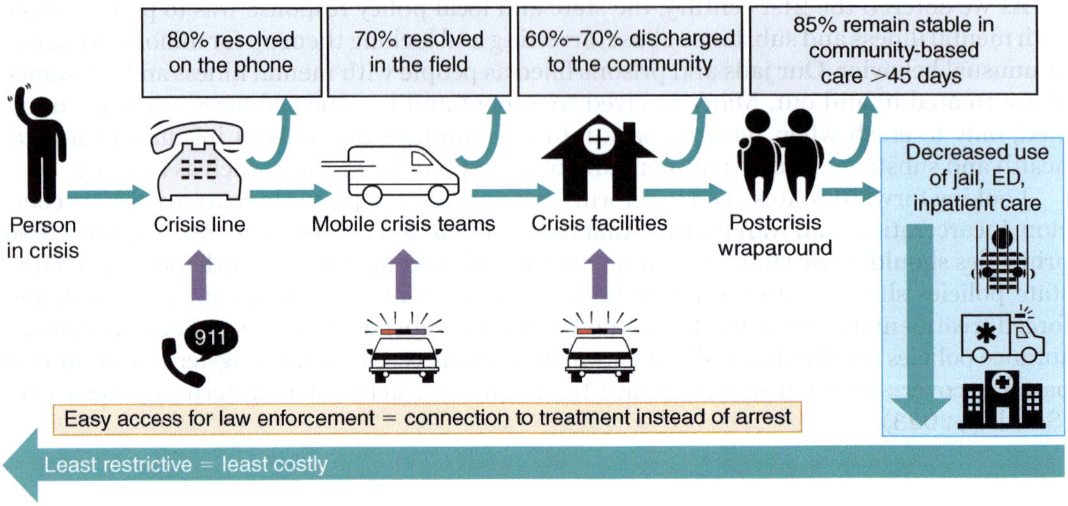

Figure 16.1 Behavioral health crisis continuum of care.
Source: Balfour, M. E., Stephenson, A. H., Delany-Brumsey, A., Winsky, J., & Goldman, M. L. (2022). Cops, clinicians, or both? Collaborative approaches to responding to behavioral health emergencies. *Psychiatric Services, 73*(6), 658–669. https://doi.org/10.1176/appi.ps.202000721

The three components of the behavioral crisis continuum of care operate to de-escalate, stabilize, and connect people having a mental health crisis to community-based, recovery-oriented services. The continuum reduces interactions with police and decreases unnecessary incarceration and hospitalization.

Recent federal law supports states that want to shift state policy to a behavioral health crisis continuum of care response. In 2020, Congress designated 988 as a new nationwide mental health crisis hotline and authorized states to impose cell phone bill surcharges to support local 988 call centers and mental health crisis–related services (Interconnection, 2023). In 2021, the American Rescue Plan Act (ARPA) authorized planning grants and enhanced Medicaid funding to help states transition to 988 and create and improve mobile crisis services to better align the delivery of mobile crisis services with SAMHSA guidelines (Saunders, 2023). In 2023, Congress allocated additional grants to states for mobile crisis response teams (see SAMHSA, 2022).

States have begun to shift state policy toward a behavioral health continuum of care crisis response. In Illinois, legislation now requires the state's department of mental health to develop a mobile crisis team capacity sufficient to offer services 24r hours a day, 7 days a week. The law prohibits police from responding to a mental health crisis, except if the person is suspected of committing a crime or presents a threat of physical injury to themselves or others (Community Emergency Services and Support Act, 2024; Watson & El-Sabawi, 2023). Virginia passed a bill that requires the state to develop a crisis continuum of care and local protocols for mobile crisis response to mental health crises whenever possible (Crisis Intervention Teams, 2009; Watson & El-Sabawi, 2023).

A key challenge for states will be finding funds to support the creation and expansion of mobile crisis teams, crisis facilities, and follow-up services. Federal dollars support 988 nationally, but states are responsible for long-term funding for the local 988 crisis call centers and continuum of care services. As of March 2024, eight states have authorized cell phone fees to support 988 services, eight states have strengthened state laws mandating that commercial health insurance plans cover crisis care services, and 30 states have passed appropriations to support at least one of the three core mental health crisis care services

(National Alliance on Mental Illness [NAMI], 2024). As of September 12, 2024, 21 states have federal approval to receive enhanced Medicaid funding for mobile crisis teams under ARPA (Centers for Medicare & Medicaid Services [CMS], 2025). Another 19 states report using regular Medicaid funding for mobile crisis services (KFF, 2022b).

The rest of this chapter focuses on how states can shape commercial insurance and Medicaid to cover mental health services better. Here are a couple questions to consider as you proceed through the chapter:

- What policy options might states have to leverage and require commercial insurance and Medicaid to pay for mobile crisis teams, crisis facilities, and follow-up care?
- What policy options would you recommend for your state and why?

SHAPING STATE POLICY TO PROMOTE COMMUNITY-BASED MENTAL HEALTH TREATMENT BY EXPANDING ACCESS TO HEALTH INSURANCE

Insurance coverage plays a critical role in access to and financing of community-based mental health treatment. State policy plays a crucial role in shaping the mental health and substance use coverage that Medicaid and commercial insurance offer. Medicare is also an essential source of health insurance, but because it is a fully federal program, state policy plays a much less significant role.

The Affordable Care Act (ACA) made health coverage more accessible and affordable and has resulted in a dramatic expansion of health insurance coverage for people with mental illness and substance use disorder. However, policies in some states leave nearly 1.5 million low-income adults in the Medicaid coverage gap without insurance to pay for mental health care and other treatment.

Increasing Access to Health Insurance by Closing the Medicaid Coverage Gap

Before the ACA, Medicaid limited eligibility to narrow categories of low-income adults, such as pregnant women, families with children, seniors, and people with disabilities. In many states, adults with mental illness who did not have or were waiting on a disability determination were left ineligible for Medicaid no matter how low their income or how severe their condition was. Instead of being able to access community-based preventive care and early treatment, low-income adults had to wait until their mental illness became so severe, it resulted in a permanent and total disability. With the ACA, millions of people with mental illness are now eligible for Medicaid, the nation's largest payer of mental health services (NAMI, 2024).

The ACA's Medicaid expansion offers coverage to nearly all low-income adults with incomes up to 138% of the federal poverty line: $20,783 for an individual in 2024 (KFF, 2022a). Medicaid expansion has narrowed long-standing gaps in insurance coverage, particularly for people of color and low-wage workers long excluded from employer-sponsored insurance. Dozens of studies show that Medicaid expansion improves access to care and outcomes for mental health and substance use disorder care (Guth & Ammula, 2021).

Yet, as of 2024, 10 states have failed to adopt Medicaid expansion, leaving nearly 1.5 million uninsured adults in the coverage gap because they do not qualify for Medicaid and earn too little to be eligible for federal tax benefits that help people pay for commercial insurance purchased through an exchange (Rudowitz et al., 2024). Eight of the 10 nonexpanding states are in the South, and nine of 10 people in the coverage gap live in these eight Southern states (see Drake et al., 2024). These nonexpanding Southern states have stingy Medicaid and other social programs, high poverty rates, and the history of slavery and Jim Crow laws that have led to today's race-based health disparities, including mental health disparities (**Figure 16.2**).

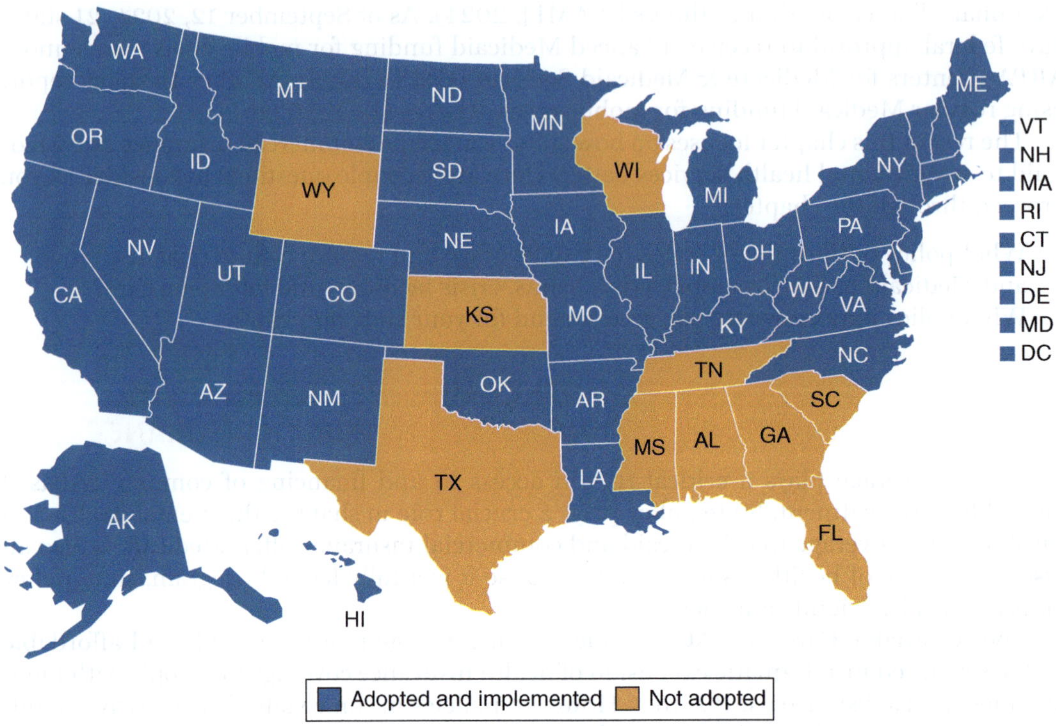

Figure 16.2 Status of state medicaid expansion decisions.

Source: KFF. (2024, July 15). *Status of state Medicaid expansion decisions: Interactive map.* https://www.kff.org/affordable-care-act/issue-brief/status-of-state-medicaid-expansion-decisions-interactive-map/

Why have these states not expanded Medicaid? Some policy makers in nonexpanding states claim states cannot afford to expand Medicaid. However, Medicaid expansion has proved to be a financial gain for states. The federal government covered 100% of the cost of the expansion in the early years of the ACA, and since 2020 has covered 90% of the cost.

Many studies show that states have offset the state costs for Medicaid expansion through state cost savings in other areas, including previously state-funded mental health services. Numerous studies have found that Medicaid expansion brings revenue gains and economic growth for states (Ammula & Guth, 2023). Moreover, in 2021, Congress enacted ARPA, which provides additional financial incentives for the remaining states to expand Medicaid, new funding that has helped reignite expansion discussions in nonexpanding states (Rudowitz et al., 2024).

Seven of the last eight states to adopt expansion did so not through the state legislature but through a ballot measure and direct vote of the people. However, most of the remaining 10 nonexpansion states do not have a ballot initiative process, meaning that future expansion efforts will need to focus on building bipartisan support in state legislatures (Drake et al., 2024).

SHAPING STATE POLICY TO IMPROVE COMMERCIAL HEALTH INSURANCE COVERAGE FOR MENTAL HEALTH TREATMENT

Commercial insurance—the kind offered by private for-profit companies to individuals, families, and small and large employers—also provides an essential source of coverage for people seeking community-based mental health treatment. In 2022, commercial insurance covered 65% of children and nonelderly adults: more than 174 million people (KFF, 2022a). In 2020, commercial insurance covered 58% of nonelderly adults diagnosed with mental illness or substance use disorder—more than 37 million people (Saunders & Rudowitz, 2022).

States play a crucial role in regulating certain commercial health plans. States can legislate the coverage offered by health plans in the individual and small group market, including plans offered on the ACA health insurance exchanges. States can also regulate the coverage offered to state and local government employees. However, a federal law, the Employee Retirement Income Security Act of 1974, known as ERISA, preempts state laws that seek to regulate employee benefit plans. ERISA prevents states from enforcing state health insurance mandates against private employers who self-fund their employee benefit plans rather than purchasing a plan from an insurance company, the form of coverage used by most large employers (Other Laws, 2024; **Box 16.1**).

Box 16.1 WHAT IS ERISA?

- **Why did Congress enact ERISA?**
  ERISA, the federal Employee Retirement and Income Security Act, was enacted in 1974 primarily to regulate employee pension funds. Although the law was originally enacted to protect employee pension funds, it also affects employer-sponsored health insurance. ERISA prevents states from directly regulating employee welfare benefits, including *self-funded* employer-sponsored health plans.
- **Which employers does ERISA apply to?**
  ERISA governs employer-sponsored health plans, except those offered by a church or a governmental entity for its employees. ERISA does not govern health insurance provided by a church or a governmental entity. ERISA also does not govern public health insurance plans (such as Medicaid or Medicare) or private health insurance bought in the nongroup market.
- **What is a *self-funded* employer-sponsored plan?**
  Employers providing health benefits for workers and their families can fund those benefits in one of two ways.
  - *Insured plans:* Employers may purchase a health insurance plan from a state-licensed health insurer. The employer pays premiums to the health insurer, and the insurer pays for the care provided to employees and their families. This is called an "insured plan."
  - *Self-funded plans:* Employers can pay directly with their own assets for the healthcare their enrollees use. Employees enroll in a health plan, but the employer is responsible for paying the healthcare costs, not just the insurance premiums. This is called a "self-funded plan."
- **When does ERISA prohibit state regulation of employer-sponsored health plans?**
  Most large employers self-fund their health benefit plans. Under ERISA, states may regulate health insurers and the plans they sell to employers. However, ERISA prohibits states from regulating how employers structure their employee benefit plans, including self-funded health plans.

ERISA, Employee Retirement Income Security Act.

Source: Adapted from Claxton, G., Rae, M., & Winger, A. (2004, May 28). *Employer-sponsored health insurance 101*. KFF. https://www.kff.org/health-policy-101-employer-sponsored-health-insurance/?entry=table-of-contents-introduction

States have various options for shaping state laws to improve the mental health coverage offered by commercial plans they regulate. Many states have used this authority to expand the coverage for mental health services provided by the commercial health plans they regulate.

State Mental Health Mandates to Require Health Plans to Cover all Medically Necessary Mental Health Services

For decades, commercial health insurance plans, particularly those offered in the individual and small-group market, did not cover mental health services. However, that changed with the passage of the ACA. The ACA now requires that non-grandfathered health plans (those offered since the passage of the ACA) in the individual and small-group markets must cover 10 essential health benefits, including "mental health and substance use disorder services, including behavioral health treatment" (Comprehensive Health Insurance Coverage, 2010). The ACA does not define the coverage that plans must offer for mental health, substance use disorder, or behavioral health treatment. Federal regulations give states the authority to pick a benchmark plan to define the scope of coverage that must be offered. Still, many times benchmark plans have vague standards or limited mental health coverage (see CMS, 2024).

Insurers continue to use a variety of cost-containment tools to restrict coverage for mental health and substance use disorders. Some plans still limit covered services to acute or short-term treatment. Some exclude specific types of mental health treatments and services, refusing to cover care for conditions such as autism. Others narrowly restrict the number or types of providers in their networks, excluding peer recovery specialists or specialized behavioral counselors. Still others impose overly restrictive definitions of medical necessity and burdensome prior authorization and step therapy requirements that prevent people from accessing care recommended by their providers (see Lawrence, 2020).

Numerous states have stepped up to enact laws to prevent these and other insurance practices that restrict coverage for mental health and substance use treatment. Some states specify coverage of specific services, such as autism. Others have passed state mental health parity laws expanding upon the requirements in federal law that prohibit certain health plans from using more stringent requirements for coverage of mental health conditions than they apply to physical health. Others require insurers to cover all diagnoses listed in the American Psychiatric Association's *Diagnostic and Statistical Manual of Mental Health Disorders* (Kirby & Slone, 2022). At least four states—Louisiana, Massachusetts, New Jersey, and Wyoming—enacted bills in 2022 and 2023 requiring private insurers to reimburse for services provided through psychiatric collaborative care models. This innovative, integrated care model includes teams of primary care providers, psychiatric consultants, and care managers who coordinate the patients' behavioral health needs in the community (Pitsor, 2023).

At least 17 states have passed legislation prohibiting insurers from limiting benefits or coverage for mental health and substance use disorders to short-term or acute treatment. These states require insurers to cover the full range of medically necessary services according to the standards of care and practice generally recognized by healthcare providers in psychiatry, addiction medicine, and similar specialties (Kirby & Slone, 2022; The Kennedy Forum, 2020).

State Policies to Enforce Parity in Insurance Coverage for Mental and Physical Healthcare

Federal law prohibits most commercial health insurance plans—individual, small group, and large employer—from imposing more stringent limits on mental health and substance use benefits than they do on other medical benefits. These so-called mental health parity requirements address the following three different types of cost containment strategies used by health plans:

- Financial requirements, such as deductibles and copayments
- Quantitative treatment limits, such as the number of covered visits or days of coverage
- Nonquantitative treatment limits, such as prior authorizations, drug formularies, and provider networks (Comprehensive Health Insurance Coverage, 2010; Parity in Mental Health and Substance Use Disorder Benefits, 2024; Volk et al., 2022)

State insurance departments have primary responsibility for enforcing these federal mental health parity requirements for individual and group plans sold by insurers, including ACA marketplace plans. However, three states have opted for the federal government to assume this enforcement authority: Missouri, Texas, and Wyoming. The federal government oversees mental health parity compliance for all self-funded employer-sponsored plans, typically large-employer plans (Kona, 2023).

State enforcement of financial and quantitative treatment requirements has generally proven to be effective. Still, states have struggled to identify and correct differences in insurers' use of nonquantitative treatment limits, including insurers' use of differing standards for medical necessity and inconsistent prior authorization requirements (Volk et al., 2022).

Many have called for additional federal guidance and resources to help states, and new federal regulations are pending (Kona, 2023). Since 2018, at least 17 states have enacted legislation bolstering mental health parity reporting and oversight (Pitsor, 2023). For example, since 2022, Georgia requires insurers to submit parity compliance reports to the department of insurance and has established a streamlined process for reporting parity violations. Massachusetts now requires the insurance commissioner to conduct market examinations every 4 years and has improved its processes for submitting and investigating consumer complaints, and New Hampshire established reporting requirements specifically for nonquantitative treatment limits (Pitsor, 2023).

SHAPING STATE MEDICAID POLICY TO EXPAND COVERAGE FOR COMMUNITY-BASED MENTAL HEALTH TREATMENT

Medicaid plays a crucial role in covering and financing care for people with mental illness and substance use disorder. In 2020, nearly 40% of the nonelderly adults covered by Medicaid, almost 14 million people, had a mental health or substance use disorder or both (Guth et al., 2023).

Historically, states paid for state-provided mental health services—typically acute care in institutions—through state tax dollars. However, states have increasingly shifted to using Medicaid to cover mental health and substance abuse care for low-income adults and children. Medicaid is a joint federal–state program. States do not have to participate in Medicaid, but states that do (and all states do) are guaranteed a federal match of at least 50%, and up to 90% for some services and populations. States also have great flexibility to design and administer their Medicaid programs, subject to federal standards.

Medicaid's flexibility and federal funding have helped states expand community-based mental health services for low-income patients. Medicaid is now the country's single largest payer for mental health and substance use services, financing 26% of all such spending (CMS, 2023; Medicaid and CHIP Payment and Access Commission [MACPAC], 2015). Most states use private managed care plans to deliver Medicaid mental health and substance use treatment services (Guth et al., 2023).

Mental health services are not a specifically defined category of Medicaid benefits. However, federal law mandates that states must cover many types of mental health services, and states have broad authority to cover many other optional mental health services. States may also seek waivers to cover even more types of services and social supports.

For children, coverage is comprehensive: Medicaid's Early and Periodic Screening, Diagnostic, and Treatment (EPSDT) benefit requires that states cover age-appropriate child screenings for both mental and physical health needs and any medically necessary care "to correct or ameliorate" a condition that can be covered by Medicaid, even if it is an optional service not covered for adults (MACPAC, n.d.). In 2022, the federal government released updated guidance for state Medicaid programs that emphasizes how states can cover mental health and substance use disorder services under EPSDT, highlighting a variety of Medicaid strategies states can use to expand and strengthen behavioral health services for children (Tsai, 2022). Medicaid can also provide school-based care, including mental health care and substance use disorder treatment for children and adolescents in a school setting. Schools are uniquely positioned to increase health equity by reducing disparities in access to care and to help ensure that all children have access to the preventive, screening, and treatment services they need (Tsai, 2022).

All state Medicaid programs cover outpatient mental health treatments, including psychiatric services, prescription drugs, case management, counseling, outpatient substance use treatment, and preventive screenings for adults. Many state Medicaid programs also cover a variety of evidence-based, innovative, community-based, recovery-oriented mental health services. One example is Medicaid coverage for behavioral crisis continuum of care services, such as mobile crisis teams and crisis stabilization services (MACPAC, 2021).

Another example is Medicaid coverage for assertive community treatment (ACT) for adults, a community-based service delivery model for people with severe and persistent mental illness that dramatically reduces unnecessary institutionalization and incarceration of people with severe mental health illness (MACPAC, 2021; Swadley, 2023). ACT teams are interdisciplinary groups of 10 to 12 mental health and rehabilitation professionals who work collaboratively to deliver comprehensive, individualized, and integrated treatment, rehabilitation, and support services. ACT teams deliver services where needed—at home, on the street, or in other community settings—and are available 24 hours a day, 7 days a week (Title IV-E Prevention Services Clearinghouse, 2023).

States have also used the flexibility allowed under federal law to cover peer support services under Medicaid. Peer support workers are people who have personal, lived experience with behavioral health challenges. Like community health workers, peer support persons help Medicaid enrollees navigate the healthcare and social service systems and provide emotional support. Peer support workers are an essential approach to growing the behavioral workforce (Guth et al., 2023).

Finally, the federal government has begun partnering with states to identify ways that state Medicaid programs can use Medicaid to address the social determinants of health that cause and exacerbate mental health and substance use disorders. States have begun using Medicaid to help with supportive housing, food, transportation, and related social services (Hinton & Diana, 2024). The resources that Medicaid can provide to address the upstream social determinants of health are relatively modest in light of the crushing social needs. Still, it is vital for state Medicaid programs to acknowledge the need for upstream solutions to the causes of mental health inequities.

SUMMARY

Historically, state policies have contributed to mental health inequities. Looking forward, states need to reform their policies to replace old patterns of state coercion, incarceration, and warehousing that have contributed to mental health inequities. This chapter offers examples of how states have begun to shift state policies away from the police toward an evidence-based behavioral health continuum of care crisis response model that offers local crisis call centers, mobile crisis teams, and crisis stabilization facilities. However, a key challenge states face is finding funding to support the creation and expansion of mobile crisis teams, crisis facilities, and follow-up services. This chapter shows how states can use state policy to shape commercial insurance and Medicaid to cover mental health services better, focusing on the policy options states have to leverage and require commercial insurance and Medicaid to pay for behavioral health crisis continuum of care services.

DISCUSSION QUESTIONS

1. States operate within a federal system in which federal law authorizes, influences, funds, and constrains state lawmaking. As you read this chapter, when did federalism interact to constrain state lawmaking to shape state policy to address mental health inequities? What examples can you give? When did federalism encourage state lawmaking to address mental health inequities? What examples can you give?
2. Expanding Medicaid in the states that have yet to expand will likely require bipartisan support in the state legislature. If you were representing advocates interested in addressing mental health inequities and improving access to mental health services, what arguments might be most persuasive to such legislators?
3. States can regulate only certain types of commercial health insurance. Who gets left out when states pass state mental health mandates? In a federal system, what level of government will need to pass legislation to address mental health inequities and ensure these people access to commercial insurance that meets their mental health needs?
4. What kind of law might a state pass to ensure that people with commercial insurance have access to mobile crisis teams and crisis facilities?
5. States have great flexibility to use Medicaid to pay for recovery-oriented, community-based mental health and substance use disorder care, but many states do not take full advantage of that flexibility. What barriers might inhibit states from using Medicaid to the max?

REFERENCES

Ammula, M., & Guth, M. (2023, January 18). *What does the recent literature say about Medicaid expansion?: Economic impacts on providers.* KFF. https://www.kff.org/affordable-care-act/issue-brief/what-does-the-recent-literature-say-about-medicaid-expansion-economic-impacts-on-providers/

Burt, R. A. (2001). Promises to keep, miles to go: Mental health law since 1972. In L. E. Frost & R. J. Bonnie (Eds.), *The evolution of mental health law* (pp. 11–30). American Psychological Association. https://doi.org/10.1037/10414-001

Centers for Medicare & Medicaid Services. (2023, July). *Mental health and substance use disorder action plan.* U.S. Department of Health and Human Services (HHS). https://www.medicaid.gov/medicaid/benefits/behavioral-health-services/index.html

Centers for Medicare & Medicaid Services. (2024, June 26). *Information on essential health benefits (EHB) benchmark plans.* U.S. Department of Health and Human Services (HHS). https://www.cms.gov/marketplace/resources/data/essential-health-benefits

Centers for Medicare & Medicaid Services. (2025). State options to provide qualifying community-based mobile crisis intervention services. https://www.medicaid.gov/medicaid/benefits/behavioral-health-services/state-option-provide-qualifying-community-based-mobile-crisis-intervention-services.

Community Emergency Services and Support Act. (2024). 50 Ill. Comp. Stat. Ann. § 754/30. https://ilga.gov/legislation/ilcs/ilcs3.asp?ActID=4210

Crisis Intervention Teams. (2009). Va. Code Ann. § 9.1-187-9.1-190. https://law.justia.com/codes/virginia/title-9-1/chapter-1/

Davoli, J. I. (2003). No room at the inn: how the federal Medicaid program created inequities in psychiatric hospital access for the indigent mentally ill. *American Journal of Law & Medicine, 29*(2–3), 159–183. https://doi.org/10.1017/S0098858800002793

Drake, P., Tolbert, J., Rudowitz, R., & Damico, A. (2024, February 26). *How many uninsured are in the coverage gap and how many could be eligible if all states adopted the Medicaid expansion?* KFF. https://www.kff.org/medicaid/issue-brief/how-many-uninsured-are-in-the-coverage-gap-and-how-many-could-be-eligible-if-all-states-adopted-the-medicaid-expansion/

Essential Health Benefits Requirements. (2010). 42 U.S.C. § 18022(b). https://www.govregs.com/uscode/expand/title42_chapter157_subchapterIII_partA_section18022

Guth, M., & Ammula, M. (2021). *Building on the evidence base: Studies on the effects of Medicaid expansion, February 2020 to March 2021.* KFF. https://www.kff.org/report-section/building-on-the-evidence-base-studies-on-the-effects-of-medicaid-expansion-february-2020-to-march-2021-appendix-a/

Guth, M., Saunders, H., Corallo, B., & Moreno, S. (2023, March 17). *Medicaid coverage of behavioral health services in 2022: Findings from a survey of state Medicaid programs.* KFF. https://www.kff.org/mental-health/issue-brief/medicaid-coverage-of-behavioral-health-services-in-2022-findings-from-a-survey-of-state-medicaid-programs/

Hinton, E., & Diana, A. (2024, January 29). *Medicaid authorities and options to address social determinants of health.* KFF. https://www.kff.org/medicaid/issue-brief/medicaid-authorities-and-options-to-address-social-determinants-of-health-sdoh/

Hylton, A. (2024). *Madness: Race and insanity in a Jim Crow asylum.* Legacy Publishers.

Interconnection. (2023). 47 U.S.C. § *251*(e)(4). https://www.govinfo.gov/app/details/USCODE-2011-title47/USCODE-2011-title47-chap5-subchapII-partII-sec251.

KFF. (2022a). *Health insurance coverage of nonelderly 0–64.* https://www.kff.org/other/state-indicator/nonelderly-0-64/?dataView=1&currentTimeframe=0&sortModel=%7B%22colId%22:%22Location%22,%22sort%22:%22asc%22%7D

KFF. (2022b). *State health facts Medicaid behavioral health services: Mobile crisis.* https://www.kff.org/other/state-indicator/medicaid-behavioral-health-services-mobile-crisis/?currentTimeframe=0&print=true&sortModel=%7B%22colId%22:%22Location%22,%22sort%22:%22asc%22%7D

Kirby, J., & Slone, S. (2022). *Mental health insurance and parity: State legislative and enforcement activities.* Council of State Governments. https://www.csg.org/2022/04/28/mental-health-insurance-parity-state-legislative-and-enforcement-activities/

Kona, M. (2023, September 23). *New federal rules seek to strengthen mental health parity.* Health Affairs Forefront. https://www.healthaffairs.org/content/forefront/new-federal-rules-seek-strengthen-mental-health-parity

Lawrence, M. B. (2020). Parity is not enough! Mental health, managed care, and Medicaid. *The Journal of Law, Medicine & Ethics, 48*(3), 480–484. https://doi.org/10.1177/1073110520958872

Medicaid and CHIP Payment and Access Commission. (2015, July). *Report to Congress on Medicaid and CHIP.* HHS. https://www.macpac.gov/wp-content/uploads/2015/06/June-2015-Report-to-Congress-on-Medicaid-and-CHIP.pdf

Medicaid and CHIP Payment and Access Commission. (2021, July). *State coverage policies of mental health services for adults.* HHS. https://www.macpac.gov/publication/state-coverage-policies-of-mental-health-services-for-adults/

Medicaid and CHIP Payment and Access Commission. (n.d.). *Behavioral health benefits.* HHS. https://www.macpac.gov/subtopic/behavioral-health-benefits/

National Alliance on Mental Illness. (2024). *988 Crisis response state legislation map.* https://reimaginecrisis.org/map/

Other Laws, 29 U.S.C. § 1144. (2024). https://codes.findlaw.com/us/title-29-labor/29-usc-sect-1144/

Parity in Mental Health and Substance Use Disorder Benefits, 26 C.F.R. § 54.9812. (2024). https://www.ecfr.gov/current/title-26/chapter-I/subchapter-D/part-54/section-54.9812-1

Pitsor, J. (2023, May 15). *States seek to lower costs, increase coverage of mental health care.* National Conference of State Legislatures. https://www.ncsl.org/state-legislatures-news/details/states-seek-to-lower-costs-increase-coverage-of-mental-health-care#:~:text=State%20lawmakers%20are%20pursuing%20various,protections%20to%20mental%20health%20emergencies

Rudowitz, R., Tolbert, J., Hinton, E., & Burns, A. (2024, January 30). *Medicaid: What to watch in 2024.* KFF. https://www.kff.org/medicaid/issue-brief/medicaid-what-to-watch-in-2024/

Saunders, H. (2023, November 30). *A look at state take-up of ARPA mobile crisis services in Medicaid.* KFF. https://www.kff.org/medicaid/issue-brief/a-look-at-state-take-up-of-arpa-mobile-crisis-services-in-medicaid/

Saunders, H., & Rudowitz, R. (2022, June 6). *Demographics and health insurance coverage of nonelderly adults with mental illness and substance use disorders in 2020.* KFF. https://www.kff.org/medicaid/issue-brief/demographics-and-health-insurance-coverage-of-nonelderly-adults-with-mental-illness-and-substance-use-disorders-in-2020/

Substance Abuse and Mental Health Services Administration. (2020). *National guidelines for behavioral health crisis best practice toolkit.* HHS. https://www.samhsa.gov/sites/default/files/national-guidelines-for-behavioral-health-crisis-care-02242020.pdf

Substance Abuse and Mental Health Services Administration. (2022). *Cooperative agreements for innovative community crisis response partnerships.* HHS. https://www.samhsa.gov/grants/grant-announcements/sm-22-016.

Swadley, H. (2023). The structural harms of providing mental health services through the bipartisan safer communities act. *Nebraska Law Review, 102*(1), 52–92.

The Kennedy Forum. (2020, December 10). *New model state parity legislation named in honor of former U.S. Rep. Jim Ramstad*. The Kennedy Forum. https://www.thekennedyforum.org/press-releases/new-model-state-parity-legislation-named-in-honor-of-former-u-s-rep-jim-ramstad/

Title IV-E Prevention Services Clearinghouse. (2023). *Assertive community treatment*. https://preventionservices.acf.hhs.gov/programs/619/show

Tsai, D. (2022, August 18). *CMCS informational bulletin*. Centers for Medicare & Medicaid Services. https://www.medicaid.gov/sites/default/files/2022-08/sbscib08182022_2.pdf

Volk, J., Schwab, R., Kona, M., & Walsh-Alker, E. (2022, October). *A review of state efforts to enforce mental health parity: Lessons for policymakers and regulators*. Georgetown University Health Policy Institute Center on Health Insurance Reforms. https://www.rwjf.org/content/dam/farm/reports/issue_briefs/2022/rwjf470267

Watson, A., & El-Sabawi, T. (2023). Expansion of the police role in responding to mental health crises over the past fifty years: Driving factors, race inequities and the need to rebalance roles. *Law and Contemporary Problems, 86*(1), 1–28. https://scholarship.law.duke.edu/lcp/vol86/iss1/2

17 SHAPING FEDERAL POLICY TO ADDRESS MENTAL HEALTH INEQUITIES

ELIZABETH PENDO

LEARNING OBJECTIVES

After reading this chapter, readers will be able to:

- Identify the federal antidiscrimination and healthcare laws that influence access to healthcare and health insurance for people with mental health conditions, substance use disorders, and other disabilities.
- Discuss the historical and current treatment of people with mental health conditions, substance use disorders, and other disabilities by the healthcare system and how assumptions, biases, and lack of knowledge contribute to mental health inequities.
- Describe how the Rehabilitation Act and the Americans with Disabilities Act address discrimination and unequal treatment in healthcare and health insurance experienced by people with mental health conditions and substance use disorders.
- Describe how the Mental Health Parity and Addiction Equity Act (MHPAEA) and the Patient Protection and Affordable Care Act address inequities in healthcare and health insurance experienced by people with mental health conditions and substance use disorders.
- Explain opportunities to further leverage federal antidiscrimination and healthcare laws and policies in order to address and eliminate mental health inequities.

INTRODUCTION

In 2023, according to the National Survey on Drug Use and Health, 58.7 million adults experienced some form of mental illness and 48.5 million people aged 12 or older experienced a substance use disorder (SUD) in the past year (Substance Abuse and Mental Health Services Administration [SAMHSA], 2024). Federal laws and policies play a significant role in influencing equitable access to healthcare and health insurance for the millions of Americans with these conditions. This chapter focuses on current federal laws in two major categories: broad disability civil rights laws, including the Americans with Disabilities Act of 1990 (ADA, 2008) and the Rehabilitation Act of 1973 (Rehabilitation Act, 1973), and laws relating to healthcare services and health insurance coverage, including the Mental Health Parity and Addiction Equity Act (MHPAEA) of 2008 (Paul Wellstone and Pete Domenici MHPEA, 2008) and the Patient Protection and Affordable Care Act of 2010 (ACA; Patient Protection and Affordable Care Act, 2010). Together, the laws examined in this chapter can address inequities in access to and coverage of healthcare services experienced by people with mental health conditions and SUDs, which often are rooted in policies, practices, and beliefs that reflect long-standing stigma, unequal treatment, and discrimination. The chapter concludes by highlighting opportunities to leverage federal laws and policies to make further progress toward addressing and eliminating mental health inequities.

FEDERAL ANTIDISCRIMINATION LAWS

In 1990, Congress enacted the ADA to provide a clear and comprehensive national mandate for eliminating widespread discrimination against individuals with disability and to establish enforceable standards to address discrimination. The landmark civil rights law expands the protections of an earlier law, Section 504 of the Rehabilitation Act, which bans disability discrimination in programs and activities that receive federal financial assistance. The ADA applies across many areas of American life, including healthcare and health insurance. There are other federal laws that address disability discrimination in areas such as education, housing, air travel, voting, and telecommunications (U.S. Department of Justice [DOJ], 2009).

Although there are differences between the Rehabilitation Act and the ADA, Section 504 and ADA Title II are generally understood to impose substantially the same requirements (Nondiscrimination in Health Programs and Activities, 2024). The requirements of the ADA are summarized in **Table 17.1**.

Nearly all healthcare providers and institutions are governed by the ADA or Section 504 of the Rehabilitation Act. Section 504 of the Rehabilitation Act prohibits discrimination against people with disabilities in programs and activities that receive federal financial assistance, which includes mental health and substance use treatment programs, hospitals and health clinics, treatment facilities, and nursing homes. Title II of the ADA applies to state and local government programs, services, and activities, which include state Medicaid programs and healthcare services provided by public hospitals and clinics. Title III of the ADA applies to places of public accommodations, which include private physician's offices and private hospitals, private nursing homes, and private treatment programs open to the public, regardless of federal funding.

Table 17.1 SUMMARY OF AMERICANS WITH DISABILITIES ACT REQUIREMENTS

TITLE	COVERED ENTITIES AND REQUIREMENTS
Title I (Employment)	Requires equal access to employment opportunities and benefits, including employer-sponsored health insurance. Requires that employers provide reasonable accommodations for applicants and employees with disabilities.
Title II (Public entities)	Bars disability discrimination in state and local government services, programs, and activities, such as healthcare services and programs, public education, transportation, recreation, social services, courts, and voting. Requires reasonable modifications to ensure that people with disabilities can participate in and enjoy these services, programs, and activities.
Title III (Public accommodations)	Bars disability discrimination by private places of public accommodation, such as private clinical practices, restaurants, retail establishments, and other businesses open to the public. Requires reasonable modifications to afford access to people with disabilities.
Title IV (Telecommunications)	Requires telephone and television access for people with hearing and speech disabilities.
Title V (Miscellaneous provisions)	Includes provisions that apply to the ADA as a whole, including direction to specific federal agencies to provide information and guidance about the requirements of the law.

ADA, Americans with Disabilities Act.

Source: Adapted from U.S. Department of Justice Civil Rights Division. (2009). *A guide to disability rights laws*. https://www.ada.gov/cguide.htm

The ADA and the Rehabilitation Act protect individuals who meet the statutory definition of *disability*, which includes people with mental health conditions and SUDs. The statutes and regulations define *disability* with respect to an individual as a physical or mental impairment that substantially limits one or more major life activities, a record of such impairment, or being regarded as having such an impairment (Definition of Disability, 2008). The ADA was amended in 2008 to clarify that the definition of *disability* should be construed in favor of broad coverage. Regulations implementing the amendments to the ADA provide mental health conditions such as bipolar disorder, major depression, obsessive-compulsive disorder, posttraumatic stress disorder, and schizophrenia, among other conditions, will consistently meet the definition of *disability* (Definitions, 2011). In addition, federal agencies tasked with enforcing these laws in healthcare also have affirmed that an SUD is a disability if the impairment substantially limits a major life activity, which includes major bodily functions (e.g., caring for oneself, learning, concentrating, thinking, communicating, working, or the operation of major bodily functions, including neurological and brain functions; Definition of "Disability," 2016a, 2016b) Individuals with a history of mental health conditions or SUDs, or who are incorrectly assumed to have these conditions, are also protected under these laws.

The ADA excludes individuals who are currently engaged in illegal drug use, although there is an exception for people who are participating in, or have participated in, a rehabilitation program and are no longer engaged in illegal use of drugs. With respect to healthcare, however, the Rehabilitation Act specifically provides that the current use of illegal drugs is not a basis to deny hospital, outpatient facility, drug rehabilitation, vocational rehabilitation program treatment, and other covered programs and services if the individual is otherwise entitled to such services (Dineen & Pendo, 2021; U.S Department of Health and Human Services [HHS], 2018a, 2018b).

Healthcare Services and Programs

People with mental health and substance use conditions report unmet needs and barriers to needed healthcare programs and services. According to the National Survey on Drug Use and Health, in 2023, 23% of adults with mental illness in the past year received mental health services. Among people who did not receive treatment, one of the most common reasons given was perceived cost. Lack of knowledge about how or where to access treatment was also reported (SAMHSA, 2024; **Figure 17.1**).

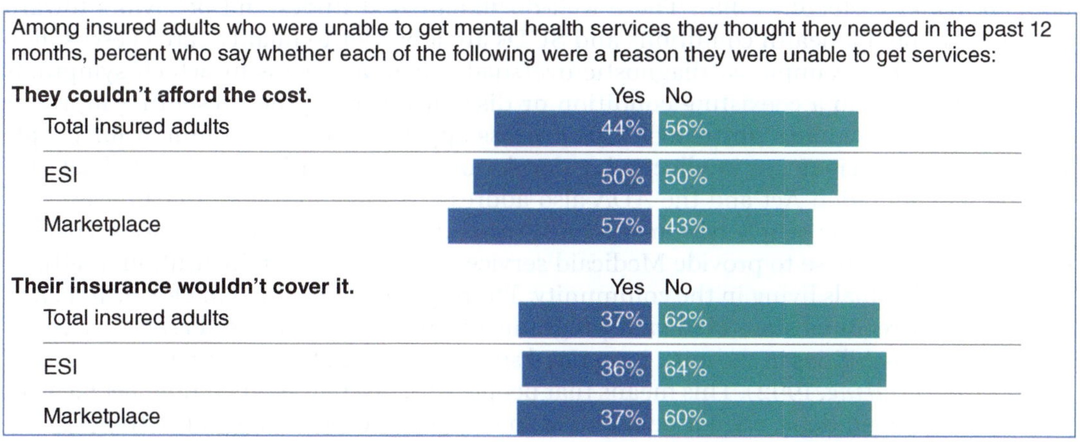

Figure 17.1 Many adults who did not get needed mental health services say cost or lack of coverage was the reason they did not get care.

ESI, employer-sponsored insurance.

The survey also estimates that only 23.6% of people aged 12 and older who experienced SUD in the past year received SUD treatment. Among the reasons given for not receiving treatment were not knowing how or where to get treatment, perceived cost of treatment, concerns about what people would think or say if they got treatment, and not having health insurance coverage for substance use treatment.

The ADA and the Rehabilitation Act were intended to address a wide range of barriers to care. These laws prohibit exclusion from or refusal to provide healthcare services based on disability (Activities, 1992; General Prohibitions Against Discrimination, 2016) Instead, healthcare services must be delivered in a way that ensures equal access to people with disabilities, subject to some limitations. Despite these legal protections, people with mental health conditions, SUDs, or other disabilities continue to face significant barriers to healthcare services. For example, some healthcare providers continue to refuse to treat individuals on the basis of SUD (Dineen & Pendo, 2021).

These laws also require that treatment decisions for individuals with mental health conditions and other disabilities be made based on an individualized assessment of the patient's needs. During the COVID-19 pandemic, concerns arose regarding medical resource allocation policies and practices that disadvantaged people with disabilities. In response to these concerns, the HHS Office for Civil Rights (OCR) issued a statement affirming that people with disabilities should not be denied medical care on the basis of "stereotypes, assessments of quality of life," or "judgments about a person's relative 'worth' based on the presence or absence of disabilities or age." Instead, decisions concerning whether an individual is a candidate for treatment should be "based on an individualized assessment of the patient based on the best available objective medical evidence" (HSS OCR, 2020, p. 1). The OCR statement also emphasizes other legal requirements, including the obligation to make reasonable modifications to address the needs of individuals with disabilities.

The requirement of individualized assessment has the potential to interrupt long-standing negative assumptions, attitudes, and biases about people with mental health and substance use conditions. Studies have documented stigma and bias against people with mental illness, including the stigmatizing attitudes and beliefs of clinicians (Henderson et al., 2014; Stone et al., 2019). For example, one study noted that clinicians viewed people with serious mental illness as more dangerous than other patients (Stone et al., 2019). Although a healthcare entity may impose legitimate safety requirements necessary for safe operation, the ADA requires that those requirements be based on actual risks and not speculation, stereotypes, or generalizations about people with disabilities even if held in good faith (*Bragdon v. Abbott*, 1998). These well-documented attitudes and behaviors toward people with mental health conditions and SUDs are a barrier to quality care (Pescosolido et al., 2021). One example is "diagnostic overshadowing," a process by which symptoms are misattributed to a coexisting condition or disability, leaving the presenting injury or disease undiagnosed and untreated. This process appears especially common for people with mental health issues or intellectual or developmental disabilities (Molloy et al., 2020).

The Rehabilitation Act and the ADA also address systemic barriers in healthcare programs experienced by people with mental health conditions and other disabilities. Historically, some states chose to provide Medicaid services to individuals in institutional settings but not to individuals living in the community. The Supreme Court held in *Olmstead v. L.C.* that the ADA requires state Medicaid programs to provide community-based services to persons with disabilities in the most integrated setting appropriate to their needs (*Olmstead v. L.C. ex rel. Zimring*, 1992). This means that people with disabilities, including people with mental health conditions, cannot be required to live in institutions or group settings to obtain the healthcare and other services they need. The DOJ, OCR, and advocacy groups have taken actions to enforce the *Olmstead* decision and the ADA's integration mandate (Pendo & Iezzoni, 2020).

Health Insurance

Prior to the ACA, many people with disabilities faced challenges obtaining adequate and affordable health insurance. In 2009, the National Council on Disability (NCD) published *The Current State of Health Care for People with Disabilities*, an evaluation of decades of research on health inequities and barriers experienced by people with disabilities. The report found that the complex, fragmented, and often overly restrictive U.S. health insurance system leaves some people with disabilities with no healthcare coverage and others with exclusions, limits, and cost-sharing obligations that prevent them from obtaining needed services, including mental health and rehabilitative care. Many disabled individuals were therefore denied private health insurance or charged higher prices, often with coverage limitations and exclusions, including for mental health services (NCD, 2009).

Although the ADA generally applies to health insurance policies, cases brought under the ADA challenging policies that, for example, provide less coverage for treatment of mental conditions than for treatment of physical conditions, have encountered serious obstacles (Clark et al., 2022). One of the most significant obstacles is the ADA's "safe harbor" provision, which permits some plans to have terms that treat individuals with disability differently on the basis of underwriting, classifying, or administering risks (ADA, 2008, § 12201(c)). The ACA's insurance reforms, discussed in the next section, address some of these obstacles.

FEDERAL HEALTHCARE LAWS

The MHPAEA and the many provisions of the landmark ACA each address mental health inequities. Although these laws are relatively recent, there have been many federal laws and policies directed to mental health and mental health care dating back to the mid-1900s (Dawes, 2016).

The Mental Health Parity and Addiction Equity Act

In response to the gaps and inequities in health insurance coverage of mental health conditions described above, in 1996, the federal government enacted the Mental Health Parity Act (Mental Health Parity Act, 1996). The 1996 act requires group health plans to impose the same aggregate lifetime and annual dollar limits for mental health benefits as for medical or surgical benefits. However, the 1996 act did not apply to substance use benefits and did not require other provisions and restrictions, such as copayments, limits on inpatient days, and limits on the number of visits, to be the same for mental health benefits as for medical or surgical benefits.

In 2008, Congress extended mental health parity requirements through the MHPAEA (Paul Wellstone and Pete Domenici MHPAEA, 2008). The 2008 act requires insurers and employers that choose to offer mental health and substance use benefits to treat those benefits in the same manner as medical or surgical benefits. For example, limits on the frequency of treatment, number of visits, days of coverage, or other limits on the scope or duration of treatment must be applied equally to mental health and substance use benefits as to medical or surgical benefits. Additionally, requirements such as copayments and coinsurance cannot be greater for mental health or substance use benefits than for medical or surgical benefits. Finally, if a health plan allows patients to go out of network for medical or surgical benefits, it must also do so for mental health or substance use benefits.

The Patient Protection and Affordable Care Act

The ACA was intended to ensure that all Americans, including people with disabilities, would have access to comprehensive, affordable, and nondiscriminatory healthcare and health coverage (ACA, 2010). The ACA has many different provisions addressing the healthcare system, including policies intended to expand access to public and private insurance coverage, enhance healthcare quality, improve healthcare delivery systems, control healthcare costs, and identify and eliminate health inequities. Many provisions have the potential to improve access to care and coverage for people with mental health disorders and SUDs (Beronio et al., 2014).

Insurance Reforms

The ACA imposed significant new requirements for health plan access and content and explicit protections against discrimination in health plan benefit design. As discussed previously, prior to the ACA, many insurers evaluated the health status, health history, and other risk factors of applicants to determine whether and under what terms to issue coverage, a process called "medical underwriting." As a result, many health insurers were allowed to exclude or restrict coverage for individuals with preexisting conditions, such as cancer, asthma, and mental disorders such as bipolar disorder or eating disorder (Claxton et al., 2016). The ACA severely restricted the practice of medical underwriting. Under the ACA, insurers are banned from denying coverage or benefits or charging higher premiums because of a patient's preexisting condition or health status (Fair Health Insurance Premiums, 2010; **Figure 17.2**).

The ACA also closed an important gap in the MHPAEA by requiring coverage of mental health and substance use benefits as "essential health benefits." Under the 2008 MHPAEA, plans were not required to provide coverage of mental health and substance use services, only to provide parity in the event the plan provided coverage of mental health or substance use services. Under the ACA, however, health plans in the individual and small-group markets must cover a package of 10 "essential health benefits" (EHB), including mental health and SUD services and behavioral health treatment (Essential Health Benefits Requirements, 2014). The ACA's EHB requirements are shown in **Box 17.1**.

As a result, all health insurance plans in the individual and employer market must include coverage for treatment of mental health and substance use conditions. In order to satisfy the EHB requirement, insurers must comply with the Parity Act (Frank et al., 2014).

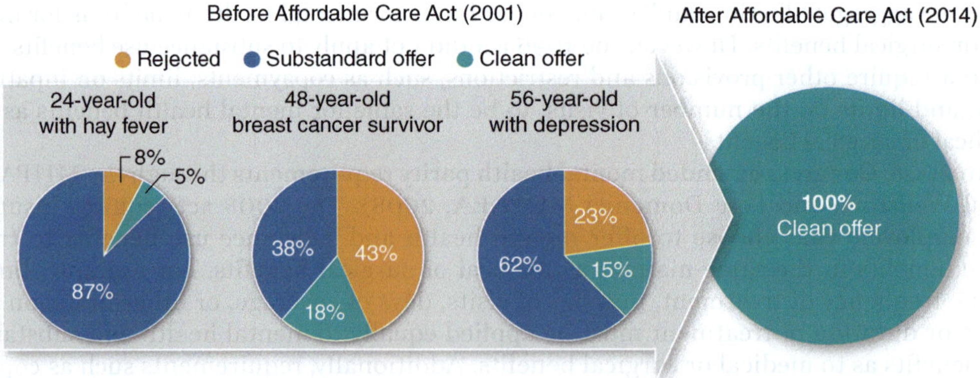

Figure 17.2 Insurer responses to hypothetical applications for individual health insurance before and after the Affordable Care Act.

Note: A substandard offer includes offers that impose premium increases or other benefits limits like exclusions of coverage for specific conditions or body parts.

Source: KFF. (2020). *How health insurers responded to applicants with pre-existing conditions before and after the Affordable Care Act.* https://www.kff.org/affordable-care-act/slide/how-health-insurers-responded-to-applicants-with-pre-existing-conditions-before-and-after-the-affordable-care-act/

Box 17.1 AFFORDABLE CARE ACT ESSENTIAL HEALTH BENEFITS REQUIREMENTS

Non-grandfathered health plans in the individual and small-group markets are required to cover essential health benefits, which include items and services in the following 10 benefit categories:

- Ambulatory patient services
- Emergency services
- Hospitalization
- Maternity and newborn care
- Mental health and substance use disorder services, including behavioral health treatment
- Prescription drugs
- Rehabilitative and habilitative services and devices
- Laboratory services
- Preventive and wellness services and chronic disease management
- Pediatric services, including oral and vision care

Source: Adapted from Essential Health Benefits Requirements, 42 U.S.C. § § 18022. (2014). https://uscode.house.gov/view.xhtml?req=(title:42%20section:18022%20edition:prelim)

Antidiscrimination Provision

The ACA also includes an overarching antidiscrimination provision, Section 1557. Section 1557 affirms and expands the reach of existing laws, including the Rehabilitation Act, to provide additional protections against discrimination on the basis of race, color, national origin, sex, age, or disability in healthcare programs, activities, and settings that receive federal funds (Nondiscrimination, 2010).

OPPORTUNITIES TO SHAPE FEDERAL POLICY TOWARD MENTAL HEALTH EQUITY

The requirements of the federal antidiscrimination and healthcare laws examined in this chapter are strong tools to address inequities in access to healthcare services and health insurance experienced by people with mental health conditions and SUDs. This section highlights opportunities to leverage these laws and policies to make further progress toward assessing and addressing mental health inequities.

Robust Enforcement of Existing Laws

To be effective, the laws discussed in this chapter require robust and equitable enforcement by multiple federal agencies. Given the structure and overlapping goals of these laws, coordination among departments and agencies on enforcement efforts is warranted.

The HHS OCR is responsible for enforcing Title II of the ADA, Section 504 of the Rehabilitation Act, and Section 1557 of the ACA. The DOJ is also charged with enforcing Section 504, Title II and Title III of the ADA, and Section 1557 of the ACA. These agencies have broad authority to investigate, mediate, litigate, and settle individual and class-based claims under these laws. Private individuals and groups also are entitled to bring disability discrimination actions pursuant to these laws, with certain limitations. Experts often claim that disability antidiscrimination laws are underenforced and, consequently, their promises have gone unrealized, particularly in healthcare settings and for people with SUDs (Dineen & Pendo, 2021; NCD, 2009). Over the past several years, however, these agencies have increased enforcement activity aimed at protecting individuals with SUDs in healthcare settings (Dineen & Pendo, 2021).

Multiple federal agencies enforce the provisions of the 2008 MHPAEA, as well, based on the type of insurance plan. For example, the U.S. Department of Labor and the Internal Revenue Service are charged with enforcement for private, self-insured plans offered by employers, and state insurance commissioners are charged with enforcement for plans sold in the individual and small-group markets. Research has identified the lack of multidepartment and multiagency coordination as an issue (Barry et al., 2016). To encourage coordination in enforcement efforts, an interagency parity task force was established in 2016 to ensure that executive departments and agencies work together to achieve the promise of federal parity protections (Mental Health and Substance Use Disorder Parity Task Force, 2016). In 2024, the agencies issued a new rule implementing the MHPAEA that strengthens the law by making it easier to recognize and remedy lack of compliance with parity requirements (Requirements Related to the MHPAEA, 2024). The new rule requires plans to collect, evaluate, and analyze types of data relevant to the parity requirements.

Educational Initiatives

Given the pervasive stigma, stereotypes, and false beliefs associated with mental health conditions and SUDs, and disabilities generally, successful enforcement efforts of federal antidiscrimination laws must be accompanied by effective education of healthcare providers, entities, and systems. Research demonstrates a lack of knowledge of, and noncompliance with, disability antidiscrimination laws in healthcare settings (Lagu et al., 2022). Studies have found that many physicians know little about their legal responsibilities under the ADA (Agaronnik et al., 2019), including the statute's accommodation requirements (Iezzoni et al., 2022), and hold negative beliefs about people with disabilities (Lagu et al., 2022). A recent study in the context of patients with SUDs concluded that 20% to 51% of healthcare providers had negative attitudes and beliefs about patients with SUDs, and that SUD training and clinical experience with SUD patients were associated with less negative attitudes (Cazalis et al., 2023).

One promising sign is the expanded efforts of the OCR and DOJ to educate healthcare professionals about their obligations to people with SUD under existing antidiscrimination law. In 2018, the OCR issued guidance clarifying the federal civil rights protections for people with SUD (HHS, 2018a, 2018b). In 2022, the DOJ issued similar guidance concerning the ADA's protections for people in treatment for or recovery from opioid use disorder (OUD) and other types of SUDs (DOJ, 2022).

Research to Drive Policy

Federal agencies, laws, and policies also play a large role in supporting mental health equity research. For example, the National Institute of Mental Health (NIMH), part of the National Institutes of Health (NIH) within HHS, is the lead federal agency for research on mental disorders. SAMHSA is the federal agency charged with leading U.S. behavioral health efforts and making information, services, and research concerning mental health and substance use conditions more accessible. NIMH also supports research and educates the public about findings. Federal laws and policies, including the ACA, also direct data collection efforts to support health equity efforts (Pendo & Iezzoni, 2020).

It is also critical to continue to research the impact and effectiveness of the federal laws discussed in this chapter. For example, additional research on the impact and implementation of the 2008 MHPAEA, as extended by the parity provisions of the ACA, is needed to better identify the effectiveness of the laws and progress toward parity (Barry et al., 2016). Notably, the 2024 rule implementing the MHPAEA requires plans to collect, evaluate, and analyze specific types of data relevant to the parity requirements of the law (Requirements Related to the MHPAEA, 2024). People with disabilities generally, and people with mental health disorders and SUDs specifically, also must be included in health equity research and programming more broadly (NCD, 2022; Pendo & Iezzoni, 2020). For example, until recently, people with disabilities were not recognized as a health disparity population under the Minority Health and Health Disparities Research and Education Act of 2000 (Minority Health and Health Disparities Research and Education Act, 2000). Recognition as a health disparity population is important because the act directs the NIH National Institute on Minority Health and Health Disparities to conduct and support research with respect to minority health conditions and other populations with health disparities. Fortunately, on September 26, 2023, NIH designated people with disabilities as a population with health disparities (NIH, 2023).

SUMMARY

Federal laws and policies play a significant role in ensuring access to healthcare and health insurance for people with mental health and substance use conditions. This chapter examines current laws in two major categories: broad disability civil rights laws that protect people with disabilities, and healthcare laws addressing the delivery and coverage of services. Together, these laws can address mental health inequities experienced by people with mental health conditions and SUDs, which are rooted in policies, practices, and beliefs that reflect long-standing stigma, unequal treatment, and discrimination. Although progress has been made, there are opportunities to leverage federal laws and policies to make further progress toward addressing mental health inequities.

DISCUSSION QUESTIONS

1. What do you believe are common challenges or objections to recognizing mental health and substance use conditions as disabilities protected under federal antidiscrimination laws?
2. How effective have federal antidiscrimination laws been in addressing discrimination and unequal treatment in healthcare and health insurance experienced by people with mental health conditions, SUDs, and other disabilities, and why?
3. What do you believe are some of the most common assumptions and biases surrounding those with mental health conditions, SUDs, and other disabilities, and how do you believe those beliefs contribute to inequities in specific settings, such as healthcare, health insurance, employment, state and local services, and private business open to the public?
4. Prior to mental health parity laws, why do you think that insurers offered less coverage for treatment of mental health and substance use conditions than for physical conditions?
5. What do you believe is the most significant opportunity to further leverage federal antidiscrimination and healthcare laws and policies to address and eliminate mental health inequities and why?

REFERENCES

Activities, 28 C.F.R. § 36.202(a) (1992). https://www.ecfr.gov/current/title-28/chapter-I/part-36/subpart-B/section-36.202

Agaronnik, N. D., Pendo, E., Campbell, E. G., Ressalam, J., & Iezzoni, L. I. (2019). Knowledge of practicing physicians about their legal obligations when caring for patients with disability. *Health Affairs, 38*(4), 545–553. https://doi.org/10.1377/hlthaff.2018.05060

Americans with Disabilities Act, 42 U.S.C. § 12101 et seq. U.S.C. (2008). https://www.ada.gov/law-and-regs/ada/

Barry, C. L., Goldman, H. H., & Huskamp, H. A. (2016). Federal parity in the evolving mental health and addiction care landscape. *Health Affairs, 35*(6), 1009–1016. https://doi.org/10.1377/hlthaff.2015.1653

Beronio, K., Glied, S., & Frank, R. (2014). How the Affordable Care Act and Mental Health Parity and Addiction Equity Act greatly expand coverage of behavioral health care. *The Journal of Behavioral Health Services & Research, 41*(4), 410–428. https://doi.org/10.1007/s11414-014-9412-0

Bragdon v. Abbott, 524 U.S. 624 (1998). https://supreme.justia.com/cases/federal/us/524/624/

Cazalis, A., Lambert, L., & Auriacombe, M. (2023). Stigmatization of people with addiction by health professionals: Current knowledge. A scoping review. *Drug and Alcohol Dependence Reports, 9*, 100196. https://doi.org/10.1016/j.dadr.2023.100196

Clark, B. R., Fuse Brown, E. C., Gatter, R., McCuskey, E. Y., & Pendo, E. (2022). *Health law: Cases, materials and problems* (8th ed.). West Academic.

Claxton, G., Cox, C., Damico, A., Levitt, L., & Pollitz, K. (2016). *Pre-existing conditions and medical underwriting in the individual insurance market prior to the ACA* [Issue brief]. KFF. https://www.kff.org/health-reform/issue-brief/pre-existing-conditions-and-medical-underwriting-in-the-individual-insurance-market-prior-to-the-aca/

Dawes, D. E. (2016). *150 Years of ObamaCare*. Johns Hopkins University Press.

Definition of Disability, 42 U.S.C. §12102 (2008). https://codes.findlaw.com/us/title-42-the-public-health-and-welfare/42-usc-sect-12102/

Definition of "Disability," 28 C.F.R. § 35.108(b)(2) (2016a). https://www.govinfo.gov/content/pkg/CFR-2024-title28-vol1/pdf/CFR-2024-title28-vol1-sec35-108.pdf

Definition of "Disability," 28 C.F.R. § 36.105(b)(2) (2016b). https://www.govinfo.gov/content/pkg/CFR-2017-title28-vol1/pdf/CFR-2017-title28-vol1-sec36-105.pdf

Definitions, 29 C.F.R. § 1630.2 (2011). https://www.law.cornell.edu/cfr/text/29/1630.2

Dineen, K. K., & Pendo, E. (2021). Substance use disorder discrimination and the CARES act: Using disability law to inform. Part 2. Rulemaking. *Arizona State Law Journal, 52*, 1143.

Essential Health Benefits Requirements, 42 U.S.C. § § 18022 (2014). https://www.govinfo.gov/app/details/USCODE-2010-title42/USCODE-2010-title42-chap157-subchapIII-partA-sec18022

Fair Health Insurance Premiums, 42 U.S.C. § § 300gg (2010). https://www.govinfo.gov/app/details/USCODE-2015-title42/USCODE-2015-title42-chap6A-subchapXXV-partA-subpart1-sec300gg

Frank, R. G., Beronio, K., & Glied, S. A. (2014). Behavioral health parity and the Affordable Care Act. *Journal of Social Work in Disability & Rehabilitation, 13*(1–2), 31–43. https://doi.org/10.1080/1536710X.2013.870512

General Prohibitions against Discrimination, 28 C.F.R. § 35.130(b) (2016). https://www.ecfr.gov/current/title-28/chapter-I/part-35

Henderson, C., Noblett, J., Parke, H., Clement, S., Caffrey, A., Gale-Grant, O., Schulze, B., Druss, B., & Thornicroft, G. (2014). Mental health-related stigma in health care and mental health-care settings. *The Lancet Psychiatry, 1*(6), 467–482. https://doi.org/10.1016/S2215-0366(14)00023-6

Iezzoni, L. I., Rao, S. R., Ressalam, J., Bolcic-Jankovic, D., Agaronnik, N. D., Lagu, T., Pendo, E., & Campbell, E. G. (2022). US physicians' knowledge about the Americans with Disabilities Act and accommodation of patients with disability: Study examines what physicians know about the Americans with Disabilities Act and what is done to accommodate patients with a disability. *Health Affairs, 41*(1), 96–104. https://doi.org/10.1377/hlthaff.2021.01136

Lagu, T., Haywood, C., Reimold, K., DeJong, C., Walker Sterling, R., & Iezzoni, L. I. (2022). 'I am not the doctor for you': Physicians' attitudes about caring for people with disabilities. *Health Affairs, 41*(10), 1387–1395. https://doi.org/10.1377/hlthaff.2022.00475

Mental Health and Substance Use Disorder Parity Task Force. (2016, March 29). Presidential Memorandum. *Whitehouse.Gov*. https://obamawhitehouse.archives.gov/the-press-office/2016/03/29/presidential-memorandum-mental-health-and-substance-use-disorder-parity

Mental Health Parity Act of 1996, Pub. L. No. 104–204, secs. 701–03, 110 Stat. 2944 (codified as amended at 29 U.S.C. § 1185a (2006 & Supp. IV 2010) and 42 U.S.C. § 300gg-26 (2006 & Supp. IV 2010)), U.S.C. (1996).

Minority Health and Health Disparities Research and Education Act, Pub. L. No. 106–525 (2000). https://www.govinfo.gov/content/pkg/PLAW-106publ525/pdf/PLAW-106publ525.pdf

Molloy, R., Munro, I., & Pope, N. (2020). Understanding the experience of diagnostic overshadowing associated with severe mental illness from the consumer and health professional perspective: A qualitative systematic review protocol. *JBI Evidence Synthesis, 19*(6), 1362–1368. https://doi.org/10.11124/JBIES-20-00244

National Council on Disability. (2009). *The current state of health care for people with disabilities.* https://www.ncd.gov/report/the-current-state-of-health-care-for-people-with-disabilities/

National Council on Disability. (2022). *Health equity framework for people with disabilities* [Policy brief]. https://www.ncd.gov/report/framework-to-end-health-disparities-of-people-with-disabilities/

National Institutes of Health. (2023, September 26). *NIH designates people with disabilities as a population with health disparities* [News release]. https://www.nih.gov/news-events/news-releases/nih-designates-people-disabilities-population-health-disparities

Nondiscrimination, Pub. L. No. 111–148, title I, Section 1557, 42 U.S.C. § 18116 ("Section 1557") (2010).

Nondiscrimination in Health Programs and Activities, 89 Fed. Reg 37522 (2024). https://www.govinfo.gov/content/pkg/FR-2024-05-06/pdf/2024-08711.pdf

Olmstead v. L.C. Ex Rel. Zimring, 527 U.S. 581 (1999). https://tile.loc.gov/storage-services/service/ll/usrep/usrep527/usrep527581/usrep527581.pdf

Patient Protection and Affordable Care Act, Pub. L. No. 111- 148 § 4203, 124 Stat. 119, 570 (2010) (codified as amended at 29 U.S.C. § 794f [2010]). (2010). https://www.govinfo.gov/content/pkg/PLAW-111publ148/html/PLAW-111publ148.htm

Paul Wellstone and Pete Domenici Mental Health Parity and Addiction Equity Act of 2008, in Emergency Economic Stabilization Act of 2008, Pub. L. No. 110-343, Secs. 511–12, 122 Stat. 3765, 3881–93 (Codified as Amended at 29 U.S.C. § 1185a [2006 & Supp. IV 2010] and 42 U.S.C. § 300gg-26 [2006 & Supp. IV 2010]), Pub. L. No. 110–343, secs. 511–12, 122 Stat. 3765, 3881– 93 (codified as amended at 29 U.S.C. § 1185a [2006 & Supp. IV 2010] and 42 U.S.C. § 300gg- 26 [2006 & Supp. IV 2010]) (2008).

Pendo, E., & Iezzoni, L. I. (2020). *The role of law and policy in achieving healthy people's disability and health goals around access to health care, activities promoting health and wellness, independent living and participation, and collecting data in the United States.* Department of Health and Human Services, Office of Disease Prevention and Health Promotion. https://health.gov/our-work/national-health-initiatives/healthy-people/healthy-people-2020/healthy-people-2020-law-and-health-policy/disability-and-health

Pescosolido, B. A., Halpern-Manners, A., Luo, L., & Perry, B. (2021). Trends in public stigma of mental illness in the US, 1996–2018. *JAMA Network Open, 4*(12), e2140202. https://doi.org/10.1001/jamanetworkopen.2021.40202

Rehabilitation Act, 29 U.S.C. § 701 et seq. (1973). https://uscode.house.gov/view.xhtml?req=(title:29%20section:701%20edition:prelim)

Requirements Related to the Mental Health Parity and Addiction Equity Act, 89 Fed. Reg. 77586 (codified at 26 C.F.R. Part 54, 29 C.F.R. Part 2590, and 45 C.F.R. Parts 146 and 147) 77586 (2024). https://www.federalregister.gov/documents/2024/09/23/2024-20612/requirements-related-to-the-mental-health-parity-and-addiction-equity-act

Stone, E. M., Chen, L. N., Daumit, G. L., Linden, S., & McGinty, E. E. (2019). General medical clinicians' attitudes toward people with serious mental illness: A scoping review. *The Journal of Behavioral Health Services & Research, 46*(4), 656–679. https://doi.org/10.1007/s11414-019-09652-w

Substance Abuse and Mental Health Services Administration. (2024). *Key substance use and mental health indicators in the United States: Results from the 2023 National Survey on Drug Use and Health* (HHS Publication No. PEP24-07-021, NSDUH Series H-59; pp. 1–146). Substance Abuse and Mental Health Services Administration. https://www.samhsa.gov/data/report/2023-nsduh-annual-national-report

U.S. Department of Health and Human Services, Office for Civil Rights. (2018a, October 25). *Fact sheet, drug addiction and federal disability rights law.* https://public3.pagefreezer.com/content/HHS.gov/20-06-2023T05:11/https://www.hhs.gov/sites/default/files/drug-addiction-aand-federal-disability-rights-laws-fact-sheet.pdf [https://perma.cc/NDH6-YXSB]

U.S. Department of Health and Human Services, Office for Civil Rights. (2018b, October 25). *Fact sheet, nondiscrimination and opioid use disorder.* https://public3.pagefreezer.com/content/HHS.gov/20-06-2023T05:11/https://www.hhs.gov/sites/default/files/fact-sheet-nondiscrimination-and-opioid-use.pdf [https://perma.cc/E4UD-JJK4]

U.S. Department of Health and Human Services, Office for Civil Rights. (2020, March 28). *Bulletin: Civil rights, HIPAA, and the coronavirus disease 2019 (COVID-19).* https://www.justice.gov/file/1263421/download

U.S. Department of Justice, Civil Rights Division, Disability Rights Section. (2009). *A guide to disability rights laws.* https://www.ada.gov/cguide.htm

18 THE ROLE OF PAYMENT POLICY IN ACHIEVING MENTAL HEALTH EQUITY

STEVEN S. SHARFSTEIN AND JOSHUA M. SHARFSTEIN

LEARNING OBJECTIVES

After reading this chapter, readers will be able to:

- Describe shifts in who pays for mental health care across U.S. history, with implications for equity in access to quality care.
- Identify key moments in U.S. history when the federal government could have taken on a more fundamental role in advancing equity in mental health care.
- Explain the gaps in private insurance coverage that led to battles over mental health parity.
- Discuss options for reform of mental health payment to improve equity.
- Envision an expanded partnership between the federal and state governments to improve mental health equity through a fundamental reform of financing mental health care.

INTRODUCTION

The past is never dead. It isn't even past.

—William Faulkner (1951)

The U.S. mental health crisis is characterized by surging rates of depression and anxiety among children and young adults, growing numbers of older adults with mental illness, and high levels of suicide and overdose. It is also characterized by profound disparities by race, ethnicity, geography, and economic disadvantage. A common theme is inadequate access to care and treatment, and at the core of inadequate access are unsuccessful approaches to paying for services. Attention to financing is essential both to understanding the causes of the nation's predicament and designing fundamental reforms to achieve mental health equity.

THE PAST: ORIGINS OF INEQUITY

Attempting to diagram how the United States pays for mental health care today is a futile endeavor. It is extraordinarily difficult to map the intersecting and overlapping responsibilities between 50 states and the federal government, between the public and private sectors, and among health, social services, and criminal justice. Moreover, as soon as one payer attempts to describe these relationships, another is likely to disagree.

A more productive way to approach payment policy is to begin with some history. For more than 150 years, the defining question of mental health payment has not been "what's covered" or "how much?" but rather, "who pays?"—the fundamental issue of responsibility. Is mental health care fundamentally a public or private responsibility? If public, what are the fundamental roles of the federal, state, and local governments?

Through much of the early to mid 19th century, mental health care was primarily a family responsibility. In the early to mid 19th century, cities and towns held people with mental illness along with others in jails, workhouses, and poorhouses. Beginning at the end of the 19th century, responsibility began to shift to states, which established large asylums for adults and child welfare and juvenile justice systems for youth. Until the middle of the 20th century, by law in many states, these systems were racially segregated.

About 60 years ago, states began to reduce their commitment to large mental asylums and eventually discharged tens of thousands of long-term patients. In part, this movement was based on the erroneous expectation that the federal government would step up and fund mental health care in community settings. In recent years, struggles over "parity" represent a financial tug-of-war between the government and private insurance companies. Over more than 150 years of such struggles, people with mental illness—particularly those with serious and persistent disorders—have often lost ground. For those without power because of income, race and ethnicity, geography, and other characteristics, progress has been halting, and many still suffer devastating and unnecessary consequences of their illness.

The earliest systems of care for individuals with mental illness date back in the 18th century to town jails and poorhouses. Prior to their establishment, many individuals with serious mental illness were cared for in private homes, locked away in attics and basements. The social stigma of a family member with mental illness was profound, as families let their siblings, parents, and children suffer in local institutions. Life for people with mental illness remained cruel, with the cruelty often compounded by racism and prejudice.

Recognizing the inhumanity of this approach, reformer Dorothea Dix crusaded in the 19th century to pull people with mental illness into new state asylums, which would be designed for tranquility and recovery (Gollaher, 1995). Over nearly 40 years, she lobbied legislatures in 18 states to establish 32 asylums at state expense. She then sought to establish a system of asylums run by the federal government. However, after Dix convinced Congress in 1854 to pass the "12 Million, 500,000 Acres Act," which would have provided support for this effort, President Franklin Pierce issued an emphatic veto (**Box 18.1**). He stated that the federal government should not become "the great almoner of public charity" throughout the United States and declared that states, localities, and private individuals and families were responsible for the sick and disabled (Foley & Sharfstein, 1983).

As a consequence of President Pierce's veto, states retained the responsibility of creating asylums for people with severe and persistent mental illness. Initially established as small facilities that provided individualized care and treatment, state mental institutions expanded over time to accommodate the many referrals from localities seeking to shift the cost

Box 18.1 PRESIDENT FRANKLIN PIERCE VETOES FEDERAL SUPPORT FOR MENTAL HEALTH

I cannot find any authority in the Constitution for making the Federal Government the great almoner of public charity throughout the United States.

— President Franklin Pierce, upon vetoing legislation to provide federal support for mental institutions

Source: Holt, M. F. (2010). *Franklin Pierce*. Henry Holt and Company, LLC.

from local to state tax dollars. As individualized treatment called "moral treatment" gave way to "economies of scale," therapeutic optimism was replaced by pessimism about the potential for improvement, and custodial care. By 1950, there were nearly 600,000 beds in state-run psychiatric facilities—and scandals about the quality of care and safety appeared regularly in news headlines.

Exposés in books and newspapers, including *Life Magazine* and the *New York Post*, led psychiatric hospitals to become known as "the shame of the states" (Deutsch, 1948). This shame was especially well deserved for segregated facilities responsible for Black Americans. In Maryland, the *Baltimore Sun* published a series in 1949 titled "Maryland's Shame," which illuminated awful conditions across the state's psychiatric hospitals. The series detailed the conditions at the Crownsville Hospital, which poorly served Black Marylanders for dozens of years. The report found that "thousands of state-supported patients live like animals. Some roll in their own excrement on the floor at night. Others sleep on thin, reeking mattresses on equally reeking floors because there aren't enough beds" (Schoeberlein, 2003, p. 59).

The outcry that followed, however, led to only temporary increases in funding. In Maryland as elsewhere, what states sought above all was to evade responsibility by reducing the number of patients in their facilities and shifting the cost of care to the federal government. The adoption of the disability provisions of the Social Security Act in 1952 and the subsequent passage of Medicare and Medicaid in the 1960s provided that opportunity (Geller, 2019).

For the first time since President Pierce's veto, the federal government began to take on a greater share of health costs. One notable limitation, however, was to be found in the Medicaid program's approach to mental illness. To avoid states charging the federal government for care in state mental hospitals, Congress had prohibited the use of federal funds to care for patients in "institutions of mental disease," a definition designed to include the state institutions (Congressional Research Service, 2023).

Slowly at first, and then more quickly, states began discharging hundreds, then thousands, then tens of thousands of patients with mental illness. These steps were heralded by a growing movement to allow people to live in less restrictive environments. However, key questions remained unanswered, including who would take responsibility and pay for the care they would receive in the community.

States did not necessarily shift savings from closing state hospitals back into the mental health system. Nor did the federal government provide necessary, sustained investments in community services. President John F. Kennedy championed legislation in 1963 that provided capital funds for the construction and operating funds of community-based mental health centers (Erickson, 2021). However, the support for program operations that accompanied these grants was designed to phase out over an 8-year period. Unfortunately, the envisioned rise of public and private insurance payments to fill the gap never fully materialized, nor did new commitments of state funding. Many mental health centers constructed with federal support closed (Foley & Sharfstein, 1983).

By the late 1970s, the results of deinstitutionalization were becoming starkly apparent in streets and jails across the nation. Cities saw thousands of individuals with untreated serious mental illness trying and often failing to live successfully on their own. After her husband's election to the presidency in 1976, First Lady Rosalynn Carter made improving care for people with serious mental illness her top priority and advocated for the passage of legislation, known as The Mental Health Systems Act of 1980, that aimed to create a more robust federal financing system for mental health (Carter Center, 2023). This effort, however, ran headlong into the election of President Ronald Reagan, who declined to provide funding for the community services authorized in the law. In his distaste for federal funding of healthcare, Reagan was the reincarnation of Franklin Pierce (Torrey, 2013).

Reagan's enthusiasm for private sector solutions, however, offered little to individuals with severe mental illness, few of whom were able to be employed with health benefits. Private insurers restricted care for mental health services by imposing large deductibles, increased copayments, and lifetime limits. These restrictions were far more stringent for mental health care than for physical health services (Barry et al., 2010). As people developed serious mental illness, many paid thousands of dollars out of pocket for treatment—until they lost their jobs and, as a result, their private insurance.

Starting in the 1990s, the federal government began to ask private and public insurers such as Medicare to do their share under the banner of "parity." Congress passed laws to increase spending by private employers and insurance companies on mental health care. These included the Mental Health Parity Act of 1996, which blocked annual or lifetime dollar limits on mental health coverage in large-group plans, and the Mental Health Parity and Addiction Equity Act of 2008, which prevents insurance plans that cover mental health and addiction services from imposing limitations that are not equivalent to those imposed on physical health services. The Affordable Care Act of 2010 expanded the parity provisions even further to include Health Maintenance Organizations and small insurance plans and made mental health care an "essential service" for health plans purchased through exchanges.

Unfortunately, these laws did not fundamentally alter the dynamics of payment for mental health care; private insurers never fully embraced their role as responsible for individuals with these conditions, many of whom might not remain their enrollees in future years. Moreover, because the laws did not stop insurers from applying intense utilization review to mental health care, enforcement has been a major challenge. Especially restrictive is coverage for the care of children and adolescents, which has constricted the capacity of community-based mental health services. One consequence is the wide and inappropriate use of child welfare and juvenile justice facilities for this population. In one national survey conducted in 2004 by Congressman Henry A. Waxman and Senator Susan Collins, two thirds of juvenile detention centers reported holding youth without charges (Pear, 2004). Even the Affordable Care Act, which increased private insurance coverage and labeled mental health care an essential health benefit, has left many gaps in place (Pestaina, 2022).

THE PRESENT: THE GAPS IN A SPLINTERED SYSTEM

As a consequence of this unfortunate history, funding for care of people with serious and persistent mental illness remains highly fragmented. Today, payment is not just split, it is splintered, and as a result, there is often little clarity over who has the fundamental responsibility to support essential care.

According to a report from the Agency for Health Care Research and Quality, there is no majority payer for mental health care in the United States. In 2019, the most recent year for which data are available, private insurance covered 32%, Medicaid covered 26%, Medicare covered 19%, and out-of-pocket costs covered 14%. Other payers paid for the remainder (Soni, 2022).

The picture becomes even more diffuse when costs that are complementary to clinical care are considered. The federal government through the Substance Abuse Mental Health Services Administration provides modest "block grants" for community services to states; these are used for an array of prevention and clinical services. Social Security Administration disability programs provide a minimal level of income support to individuals who can navigate its complicated enrollment process. Housing departments—as well as a few state Medicaid programs operating under waivers—may cover some of the costs of supported housing for individuals who cannot care for themselves. State governments themselves pay for psychiatric care in state mental institutions, which increasingly have become forensic facilities for court-ordered care.

This splintered approach to funding has been particularly damaging to Black, Hispanic, and low-income Americans with mental illness. Substantially fewer Black and Hispanic Americans with mental illness report receiving treatment than their White counterparts (Substance Abuse and Mental Health Services Administration [SAMHSA], 2022). Only about half of Black Americans with serious mental illness receive any care over the course of a year (SAMHSA, 2022). Reflecting the toxic mix of the stigma of mental illness and racism, many affected children in disadvantaged groups who need clinical care find themselves kicked out of school, arrested, or placed out of the home as a result of inadequate coverage of effective treatment.

Today, millions of Americans, disproportionately poor, Black, and Hispanic, cycle between community services inadequately funded by the federal government and hospitals inadequately funded by states. It would not be uncommon for someone with serious mental illness to seek care at a crowded outpatient treatment program, be hospitalized in a state-run facility, be discharged to the streets, and then receive intermittent attention only when jailed for property crimes (see **Box 18.2**). Despite generating many tens of thousands of dollars in costs across multiple systems, few if any of these resources are devoted to maintaining their well-being over time. As a direct consequence, jails have become the nation's largest providers of psychiatric care (**Box 18.3**). The Los Angeles County Detention Center is considered the largest mental hospital in the nation, holding 1,400 people a day (Montagne, 2008). Recently, the Rikers Island jail became the largest mental institution in New York (Ransom & Harris, 2023).

Box 18.2 EXAMPLE CASE OF INADEQUATE FINANCING FOR NEEDED CARE

E. C. is a 52-year-old divorced, employed African American mother of two adult children who suffers from major depression and struggles with her private insurer for payment for her outpatient psychiatric treatment. She has experienced two denials based on lack of "medical necessity" as determined by the payer. Her 22-year-old son, living at home, has been diagnosed with paranoid schizophrenia for 3 years, cycling in and out of hospitals supported by Medicaid. The state program, however, restricts payments for outpatient care, housing, or other necessary supports. He has had periods of homelessness and incarceration, which always cause setbacks in his ability to care for himself. The stress of his illness and lack of care is a major contributor to her depression. She spends much of her time arguing with her payer for her treatment and the state Medicaid program for her son's care.

Box 18.3 THE UNFORTUNATE USE OF JAILS AS MENTAL HOSPITALS

> *If you have someone diagnosed with a mental illness, can you think of a worse place to put them than a jail?*
>
> —Tom Dart, Sheriff of Cook County, Illinois

Source: Ford, M. (2015, June 8). America's largest mental hospital is a jail. *The Atlantic*. https://www.theatlantic.com/politics/archive/2015/06/americas-largest-mental-hospital-is-a-jail/395012/

THE FUTURE OF PAYMENT POLICY

If the history of mental health payment policy has been defined by "who pays," and if the best the answer to this question today might be "everyone and nobody at once," then a vision for the future must begin with the fundamental issue of responsibility.

The least disruptive answer would be to build on the current system. That would mean asking more of the agencies and entities now paying for care. To strengthen Medicaid and Medicare coverage, Congress could end the Institution for Mental Diseases (IMD) exclusion that bars the federal government from paying for the care of adults in state psychiatric hospitals. To enhance private insurance and Medicaid coverage, stronger enforcement of parity laws could be paired with ongoing monitoring of disparities in access to care by race, ethnicity, income, and geography. Especially for those with less serious disorders, such an approach could help to make equity a critical value in financing, alongside parity. It would be particularly important to scrutinize utilization review, to be sure that management of care for the treatment of mental illness supports access to effective treatment and does not undermine whatever coverage people may be entitled to by their insurance.

Such incremental improvements alone, however, would still leave major gaps in access to care and services for serious and persistent mental illness. That is in part because of the churn that leaves individuals cycling between different sources of coverage. It is also because many individuals with serious mental illness require more than clinical services, including income support through disability, housing, and supported employment. It is difficult to imagine undoing the criminalization of mental illness by changing reimbursement rules and benefit packages alone.

A second possible answer to "who pays" would be the federal government. Nearly 40 years ago, Talbott and Sharfstein proposed a comprehensive reform of the Social Security titles and other federal programs that merges them into one new Social Security title to pay for care and treatment of individuals with severe and persistent mental illness (Talbott & Sharfstein, 1986). The benefits could include disability payment, housing vouchers, and case management alongside specialty clinical treatment. Eligibility could extend to individuals with substance use disorders, many of whom have co-occurring mental illness, and few of whom today have robust access to effective treatment. Such an approach would be far more humane in design than our current system, but there would be major operational and political challenges. It would be a monumental task to administer such a program centrally, given the disparate conditions that exist across the country.

A third answer would be for the states to administer a new federal program or a substantially expanded Medicaid effort. States would have the responsibility of supporting people with serious mental illness—not just through clinical care, but also with income support, housing, and other services. The federal government would set expectations and standards in exchange for the new resources. States would blend in their resources and bring together services and staffing now spread between state psychiatric hospitals, community mental health centers, Medicaid, Medicare, housing, jails, and prisons. States could then develop and implement innovative models of value-based payment and comprehensive care with standards for quality.

As part of such a transformation, the federal government should not simply provide a "block grant" and leave implementation to the states. The federal government should provide its share of resources as an entitlement program, require states to measure key outcomes at the population level, and provide robust technical assistance and sharing of best practices. Public dashboards on suicides, overdoses, and homelessness of individuals with chronic mental illness and addiction could provide breakdowns of data by race, ethnicity, gender, and geography. For children, state programs could be focused on such measures as reducing dropout, improving school success, and linking adolescents to jobs and careers.

State-run comprehensive systems could allow individuals with mental illness and addiction to play a central role in the design and delivery of services. One mechanism could be a services voucher, which individuals could bring to licensed programs that would then provide income support, housing, and clinical care. To enhance the accountability of providers, individuals could be permitted to switch systems at designated time points. Community-based organizations could participate by offering services that might not be reimbursable under traditional insurance programs but can be shown to improve outcomes. Such services might facilitate skills development, job training and supported employment, and other asset-based programs.

Is such a major transformation possible? Other countries have demonstrated that similar efforts at consolidating treatment, care, and support can work. Single-payer systems in Canada, the United Kingdom, and other Western countries are examples of far better utilization of resources for care and treatment rather than management of downstream complications of homelessness and crime.

Is such change likely in the United States? Although wholesale reform is not likely to be on the agenda in the short term, states can take several steps toward this vision today. Medicaid programs can carve out financing streams for individuals with severe mental illness and addiction and pay special attention to the "dual eligible population" of Medicaid enrollees who are also part of the Medicare program. Promising models include New York's Health and Recovery Plans, which combine payment for medical, mental health, and addiction services with access to Medicaid waiver programs for housing, health homes, and other benefits (New York State Office of Mental Health, n.d.). Health departments can work with housing agencies to further develop models that provide a capitated amount for supported housing and mental health treatment for individuals who have experienced homelessness. Public health agencies can monitor not only outcomes of mental illness and addiction, including incarceration, but also protective factors, such as employment. Criminal justice agencies can scale up diversion programs, sharing budgetary support with service providers incentivized to keep people out of harm's way. An incremental step for Congress would be to authorize states to propose models of more effective systems in exchange for greater federal flexibility in the use of existing funding streams. Such a step would be analogous to an Innovation Center for mental health and addiction.

SUMMARY

Achieving mental health equity in the United States requires reform of a fractured system of financing for psychiatric and other essential services. It is a system that developed as a result of serial efforts by many agencies and entities to evade, rather than assume, responsibility for supporting some of the most vulnerable members of society. Overcoming this legacy requires a common vision for federal leadership and standard setting with flexibility and accountability for state and local agencies and private payers.

DISCUSSION QUESTIONS

1. Why do the authors say it is important to ask "who pays" when assessing equity in payment policy for mental health services?
2. How does the history of mental health payment help make sense of inequity in access to care today?
3. Why do you think public agencies and private insurers have been reluctant to take responsibility for funding mental health services?
4. What role does stigma play in undermining coherence of payment policy for serious mental illness, and what are the implications of stigma for equity?
5. How could a state, with federal support, design payment for a new system of care for people with serious mental illness that prioritizes equity?

ACKNOWLEDGMENT

The authors acknowledge Michael Friedman for his review.

REFERENCES

Barry, C. L., Huskamp, H. A., & Goldman, H. H. (2010). A political history of federal mental health and addiction insurance parity. *Milbank Quarterly, 88*(3), 404–433. https://doi.org/10.1111/j.1468-0009.2010.00605.x

Carter Center. (2023, December). Rosalynn Carter's leadership in mental health. *The Carter Center*. https://www.cartercenter.org/health/mental_health/rosalynn-carter-mental-health-leadership.html

Congressional Research Service. (2023, October 23). *Medicaid's Institution for Mental Disease (IMD) exclusion.*

Deutsch, A. (1948). *Shame of the states*. Harcourt, Brace and Company. https://www.congress.gov/crs_external_products/IF/PDF/IF10222/IF10222.15.pdf

Erickson, B. (2021). Deinstitutionalization through optimism: The Community Mental Health Act of 1963. *American Journal of Psychiatry Residents' Journal, 16*(4), 6–7. https://doi.org/10.1176/appi.ajp-rj.2021.160404

Faulkner, W. (1951). *Requiem for a nun*. Random House.

Foley, H., & Sharfstein, S. S. (1983). *Madness and government: Who cares for the mentally ill*. American Psychiatric Press.

Geller, J. (2019, March 14). The rise and demise of America's psychiatric hospitals: A tale of dollars trumping sense. *Psychiatric News*. https://psychiatryonline.org/doi/10.1176/appi.pn.2019.3b29

Gollaher, D. (1995). *Voice for the mad: The life of Dorothea Dix*. Free Press.

Montagne, R. (2008, August 13). Inside the nation's largest mental institution. *National Public Radio*. https://www.npr.org/2008/08/13/93581736/inside-the-nations-largest-mental-institution

New York State, Office of Mental Health. (n.d.). *Health and recovery plans (HARPS)*. https://omh.ny.gov/omhweb/bho/harp.html

Pear, R. (2004, July 8). Many youths reported held awaiting mental help. *The New York Times*. https://www.nytimes.com/2004/07/08/us/many-youths-reported-held-awaiting-mental-help.html

Pestaina, K. (2022, August 18). *Mental health parity at a crossroads*. KFF. https://www.kff.org/mental-health/issue-brief/mental-health-parity-at-a-crossroads/

Ransom, J., & Harris, A. J. (2023, December 29). How Rikers Island became New York's largest mental institution. *The New York Times*. https://www.nytimes.com/2023/12/29/nyregion/nyc-rikers-homeless-mental-illness.html

Schoeberlein, R. W. (2003). Maryland's shame: Photojournalism and mental health reform, 1935–1949. *Maryland Historical Magazine, 98*(1), 35–72.

Soni, A. (2022). *Healthcare expenditures for treatment of mental disorders: Estimates for adults ages 18 and older, U.S. civilian noninstitutionalized population, 2019* (AHRQ Statistical Brief #539). Agency for Health Research and Quality. https://meps.ahrq.gov/data_files/publications/st539/stat539.shtml

Substance Abuse and Mental Health Services Administration. (2022). *2022 national survey on drug use and health: Among the Black or African American population aged 12 or older*. https://www.samhsa.gov/data/sites/default/files/reports/rpt44472/2022-nsduh-pop-slides-black.pdf

Talbott, J. A., & Sharfstein, S. S. (1986). A proposal for future funding of chronic and episodic mental illness. *Hospital and Community Psychiatry, 37*(11), 1126–1130. https://doi.org/10.1176/ps.37.11.1126

Torrey, E. F. (2013, September 29). Ronald Reagan's shameful legacy: Violence, the homeless, mental illness. *Salon*. https://www.salon.com/2013/09/29/ronald_reagans_shameful_legacy_violence_the_homeless_mental_illness/

Part V

FROM POLICY, TO PRACTICE, TO RESULTS

19 CONCEPTUAL APPROACHES TO ADDRESSING THE POLITICAL DETERMINANTS OF MENTAL HEALTH

CATHERINE K. ETTMAN

LEARNING OBJECTIVES

After reading this chapter, readers will be able to:

- Discuss economic and social contexts that contribute to different mental health indicators.
- Identify two theoretical approaches that can be leveraged to shift political determinants of mental health.
- Identify policies within and outside the medical system that can improve population mental health.
- Consider a range of policies that can be implemented to improve mental health from prevention to treatment.
- Understand how public support and empiric evidence for actions to address mental health concerns relate to each other.

INTRODUCTION

Mental Health Overview

Poor mental health and addiction are common and costly, and their effects reverberate across the life course, not only for impacted individuals but also for their families, communities, and employers. In the United States, more than 21 million adults experience a depressive episode annually (Substance Abuse and Mental Health Services Administration [SAMHSA], 2022), 40 million experience an anxiety disorder (Anxiety and Depression Association of America, 2022), 46.3 million adults and adolescents struggle with substance misuse (SAMHSA, 2022), and more than 49,000 die by suicide (Centers for Disease Control and Prevention, 2023). Although attempts to estimate costs may not cover the full range of cost to society of ill mental health, annual estimates are $326 billion for major depressive disorder (Greenberg et al., 2021), $48.7 billion for anxiety disorders (Shirneshan, 2013), $249 billion for inappropriate use of alcohol (Sacks et al., 2015), $471 billion for opioid use disorder (Florence et al., 2021), $550 billion for fatal drug overdose in the United States (Florence et al., 2021), $281.6 billion for schizophrenia (Murphy et al., 2021), and $502.7 billion for suicide (Rockett et al., 2023). In the wake of the COVID-19 pandemic, depression and anxiety rates remain elevated and opioid deaths have surged (Gomes et al., 2023). Although mental health has long been an important feature of health, its urgency has risen to national levels, creating an opportunity for action.

Social and Political Forces That Shape Health

The causes of poor mental health and substance misuse are complex and many, including a combination of personality (Hengartner, 2015), genetics (Hyman, 2000), environment (Tost et al., 2015), and stressors (Pearlin et al., 1981). Over time, there has been a growing understanding that health, including mental health, is largely the result of context and environmental factors (Braveman & Gottlieb, 2014; Dawes & Williams, 2020; Galea, 2017). Rooted in Bronfenbrenner's ecological systems theory (Bronfenbrenner, 1977), whereby the individual is a product of their changing environment, this understanding has evolved to include a social–ecological model (Kaplan, 2004) whereby an individual's health is the product of multiple concentric influences of interpersonal relationships, family, neighborhood, community, city, state, and national environments. Although previous efforts may have focused on targeting specific genes that cause mental illness, few have been found, with a growing awareness of the importance of social and environmental factors on mental health (Insel, 2022). By focusing on the root causes of poor health, researchers, practitioners, and policy makers can improve, address, and maintain population mental health. Additionally, understanding different levels of influence allows for different levels of intervention. Where gridlock may prevent federal policies for certain topics, cities and states can innovate (Hearne et al., 2023). Policies across levels and sectors, including private (Maani et al., 2020) and nonprofit, can influence mental health (**Table 19.1**).

Mental Health Inequities

One cause for urgency in addressing poor mental health and addiction is that they are distributed unequally across society. Disparities in mental health indicators vary across conditions and demographic characteristics such as gender, race and ethnicity, and economic status. For example, women are diagnosed with higher rates of mood disorders than men (Salk et al., 2017); however, men are more likely to die by opioid overdose and by suicide (Butelman et al., 2023; KFF, 2023). The relationship between race and ethnicity and mental health is more complex, with many studies citing a similar or lower prevalence of mental illness in minoritized populations than White populations (Ettman et al., 2022). Competing hypotheses that explain these paradoxical findings suggest either that there are protective factors such as religiosity, resilience, and positivity that protect racial and ethnic minority groups or that there is underreporting of poor mental health in these groups due to stigma, screening instruments that may not be culturally relevant, and systemic racism that contributes to underuse of mental health services.

Although the opioid overdose epidemic initially emerged primarily among White men, from 2007 and 2019, there were notable increases in overdose deaths experienced by racial and ethnic minorities (Abdalla & Galea, 2022). As of 2023, overdose death rates in the United States were highest in American Indian and Alaska Natives followed by Black

Table 19.1 SOCIAL–ECOLOGICAL DRIVERS OF MENTAL HEALTH

LEVEL	VARIABLE	EVIDENCE
Individual	Personality	Hengartner (2015)
Community	Stressors	Pearlin et al. (1981)
Local, state, or national	Environment	Tost et al. (2015)

Sources: Adapted from Bronfenbrenner, U. (1979). *The ecology of human development: Experiments by nature and design*. Harvard University Press; Kaplan, G. A. (2004). What's wrong with social epidemiology, and how can we make it better? *Epidemiologic Reviews*, *26*(1), 124–135. https://doi.org/10.1093/epirev/mxh010

persons (Han et al., 2022). Although suicide rates are higher overall for White persons, the rates of suicide decreased for White persons between 2018 and 2020 while increasing for Hispanic and Black persons between 2000 and 2020 (Curtin et al., 2022). Racial and ethnic minorities are more likely to present more serious levels of mental illness when they interact with the medical system and are more likely to face barriers in access to treatment when they do (U.S. Department of Health and Human Services [HHS], 2001), which contributes to growing mental health disparities between groups (Maura & Weisman de Mamani, 2017; HHS, 2001). Finally, there is a well-documented gradient between socioeconomic status and mental health. Although income is the most documented economic indicator of mental health (Baptiste-Roberts & Hossain, 2018; Ettman et al., 2023c), there is also a link between lower wealth and higher levels of depressive symptoms and substance abuse–related problems. Persons with fewer financial assets (including income and family savings) have fewer resources to pool in the face of unexpected stressors, such as job loss, and are the very populations more likely to be affected by stressors that lead to poor mental health, as seen during the start of the COVID-19 pandemic (Ettman et al., 2021). Poverty, which has increased since the COVID-19 pandemic, has deep connections with mental illness and threatens to deepen mental health disparities between people with and without assets (Marbin et al., 2022).

TWO CONCEPTUAL APPROACHES FOR CONSIDERING THE POLITICAL DETERMINANTS OF MENTAL HEALTH

Two conceptual approaches may facilitate discussion and action to advance the political determinants of mental health: the policy, context, and care framework for population mental health and the policy evidence and values framework for mental health.

The Policy, Context, and Care Framework for Population Mental Health

The first framework that can inform and organize efforts to address population mental health is called the policy, context, and care framework. Action can range from prevention to treatment and can be organized into three categories: policies and regulations (which shape all else), social and economic context, and the provision of mental health care. A visual is provided in **Figure 19.1** that highlights different levels of intervention to address the political determinants of mental health.

Prevention techniques centered around mental health can effectively avoid poor and extreme outcomes. Policies can specifically target mental health or they can target the determinants that shape mental health. As an example of the former, one of the most cost-effective population-level interventions identified by the World Health Organization in reducing suicide deaths in lower income countries was the limiting of access to chemicals, such as those found in pesticides, that could be used to commit suicide (World Health Organization, 2021). Bans and restrictions on the sale of deadly pesticides have been followed with reductions in suicide mortality related to pesticides in India, Denmark, and the United States (Gunnell et al., 2017). Preventive approaches can improve outcomes throughout the life course, making them a high-yield investment (McDaid et al., 2017).

Policies that do not explicitly relate to mental health (or even health at all) can still have a major impact on mental well-being. Examples of prevention policies that can improve mental health include policies that reduce homelessness (Gutwinski et al., 2021; Roy et al., 2024); improve access to active transportation (e.g., cycling, through the construction of bike lanes; Ma et al., 2021); increase access to healthy food options (Pourmotabbed et al., 2020), such as through the Supplemental Nutrition Assistance Program (SNAP); and improve economic mobility (e.g., through income transfers; McGuire et al., 2022). Regulations and policies that promote public health trickle down to mental health and form the

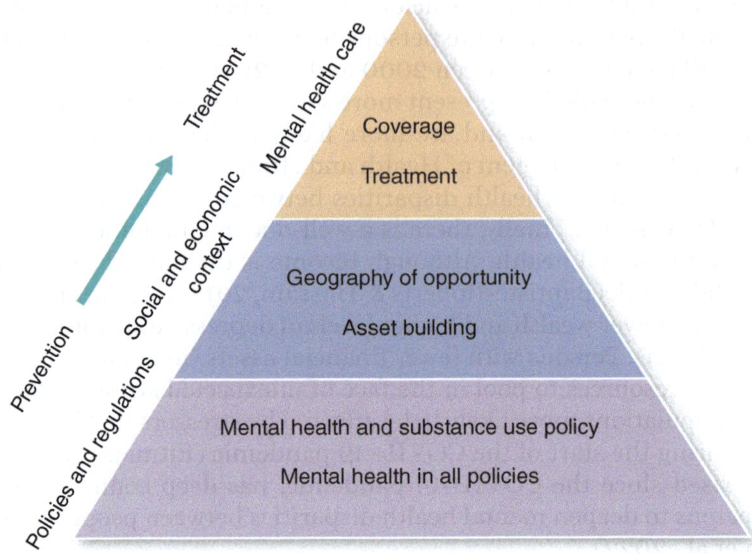

Figure 19.1 The policy, context, and care framework for population mental health.
Source: Adapted from Ettman, C. K., & Galea, S. (2023). The potential influence of AI on population mental health. *JMIR Mental Health, 10*(1), e49936. https://doi.org/10.2196/49936

foundation of efforts to improve mental health. Moving forward, regulations and policies around patient privacy will become an increasing concern, particularly as technology and digital advances, including the use of artificial intelligence, facilitate the rapid analysis of large sets of data, including sensitive patient behavior data (Ettman & Galea, 2023).

Beyond policy decisions, social and economic factors influence mental well-being, and actions taken to improve that context can improve mental health. Ample evidence shows the relation of economic context and geography of opportunity on mental health (Osypuk, 2013). Economic recessions, which often come with job loss, unemployment, and unstable housing are associated with worse mental health (Frasquilho et al., 2016), drug use (Nagelhout et al., 2017), and suicide (Mathieu et al., 2022). The COVID-19 pandemic upended access to institutional support such as education, religious engagement, community engagement, public places, and employment, which together contributed to ill mental health in the years that followed (Ettman et al., 2023a). The COVID-19 pandemic exacerbated underlying gaps in mental health that existed before the pandemic (Galea, 2022). In this way, maintaining access to social support, ensuring employment opportunities, and providing opportunities to build assets can help prevent poor mental health as well as lessen its ill effects (**Table 19.2**).

Finally, policies can address treatment of poor mental health and substance misuse. These policies, although considered more proximal to experiencing mental illness, are critical not only for maintaining mental health but also preventing serious mental illness from worsening. Despite poor mental health being common, about half of adults with a mental illness have received mental health treatment in the preceding 12 months (SAMHSA, 2024). Lack of treatment may be a result of stigma, high out-of-pocket costs, or lack of providers, as examples. Policies that improve access to healthcare in general can improve mental health. Treatment, particularly for patients with serious mental illness and substance misuse, can be effective at helping patients lead functional lives and can be lifesaving. Additional efforts to cover mental and behavioral health treatment, which have not always been fully covered by health insurance, can ensure that populations have access to resources that can help.

Table 19.2 EXAMPLES OF POLICIES THAT MAY IMPROVE POPULATION MENTAL HEALTH THROUGH PREVENTION

GOAL	POLICY ACTION	CITATION
Reduce suicide deaths through reducing access to lethal means.	Limit access to certain pesticides (with lethal chemicals) from stores where they could easily be purchased.	Gunnell et al. (2017)
Improve mental health by reducing homelessness.	Reduce homelessness by providing housing support and implementing critical time and case management interventions.	Gutwinski et al. (2021) Roy et al. (2024)
Lessen psychological distress and increase life satisfaction through improving active transportation options.	Construct bicycling infrastructure, such as cycling superhighways, to facilitate regular transport to places of employment.	Ma et al. (2021)
Reduce depression and stress through access to healthy food.	Address food insecurity through healthcare or public services that adhere to established dietary guidelines.	Pourmotabbed et al. (2020)
Improve mental health and subjective well-being through economic mobility.	Provide income through conditional and unconditional cash transfer programs.	McGuire et al. (2022)
Improve mental health of the mother and child by providing savings accounts for children.	Provide funds to newborn children in accounts to be used for educational expenses or other wealth-building activities.	Sherraden et al. (2015)

Later in this chapter, we explore policy efforts to improve coverage of mental health services through mental health parity efforts. Programs that expand access to medical insurance such as Medicare and Medicaid can improve health outcomes overall as a result of timely treatment and preventive care, as well as increased funding for certain beneficial therapies (Cuellar & Markowitz, 2007). For example, the expansion of Medicaid spurred by the Affordable Care Act was linked with better mental well-being (Winkelman & Chang, 2018). Thus, the policy, context, and care framework on population mental health can inform how policies shape mental health.

The Policy Evidence and Values Framework for Mental Health

The second framework to consider in shifting political determinants of mental health features the intersection of evidence and values. In his Multiple Streams Framework, John Kingdon proposed three process streams that must be aligned for a "policy window" to open: a problem must be clearly identified, a policy should be proposed, and the politics must be favorable to the idea (Kingdon & Thurber, 2011). Although problems in mental health and substance use have been clearly articulated, there is less consensus on the policies that should be enacted to treat them, in part shaped by public support. For policies to be successfully passed, implemented, and kept, they must have public support, which is in part shaped by the values of a society. Although evidence is mounting on interventions that can help to prevent or improve poor mental health or substance misuse, whether they are implemented depends in large part on social values, which shift over time. The policy evidence and values framework has been proposed by Sandro Galea to address public health broadly (Galea, 2017); here, we apply this framework to mental health in particular. **Figure 19.2**

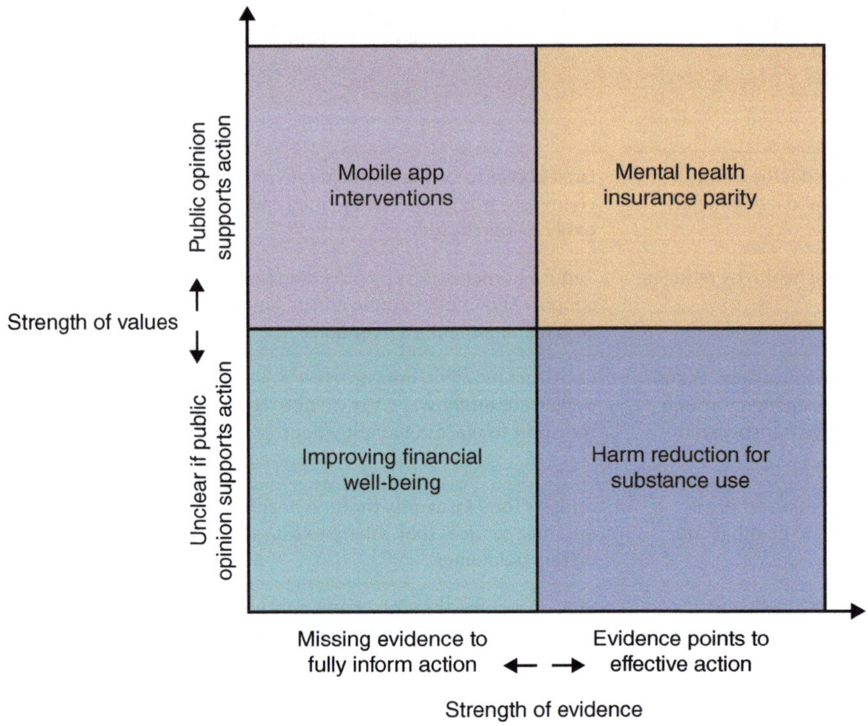

Figure 19.2 The policy evidence and values framework for mental health.
Source: Adapted from Galea, S. (2017). *Healthier: Fifty thoughts on the foundations of population health*. Oxford University Press.

shows the intersection of strength of evidence for policies and strength of values supporting these actions, with four examples reflecting 2024 values and evidence.

The framework has on the x-axis the strength of empiric evidence of an action area to improve mental health or health services utilization; on the y-axis lies the strength of public support (or disfavor) for a given action. Although a policy may have strong evidence to point to its efficacy, it may not have enough support from the public for policy makers to pursue it, reflecting values at the time; conversely, a policy action may have high public support and popularity but low evidence justifying its enaction. It is the work of researchers, practitioners, and policy makers (as discussed later) to communicate the scientific evidence to support policy actions and to be aware of how values shape what is ultimately accepted and successful, sustainable policy. Following are examples of each action.

High Public Support, High Evidence of Efficacy: Mental Health Parity

The top right quadrant of the policy evidence and values framework for mental health represents actions that have both ample evidence of their effectiveness and ample public support. In the mental health space, mental health parity, whereby insurance coverage for mental health should be reimbursed at a rate no less than that of physical health, is an example of a policy that both has evidence to support its efficacy and is largely supported by the public. Almost 70% of U.S. adults support insurance parity for mental health and substance use treatment with physical health (Barry & McGinty, 2014). There is ample evidence, starting with the RAND Health Insurance Study, that increased mental health insurance coverage is associated with increased use of mental health services across a range of mental health conditions, including autism spectrum disorder (Manning et al., 1986; Stuart et al., 2017). Mental health parity reduces out-of-pocket costs for consumers related to mental health treatment. This literature is consistent with a deep body of work that shows that health insurance coverage is associated with increased healthcare use across all conditions, including mental health and substance use (Buchmueller et al., 2005; Docrat et al., 2020).

Low Public Support, High Evidence: Harm Reduction Strategies for Substance Use

The bottom right quadrant represents policies that have ample evidence of efficacy but have low or mixed public support. Efforts to reduce or minimize the harms of unhealthy behavior have strong empiric evidence supporting their efficacy in reducing overdose deaths and infectious disease transmission (Kimber et al., 2010; Levengood et al., 2021; Logan & Marlatt, 2010; Puzhko et al., 2022; Ritter & Cameron, 2006). A review of needle exchange programs showed reductions in spread of certain blood-borne diseases, more responsible needle use, and more entry into treatment, all without an associated rise in use of drugs (Strathdee & Vlahov, 2001). Another study found that needle exchange programs could provide a large decrease in healthcare expenditures related to HIV (Gold et al., 1997). Naloxone distribution, another harm reduction strategy, has been associated with a reduction in deaths related to opioid overdose (Chimbar & Moleta, 2018; Walley et al., 2013). Despite the evidence in support of harm reduction strategies, many have low public support. For example, among U.S. adults, only 29% are in favor of safe consumption sites and 39% are in favor of needle exchange programs in their communities (McGinty et al., 2018), despite strong evidence for their success. A lack of public support can even lead to outcomes such as the banning of harm reduction programs. In 2018, the city of Philadelphia voiced their formal support for privately run safe injection sites (Feldman, 2018). This policy was so at odds with public opinion that, over the following years, a legal battle would ensue across multiple courts and a council decision resulted in an effective ban on the sites in Philadelphia in 2023 (Ovalle, 2023). Thus, despite evidence of efficacy in harm reduction interventions, low public support can stymie or reverse policy efforts (Lofaro & Miller, 2021).

High Public Support, Low Evidence of Efficacy: Mobile Apps

In the top left quadrant sit actions that have high public support and low or mixed evidence of efficacy. As the world shifted to telehealth during the COVID-19 pandemic, and as some restrictions were lifted to accommodate virtual delivery of care (Wallace & Pestaina, 2023), use of mobile mental health apps soared. Mental health was particularly receptive to virtual treatment, as seen by high levels of telehealth use in psychiatry several years after in-person medical appointments returned (Ettman et al., 2023b). Mobile health is a subset of telehealth that is delivered via phone, and phone apps have captured the excitement of businesses and the public. The year 2020 saw the introduction of 90,000 health apps into the market, and between 20% and 25% of adults had downloaded a mental health app (Leventhal, 2023). It is estimated that $4.4 billion was invested in mobile mental health apps in 2021 alone (Gold, 2022). Many businesses offer memberships or access to mental health apps as benefits, and the wellness industry reported $880 million in revenue in 2024 across 125 million wellness apps (Wylie, 2025). Mental health apps are often viewed favorably by users (Chan & Honey, 2022), although there appears to be disagreement about utility between patients and providers using apps (Hudson et al., 2022). Despite the high uptake of mobile apps, there is little evidence about their efficacy in improving mental health, and systematic reviews have shown mixed evidence (Lecomte et al., 2020; Marshall et al., 2020), with many apps using non–evidence-based approaches to treat patients (Koh et al., 2022). Although apps may hold promise in their accessibility, more work is to be done to assess the efficacy and safety of these interventions.

Low Public Support, Low Evidence of Efficacy: Financial Well-Being to Improve Mental Health

In the bottom left quadrant lie actions that have low public favor or disfavor and relatively low evidence of their efficacy. One example of this type of intervention would be efforts to improve mental health through improving financial well-being. Financial well-being interventions may range from financial literacy education to policies that remove medical debt from credit scores, as has been initiated by the three credit rating agencies removing medical debt below $500 from credit scores (Holzhauer, 2023). In September 2023, President Biden's administration proposed banning all medical debt from inclusion in credit scores (Levey, 2023). Although programs such as guaranteed income, which is one approach to alleviate financial strain, are gaining evidence for their effects on health, as of 2020, 54% of Americans said they would not support a guaranteed income initiative (Gilberstadt, 2020). Another policy that could potentially alleviate financial strain, and poverty, would be the delivery of "baby bonds" whereby low-income children would be provided with a bond at birth that would increase in value over their childhood so that they would start their adult life with assets (Brown et al., 2023). One survey on behalf of the American Civil Liberties Union found that 54% to 61% of people support the action, depending on how the policy is described (Brown et al., 2023). Although bills have been considered in Congress related to baby bonds with support from both parties, none has been enacted (Sherraden et al., 2018), and they have received little media attention relative to other economic interventions, such as Universal Basic Income (UBI), which garners stronger reactions from the public in both directions (Gilberstadt, 2020). Singapore, Canada, the United Kingdom (discontinued), Korea, Israel, Maine, Rhode Island, Nevada, Connecticut, San Francisco, St. Louis, and New York City have piloted baby bond programs (Sherraden et al., 2018). A randomized controlled trial in Oklahoma tested whether starting a 529 account for children with $1,000 (and matching contributions to those under a certain income threshold) would be beneficial (Sherraden et al., 2015); the study found that the accounts improved maternal and child mental well-being, among other pro-social benefits (Sherraden et al., 2015). The public perception of policies that improve financial literacy or change underlying credit scores, which influence a host of financial outcomes and may be predictive of health (Dean & Nicholas, 2018), may be more positively received by the public than other policies, such as UBI. Therefore, they may serve as an example of a policy in which evidence could help to bring attention to the upsides of such an intervention. More work should be done in evaluating the mental health impacts of various financial well-being efforts as they evolve.

SUMMARY

There is a growing awareness of the importance of mental health. Although stigma remains a challenge to the treatment of mental health, particularly for persons with addiction and schizophrenia, views are changing (Pescosolido et al., 2021). Although some adults still associate addiction with "bad character," there has been a cultural shift in the United States that acknowledges that mental illness and substance dependence are health concerns. Changes in attitudes around mental health may be a result of national efforts, such as the 1999 U.S. Surgeon General's Report (HHS, 1999), and more recent injection of mental health into the national conversation by high-profile athletes, popular television and movie stars, and even political figures. Together, these cultural forces have helped to create awareness for mental health, which is a necessary component of policy change. It is possible that the world is more receptive than ever to prioritizing mental health. This chapter presents two conceptual approaches that can help organize our approach to shifting the political determinants of mental health. These approaches can inform policies across sectors that improve population mental health.

DISCUSSION QUESTIONS

1. What policies can improve mental health within and outside the medical system?
2. What steps can different sectors take in both the prevention and treatment of poor mental health and substance misuse?
3. What are some examples of actions that have high evidence of efficacy in improving mental health but low public support?
4. How can protecting the public's mental health serve as motivation for policies that improve access to assets?
5. How can policies across sectors reduce mental health inequities?

ACKNOWLEDGMENT

The author would like to thank Priya Dohlman and Isabel Galea for research assistance with this chapter.

REFERENCES

Abdalla, S. M., & Galea, S. (2022). Invited commentary: Toward a better understanding of disparities in overdose mortality. *American Journal of Epidemiology*, *191*(7), 1280-1282. https://doi.org/10.1093/aje/kwac053

Anxiety and Depression Association of America. (2022). *Facts & statistics*. https://adaa.org/understanding-anxiety/facts-statistics

Baptiste-Roberts, K., & Hossain, M. (2018). Socioeconomic disparities and self-reported substance abuse-related problems. *Addiction & Health*, *10*(2), 112–122. https://doi.org/10.22122/ahj.v10i2.561

Barry, C. L., & McGinty, E. E. (2014). Stigma and public support for insurance parity and government spending on mental health: Findings from a 2013 national opinion survey. *Psychiatric Services (Washington, D.C.)*, *65*(10), 1265–1268. https://doi.org/10.1176/appi.ps.201300550

Braveman, P., & Gottlieb, L. (2014). The social determinants of health: It's time to consider the causes of the causes. *Public Health Reports (Washington, D.C.)*, *129*(Suppl 2), 19–31. https://doi.org/10.1177/00333549141291S206

Bronfenbrenner, U. (1977). Toward an experimental ecology of human development. *American Psychologist*, *32*(7), 513–531. https://doi.org/10.1037/0003-066X.32.7.513

Brown, M., Biu. O., Harvey, C., & Shanks, T. (2023). *The state of baby bonds*. Urban Institute. https://www.urban.org/sites/default/files/2023-02/The%20State%20of%20Baby%20Bonds.pdf

Buchmueller, T. C., Grumbach, K., Kronick, R., & Kahn, J. G. (2005). Book review: The effect of health insurance on medical care utilization and implications for insurance expansion: A review of the literature. *Medical Care Research and Review*, *62*(1), 3–30. https://doi.org/10.1177/1077558704271718

Butelman, E. R., Huang, Y., Epstein, D. H., Shaham, Y., Goldstein, R. Z., Volkow, N. D., & Alia-Klein, N. (2023). Overdose mortality rates for opioids and stimulant drugs are substantially higher in men than in women: State-level analysis. *Neuropsychopharmacology*, *48*(11), 11. https://doi.org/10.1038/s41386-023-01601-8

Centers for Disease Control and Prevention. (2023, December 4). *Suicide data and statistics, suicide prevention.* https://www.cdc.gov/suicide/suicide-data-statistics.html

Chan, A. H. Y., & Honey, M. L. L. (2022). User perceptions of mobile digital apps for mental health: Acceptability and usability—An integrative review. *Journal of Psychiatric and Mental Health Nursing*, *29*(1), 147–168. https://doi.org/10.1111/jpm.12744

Chimbar, L., & Moleta, Y. (2018). Naloxone effectiveness: A systematic review. *Journal of Addictions Nursing*, *29*(3), 167–171. https://doi.org/10.1097/JAN.0000000000000230

Cuellar, A. E., & Markowitz, S. (2007). Medicaid policy changes in mental health care and their effect on mental health outcomes. *Health Economics, Policy and Law*, *2*(1), 23–49. https://doi.org/10.1017/S1744133106006268

Curtin, S. C., Brown, K. A., & Jordan, M. E. (2022). *Suicide rates for the three leading methods by race and ethnicity: United States, 2000–2020* (No. 450; NCHS Data Brief). Centers for Disease Control and Prevention. https://doi.org/10.15620/cdc:121798

Dawes, D. E., & Williams, D. R. (2020). *The political determinants of health* (1st ed.). Johns Hopkins University Press.

Dean, L. T., & Nicholas, L. H. (2018). Using credit scores to understand predictors and consequences of disease. *American Journal of Public Health*, *108*(11), 1503–1505. https://doi.org/10.2105/AJPH.2018.304705

Docrat, S., Besada, D., Cleary, S., & Lund, C. (2020). The impact of social, national and community-based health insurance on health care utilization for mental, neurological and substance-use disorders in low- and middle-income countries: A systematic review. *Health Economics Review*, *10*(1), 11. https://doi.org/10.1186/s13561-020-00268-x

Ettman, C. K., Abdalla, S. M., Cohen, G. H., Sampson, L., Vivier, P. M., & Galea, S. (2021). Low assets and financial stressors associated with higher depression during COVID-19 in a nationally representative sample of US adults. *Journal of Epidemiology and Community Health, 75*(6), 501–508. https://doi.org/10.1136/jech-2020-215213

Ettman, C. K., Badillo-Goicoechea, E., & Stuart, E. A. (2023a). Evolution of depression and anxiety during the COVID-19 pandemic and across demographic groups in a large sample of U.S. adults. *AJPM Focus, 2*(4), 100140. https://doi.org/10.1016/j.focus.2023.100140

Ettman, C. K., & Galea, S. (2023). The potential influence of AI on population mental health. *JMIR Mental Health, 10*(1), e49936. https://doi.org/10.2196/49936

Ettman, C. K., Koya, S. F., Fan, A., Robbins, G., Shain, J., Cozier, Y., Abdalla, S. M., & Galea, S. (2022). More, less, or the same: A scoping review of studies that compare depression between Black and White U.S. adult populations. *SSM - Mental Health, 2*, 100161. https://doi.org/10.1016/j.ssmmh.2022.100161

Ettman, C. K., Lupton Brantner, C., Albert, M., Goes, F., Mojtabai, R., Spivak, S., Stuart, E., & Zandi, P. (2023b). Trends in telehealth and in-person psychiatric care from 2017–2022 among patients with depression in a large US academic medical system. *Psychiatric Services, 75*(2), 178–181. https://doi.org/10.1176/appi.ps.20230064

Ettman, C. K., Subramanian, M., Fan, A. Y., Adam, G. P., Abdalla, S. M., Galea, S., & Stuart, E. A. (2023c). Assets and depression in U.S. adults during the COVID-19 pandemic: A systematic review. *Social Psychiatry and Psychiatric Epidemiology, 59*(4), 571–583. https://doi.org/10.1007/s00127-023-02565-2

Feldman, N. (2018, January 23.) *Funders, operators sought to start safe drug-injection sites in Philly*. WHYY. https://whyy.org/segments/funders-operators-sought-start-safe-drug-injection-sites-philly/

Florence, C., Luo, F., & Rice, K. (2021). The economic burden of opioid use disorder and fatal opioid overdose in the United States, 2017. *Drug and Alcohol Dependence, 218*, 108350. https://doi.org/10.1016/j.drugalcdep.2020.108350

Frasquilho, D., Matos, M. G., Salonna, F., Guerreiro, D., Storti, C. C., Gaspar, T., & Caldas-de-Almeida, J. M. (2016). Mental health outcomes in times of economic recession: A systematic literature review. *BMC Public Health, 16*, 115. https://doi.org/10.1186/s12889-016-2720-y

Galea, S. (2017). *Healthier: Fifty thoughts on the foundations of population health*. Oxford University Press.

Galea, S. (2022). *The contagion next time*. Oxford University Press.

Gilberstadt, H. (2020, August 19). More Americans oppose than favor the government providing a universal basic income for all adult citizens. *Pew Research Center*. https://www.pewresearch.org/short-reads/2020/08/19/more-americans-oppose-than-favor-the-government-providing-a-universal-basic-income-for-all-adult-citizens/

Gold, A. (2022, May 2). *Mental health app boom raises alarms*. Axios. https://www.axios.com/2022/05/02/mental-health-app-boom-raises-alarms

Gold, M., Gafni, A., Nelligan, P., & Millson, P. (1997). Needle exchange programs: An economic evaluation of a local experience. *CMAJ, 157*(3), 255–262.

Gomes, T., Ledlie, S., Tadrous, M., Mamdani, M., Paterson, J. M., & Juurlink, D. N. (2023). Trends in opioid toxicity–related deaths in the US before and after the start of the COVID-19 pandemic, 2011–2021. *JAMA Network Open, 6*(7), e2322303. https://doi.org/10.1001/jamanetworkopen.2023.22303

Greenberg, P. E., Fournier, A.-A., Sisitsky, T., Simes, M., Berman, R., Koenigsberg, S. H., & Kessler, R. C. (2021). The economic burden of adults with major depressive disorder in the United States (2010 and 2018). *Pharmacoeconomics, 39*(6), 653–665. https://doi.org/10.1007/s40273-021-01019-4

Gunnell, D., Knipe, D., Chang, S.-S., Pearson, M., Konradsen, F., Lee, W. J., & Eddleston, M. (2017). Prevention of suicide with regulations aimed at restricting access to highly hazardous pesticides: A systematic review of the international evidence. *The Lancet Global Health, 5*(10), e1026–e1037. https://doi.org/10.1016/S2214-109X(17)30299-1

Gutwinski, S., Schreiter, S., Deutscher, K., & Fazel, S. (2021). The prevalence of mental disorders among homeless people in high-income countries: An updated systematic review and meta-regression analysis. *PLoS Medicine, 18*(8), e1003750. https://doi.org/10.1371/journal.pmed.1003750

Han, B., Einstein, E. B., Jones, C. M., Cotto, J., Compton, W. M., & Volkow, N. D. (2022). Racial and ethnic disparities in drug overdose deaths in the US during the COVID-19 pandemic. *JAMA Network Open, 5*(9), e2232314. https://doi.org/10.1001/jamanetworkopen.2022.32314

Hearne, S., Pollack Porter, K., & Forrest, K. (2023). *Policy engagement*. APHA Press.

Hengartner, M. P. (2015). The detrimental impact of maladaptive personality on public mental health: A challenge for psychiatric practice. *Frontiers in Psychiatry, 6*, 87. https://www.frontiersin.org/articles/10.3389/fpsyt.2015.00087

Holzhauer, B. (2023, January 19). *As of July 1, your medical debt may no longer hurt your credit score—Here's why*. https://www.cnbc.com/select/medical-debt-credit-report/

Hudson, G., Negbenose, E., Neary, M., Jansli, S. M., Schueller, S. M., Wykes, T., & Jilka, S. (2022). Comparing professional and consumer ratings of mental health apps: Mixed methods study. *JMIR Formative Research, 6*(9), e39813. https://doi.org/10.2196/39813

Hyman, S. E. (2000). The genetics of mental illness: Implications for practice. *Bulletin of the World Health Organization, 78*(4), 455–463. https://iris.who.int/handle/10665/268111

Insel, T. R. (2022). *Healing: Our path from mental illness to mental health.* Penguin Press.

Kaplan, G. A. (2004). What's wrong with social epidemiology, and how can we make it better? *Epidemiologic Reviews, 26*(1), 124–135. https://doi.org/10.1093/epirev/mxh010

KFF. (2023, January). Suicide deaths and rate by gender. https://www.kff.org/other/state-indicator/suicide-rate-by-gender/

Kimber, J., Palmateer, N., Hutchinson, S., Hickman, M., Goldberg, D., & Rhodes, T. (2010). In T. Rhodes & D. Hedrich (Eds.), *Harm reduction among injecting drug users—Evidence of effectiveness* (pp. 115–163). European Monitoring Centre for Drugs and Drug Addiction. https://doi.org/10.2810/29497

Kingdon, J. W., & Thurber, J. A. (2011). *Agendas, alternatives, and public policies* (2nd ed.). Longman.

Koh, J., Tng, G. Y. Q., & Hartanto, A. (2022). Potential and pitfalls of mobile mental health apps in traditional treatment: An umbrella review. *Journal of Personalized Medicine, 12*(9), 1376. https://doi.org/10.3390/jpm12091376

Lecomte, T., Potvin, S., Corbière, M., Guay, S., Samson, C., Cloutier, B., Francoeur, A., Pennou, A., & Khazaal, Y. (2020). Mobile apps for mental health issues: Meta-review of meta-analyses. *JMIR MHealth and UHealth, 8*(5), e17458. https://doi.org/10.2196/17458

Levengood, T. W., Yoon, G. H., Davoust, M. J., Ogden, S. N., Marshall, B. D. L., Cahill, S. R., & Bazzi, A. R. (2021). Supervised injection facilities as harm reduction: A systematic review. *American Journal of Preventive Medicine, 61*(5), 738–749. https://doi.org/10.1016/j.amepre.2021.04.017

Leventhal, R. (2023, February 21). *Most US consumers are mobile health app users.* Insider Intelligence. https://www.insiderintelligence.com/content/nearly-two-thirds-of-us-consumers-mobile-health-app-users

Levey, N. N. (2023, September 21). Biden administration to ban medical debt from Americans' credit scores. *KFF Health News.* https://kffhealthnews.org/news/article/medical-debt-credit-score-ban-biden-administration/

Lofaro, R. J., & Miller, H. T. (2021). Narrative politics in policy discourse: The debate over safe injection sites in Philadelphia, Pennsylvania. *Contemporary Drug Problems, 48*(1), 75–95. https://doi.org/10.1177/0091450921993821

Logan, D. E., & Marlatt, G. A. (2010). Harm reduction therapy: A practice-friendly review of research. *Journal of Clinical Psychology, 66*(2), 201–214. https://doi.org/10.1002/jclp.20669

Ma, L., Ye, R., & Wang, H. (2021). Exploring the causal effects of bicycling for transportation on mental health. *Transportation Research Part D: Transport and Environment, 93,* 102773. https://doi.org/10.1016/j.trd.2021.102773

Maani, N., Collin, J., Friel, S., Gilmore, A. B., McCambridge, J., Robertson, L., & Petticrew, M. P. (2020). Bringing the commercial determinants of health out of the shadows: A review of how the commercial determinants are represented in conceptual frameworks. *European Journal of Public Health, 30*(4), 660–664. https://doi.org/10.1093/eurpub/ckz197

Manning, W., Wells, K., Duan, N., Newhouse, J., & Ware, J. (1986). How cost sharing affects the use of ambulatory mental health services. *JAMA, 256*(14), 1930–1934.

Marbin, D., Gutwinski, S., Schreiter, S., & Heinz, A. (2022). Perspectives in poverty and mental health. *Frontiers in Public Health, 10,* 975482. https://doi.org/10.3389/fpubh.2022.975482

Marshall, J. M., Dunstan, D. A., & Bartik, W. (2020). Clinical or gimmickal: The use and effectiveness of mobile mental health apps for treating anxiety and depression. *Australian & New Zealand Journal of Psychiatry, 54*(1), 20–28. https://doi.org/10.1177/0004867419876700

Mathieu, S., Treloar, A., Hawgood, J., Ross, V., & Kõlves, K. (2022). The role of unemployment, financial hardship, and economic recession on suicidal behaviors and interventions to mitigate their impact: A review. *Frontiers in Public Health, 10,* 907052. https://doi.org/10.3389/fpubh.2022.907052

Maura, J., & Weisman de Mamani, A. (2017). Mental health disparities, treatment engagement, and attrition among racial/ethnic minorities with severe mental illness: A review. *Journal of Clinical Psychology in Medical Settings, 24*(3), 187–210. https://doi.org/10.1007/s10880-017-9510-2

McDaid, D., Hewlett, E., & Park, A.-L. (2017). *Understanding effective approaches to promoting mental health and preventing mental illness* (OECD Health Working Papers 97). Organisation for Economic Co-operation and Development. https://read.oecd-ilibrary.org/social-issues-migration-health/understanding-effective-approaches-to-promoting-mental-health-and-preventing-mental-illness_bc364fb2-en

McGinty, E. E., Barry, C. L., Stone, E. M., Niederdeppe, J., Kennedy-Hendricks, A., Linden, S., & Sherman, S. G. (2018). Public support for safe consumption sites and syringe services programs to combat the opioid epidemic. *Preventive Medicine, 111,* 73–77. https://doi.org/10.1016/j.ypmed.2018.02.026

McGuire, J., Kaiser, C., & Bach-Mortensen, A. M. (2022). A systematic review and meta-analysis of the impact of cash transfers on subjective well-being and mental health in low- and middle-income countries. *Nature Human Behaviour, 6*(3), 3. https://doi.org/10.1038/s41562-021-01252-z

Murphy, T., Krasa, H., Lavigne, G., Frangiosa, T., Palsgrove, A., Stalters, L., Than, K.-S., Birch, K., Ching, K., Shafrin, J., Chou, J., & Baumgardner, J. (2021). *Societal costs of schizophrenia & related disorders.* Schizophrenia & Psychosis Action Alliance. https://sczaction.org/wp-content/uploads/2021/11/571-012_WhitePaper_Report_FINAL_updated_11.09.21.pdf

Nagelhout, G. E., Hummel, K., de Goeij, M. C. M., de Vries, H., Kaner, E., & Lemmens, P. (2017). How economic recessions and unemployment affect illegal drug use: A systematic realist literature review. *International Journal of Drug Policy, 44*, 69–83. https://doi.org/10.1016/j.drugpo.2017.03.013

Osypuk, T. L. (2013). Future research directions for understanding neighborhood contributions to health disparities. *Revue D'epidemiologie Et De Sante Publique, 61*(Suppl 2), S61–S68. https://doi.org/10.1016/j.respe.2013.03.040

Ovalle, D. (2023, September 14). Philadelphia council bans safe-injection sites in most of the city. *Washington Post.* https://www.washingtonpost.com/health/2023/09/14/safe-injection-site-philadelphia-opioids/

Pearlin, L. I., Menaghan, E. G., Lieberman, M. A., & Mullan, J. T. (1981). The stress process. *Journal of Health and Social Behavior, 22*(4), 337. https://doi.org/10.2307/2136676

Pescosolido, B. A., Halpern-Manners, A., Luo, L., & Perry, B. (2021). Trends in public stigma of mental illness in the US, 1996–2018. *JAMA Network Open, 4*(12), e2140202. https://doi.org/10.1001/jamanetworkopen.2021.40202

Pourmotabbed, A., Moradi, S., Babaei, A., Ghavami, A., Mohammadi, H., Jalili, C., Symonds, M. E., & Miraghajani, M. (2020). Food insecurity and mental health: A systematic review and meta-analysis. *Public Health Nutrition, 23*(10), 1778–1790. https://doi.org/10.1017/S136898001900435X

Puzhko, S., Eisenberg, M. J., Filion, K. B., Windle, S. B., Hébert-Losier, A., Gore, G., Paraskevopoulos, E., Martel, M. O., & Kudrina, I. (2022). Effectiveness of interventions for prevention of common infections among opioid users: A systematic review of systematic reviews. *Frontiers in Public Health, 10*, 749033. https://doi.org/10.3389/fpubh.2022.749033

Ritter, A., & Cameron, J. (2006). A review of the efficacy and effectiveness of harm reduction strategies for alcohol, tobacco and illicit drugs. *Drug and Alcohol Review, 25*(6), 611–624. https://doi.org/10.1080/09595230600944529

Rockett, I. R. H., Ali, B., Caine, E. D., Shepard, D. S., Banerjee, A., Nolte, K. B., Connery, H. S., Larkin, G. L., Stack, S., White, F. M. M., Jia, H., Cossman, J. S., Feinberg, J., Stover, A. N., & Miller, T. R. (2023). Escalating costs of self-injury mortality in the 21st century United States: An interstate observational study. *BMC Public Health, 23*(1), 285. https://doi.org/10.1186/s12889-023-15188-8

Roy, R., Raman, K. J., Raj, E. A., & Varambally, S. (2024). Outcomes of psychosocial interventions for homeless individuals with mental illness: A systematic review. *The International Journal of Social Psychiatry, 70*(5), 841–849. https://doi.org/10.1177/00207640231217173

Sacks, J. J., Gonzales, K. R., Bouchery, E. E., Tomedi, L. E., & Brewer, R. D. (2015). 2010 National and state costs of excessive alcohol consumption. *American Journal of Preventive Medicine, 49*(5), e73–e79. https://doi.org/10.1016/j.amepre.2015.05.031

Salk, R. H., Hyde, J. S., & Abramson, L. Y. (2017). Gender differences in depression in representative national samples: Meta-analyses of diagnoses and symptoms. *Psychological Bulletin, 143*(8), 783–822. https://doi.org/10.1037/bul0000102

Sherraden, M., Cheng, L.-C., Ssewamala, F. M., Kim, Y., Loke, V., Zou, L., Chowa, G., Ansong, D., Johnson, L., Lee, Y., Grinstein-Weiss, M., Clancy, M. M., Huang, J., Beverly, S. G., Nam, Y., & Han, C.-K. (2018). International child development accounts. In M. Sherraden, L.-C. Cheng, F. M. Ssewamala, Y. Kim, V. Loke, L. Zou, G. Chowa, D. Ansong, L. Johnson, Y. Lee, M. Grinstein-Weiss, M. M. Clancy, J. Huang, S. G. Beverly, Y. Nam, & C.-K. Han (Eds.), *Encyclopedia of social work.* NASW Press and Oxford University Press. https://doi.org/10.1093/acrefore/9780199975839.013.1261

Sherraden, M., Clancy, M., Nam, Y., Huang, J., Kim, Y., Beverly, S. G., Mason, L. R., Wikoff, N. E., Schreiner, M., & Purnell, J. Q. (2015). Universal accounts at birth: building knowledge to inform policy. *Journal of the Society for Social Work and Research, 6*(4), 541–564. https://doi.org/10.1086/684139

Shirneshan, E. (2013). *Cost of illness study of anxiety disorders for the ambulatory adult population of the United States* [Doctoral dissertation]. University of Tennessee Health Science Center. https://doi.org/10.21007/etd.cghs.2013.0289

Strathdee, S. A., & Vlahov, D. (2001). The effectiveness of needle exchange programs: A review of the science and policy. *AIDScience, 1*(16). http://aidscience.org/articles/aidscience013.asp

Stuart, E. A., McGinty, E. E., Kalb, L., Huskamp, H. A., Busch, S. H., Gibson, T. B., Goldman, H., & Barry, C. L. (2017). Increased service use among children with autism spectrum disorder associated with mental health parity law. *Health Affairs, 36*(2), 337–345. https://doi.org/10.1377/hlthaff.2016.0824

Substance Abuse and Mental Health Services Administration. (2022). *Key substance use and mental health indicators in the United States: Results from the 2021 national survey on drug use and health* (Publication Number PEP22-07-01-005). https://www.samhsa.gov/data/sites/default/files/reports/rpt39443/2021NSDUHFFRRev010323.pdf

Substance Abuse and Mental Health Services Administration. (2024). *Key substance use and mental health indicators in the United States: Results from the 2023 national survey on drug use and health.* https://www.samhsa.gov/data/report/2023-nsduh-annual-national-report

Tost, H., Champagne, F. A., & Meyer-Lindenberg, A. (2015). Environmental influence in the brain, human welfare and mental health. *Nature Neuroscience, 18*(10), 10. https://doi.org/10.1038/nn.4108

U.S. Department of Health and Human Services. (1999). *Mental health: A report of the Surgeon General.* U.S. Department of Health and Human Services, Substance Abuse and Mental Health Services Administration, Center for Mental Health Services, National Institutes of Health, National Institute of Mental Health.

U.S. Department of Health and Human Services. (2001). *Mental health: Culture, race, and ethnicity: A supplement to mental health: A report of the Surgeon General.* Substance Abuse and Mental Health Services Administration, Center for Mental Health Services. http://www.ncbi.nlm.nih.gov/books/NBK44243/

Wallace, R., & Pestaina, K. (2023, June 20). Rise in use of mental health apps raises new policy issues. *KFF.* https://www.kff.org/mental-health/issue-brief/rise-in-use-of-mental-health-apps-raises-new-policy-issues/

Walley, A. Y., Xuan, Z., Hackman, H. H., Quinn, E., Doe-Simkins, M., Sorensen-Alawad, A., Ruiz, S., & Ozonoff, A. (2013). Opioid overdose rates and implementation of overdose education and nasal naloxone distribution in Massachusetts: Interrupted time series analysis. *BMJ, 346*, f174. https://doi.org/10.1136/bmj.f174

Winkelman, T. N. A., & Chang, V. W. (2018). Medicaid expansion, mental health, and access to care among childless adults with and without chronic conditions. *Journal of General Internal Medicine, 33*(3), 376–383. https://doi.org/10.1007/s11606-017-4217-5

World Health Organization. (2021). *WHO menu of cost-effective interventions for mental health.* https://iris.who.int/bitstream/handle/10665/343074/9789240031081-eng.pdf

Wylie, L. (2025, April 7). *Wellness app revenue and usage statistics.* https://www.businessofapps.com/data/wellness-app-market/

20 ECOLOGICAL AND SYSTEMIC APPROACHES TO ADVANCE MENTAL HEALTH EQUITY

BRIAN SMEDLEY

LEARNING OBJECTIVES

After reading this chapter, readers will be able to:

- Identify examples of the structural and political determinants of health associated with mental and behavioral health challenges among Black Americans.
- Discuss why place—of residence, education, and work—is an important determinant of health and mental health.
- Describe how "redlining" is associated with present-day disadvantage for neighborhoods that faced this form of discrimination.
- Provide examples of "people-based" and "place-based" policy strategies to reduce concentrated neighborhood economic disadvantage, and how these strategies may impact residents' mental health.
- Describe how housing mobility programs may reduce neighborhood poverty concentration.

INTRODUCTION

Many U.S. people of color have a higher burden of stress and associated mental and behavioral health challenges relative to White Americans. These inequities were starkly revealed in 2020 with the dual pandemics of COVID-19 and resurgent expressions of racism (e.g., the murder of George Floyd), both of which were associated with sharp increases in mental health symptomatology among people of color. The American Psychological Association's (APA) *Stress in America* survey, conducted in 2020 during the height of the pandemic, brings these inequities into sharp relief. The survey found that two in three Black adults (67%) cited discrimination as a significant source of stress in their lives, compared with 55% of Black adults who cited this in May to June of 2019. More than two in five U.S. adults (45%) said being their race is difficult in today's society, with more than three in four Black adults (78%) agreeing with this statement. Three in five U.S. adults (60%) reported that police violence toward minorities is a significant source of stress in their life; fewer than two in five (36%) said the same when APA first started tracking this data point during the 2016 annual *Stress in America* survey. Black adults are the most likely to report this source of stress (79% vs. 44% Native American, 55% White, 61% Asian, and 72% Hispanic; APA, 2020).

Unlike broader health inequities, however, researchers and policy makers seeking to reduce mental health inequities have been slow to address ecological and systemic factors underlying these inequities. Specifically, although many ecological models of population mental health acknowledge the importance of contextual and neighborhood factors in shaping mental health symptomatology, researchers have rarely conceptualized and tested interventions aimed at improving community conditions for positive mental health. Yet, as has been well established in the literature regarding life expectancy and overall health status, *place* matters for mental health (Williams & Collins, 2001). For Black Americans and other people of color in the United States, however, the places and spaces where people live, work, and play are often not conducive to healthy development. This fact is a result of policies and practices that have served to marginalize and exclude these populations from health-enhancing resources and economic opportunities (Penner et al., 2023).

To address these challenges, we must confront our nation's history of racism, which includes socioeconomic inequities resulting from 200 years of chattel slavery and 100 subsequent years of Jim Crow segregation, neither of which has been remedied. One major mechanism of racial subordination has been the practice—originally, by law, and more recently entrenched by persistent discrimination—of residential, occupational, and school segregation, which shapes exposure to health risks and resources, in addition to socioeconomic opportunity (Rothstein, 2017). Indeed, levels of Black–White residential segregation have declined little since modest initial progress toward desegregation following the 1965 Fair Housing Act (Logan & Stults, 2021). School segregation is similarly holding relatively steady in the 70 years since the U.S. Supreme Court declared public school segregation unconstitutional (Owens et al., 2023). Because of its foundational role in shaping exposure to health and mental health risks, racial and economic segregation are forms of structural racism that must be addressed to promote mental health equity. A combination of investments in places that have been historically and purposefully segregated and economically marginalized, such as those localities formerly "redlined" by the U.S. government, as well as investments to expand housing choice, particularly for those families who could benefit from living in communities with greater economic integration, are needed to correct this structural injustice (Smedley, 2019).

This chapter argues that Black mental health, like overall health, is powerfully shaped by place—of residence, education, and work. Racial segregation of these spaces has been often associated with greater exposure to health risks and access to fewer health-enhancing resources (e.g., healthy food retail environments). But because segregation's origins can be found in U.S. law and policy, and because less formal, "de facto" forms of segregation persist across U.S. society, they must be addressed with robust, race-conscious policy. This chapter offers examples of policy strategies that can begin to address the health challenges associated with racially segregated and economically disinvested places.

RACIAL SEGREGATION AND NEIGHBORHOOD POVERTY CONCENTRATION

Racial segregation in housing is not only the result of racism, it also is a major cause of racial inequalities in almost all facets of Black Americans' lives, including their health and healthcare. One measure of the level of segregation between Black and White people is the dissimilarity index, which is the percentage of people in each of two racial groups in a defined geographic area (e.g., a census tract, city, or region) who would need to move to create complete integration. An index of 100 indicates complete segregation, whereas an index of zero indicates full integration. Although the national Black–White dissimilarity index fell from 59 in 2010 to 55 in 2020, this level of segregation is still in the moderate to high range. Black and White people remain largely segregated, particularly in our largest cities: Milwaukee, Philadelphia, Chicago, Detroit, and Cleveland all have dissimilarity indexes of 74 or higher, indicating that three fourths of Black and White residents of these cities would need to move to create complete integration (Logan & Stults, 2021). This phenomenon is not limited to major cities, however: Most Americans live in neighborhoods where the clear majority of their neighbors are of the same race or ethnicity as them. And by some measures, segregation is worsening: The Roots of Structural Racism Project of the Othering and Belonging Institute found that 54% of metropolitan areas were more segregated in 2020 than in 1990, using a Divergence Index, which accounts for localized trends in racial diversity (Menendian et al., 2021).

Residential segregation in the United States has not always been bad for the health of segregated residents. Historically, ethnic enclaves have served as a source of support, particularly for new arrivals to this country. However, for Black, Latinx, and American Indian people, residential segregation is associated with high levels of neighborhood poverty concentration, which is often exacerbated by purposeful economic marginalization in our recent history (e.g., "redlining," discussed later). This concentration of poverty increases exposure to health risks, such as sources of air, water, and soil pollution, while constraining access to health-enhancing resources, such as access to safe parks and green space (Center for American Progress, 2021).

Of course, not all majority-Black neighborhoods are characterized by high levels of concentrated poverty. Many predominantly Black neighborhoods have wealthy Black residents, and these neighborhoods are well resourced. Nevertheless, the residents of predominantly Black neighborhoods are much more likely to be poor than residents of predominantly White neighborhoods. Poor Black Americans are 3 times more likely than poor White Americans to live in neighborhoods where the poverty level is characterized by demographers as "extreme" (i.e., where 40% or more of residents live below poverty). And a large percentage of middle- and upper-income Black Americans also live in low-income, racially segregated neighborhoods. Middle-class Black families are much more likely to live in high-poverty areas than are *low-income* White families (Logan & Stults, 2021). Even relatively affluent Black families (with incomes of more than $75,000) are more than twice as likely as relatively affluent White families to live in high-poverty neighborhoods. For example, in Detroit and Cleveland, over 25% of affluent Black families live in high-poverty, predominantly Black neighborhoods (Logan, 2011). Some of these higher income Black families may have chosen to live in neighborhoods with people who are racially similar to them. But the realities of pervasive racism and de facto housing segregation that still exist in the United States limit many Black families' choices of where they might live and be accepted by their neighbors much more than White families with comparable incomes.

A Brief History of U.S. Segregation

A powerful myth in the United States is that racial segregation arises from the unintended consequences of economic forces—Black people, on average, have lower incomes and less wealth than White Americans (in itself the consequence of persistent racial discrimination and segregation) and therefore are more likely to live in poor neighborhoods. This is at once obvious and evident, but as noted earlier, poor White Americans are much *less* likely to live in high-poverty neighborhoods than similarly poor—or even more economically advantaged—Black Americans. The reality is that our current housing patterns are powerfully shaped by our history.

From roughly the end of the Reconstruction era to the mid-1960s, federal, state, and local governments systematically imposed residential segregation with policies and practices such as racial zoning, including the use of racial and religious covenants to prevent homeowners from selling properties to minoritized groups. Many local governments sought to cite federally subsidized (and federally approved) public housing in ways that purposefully segregated communities, particularly by concentrating public housing in already low-income communities. These governments also approved subsidies for builders to create Whites-only suburbs, and tax exemptions for racially discriminatory organizations, under the assumption that racial exclusion protected investors. As pernicious, but less widely acknowledged, was their complicity in violent resistance to African Americans in White neighborhoods by dampening law enforcement responses (Rothstein, 2017).

At the federal level, government compounded the economic isolation of segregation by creating a policy of disinvestment now known as redlining. Beginning in the 1930s, the former federal Home Ownership Loan Corporation (HOLC) was tasked with financially backing the then relatively nascent home mortgage loan industry. They assigned levels of risk for mortgage default to various neighborhoods in cities around the country, but the risk assigned was based solely on the demographic composition of the neighborhoods. Black neighborhoods were routinely assigned a risk level of "red" (which was the color used on HOLC maps); yellow indicated less risk (and fewer non-White persons), followed by blue and green, the lowest risk ratings. These risk assignments not only determined who received a federally backed home loan, but they also signaled to other investors and businesses which communities were considered economically viable—further dampening investment (Rothstein, 2017).

Although these risk assignments were made more than 80 years ago, they have had lasting impacts. The National Community Reinvestment Coalition (NCRC) in their report, *The Persistent Structure of Segregation and Economic Inequality,* found that three of four neighborhoods redlined on HOLC maps 80 years ago continue to struggle economically. Nationally, nearly two thirds of neighborhoods deemed "hazardous" in the 1930s continue to be inhabited by mostly racial and ethnic minority residents. Cities with more of these neighborhoods have significantly greater economic inequality. Conversely, 91% of areas classified as "best" in the 1930s remain middle to upper income today, and 85% of them are still predominantly White (NCRC, 2018). Their effect has been to advantage White families in access to property and wealth while maintaining stable, intergenerational places of disadvantage for Black families.

Readers interested in a more in-depth history of racial residential segregation and its relationship to high Black infant mortality rates should read Barnett et al. (2024), "A History of the Impacts of Discriminatory Policies on Housing and Maternal and Infant Health in an Ohio Neighborhood," which documents the history of de jure segregation and economic disinvestment in Linden, a predominantly Black neighborhood in Columbus, Ohio. Like many predominantly Black neighborhoods around the country, Linden faces a high concentration of health risks resulting from state and local policies that excluded and isolated Linden's residents from the opportunities for good health and economic well-being (Barnett et al., 2024).

Neighborhoods and Health

Although the research cited here helps to explain the systemic disadvantages Black Americans and other people of color face from persistent segregation, it does little to explain the mechanisms through which neighborhoods shape health. Several studies have found an association between aspects of a neighborhood's quality (e.g., poverty concentration) and the physical and mental health of its residents. Aspects of the built environment, such as housing quality and density, are among the factors that shape mental health that are typically worse in segregated, predominantly Black neighborhoods (Pearson et al., 2023). Similarly, the retail food environment—including the cost, quality, and nutritious value of what is for sale, and by what kinds of vendors—is typically less healthy in these neighborhoods (Hirsch et al., 2023). Black neighborhoods are more often exposed to sources of air, water, and soil pollution than predominantly White neighborhoods (Tessum et al., 2021). To compound these challenges, predominantly Black neighborhoods experience suppressed property values, which, combined with business disinvestment from inner-city neighborhoods, generate far less local tax revenue than White neighborhoods (Penner et al., 2023). This, in turn, sharply affects the quality of local services and schools. And although local governments have policy levers such as zoning and land use regulations that could be used to promote economic integration, in an increasing number of states, local jurisdictions are being prohibited from taking such actions by state governments (Arcaya et al., 2024).

WHAT IS NEEDED

To address the structural and ecological factors associated with segregation and mental health, we need comprehensive interventions applied across levels, which can produce "synergistic" effects (Boyd et al., 2023). Such an approach is needed because structural inequities "are produced and maintained by complex interactions" (Boyd et al., 2023) among social, economic, and political determinants of heath, all of which are ultimately shaped by the United States' history of Indigenous genocide, chattel slavery, and Jim Crow segregation. In this section, we explore the need for both people- and place-based strategies to be applied simultaneously to reduce risks associated with concentrated neighborhood poverty.

People-Based Strategies: Expanding Housing Choice

A considerable source of stress for low-income families is housing—particularly issues related to location, quality, and affordability. Research has identified several ecological and structural factors that shape mental health, including many risks concentrated in high-poverty neighborhoods. These include issues such as stress from housing costs; the vicarious impacts of police violence against community members; violence in schools, homes, and the community; and the physical infrastructure of neighborhoods, all of which are implicated in mental health symptomatology (Arcaya et al., 2024). Several studies have examined whether housing-related interventions can ameliorate these conditions.

Housing affordability remains a significant source of stress for many low-income families. Nearly 90% of poor households pay more than 30% of their monthly income for housing, and 75% have a housing cost burden of about half of family income (Newman et al., 2024). The federal Housing Choice Voucher program was intended to address these challenges, but despite annual costs of $25 billion, the program currently serves only 25% of eligible households, including 1.3 million families and 2.2 million children in 2019 (Government Accountability Office, 2024). Demand for portable rent vouchers far exceeds supply—a deficit that Congress must correct, as noted later—but this imbalance creates opportunities for researchers to study the effects of family relocation for health and well-being.

In one of the first large-scale studies of the potential of portable housing vouchers to help expand housing options for low-income families, the U.S. Department of Housing and Urban Development funded the Moving to Opportunity (MTO) experiment, which randomly selected low-income families living in public housing in some of the country's most disadvantaged neighborhoods to experimental and control conditions. (Such random assignment was possible only because of the large number of families on waiting lists to receive vouchers.) In the experimental condition, families received rent vouchers that enabled them to move into private housing in less distressed, lower poverty neighborhoods. Ten to 15 years later, they were compared with families who were given rent vouchers for public housing in the same neighborhoods where they currently lived, as well as to families who received no vouchers at all. On follow-up, the adults in families that moved showed improvements in their health, such as lower diabetes rates and improved mental health. Female children in the experimental group showed improvement in their mental health, but older boys did not. However, if the children were relatively young when their family was able to move, there were economic and educational benefits for them as adults. Their incomes as adults were 31% higher than children in the other groups, and they were also more likely to attend college. However, this was not true for the adults or children who were older when they moved. Overall, this study suggested that the longer a person lives in a disadvantaged neighborhood, the harder it is to reverse its impact on their lives. This is because the poverty in many segregated Black neighborhoods combines with other aspects of these neighborhoods to create enduring threats to their residents' health (Chetty et al., 2016).

Additional evidence of the health and mental health benefits of expanded housing choice and security is provided by the Housing and Children's Healthy Development study. This research, conducted in the Cleveland, Ohio, and Dallas, Texas, metropolitan areas, is a randomized controlled trial to examine the impact of portable housing vouchers on low-income Black parents' and children's health and mental health. To date, this study has completed two waves of data collection involving families randomly assigned to an experimental or control condition. As with the MTO study, families in the experimental condition received portable housing vouchers to support rental housing costs, whereas those in the control condition received no housing assistance. This randomization was possible because of the large number of families on waiting lists to receive housing vouchers. In the first wave of the study, 895 primary caregivers and more than 1,200 children aged 3 to 10 participated in the study (Newman et al., 2024).

On follow-up, study investigators measured four indicators of family stress: mothers' self-reports of hypertension in the past year (as a physiological marker of stress), self-reported parental stress, mothers' mental health symptoms, and self-reported parent–child conflict and discipline problems in the past year. Investigators also measured housing affordability, housing conditions, and neighborhood conditions at follow-up. Results indicated that the families receiving housing vouchers experienced a 40% reduction in housing cost burdens and showed a 42% decrease in the share of families reporting insufficient space. Only 2% of families in the experimental condition reported feeling unsafe in their neighborhood in the daytime, compared with 10% of the control families, although there was no significant difference in census tract–level poverty between control and experimental group families. Importantly, parents in voucher families reported a 50% reduction in hypertension and 7% reduction in parent stress (although there was no difference between experimental and control families in family stress indicators or parent–child conflict). The investigators noted that although housing vouchers were significantly associated with improved housing affordability, quality, and neighborhood safety, it is possible that mothers' mental health and parent–children conflict were adversely affected by the COVID-19 pandemic, which coincided with the study period (Newman et al., 2024).

A comprehensive approach to advancing mental health equity should innovate and expand "people-based" investments that consider the needs of people across the life cycle. A strong start, of course, is well before birth, for example, by ensuring that girls and women of color have access to needed health and reproductive health services before conception. A universal health plan such as Medicare-for-All would provide the kind of equitable healthcare coverage to do this. Recognizing that its arrival date is unknown, Congress should continue to expand the state–federal Child Health Insurance Program, Medicaid, and other health and social supports for mothers and mothers-to-be (Penner et al., 2023).

For Black mothers who face social or economic challenges during their babies' early months, programs such as Nurse Home Visitation have been established as cost-effective interventions because they help foster healthy development and mitigate health risks. In addition, longitudinal studies point to the effectiveness of high-quality, early childhood (particularly ages 0–3) education in inoculating children in low-resource neighborhoods from some of the risks they may face. The studies suggest that the early educational and social gains these children acquire carry into adulthood, in the form of higher educational attainment, better job histories, and less involvement in criminal justice systems, among other positive outcomes. These studies used a high-quality curriculum and instruction from experienced teachers, something to which today's Head Start programs have less access. Funding for Nurse Home Visitation and Head Start should be increased to improve these programs' quality and reach. The rationale for these investments should be made clear to all Americans: this is part of what we owe to people who have faced systematic health assaults since their arrival on these shores (Penner et al., 2023).

Other people-based investments should include expanding housing choice—or specifically, the ability to choose a healthier, lower poverty neighborhood. Cited earlier, the federal MTO study provided promising evidence regarding the benefits of helping families move from high- to low-poverty neighborhoods; those that did saw improved economic and health outcomes. Housing mobility can be expanded with existing federal housing programs. Public health departments could work with Section 8 voucher holders, for example, to move children with asthma and their families from triggering homes and neighborhoods with poor air quality to neighborhoods that have fewer of these risks. Section 8 voucher holders also should be provided with the resources and support to stay in their neighborhood if they are at risk of displacement because of rising rents in communities that are experiencing economic revival.

At the federal level, leadership is needed to correct the historical wrong of the U.S. government's role in the segregation and economic marginalization of Black people. Any effort to begin to voluntarily desegregate our communities will be an important start toward that remedy. To date, however, the federal government's efforts have been incomplete and fleeting. In 2015, the Obama administration established a new rule, "Affirmatively Furthering Fair Housing," that would incentivize jurisdictions around the country to work with community and civic leaders to assess patterns of segregation in their community and develop and implement plans to address it. This rule was suspended by the subsequent administration (Penner et al., 2023).

Other strategies to expand access to affordable housing in racially and economically integrated neighborhoods include set-asides for affordable housing units in new developments, banning zoning ordinances that prohibit multifamily housing or that require all single-family homes, and promoting inclusionary zoning policies that permit developers to build multifamily units only if a share is set aside for low- and moderate-income families. Montgomery County, Maryland, for example, has an inclusionary zoning ordinance that requires developers to reserve 12% to 15% of units for moderate-income families, but goes further to purchase a third of the subsidized units for rental to low-income families. For readers interested in other creative approaches to law and policies that promote integration, Richard Rothstein's *The Color of Law* offers an array of ideas in the "Considering Fixes" chapter (Rothstein, 2017).

Place-Based Investments and Economic Stimulus

Communities around the country are experimenting with polices to stimulate investment and attract health-enhancing resources while regulating the concentration of health risks. To improve access to healthy food retail, the Obama administration launched the Fresh Food Financing Initiative, which provides financing to developers and grocers to attract grocery stores in food deserts. Modeled after a similar initiative in Pennsylvania, Fresh Food Financing Initiatives typically offer tax advantages and ease land-use restrictions to help attract grocers. In so doing, it offers a "win–win–win": not only do residents have more access to better nutritional options, they also benefit from jobs the stores create, whereas grocers stand to expand in new markets and return profits (Penner et al., 2023).

Other place-based investments that could improve health in high-poverty communities of color include infrastructure improvements to the built environment. Among the most urgent is public transit, particularly to connect disinvested communities to centers of economic activity and jobs. Infrastructure investments should also address the deficit Black communities face in opportunities for physical activity and connections to nature (e.g., improving geographic access to parks, recreational facilities, and spaces for walking and biking; Center for American Progress, 2021). Similarly, we need to ensure that all children, particularly those living in high-poverty communities, have access to high-speed internet. A study by the Joint Center for Political and Economic Studies found that Black children in the rural South are nearly twice as likely to lack access as White children, which leaves them digitally behind their peers (Harrison, 2021). However, infrastructure investments cannot be limited to digital access—Black children are still disproportionately at risk for exposure to lead, allergens, and other risks in their homes, which needs to be corrected through expansion of programs such as the U.S. Department of Housing and Urban Development's Healthy Homes Program, which provides grants and demonstration projects to comprehensively remediate health risks (U.S. Department of Housing and Urban Development, n.d.).

Other place-based investments, such as those improving infrastructure and housing, can be helpful to remedy the effects of neighborhood economic marginalization. Observing that land use and features of the built environment are associated with neighborhood characteristics such as crime rates, a study in Philadelphia asked whether structural repairs to homes of low-income owners would be associated with reduced crime in Black urban neighborhoods. A city initiative provided grants of up to $20,000 to low-income owners for structural repairs to electrical, plumbing, heating, and roofing damage. In blocks where these grants were offered, crime was more than 20% lower than in comparable blocks where grants were not offered, suggesting that scalable and sustainable place-based interventions in neighborhoods suffering from disinvestment can be part of a broader strategy toward repair (South et al., 2021).

SUMMARY

Black Americans have been exposed to an array of mental and behavioral health risks as a result of the nation's history of segregation—a structural form of racism that, operating over time and in partnership with racism operating at institutional, interpersonal, and intrapersonal levels, produces health and mental health inequities. This chapter argues that Black mental health, like overall health, is powerfully shaped by place—of residence, education, and work. Racial segregation of these spaces often has been associated with greater exposure to health risks and fewer health-enhancing resources. However, because segregation's origins can be found in U.S. law and policy, and because less formal, de facto forms of segregation persist across U.S. society, they must be addressed with robust, race-conscious policies.

A combination of investments in places and people is needed. The federal government should lead efforts to invest in places that have been historically and purposefully segregated and economically marginalized, such as localities formerly redlined by the U.S. government. Several people-based investments also offer clear, long-term benefits, as research clearly indicates. These include proven strategies such as nurse home visitation services for vulnerable mothers and infants. Other people-based investments are newer strategies that researchers should continue to study for their mental and behavioral health benefits. These include investments to expand housing choice, particularly for families who could benefit from living in communities with greater economic integration.

DISCUSSION QUESTIONS

1. Why is it important to consider implementing place- and people-based equity strategies simultaneously?
2. What opportunities do you envision for business sector leaders to engage in people- or place-based health equity work?

3. This chapter primarily addresses Black–White segregation. What are the issues facing other minoritized groups with respect to segregation? How does segregation shape mental health in these communities?
4. What are some potential challenges associated with moving families from high- to low-poverty neighborhoods, both for the families and their new communities?
5. What are some examples of people-based strategies that may advance mental health equity?

REFERENCES

American Psychological Association. (2000). *Stress in America: A national mental health crisis*. https://www.apa.org/news/press/releases/stress/2020/report-october

Arcaya, M. C., Ellen, I. G., & Steil, J. (2024). Neighborhoods and health: Interventions at the neighborhood level could help advance health equity. *Health Affairs*, *43*(2), 156–163. https://doi.org/10.1377/hlthaff.2023.01037

Barnett, K. S., Reece, J., Mosley, B. M., Baek, M., Hyder, A., Kelleher, K., Sealy-Jefferson, S., & Chisolm, D. J. (2024). A history of the impacts of discriminatory policies on housing and maternal and infant health in an Ohio neighborhood. *Health Affairs*, *43*(2), 181–189. https://doi.org/10.1377/hlthaff.2023.01045

Boyd, R. C., Castro, F. G., Finigan-Carr, N., Okamoto, S. K., Barlow, A., Elizabeth Kim, B.-K., Lambert, S., Lloyd, J., Zhang, X., Barksdale, C. L., Crowley, D. M., Maldonado-Molina, M., Obasi, E. M., & Kenney, A. (2023). Strategic directions in preventive intervention research to advance health equity. *Prevention Science*, *24*(4), 577–596. https://doi.org/10.1007/s11121-022-01462-5

Center for American Progress. (2021). *The nature gap: Confronting racial and economic disparities in the destruction and protection of nature in America*. https://www.americanprogress.org/article/the-nature-gap/

Chetty, R., Hendren, N., & Katz, L. F. (2016). The effects of exposure to better neighborhoods on children: New evidence from the Moving to Opportunity experiment. *American Economic Review*, *106*(4), 855–902. https://doi.org/10.1257/aer.20150572

Government Accountability Office. (2020). *Rental housing: As more households rent, the poorest face affordability and housing quality challenges*. GAO. https://www.gao.gov/products/gao-20-427

Harrison, D. (2021). *Affordability & availability: Expanding broadband in the Black rural South*. Joint Center for Political & Economic Studies. https://jointcenter.org/affordability-availability-expanding-broadband-in-the-black-rural-south/

Hirsch, J. A., Zhao, Y., Melly, S., Moore, K. A., Berger, N., Quinn, J., Rundle, A., & Lovasi, G. S. (2023). National trends and disparities in retail food environments in the USA between 1990 and 2014. *Public Health Nutrition*, *26*(5), 1052–1062. https://doi.org/10.1017/S1368980023000058

Logan, R. (2011). *Separate and unequal: The neighborhood gap for Blacks, Hispanics, and Asians in metropolitan America*. https://www.russellsage.org/sites/all/files/US2010/US2010_Logan_20110727.pdf

Logan, J. R., & Stults, B. (2021). *The persistence of segregation in the metropolis: New findings from the 2020 census*. Diversity and Disparities Project. Brown University. https://s4.ad.brown.edu/Projects/Diversity

Menendian, S., Gambhir, S., & Hsu, C.-W. (2021). *Roots of structural racism: The 2020 census update*. https://belonging.berkeley.edu/roots-structural-racism-2020

National Community Reinvestment Coalition. (2018). *HOLC "redlining" maps: The persistent structure of segregation and economic inequality*. https://ncrc.org/holc/

Newman, S., Leventhal, T., Holupka, C. S., & Tan, F. (2024). Experimental evidence shows that housing vouchers provided measurable benefits, including parent stress reduction. *Health Affairs*, *43*(2), 278–286. https://doi.org/10.1377/hlthaff.2023.01020

Owens, A., Reardon, S. F., Kalogrides, D., Jang, H., & Tom, T. (2022). *Trends in racial/ethnic and economic school segregation, 1991–2020*. The Segregation Index Research Brief. https://segindex.org/wp-content/uploads/2023/06/Trends-in-Racial-Ethnic-Segregation_Rnd6.pdf

Pearson, A. L., Zhou, Y., Buxton, R. T., Horton, T. H., Pfeiffer, K. A., & Beyer, K. M. M. (2023). The effects of contemporary redlining on the mental health of Black residents. *SSM Population Health*, *23*, 101462. https://doi.org/10.1016/j.ssmph.2023.101462

Penner, L. A., Dovidio, J. F., Hagiwara, N., & Smedley, B. D. (2023). *Unequal health: Anti-Black racism and the threat to America's health*. Cambridge University Press.

Rothstein, R. (2017). *The color of law: A forgotten history of how our government segregated America*. Norton.

Smedley, B. D. (2019). Toward a comprehensive understanding of racism and health inequities: A multilevel approach. In C. L. Ford, D. M. Griffith, M. A. Bruce, & K. L. Gilbert (Eds.), *Racism: Science & tools for the public health professional*. APHA Press. https://doi.org/10.2105/9780875533049ch24

South, E. C., MacDonald, J., & Reina, V. (2021). Association between structural housing repairs for low-income homeowners and neighborhood crime. *JAMA Network Open*, 4(7), e2117067. https://doi.org/10.1001/jamanetworkopen.2021.17067

Tessum, C. W., Paolella, D. A., Chambliss, S. E., Apte, J. S., Hill, J. D., & Marshall, J. D. (2021). PM2. 5 polluters disproportionately and systemically affect people of color in the United States. *Science Advances*, *7*(18), eabf4491. https://doi.org/10.1126/sciadv.abf4491

U.S. Department of Housing and Urban Development. (n.d.). *The Healthy Homes program*. https://www.hud.gov/program_offices/healthy_homes/hhi

Williams, D. R., & Collins, C. (2001). Racial residential segregation: A fundamental cause of racial disparities in health. *Public Health Reports*, *116*(5), 404–416. https://doi.org/10.1093/phr/116.5.404

21 PUBLIC MENTAL HEALTH RESEARCH CONSIDERATIONS

OCTAVIO N. MARTINEZ, JR.

LEARNING OBJECTIVES

After reading this chapter, readers will be able to:

- Define health research and describe what it entails.
- Explain the lack of diversity in clinical trials and why it is an equity issue.
- Identify at least five major barriers to inclusion and participation in clinical trials.
- Define community-engaged research.
- Explain how to achieve mental health equity in research.

INTRODUCTION

Medical research—or health research—involves the use of scientific methods to expand knowledge about diseases and conditions that affect individuals, including how to prevent, diagnose, and treat them. Medical research includes basic science research, also known as fundamental or bench research, which seeks to uncover the underlying mechanisms of diseases and their biological, chemical, or physical processes. It encompasses clinical research, which involves direct interaction with and participation of human beings to assess the safety and efficacy of medications, diagnostic and screening products, medical devices, and treatment regimens to prevent, screen, and diagnose diseases and conditions and improve the health of individuals. Medical research also includes translational research, which bridges the gap between basic research and clinical research, and of which there are two types:

- Type 1 translational research, which refers to the conversion of knowledge from basic science research into a potential clinic product for testing.
- Type 2 translational research, which typically involves a 17-year process, involves converting promising interventions in clinical research for use in clinical practice (Morris et al., 2011).

There also are two main types of clinical research: observational studies and interventional studies, the latter of which are commonly referred to as clinical trial research (see **Figure 21.1**). Observational studies involve collecting new data from study participants or analyzing existing data without the introduction of an intervention. Interventional studies—or clinical trial research—involves actively administering treatments or interventions, or implementing novel strategies to evaluate their safety and efficacy on study participants (National Library of Medicine, n.d.).

Clinical trials are a driving force in medical innovations, including those that occur in the mental health space (Martell, 2024). The gold standard in clinical trials is the explanatory randomized controlled trial (RCT), which is designed to optimize the internal validity of the study by reducing variance and removing the potential for confounding (i.e., when

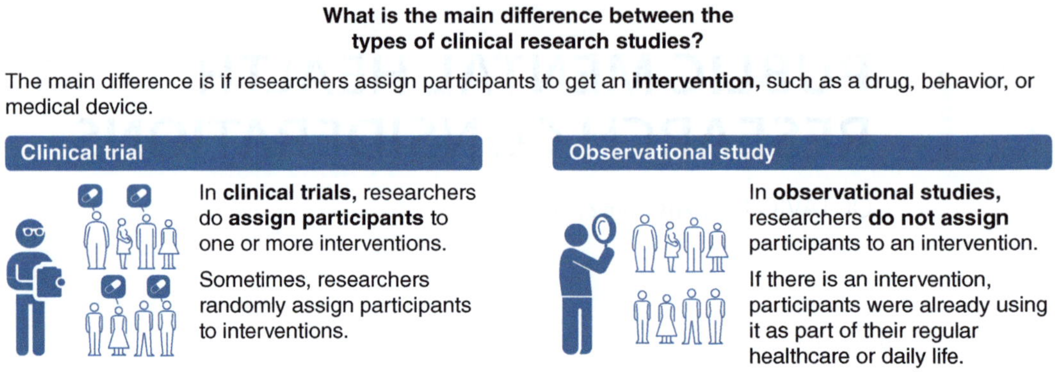

Figure 21.1 Difference between clinical trial and observational study.

a third factor warps the relationship between the intervention being investigated and the outcomes observed). Maximizing the internal validity allows an explanatory RCT to methodically investigate and accurately assess the association between the exposure to a given intervention or treatment and the observed outcome. An RCT is conducted under rigorously controlled conditions that strictly adhere to structured protocols to determine the efficacy of an intervention. This process includes restrictive inclusion and exclusion criteria and randomization of study participants, both of which can directly and negatively affect the rates of participation in clinical trials and other medical research, which can limit the generalizability of research findings.

Efficacy of a treatment or intervention in a clinical research setting does not always translate in "real-world" healthcare settings. Therein lies one of the major challenges associated with explanatory RCT: generalizability (or external validity) of research findings (Kennedy-Martin et al., 2015). To surmount this challenge, the pragmatic RCT—which is a type of RCT that uses a different design than an explanatory RCT—minimizes exclusion criteria by conducting the study in real-world healthcare settings, instead of in clinical research settings, to evaluate the effects of an intervention under normative conditions (National Academies of Science, Engineering, and Medicine [NASEM], 2016).

THE UNDERREPRESENTATION OF MINORITIZED INDIVIDUALS IN CLINICAL TRIAL PARTICIPATION

According to the latest U.S. census, racial and ethnic minorities comprise 30% to 40% of the total U.S. population, with Latinx accounting for 19%, African Americans for 14%, and Asian Americans for 6%; a smaller percentage—roughly 2%—are Indigenous Americans. Despite the growing racial and ethnic diversity in the nation, there is a dearth of racial and ethnic minorities who participate in clinical trials. In fact, according to a recent study of 32,000 individuals who participated in a U.S. clinical trial for a new drug in 2020, 11% of the participants were Latinx, 8% were Black, and 6% were Asian American (Kelsey et al., 2022). Further, the clinical trial inclusion of other racial and ethnic minority individuals—Native Hawaiians, Pacific Islanders, Alaska Natives, and Indigenous individuals—often is negligible (Ruiz-White et al., 2023; Zuckerman & Edwards, 2024).

The disproportionate underrepresentation of minoritized individuals is both persistent and stark, and may result in dangerous ramifications for public health, including mental health. When clinical trials include only small samples from racial, ethnic, and other demographic groups, the study results may not be generalizable to the larger U.S. population.

Consequently, this could lead to treatments and regimens that are put on the market yet may be less effective and safe (and possibly even dangerous) to some population groups (Heller et al., 2014).

There are several barriers to expanding racial and ethnic diversity and greater inclusion of other minoritized individuals in clinical trial research, many of which are deeply embedded in the clinical trial system. These barriers exist at multiple levels throughout any given clinical trial protocol and throughout its policies and practices. They exist at the individual/participant level, at the community level, in the design and implementation of any given clinical research trial, in the institutions and entities conducting and analyzing the research, and at the policy level that funds and governs the research. Despite this, however, clinical trial researchers and policy makers often focus solely on characteristics at the individual and community levels—specifically, the willingness to participate and issues around distrust—as the reasons behind the lack of greater inclusion of racial and ethnic minorities and other minoritized individuals in clinical trial research. Further, they seldom consider the role that other barriers play in the persistent and systemic underrepresentation of minoritized individuals and communities in clinical research trials.

It is common for clinical trial researchers and stakeholders to claim that a lack of willingness to participate is to blame for the stark underrepresentation of racial and ethnic minorities and other minoritized individuals. However, there is an overwhelming body of literature that directly contradicts this assertion (Hillyer et al., 2020). In fact, there is ample evidence that racial and ethnic minorities are as likely as Whites to be willing to participate (Byrd et al., 2011; Gadegbeku et al., 2008; Kaplan et al., 2015). Studies have also found that some racial and ethnic minority individuals are more willing than Whites to participate (Guadagnolo et al., 2009). Lastly, and perhaps more important, these studies collectively have found that the issue is not about willingness; it is about being asked, which studies confirm occurs more often for some individuals (nonminoritized) than for others (minoritized).

It is true that racial and ethnic minorities are significantly more likely than Whites to have and express issues of mistrust and distrust with the U.S. healthcare system and with those who work in it. Studies confirm that some of these trust issues have deep historical roots embedded in the structural and systemic racism and discrimination that have impacted and continue to detrimentally affect all aspects of our society, including medical research (Alvidrez & Barksdale, 2022; Collins et al., 2021). There is a long and indisputable history of unethical medical research studies conducted on racial and ethnic minorities and other minoritized individuals in the United States. In fact, these unethical practices, in the name of advancing medical research and improving human health and well-being, began long before the Tuskegee syphilis study and the medical research conducted on Henrietta Lacks, and can actually be traced back to the 1840s (Alsan & Eichmeyer, 2021; Byrd et al., 2011; Ojanuga, 1993; Skloot, 2010). During this time, James Marion Sims—a White doctor in Montgomery, Alabama, who was lauded as the "Father of Gynecology" after his death—performed numerous experiments, without anesthesia, informed consent, or basic regard for the humanity and personhood of his victims, who were enslaved Black women. Other medical experiments performed on slaves in the United States in the mid-1800s included electric shock therapy and brain surgery. (See **Table 21.1** for a list of examples of unethical medical studies and interventions conducted in the 20th century.)

The trauma caused by the awareness of these early, unethical medical experiments has proven to be transgenerational and likely has a profound impact on racial and ethnic disparities in trust in medical research that are expressed today. In fact, a 2022 Pew Research Center survey found that more than three in four African Americans (78%) "have heard" that medical researchers experimented on Black people without their knowledge or consent. This same study found that more than half of Black survey participants (55%) believe that this practice still happens today (Pew Research Center, 2024).

Table 21.1 EXAMPLES OF 20th CENTURY UNETHICAL MEDICAL STUDIES AND INTERVENTIONS

YEARS	STUDIES AND INTERVENTIONS
1932 to 1972	U.S. Public Health Service's Tuskegee syphilis study conducted on a group of nearly 400 Black men with syphilis. The purpose of the study was to observe the effects of the disease when left untreated. The men were not informed of the purpose of the experiment and were deprived appropriate treatment once discovered, i.e., penicillin.
1940s	U.S. military secretly exposed Black, Japanese American, and Puerto Rican soldiers to mustard gas to determine difference in susceptibility to the gas compared with White soldiers.
1951	Henrietta Lacks's cervical tissue cells cultured without her knowledge or consent at Johns Hopkins Hospital in Baltimore, Maryland. Her cancer cells became the source of the HeLa cell line, the first immortalized human cell line and one of the most valuable cell lines in medical research.
1956	Willowbrook hepatitis study: children were deliberately infected with mild form of hepatitis, and consent was obtained from parents without informing them about the hazards.
1963	Jewish Chronic Disease Hospital Study: cancer cells were inoculated into patients with cognitive decline without proper explanation about the risk.
1930s to 1970s	Nearly one third of childbearing women in Puerto Rico were coerced into sterilization to supposedly improve Puerto Rico's economy by reducing the population.
1960s	Sterilization of Black women in North Carolina made up 65% of all sterilizations of women, although Black women were only 25% of the population.
1960s to 1970s	U.S. Indian Health Service sterilized nearly 25% of Native American women without consent.

Other roots of distrust of medical research are based in concerns over more current and nuanced issues. These include apprehensions about the use of the health and medical information that is collected, the perceived increased risk of losing federal and other public assistance, and the impact that participation in a clinical trial may have on immigration status (Lor & Bowers, 2018; Occa et al., 2018). Current experiences that a minoritized individual has had while accessing care and treatment in the current healthcare system also have been observed as a source of distrust and mistrust in participating in medical research or a clinical trial (Corbie-Smith et al., 2002; Griffith et al., 2021). For example, research confirms that although racial and ethnic minorities may express support for medical and clinical trial research overall, their experiences with and perceptions of implicit and explicit racism in the healthcare system deter them from participating (Scharff et al., 2010).

Despite this body of literature, there is a growing body of evidence that distrust and mistrust are not always the explanation for an unwillingness to participate in clinical trial research (Ford et al., 2008; Garber et al., 2007; Webb et al., 2019; Westergaard et al., 2014). One macro-systematic review of research focusing on the perceived and real barriers to expanding diversity in clinical trials found that although trust issues are a factor, the most common barrier to the inclusion of racial and ethnic minorities in clinical trial research is the systemic and persistent absence of them being asked or given the opportunity to participate in the first place (Ford et al., 2008). Numerous studies confirm that this is driven, in large part, by implicit and explicit racial and other biases that are prevalent in and throughout the medical research realm (Adeyemi et al., 2009; Braunstein et al., 2008; Evans et al, 2010; George et al., 2014).

As included in **Box 21.1**, there are other barriers that dissuade racial and ethnic minorities from participating in clinical trial research. For example, several recent studies have

Box 21.1 BARRIERS TO DIVERSITY AND INCLUSION IN CLINICAL TRIALS

- Lack of diversity of healthcare providers and researchers
- Implicit bias of healthcare providers and researchers
- Lack of cultural humility by healthcare providers and researchers
- Lack of community engagement skills by researchers
- Poor communication skills by healthcare providers and researchers
- Trial design inaccessibility
- Physical inaccessibility of clinical trials
- Financial inaccessibility of clinical trials
- Populations of color poorly informed about clinical trials
- Community and individual mistrust of research, medical institutions, and the healthcare system

found that socioeconomic factors, such as financial inaccessibility of clinical trials, drive decision-making about clinical trial participation (Indorewalla et al., 2021). These barriers are rooted in the fact that racial and ethnic minorities and other minoritized individuals are disproportionately more likely to live at or below the federal poverty level (KFF, 2013). Thus, they are more likely to hold jobs with no or limited vacation days, earned time off, and sick days, leaving little to no time to participate in a clinical trial study. Further, minoritized individuals who have limited economic resources tend to carry heavier burdens associated with childcare and/or with providing care to an elderly or disabled family member (Indorewalla et al., 2021). In addition to contending with greater socioeconomic and financial burdens, minoritized individuals living with a mental health disorder or disease experience a disproportionately higher mental health burden, leading to physical and mental inaccessibility of clinical trials.

These dynamics—although not a reflection of an individual's willingness to participate in a clinical trial—directly affect a person's decision-making about their participation in a medical research project, as well as their ability to complete the study. In fact, a systemic review of the barriers and challenges associated with clinical trial recruitment and retention found that among racial and ethnic minorities, especially those from economically disadvantaged backgrounds, the most reported factor thwarting participation in medical research studies was competing priorities (Bonevski et al., 2014).

A great deal of blame is assigned to individual- and community-level factors and characteristics to explain (and sometimes try to justify) the exclusion of racial and ethnic minorities and other minoritized individuals from clinical trials. However, far too little emphasis has been assigned to the impact of the medical research study design on recruitment and participation. In fact, one study found that such considerations of a clinical study design (i.e., its purpose, how it is designed and funded, and who is involved at every level of the design protocol) often occur long after the study has commenced (Ford et al., 2008). This strongly suggests that understanding the causes of and designing and implementing solutions to the underrepresentation of racial and ethnic minorities and other minoritized individuals in clinical trial research should begin with reforming many of the common practices used in the clinical trial research project process. This includes cultural competence and racial sensitivity training across the entire research team and integrated into the entire participant recruitment, selection, and retention processes; strong considerations about where the research site will be located to alleviate travel-related burdens; stringent and consistently enforced ethical standards embedded into the research protocol through its entirety; and how the actual questions and information are developed and communicated (e.g., use of multilingual options and awareness of health literacy levels; Ford et al., 2008).

Minoritized individuals are woefully underrepresented in the healthcare provider and medical research workforce, which is problematic because providers and medical researchers have a direct impact on the rates of participation of minoritized individuals in clinical trial research. For many who enroll in a clinical trial, it begins with a referral from their healthcare providers, who then directly engage medical researchers leading a clinical trial. With studies finding that more than half (57%) of patients report that they prefer to receive information about clinical trials from them, healthcare providers are the most influential actor in earliest phases of clinical trial participant enrollment (NASEM, 2016). Research on racial and ethnic minority participation in clinical trials also has found that implicit and explicit racial bias, coupled with a lack of cultural competence and humility, plays a demonstrative and detrimental role in the referrals for and enrollment in clinical trial research that minoritized individuals receive and experience. These studies have found that implicit and explicit racial bias often prevents healthcare providers and medical researchers from considering and discussing clinical trial participation with racial and ethnic minorities and other minoritized individuals because of negative, discriminatory beliefs and stereotypes, such as that certain groups are less trustworthy, less compliant with treatment protocols, and/or too unintelligent to understand the purpose and benefits of clinical trial research. Expanding the racial and ethnic diversity in the healthcare provider and medical research workforces, then, would reduce the negative impact that implicit and explicit bias plays in whether a minoritized individual is given the opportunity or encouraged to enroll in a clinical trial research project (Ruiz-White et al., 2023; Yeager & Bauer-Wu, 2013).

EQUITY IN MENTAL HEALTH RESEARCH: WHY IT IS IMPORTANT AND ACTIONABLE STEPS TO ACHIEVE IT

Mental health challenges, conditions, and diseases often are considered secondary to the larger health discourse that focuses on more widely known chronic and acute conditions and diseases that affect millions of people in the United States. However, studies confirm that mental health inequities have been and remain a persistent public health challenge in the United States, particularly among minoritized individuals and communities. During the past decade, these disparities and inequities were magnified by the "dual pandemics" of COVID-19 and the resurgence of acts of racism and discrimination (e.g., the murders of Breonna Taylor and George Floyd in 2020). Although they had an effect on the mental health of all individuals, the dual pandemics had a profoundly negative impact on the mental health of African Americans and other minoritized individuals and communities. In fact, the compounded effects of the COVID-19 pandemic and increased exposure to acts of racism and discrimination led to significant increases in feelings of stress and worry and in symptoms of trauma, depression, anxiety, and stressor-related disorders among minoritized individuals (Czeisler et al., 2020; Perrigo et al., 2022; Stinson et al., 2021).

The dual pandemics also led to an expansion of efforts to reduce and eliminate mental health inequities. Despite these initiatives, however, not all people have equal and equitable access to the most advanced, high-quality treatments and care. They also do not experience similar health outcomes. This holds especially true in the world of mental health care. Further, one of the major drivers of these persistent and pervasive racial and ethnic disparities and inequities in mental health is rooted in the very place where rising treatments and interventions, and the subsequent outcomes data and evidence, are first initiated, investigated, collected, and analyzed: in mental health research.

Equity in Mental Health Research: Why It Is Important

Mental health research is fundamental to the understanding of how mental health conditions, disorders, and diseases develop and impact individuals, families, and communities, and how symptoms can be safely and effectively managed. It is a fact that treatments for mental health conditions, disorders, and diseases work. When individuals have access to appropriate treatments for a diagnosed mental health condition, they are better equipped to manage their illness, foresee and overcome associated challenges, and lead productive lives. These are the core reasons that underscore the importance of mental health research.

Although mental health research has uncovered the persistent, disproportionate, and detrimental impacts of mental health on minoritized individuals and communities, it alone has done little to meaningfully reduce and eliminate mental health disparities and inequities (Barksdale et al., 2022). This is a direct result of the absence of *equity* in and across the entire mental health research continuum. This absence has given rise to the dearth of racial and ethnic diversity across the mental health research realm and the underrepresentation of minoritized individuals in all aspects of mental health research protocols, the compounding effects of which are most evident in the lack of diversity in clinical trials. Studies confirm that the absence of racial and ethnic minorities and other minoritized individuals in clinical trials undermines the studies' ability to apply the study results to certain populations, which could give rise to missed opportunities to identify specific treatments or regimens that are both safe and efficacious in different populations. For example, in a recent meta-analysis of men with prostate cancer, in which roughly 20% of the participants were African American, investigators found that radiation therapy was more impactful in Black men than in their White cohort (Spratt et al., 2018).

The dearth of diversity in clinical trials also compromises a study's ability to achieve generalizability (Boulware et al., 2022). When generalizability is compromised, so too is the level of confidence that a particular mental health therapy or regimen will be safe and effective across all groups of people and not just those who participated in the clinical trial. Given the profound impacts of mental health inequities, steps must be taken to maximize—*not limit*—the applicability of all promising mental health therapies and regimens to all population groups.

There is ample evidence that minoritized individuals are disproportionately more likely than nonminoritized individuals to directly experience racism and other forms of discrimination in all settings, including healthcare settings; live in racially, socioeconomically, and geographically segregated communities; experience the deleterious mental and other health consequences of environmental determinants; and experience pervasive disparities in access to high-quality, evidence-based health and mental health care services and treatments (Barksdale et al., 2022; Plough & Christopher, 2021). All of these factors have a demonstratively negative impact on an individual's mental health and well-being. In fact, recent research has found that mental health disparities and inequities not only have persisted but have worsened over the past two decades driven, in large part, by sociocultural, structural, and systemic factors, especially structural and systemic racism (Barksdale et al., 2022). Further, these same factors impact the participation of minoritized individuals in mental health clinical trials and thus must be appropriately weighed and mitigated against throughout every phase of clinical trial research design.

Equity in Mental Health Research: Actionable Steps to Achieve It

Expanding diversity in mental health clinical trials is widely touted as a requisite for meaningful progress in mental health equity (Boulware et al., 2022; NASEM, 2016; Rajasimha, 2023). Research concludes that key stakeholders in the current mental health research and clinical trial community—both individually and in tandem—must make fundamental changes to research practices, policies, and protocols if the lofty—albeit worthwhile—goal of advancing mental health equity is ever to be achieved. These stakeholders are a dynamic group and include investigators, regulatory agencies, participants in clinical trials, research and academic institutions, funders and sponsors of trials, journals, and professional societies (Bryant et al., 2021). Additionally, and perhaps most germane, an institutional shift in clinical trial design has to occur in a manner that is more intentionally, appropriately, and ethically inclusive of racial and ethnic minorities and other minoritized individuals who are at disproportionately greater risk for experiencing mental health disparities and inequities (Ruiz-White et al., 2023; Zuckerman & Edwards, 2024). This shift must also ensure that minoritized individuals are not overrepresented in the clinical trials that use the U.S. Food and Drug Administration's (FDA) exceptions from informed consent (EFIC) process. Typically, this process allows clinical trial investigators to enroll critically ill individuals and patients who are in life-threatening emergency situations into trials without obtaining their immediate consent. Analyses confirm that overall, African Americans are overrepresented (29% of participants) in clinical trials that use the FDA's EFIC process. Additionally, the EFIC process has been used in the clinical trials of psychiatric drugs, especially those intended to treat schizophrenia, in which Black individuals accounted for nearly half (45%) of clinical trial participants (Ruiz-White et al., 2023).

The undeniable value and importance of greater diversity in clinical trials have gained considerable recognition, consideration, and legitimacy over the past couple of decades. Improving diversity is lauded not only as a moral imperative (because it plays a vital role in enhancing representation), but also as a medical mandate (because it demonstratively helps ensure generalizability of—and thus confidence and trust in—the data findings, results, and subsequent clinical recommendations based on outcomes from clinical trial research Heller et al., 2014). Yet, identifying and consistently incorporating effective strategies to bolster the racial and ethnic and other diversity among participants in clinical trial research continue to evade medical researchers and clinical trial investigators.

The following section includes known barriers to clinical trial participation and actionable steps—listed in no specific order—that medical researchers and clinical trial investigators should consider as they seek to increase the numbers of racial and ethnic minorities and other minoritized individuals who are recruited for, participate in, and complete a clinical trial research project. Although alone each barrier and factor contribute to the absence of minoritized individuals at every stage of a clinical trial research project, many of them are inextricably linked and tend to either reinforce and exacerbate—or mitigate and absolve—one another.

Actionable Step: Implement Meaningful Community Engagement

Evaluations of effective strategies to recruit racial and ethnic minorities and other minoritized individuals to participate in clinical trials tout community engagement as one of the most impactful (De las Nueces, 2012; Heller et al., 2014). Effective community engagement begins *well before* a clinical trial study begins and requires the investigators and affiliated institutions to build a rapport and establish trust in a community to become educated about, and make meaningful investments to help address, the needs in and of the community. Researchers need to be visible and actively engaged at community events, listen to and collaborate with community leaders and stakeholders, and ask community members to advise them on respectful language to use during communications and effective modes of dissemination, consent forms, and other vital research documents. Further, investigators and affiliated institutions must be prepared to offer compensation to community members for their time and sharing their perspectives and expertise (Alegria et al., 2022; Ruiz-White et al., 2023). Typically, investigators and other members of the research team who have long-standing and established relationships with community members and leaders are more successful in their recruitment efforts (Yancey et al., 2006).

Some clinical trials use a unidirectional community engagement approach, with pertinent information about the clinical trial and the value of clinical trial participation flowing directly from the clinical trial investigators to community members. However, evaluations suggest that a more dynamic—and thus effective—community engagement strategy is built upon a multidirectional, mutually beneficial relationship in which the community is involved—as a key decision-maker—in all aspects of the clinical trial research project. This paradigm facilitates and encourages a reciprocal flow of information whereby the investigators and affiliated institutions learn of the challenges in, and needs of, the community and the community learns about the intentions and perspectives of the researchers. Further, this engagement approach inspires both the researchers and the community members not only to embrace a sense of investment, but a sense of ownership in the clinical trial purpose, goals, design, implementation, and outcome analysis (MacFarlane, 2021). As such, a multidirectional community engagement approach has played a significant role in increasing the recruitment of underrepresented minoritized individuals and communities in past clinical research trials (MacFarlane, 2021). Outcomes research values authentic voices, champions respect and dignity, avoids exploitation, and encourages empowerment and agency from underrepresented, underserved, and underresourced communities. The resultant effect is one of mutual trust and a culture of meaningful and purposeful inclusion in which communities are regarded as co-researchers throughout all phases—including key decision-making—of a clinical trial study (Alegria et al., 2022).

Actionable Step: Bolster the Racial and Ethnic Diversity in the Medical and Clinical Trial Research Workforce

Earlier in this chapter, the deleterious impacts of implicit and explicit racial bias on the rates of clinical trial referral and enrollment among minoritized individuals were explored. Numerous studies confirm that one of the most effective strategies to mitigate the negative effects of these forms of bias is through the expansion of racial and ethnic diversity in the healthcare provider and medical research workforces. Despite their best attempts, however, efforts to attract, train, retain, and promote medical researchers from underrepresented racial and ethnic groups have and continue to fall woefully short. In fact, although racial and ethnic minorities comprise 30% to 40% of the total U.S. population, they account for less than 6% of medical research faculty members (Collins et al., 2021). A number of factors—all of which are reparable—are to blame. They include a scarcity of mentorship programs to introduce minoritized individuals to the field and a dearth of opportunities for rising minoritized clinical investigators to receive the professional and financial support needed to advance and excel as their medical research career develops. For example, medical school graduates from underrepresented racial and ethnic minority groups receive career development awards from NIH at less than half the rate of individuals from well-represented groups (Boulware et al., 2022; Ruiz-White et al., 2023).

Turning the tide will require a stronger and more consistent commitment to the creation of systemic and institutional cultures of inclusivity that embrace cultural humility, which facilitates honest and trustworthy relationships with colleagues, patients, and communities from diverse backgrounds (Yeager & Bauer-Wu, 2013). It also will require an ongoing dedication to the fair advancement of minoritized individuals within and across all health research settings (Boulware et al., 2022; Collins et al., 2021; Neblett, 2019).

Actionable Step: Integrate and Prioritize Equity Throughout Every Step and Phase of Medical and Clinical Trial Research Study Designs

Health research and clinical trial study designs have a direct impact on efforts to recruit and enroll racial and ethnic minorities and other minoritized individuals. See **Box 21.2** for different types of clinical research. Every component and procedure in clinical research designs—from the development and content of the research protocol; the recruitment,

Box 21.2 DIFFERENT TYPES OF CLINICAL RESEARCH

- *Treatment research* generally involves an intervention such as medication, psychotherapy, new devices, or new approaches to surgery or radiation therapy.
- *Prevention research* looks for better ways to prevent disorders from developing or returning. Different kinds of prevention research may study medicines, vitamins, vaccines, minerals, or lifestyle changes.
- *Diagnostic research* refers to the practice of looking for better ways to identify a particular disorder or condition.
- *Screening research* aims to find the best ways to detect certain disorders or health conditions.
- *Quality-of-life research* explores ways to improve comfort and the quality of life for individuals with a chronic illness.
- *Genetic studies* aim to improve the prediction of disorders by identifying and understanding how genes and illnesses may be related. Research in this area may explore ways in which a person's genes make them more or less likely to develop a disorder. This may lead to development of tailor-made treatments based on a patient's genetic makeup.
- *Epidemiological studies* seek to identify the patterns, causes, and control of disorders in groups of people.
- *Comparative effectiveness research* compares alternative approaches to the management of a clinical condition.

enrollment, and retention processes; and the data collection, analysis, and reporting methods to the racial and ethnic diversity of the entire clinical research design team and affiliated partners—has a significant, often determinative impact on the recruitment, enrollment, and retention of minoritized individuals and communities. As such, as investigators conceptualize, organize, and actualize clinical research designs, it is imperative that they do so with one overarching objective: to integrate and prioritize equity.

Purposeful steps must be taken at the onset of the planning process—before a study begins—to address and mitigate these negative effects and bolster the diversity in the participant pool. Before the study launches, careful consideration needs to be placed on its purpose, how it is designed and funded, and who is involved at every level of the design protocol. Additional consideration needs to be given to the causes of, and designing and implementing solutions to, the underrepresentation of racial and ethnic minorities and other minoritized individuals in clinical trial research. This should begin with reforming many of the common practices used in the clinical trial research project process, including cultural competence and racial sensitivity training across the entire research team and integrated into the entire participant recruitment, selection, and retention processes; strong considerations about where the research site will be located to alleviate travel-related burdens; stringent and consistently enforced ethical standards embedded into the research protocol through its entirety; and how the actual questions and information are developed and communicated (e.g., use of multilingual options and awareness of health literacy levels).

Actionable Step: Identify, Address and Surmount Barriers to Participation

Medical and clinical trial research designs also should account for and surmount known barriers to research recruitment, enrollment, and participation to ensure that the clinical trial is physically and financially accessible to individuals who have the willingness and interest to participate. There are barriers associated with travel logistics, language and literacy challenges, religious and cultural beliefs and customs, unfamiliarity with clinical trial research, and levels of distrust in medical research (Alegria et al., 2022; Ruiz-White et al., 2023; Yeager & Bauer-Wu, 2013).

Surmounting some of these barriers may require unorthodox solutions. For example, nontraditional sites (e.g., barber shops, beauty salons, churches, and community centers) may serve as more appropriate and convenient locations to recruit underrepresented individuals, and the use of digital health tools can be integrated to surmount geographic and travel-related barriers and allow for remote data collection. Additional elements that should be integrated in medical and clinical trial research plans include participant reimbursement for both direct and indirect costs of participating in a clinical trial; the dissemination of information that is culturally sensitive, linguistically appropriate, and available in multiple languages; collaborations with trusted patient advocacy organizations, media, and local community members and entities to raise awareness; and offering patients information about clinical trials directly with online tools designed to educate and enroll racially and ethnically diverse participants (National Institute of Mental Health [NIMH], n.d.; Pfizer, n.d.; Ruiz-White et al., 2023). See **Figure 21.2** for barriers and solutions to clinical trial participation.

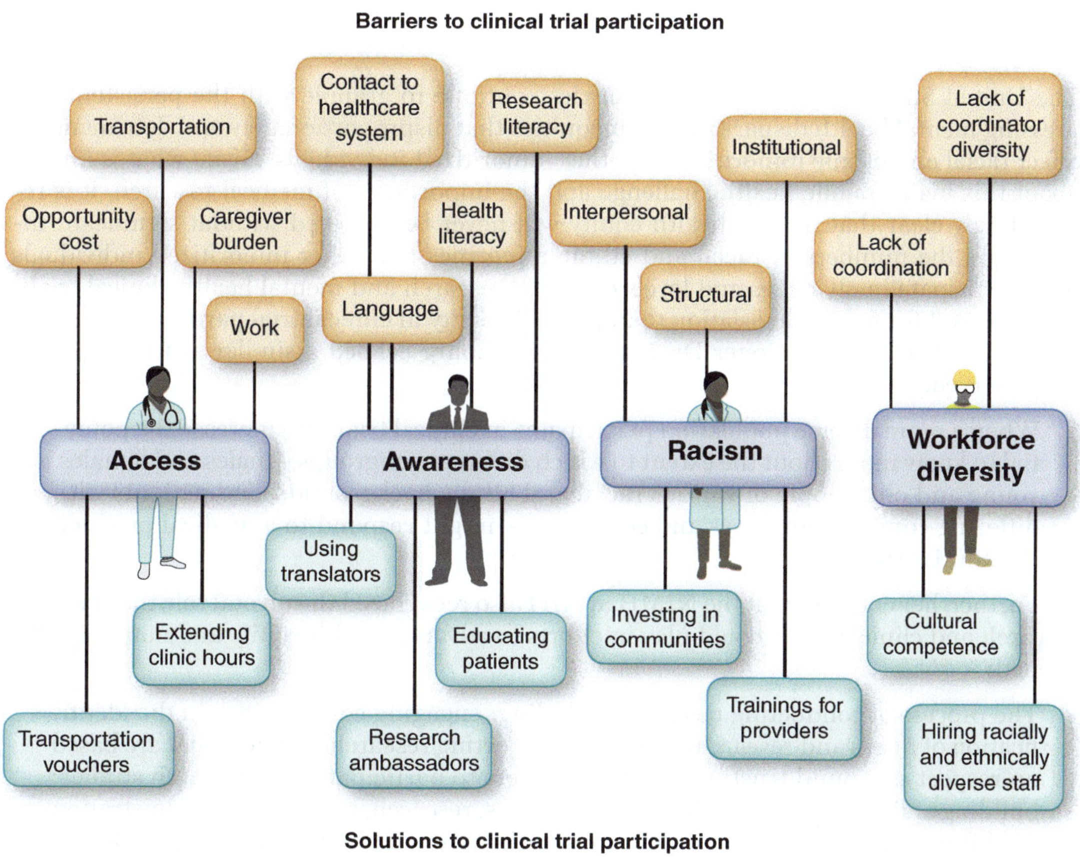

Figure 21.2 Barriers and solutions to clinical trial participation.

Source: Reopell, L., Nolan, T. S., Gray, D. M., 2nd, Williams, A., Brewer, L. C., Bryant, A. L., Wilson, G., Williams, E., Jones, C., McKoy, A., Grever, J., Soliman, A., Baez, J., Nawaz, S., Walker, D. M., Metlock, F., Zappe, L., Gregory, J., & Joseph, J. J. (2023). Community engagement and clinical trial diversity: Navigating barriers and co-designing solutions—A report from the "Health Equity through Diversity" seminar series. *PLOS ONE, 18*(2), e0281940. https://doi.org/10.1371/journal.pone.0281940

Actionable Step: Expand Data Collection and Analysis Design

Data collection and analysis involve far more than taking rudimentary head counts. In fact, data collection and analysis design—which are core elements in the larger clinical research design—are vital because they build the foundation upon which the safety and efficacy of a particular treatment or regimen is evaluated. They also are fundamental to the advancement of mental health equity because without consistently sound and valid racial and ethnic data, it is virtually impossible to meaningfully identify and measure the extent to which mental health disparities and inequities affect minoritized individuals and communities. Data that are routinely and consistently collected and analyzed can make the previously unseen and historically excluded visible, allowing for the identification of specific needs, and the creation of solutions to advance mental health equity (Kauh, 2021; NIMH, n.d.; Plough & Christopher, 2021).

It is crucial for the medical and clinical trial research communities to take the power of data steps further to advance mental health equity through their investigations. Using data to identify and measure multilevel risk and protective factors, researchers could measure community-, social-, and structural-level determinants of mental health. Together, these health equity data points, measures, and metrics will ensure accountability and regulatory compliance, and better inform efforts to advance mental health equity (Barksdale et al., 2022; Boulware et al., 2022).

SUMMARY

The United States as well as other countries continue to grapple with the persistent and pressing mental health disparities and inequities that disproportionately and detrimentally affect racial and ethnic minorities and other minoritized individuals. Given what is known about this major public health challenge and the importance of medical research, it is resoundingly clear that mental health equity will never be achieved without significant increases in the numbers of racial and ethnic minorities and other minoritized individuals who participate in all stages and levels of health research and mental health clinical trials. See **Box 21.3** for federal legislation to improve diversity in clinical trial participants.

Former FDA commissioner Dr. Margaret Hamburg echoed a similar sentiment when she observed,

> When a more diverse population participates in clinical trials, we increase the potential to know more about the extent to which different subgroups—males and females, young and old, people of various racial and ethnic backgrounds, and patients with differing comorbid diseases and conditions—might respond to a medical product. (NASEM, 2015, p. 5)

Further, her colleagues at the NIMH at NIH also recognized the pivotal role that medical research and clinical trials could play in efforts to advance health equity and noted what is needed:

> The process of conducting research, including: engaging communities in the identification of needs and research priorities; supporting research practices that are based on respect and build trust; identifying barriers to participation in research studies; building a diverse and equitable health services, research, and health administration workforce; and, including communities in the interpretation and dissemination of research findings. (NIMH, n.d.)

Mental health research and clinical trials—though they sit upstream in the fight against mental health disparities and inequities—have been one of the major drivers in the

Box 21.3 FEDERAL LEGISLATION TO IMPROVE DIVERSITY IN CLINICAL TRIAL PARTICIPANTS

- *1993 National Institutes of Health (NIH) Revitalization Act*: mandated the purposeful inclusion of racial/ethnic minorities and women in NIH-funded research.
- *2001*: NIH has described that any study proposal "should contain a description of the proposed outreach programs for recruiting women and minorities as participants."
- *2012*: Legislation that reauthorized FDA user fees, included provisions under Section 907 requiring that FDA publicly report data on the inclusion and analysis of women in FDA applications, with additional provision requiring the same for race and ethnicity.
- *2017*: NIH updated this policy to require NIH-funded phase III trials to report on race/ethnicity.
- *2020*: Food and Drug Administration released guidance to ensure purposeful eligibility criteria, loosen eligibility criteria for phase III trials, and include clinical sites located in geographic areas with a high proportion of racial and ethnic minority populations.
- *2022*: Food and Drug Omnibus Reform Act of 2022 requires pharmaceutical companies to include diverse populations in their clinical trials.

advancements that have been made within and across the mental health care continuum, the effects of which have been observed further downstream. The screenings and therapies that are now available, the preventive interventions, and the treatment regimens that are widely used literally save lives. They, therefore, should play a fundamental role in ongoing and future efforts to achieve mental health equity. However, the benefits that rise from the mental health research and clinical trial world are not experienced by every individual who is at increased risk for or currently living with a mental health disorder, condition, or disease. In too many instances, they remain inaccessible. As a direct result, the grave racial and ethnic disparities and inequities that exist across and within the mental health care continuum will continue to impede efforts to advance mental health equity. This makes identifying and implementing short- and long-term solutions to the challenges that limit the participation of minoritized individuals and communities in mental health clinical trial research an imperative.

DISCUSSION QUESTIONS

1. How would you design a clinical trial to achieve mental health equity outcomes?
2. What factors act as barriers to inclusion and participation in clinical trials; why are these barriers an equity issue?
3. How does implicit bias affect the enrollment of minoritized individuals in mental health clinical trial research?
4. Why is community engagement important to health equity research?
5. What are some of the factors that impact trust in clinical research?

ACKNOWLEDGMENT

The author acknowledges Clarissa Moreno for her review.

REFERENCES

Adeyemi, O. F., Evans, A. T., & Bahk, M. (2009). HIV-infected adults from minority ethnic groups are willing to participate in research if asked. *AIDS Patient Care and STDs, 23*(10), 859–865. https://doi.org/10.1089/apc.2009.0008

Alegria, M., Zhen-Duan, J., O'Malley, I. S., DiMarzio, K. (2022). A new agenda for optimizing investments in community mental health and reducing disparities. *American Journal of Psychiatry, 179*, 402–416. https://doi.org/10.1176/appi.ajp.21100970

Alsan, M., & Eichmeyer, S. (2021). *Experimental evidence on the effectiveness of non-experts for improving vaccine demand* (National Bureau of Economic Research Working Paper No. 28593). https://www.nber.org/papers/w28593

Alvidrez, J. L., & Barksdale, C.L. (2022). Perspectives from the National Institutes of Health on multidimensional mental health disparities research: A framework for advancing the field. *American Journal of Psychiatry, 179*(6), 417–421. https://doi.org/10.1175/appi.ajp.21100969

Barksdale, C. L., Perez-Stable, E., & Gordon, J. (2022). Innovative directions to advance mental health disparities research. *American Journal of Psychiatry, 179*(6), 397–401. https://doi.org/10.1176/appi.ajp.21100972

Bonevski, B., Randell, M., Paul, C., Chapman, K., Twyman, L., Bryant, J., Brozek, I., & Hughes, C. (2014). Reaching the hard-to-reach: A systematic review of strategies for improving health and medical research with socially disadvantaged groups. *BMC Medical Research Methodolgy, 14*(1). http://www.biomedcentral.com/1471-2288/14/42

Boulware, L. E., Corbie, G., Aguilar-Gaxiola, S., Wilkins, C. H., Ruiz, R., Vitale, A., & Egede, L. E. (2022). Combating structural inequities—Diversity, equity, and inclusion in clinical and translational research. *The New England Journal of Medicine, 386*(3), 201–203. https://doi.org/10.1056/NEJMp2112233

Braunstein, J. B., Sherber, N. S., Schulman, S. P., Ding, E. L., & Powe, N. R. (2008). Race, medical researcher distrust, perceived harm, and willingness to participate in cardiovascular prevention trials. *Medicine, 87*(1), 1–9. https://doi.org/10.1097/MD.0b013e3181625d78

Bryant, B. E., Jordan, A., & Clark, U. S. (2021). Race as a social construct in psychiatry research and practice. *JAMA Psychiatry, 79*(2), 93–94. https://doi.org/10.1001/jamapsychiatry.2021.2877

Byrd, G. S., Edwards, C. L., Kelkar, V. A., Phillips, R. G., Byrd, J. R., Pim-Pong, D. S., Starks, T. D., Taylor, A. L., McKinley, R. E., Li, Y.-J., & Pericak-Vance, M. (2011). Recruiting intergenerational African American males for biomedical research studies: A major research challenge. *Journal of the National Medical Association, 103*(6), 480–487. https://doi.org/10.1016/s0027-9684(15)30361-8

Collins, F. S., Adams, A. B., Aklin, C., et al. (2021). Affirming NIH's commitment to addressing structural racism in the biomedical research enterprise. *Cell, 184*, 3075–3079. https://doi.org/10.1016/j.cell.2021.05.014

Corbie-Smith, G., Thomas, S. B., & George, D. M. St. (2022). Distrust, race, and research. *Archives of Internal Medicine, 162*(21), 2458–2463. https://doi.org/10.1001/archinte.162.21.2458

Czeisler, M.E., Lane, R.I., Petrosky, E., Wiley, J.F., Christensen, A., Njai, R., Weaver, M.D., Robbins, R., Facer-Childs, E.R., Barger, L.K., Czeisler, C.A., Howard, M.E., & Rajaratnam, S.M.W. (2020). Mental health, substance use, and suicidal ideation during the COVID-19 pandemic-United States, June 24-30, 2020. *Morbidity and Mortality Weekly Report, 69*(32), 1049–1057.

De Las Nueces, D., Hacker, K., Di Girolamo, A., & Hicks, L.S. (2012). A systematic review of community-based participatory research to enhance clinical trials in racial and ethnic minority groups. *Health Services Research, 47*(3pt2), 1363–1386. https://doi.org/10.1111/j.1475-6773.2012.01386.x

Evans, M. K., Lepkowski, J. M., Powe, N. R., LaVeist, T., Kuczmarski, M. F., & Zonderman, A. B. (2010). Healthy aging in neighborhoods of diversity across the life span (HANDLS): Overcoming barriers to implementing a longitudinal, epidemiologic, urban study of health, race, and socioeconomic status. *Ethnicity and Disease, 20*(3), 267–275.

Ford, J. G., Howerton, M. W., Lai, G. Y., Gary, T. L., Mid, S. B., Gibbons, M. C., Tilburt, J., Baffi, C., Tanpitukpongse, T. P., Wilson, R. F, Powe, N.R., & Bass, E. B. (2008). Barriers to recruiting underrepresented populations to cancer clinical trials: A systematic review. *Cancer, 112*(2), 228–242. https://doi.org/10.1002/cncr.23157

Gadegbeku, C. A., Stillman, P. K., Huffman, M. D., Jackson, J. S., Kusek, J. W., & Jamerson, K. A. (2008). Factors associated with enrollment of African Americans into a clinical trial: Results from the African American Study of Kidney Disease and Hypertension. *Contemporary Clinical Trials, 29*(6), 837–842. https://doi.org/10.1016/j.cct.2008.06.001

Garber, M., Hanusa, B. H., Switzer, G. E., Mellors, J., & Arnold, R. M. (2007). HIV-infected African Americans are willing to participate in HIV treatment trials. *Journal of General Internal Medicine, 22*(1), 17–42. https://doi.org/10.1007/s11606-007-0121-8

George, S., Duran, N., & Norris, K. (2014). A systematic review of barriers and facilitators to minority research participation among African Americans, Latinos, Asian Americans, and Pacific Islanders. *American Journal of Public Health, 104*(2), e16–e31. https://doi.org/10.2105/AJPH.2013.301706

Griffith, D. M., Bergner, E. M., Fair, A. S., & Wilkins, C. H. (2021). Using mistrust, distrust, and low trust precisely in medical care and medical research advances health equity. *American Journal of Preventive Medicine, 60*(3), 442–445. https://doi.org/10.1016/j.amepre.2020.08.019

Guadagnolo, B. A., Petereit, D. G., Helbig, P., & Koop, D., Kussman, P., & Dunn, E. F., Patnaik, A. (2009). Involving American Indians and medically underserved rural populations in cancer clinical trials. *Clinical Trials, 6*(6), 610–617. https://doi.org/10.1177/1740774509348526

Heller, C., Balls-Berry, J.E., Nery, J.D., Erwin, P.J., Littleton, D., Kim, M., & Kuo, W.P. (2014). Strategies addressing barriers to clinical trial enrollment of underrepresented populations: A systematic review. *Contemporary Clinical Trials, 39*(2), 169–182. https://doi.org./10.1016/j.cct.2014.08.004

Hillyer, G. C., Beauchemin, M., Hershman, D. L., Kelsen, M., & Brogan, F. L., Sandoval, R., Schmitt, K. M., Reyes, A., Terry, M. B., Lassman, A. B., & Schwartz, G. K. (2020). Discordant attitudes and beliefs about cancer clinical trial participation between physicians, research staff, and cancer patients. *Clinical Trials, 17*(2), 184–194. https://doi.org/10.1177/1740774520901514

Indorewalla, K.K., O'Connor, M.K., Budson, A.E., Guess, C., & Jackson, J. (2021). Modifiable Barriers for Recruitment and Retention of Older Adults Participants from Underrepresented Minorities in Alzheimer's Disease Research. *Journal of Alzheimer's Disease, 80*(3), 927–940. https://doi.org/10.3233/JAD-201081

Kaplan, C. P., Nápoles, A. M., Narine, S., Gregorich, S., Livaudais-Toman, J., Nguyen, T., Leykin, Y., Roach, M., & Small, E. J. (2015). Knowledge and attitudes regarding clinical trials and willingness to participate among prostate cancer patients. *Contemporary Clinical Trials, 45*(Pt B), 443–448. https://doi.org/10.1016/j.cct.2015.09.023

Kauh, T. J. (2021, November 29). *Racial equity will not be achieved without investing in data disaggregation.* Health Affairs Blog. https://doi.org/10.1377/hblog20211123.426054

Kelsey, M.D., Patrick-Lake, B., Abdulai, R., Broedl, U.C., Brown, A., Cohn, E., Curtis, L.H., Komelasky, C., Mbagwu, M., Mensah, G.A., Mentz, R.J., Nyaku, A., Omokaro, S.O., Sewards, J., Whitlock, K., Zhang, X., & Bloomfield, G.S. (2022). Inclusion and diversity in clinical trials: Actionable steps to drive lasting change. *Contemporary Clinical Trials, 116.* https://doi.org/10.1016/j.cct.2022.106740

Kennedy-Martin, T., Curtis, S., Faries, D., Robinson, S., & Johnston, J. (2015). A literature review on the representativeness of randomized controlled trial samples and implications for the external validity of trial results. *Trials, 16*(1), 495. https://doi.org/10.1186/s13063-015-1023-4

KFF. (2023). *State health facts, poverty rate by race/ethnicity.* https://www.kff.org/other/state-indicator/poverty-rate-by-raceethnicity

Lor, M., & Bowers, B. J. (2018). Hmong older adults' perceptions of insider and outsider researchers: Does it matter for research participation? *Nursing Research, 67*(3), 222–230. https://doi.org/10.1097/NNR.0000000000000277

MacFarlane, A.E. (2021). Optimising individual and community involvement in health decision-making in general practice consultations and primary care settings: A way forward. *European Journal of General Practice, 26*(1), 196–201. https://doi.org/10.1080/13814788.2020.1861245

Martell, G. (2024, July 31). Clinical trials must be more equitable, here's how. *HIT Consultant.* https://hitconsultant.net/2024/07/31/clinical-trials-must-be-more-equitable-heres-how/

Morris, Z. S., Wooding, S., & Grant, J. (2011). The answer is 17 years, what is the question: Understanding time lags in translational research. *Journal of the Royal Society of Medicine, 104,* 510–520. https://doi.org/10.1258/jrsm.2011.110180

National Academies of Sciences, Engineering, and Medicine. (2016). *Strategies for ensuring diversity, inclusion, and meaningful participation in clinical trials: Proceedings of a workshop.* The National Academies Press. https://doi.org/10.17226/23530

National Institute of Mental Health. (n.d.). *NIMH strategic framework for addressing youth mental health disparities.* https://www.cmhnetwork.org/wp-content/uploads/2023/02/Youth-MH-Disparities-Framework_0.pdf

National Library of Medicine. (n.d.). *Learn about studies.* https://clinicaltrials.gov/study-basics/learn-about-studies.

Neblett, E. W. (2019). Racism and health: Challenges and future directions in behavioral and psychological research *Cultural Diversity and Ethnic Minority Psychology, 25*(1), 12–20. https://doi.org/10.1037/cdp0000253

Occa, A., Morgan, S. E., & Potter, J. N. E. (2018). Underrepresentation of Hispanics and other minorities in clinical trials: Recruiters' perspectives. *Journal of Racial and Ethnic Health Disparities, 5*(2), 322–332. https://doi.org/10.1007/s40615-017-0373-x

Ojanuga, D. (1993). The medical ethics of the 'father of gynaecology', Dr J Marion Sims. *Journal of Medical Ethics, 19,* 28–31. https://doi.org/10.1136/jme.19.1.28

Perrigo, J.L., Samek, A., & Hurlburt, M. (2022). Minority and low-SES families' experiences during the early phases of the COVID-19 pandemic crisis: A qualitative study. *Children and Youth Services Review, 140.* https://doi.org/10.1016/j.childyouth.2022.106594

Pew Research Center. (2024). *Most black Americans believe U.S. institutions were designed to hold black people back.* https://www.pewresearch.org/wp-content/uploads/sites/20/2024/06/RE_2024.06.15_Black-Americans-and-US-Institutions_REPORT.pdf

Pfizer. (n.d.). *Diversity in our clinical trials.* https://www.pfizer.com/science/clinical-trials/diversity

Plough, A., & Christopher, G. C. (2021, May 18). New commission to tackle how national health data are collected, shared, and used. *Health Affairs Blog.* https://doi.org/10.1377/hblog20210518.409206

Rajasimha, H. (2023, September 18). The future of clinical trials: Diversity, transparency, and reform. *Psychiatric Times.* https://www.psychiatrictimes.com/view/the-future-of-clinical-trials-diversity-transparency-and-reform

Ruiz-White, I., Kramer, L., Phillips, L., Wong, B., Lonergan, K., & Moreno, F. (2023). Racial and ethnic disparities in physical and mental health care and clinical trials. *The Journal of Clinical Psychiatry, 84*(4), 54–64. https://doi.org/10.4088/JCP.23ah14887

Scharff, D. P., Mathews, K. J., Jackson, P., Hoffsuemmer, J., Martin, E., & Edwards, D. (2010). More than Tuskegee: Understanding mistrust about research participation. *Journal of Health Care for the Poor and Underserved, 21*(3), 879–897. https://doi.org/10.1353/hpu.0.0323

Skloot, R. (2010). *The immortal life of Henrietta Lacks.* Crown Publishers.

Spratt, D.E., Dess, R.T., Hartman, H.E., Mahal, B.A., Jackson, W.C., Soni, P.D., Alshalalfa, M., Fishbane, N., Zumsteg, Z.S., Shipley, W.U., Pisansky, T.M., Roach, M., Zhao, S.G., Speers, C., Davicioni, E., Schipper, M., Nguyen, P.L., Schaeffer, E. M., Feng, F.Y., & Sandler, H.M. (2018). Androgen receptor activity and radiotherapeutic sensitivity in African-American men with prostate cancer: A large scale gene expression analysis and meta-analysis of RTOG trials. *International Journal of Radiation Oncology Biology Physics, 102*(3), *S3*. doi:10.1016/j.ijrobp.2018.06.104

Stinson, E.A., Sullivan, R.M., Peteet, B.J., Tapert, S.F., Baker, F.C., Breslin, F.J., Dick, A.S., Gonzalez, M.R., Guillaume, M., Marshall, A.T., McCabe, C.J., Pelham, W.E., Van Rinsveld, A., Sheth, C.S., Sowell, E.R., Wade, N.E., Wallace, A.L., & Lisdahl, K.M. (2021). Longitudinal impact of childhood adversity on early adolescent mental health during the COVID-19 pandemic in the ABCD study cohort: Does race or ethnicity moderate findings? *Biological Psychiatry: Global Open Science, 1,* 324–335. https://doi.org/10.1016/j.bpsgos.2021.08.007

Webb, F. J., Khubchandani, J., Striley, C. W., & Cottler, L. B. (2019). Black–white differences in willingness to participate and perceptions about health research: Results from the population-based healthstreet study. *Journal of Immigrant and Minority Health, 21*(2), 299–305. https://doi.org/10.1007/s10903-018-0729-2

Westergaard, R. P., Beach, M. C., Saha, S., & Jacobs, E. A. (2014). Racial/ethnic differences in trust in health care: HIV conspiracy beliefs and vaccine research participation. *Journal of General Internal Medicine, 29*(1), 140–146. https://doi.org/10.1007/s11606-013-2554-6

Yancey, A.K., Ortega, A.N., & Kumanyika, S.K. (2006). Effective recruitment and retention of minority research participants. *Annual Review of Public Health, 27*(1), 1–28. https://doi.org/10.1146/annurev.publhealth.27.021405.102113

Yeager, K. A., & Bauer-Wu, S. (2013). Cultural humility: Essential foundation for clinical researchers. *Applied Nursing Research, 26*(4), 10.1016/j.apnr.2013.06.008. https://doi.org/10.1016/j.apnr.2013.06.008

Zuckerman, M. C., & Edwards, H. A. (2024). Diversity in U.S. clinical trials for head and neck cancer: Are we improving? *Head & Neck, 47*(2), 679–686. https://doi.org/10.1002/hed.27943

22 HISTORY, HOPE, AND MENTAL WELL-BEING: EQUITY-CENTERED PUBLIC MENTAL HEALTH CONSIDERATIONS

GAIL C. CHRISTOPHER

LEARNING OBJECTIVES

After reading this chapter, readers will be able to:

- Explore three considerations for equity data in public mental health: context and history, the voice of marginalized populations, and the commitment to ending racism.
- Move from a deficit frame of mental health to a positive focus on well-being.
- Increase their understanding of the harm created by racial hierarchy.
- Increase their awareness and understanding of successful efforts in the United States to end racism and foster mental and physical health equity.
- Increase their understanding of Truth, Racial Healing & Transformation (TRHT) work in the United States as an adaptation of the globally recognized Truth and Reconciliation Commission (TRC) process.

INTRODUCTION

Mental health and well-being considerations in countries that have a history of protracted adherence to a false hierarchy of human value, such as centuries of enslavement and colonization, must encompass the history as well as healing and resilience strategies for all populations. Population mental health data systems must be transformed to reflect this understanding and to accelerate the well-being of marginalized populations. Although there has been progress in identifying mental health disparities and inequities, and the disparities in access to treatment for mental illness, progress toward centering equity and eliminating inequities requires data systems that encompass the known social and political determinants of mental and physical health. *Social Determinants of Mental Health*, edited by Michael T. Compton and Ruth S. Shim, reminds practitioners and researchers that societies, environments, and ecosystems help to shape mental health and mental illness (Compton & Shim, 2015). Such social and political factors include economic viability and full employment; quality education; affordable housing; community safety; environmental justice with limited exposure to toxins such as lead and arsenic; and the distribution of mediating and empowering factors such as access to affordable, quality food, voting rights, political power, and economic justice.

This chapter focuses on mental health as a state of overall well-being, and the capacity for resilience and coping with the vicissitudes of life and adaptation to adversity. Just as the World Health Organization's definition of health is that "health is a state of complete physical, mental and social well-being and not merely the absence of disease or infirmity," mental health is more than the absence of mental illness (World Health Organization, n.d.). The basic premise is that mental health must be viewed through a nondeficit or positive lens, which encompasses optimal opportunities for well-being. Given this positive perspective, governments, jurisdictions, and public health agencies must acknowledge that policies of racial oppression and exclusion are simply not compatible with the goals of achieving mental health and well-being. Considerations for equity and fairness require that jurisdictions uncover and acknowledge the harmful policies of the past and present and devote resources to redressing and mitigating contemporary residual effects of these harms; equitable policies must be created. Therefore, foundational systems of data and information must support these efforts. The primary consideration for equity-centered public mental health data is the context. In nations with a protracted history of oppression and marginalization of diverse groups, a commitment to truth and acknowledgment and subsequent elimination of policies that enforce racial hierarchy are required. This perspective requires a realistic appraisal of the degree to which racial hierarchy, when imposed by society, creates barriers to experiencing well-being and happiness and increases demands for energy for managing stress and distress. These increased demands take a toll on the human body throughout the life course, and these demands have neurobiological effects.

In his book *Why Zebras Don't Get Ulcers*, Robert M. Sapolsky reminds us that the stress response was not intended to be maintained on a chronic basis (Sapolsky, 1994). He explores the multiple ways in which chronic fear and distress affect all body systems, particularly cardiovascular, glucose regulation, and the health of the nervous system. In the updated version of his book, Sapolsky zeroes in on the effects of social factors such as poverty and employment instability as stress-inducing experiences. Whereas Sapolsky's comprehensive treatment on the subject compares the human response to that of other mammals and primates, the work of Bruce McEwen and Eliot Stellar aligns with Sapolsky's conclusions and introduces the concept of allostatic load to describe the cumulative burden of chronic exposures to stress and distress (McEwen & Stellar, 1993). When environmental challenges exceed the individual ability to cope, then allostatic overload ensues. Allostatic load is identified by the use of biomarkers and clinical criteria (Guidi et al., 2021). One factor for a more equitable mental health data consideration would be the prioritization of measuring clinical and social indicators of allostatic burden and overload. This could be part of a public health chronic disease prevention strategy. The Everyday Discrimination Scale has been a useful tool in documenting the clinical biomarkers associated with experiences of discrimination and the psychological impact (Lawrence et al., 2022). In addition to measuring the experiences of discrimination, chronic stress, and allostatic load, another consideration for more equitable mental health data should also include the availability of opportunities to mitigate the effects of chronic stress. Recent scientific evidence supports that a current mitigating strategy is optimizing opportunities for connection and strong relationships.

America's 19th surgeon general, Dr. Vivek Murthy, has authored a related book, *Together: The Healing Power of Human Connection in a Sometimes Lonely World*. Dr. Murthy draws from his clinical experience as a physician and extensive research on efforts throughout the globe to address the epidemic of loneliness and related stress. Murthy makes a case for loneliness as a public health concern: a root cause and contributor to many of the epidemics sweeping the world today from alcohol and drug addiction to violence to depression and anxiety. Loneliness, he argues, is affecting not only our health but also how our children experience school, how we perform in the workplace, and the sense of division and polarization in our society (Murthy, 2023). Decades of research on the effects of stress reveal that stress has a negative impact on relational capacities and subsequently a negative impact on health and mental well-being.

Societies that have embedded human value hierarchy and discriminatory barriers to opportunity for marginalized groups have generally failed to acknowledge and track the psychological and subsequent mental and physical health harms created by related norms and practices. The COVID-19 pandemic presented a unique opportunity for acknowledging the burdens experienced by marginalized groups, while at the same time exacerbating those burdens, particularly economic vulnerability. The pandemic was also accompanied by repeated exposure to extrajudicial killings of Black people by police including the brutal murder of George Floyd. This created an unprecedented moment for public protests and mobilization for racial justice, and subsequent calls for more effective strategies for centering and creating equity in public health data systems in the United States. These protests are largely attributable to the organizing capacity of the Black Lives Matter movement, which involved more than 25 million people in protests in the United States (Buchanan et al., 2020). The majority of these protesters were not Black. This catalyzed a new era of conscious awareness about the need for reparations, justice, healing, and transformation. The United States, despite its history of racial hierarchy, has never engaged in a national truth process to acknowledge and reconcile the pain associated with centuries of the denial of the humanity of Indigenous and enslaved people. The contemporary movement for health equity calls for a national truth and healing process, along with demands for reparations and policy transformation. What has emerged is leadership for action to create a health system that includes more equitable data, public health policies, and infrastructure.

The following sections describe the expanding movement for health equity and the transformation of public health data systems to support this movement.

A HISTORY OF RACIAL VIOLENCE AND MENTAL HEALTH

When considering health equity, both mental and physical, in the United States and other countries characterized by a history of institutionalized racial hierarchy, we must consider the opportunities that are provided for optimal human development throughout all life stages. We must also document the barriers to those opportunities that are societal or structural in nature. This requires information about historic and contemporary conditions.

When the history of racism in the United States is examined, the dominant lesson that emerges is violence. The decimation of Indigenous people and cultures; the centuries of enslavement; the war that ended it; the resistance to the Reconstruction efforts, which was dominated by terror, violence, and lynching of formally enslaved African Americans; and the subsequent Jim Crow era that stretched from the 19th century until the 1960s were maintained through systematic violent actions. In their book *Black Rage*, psychiatrists William H. Grier and Price M. Cobbs leveraged the momentum of the civil rights era and provided the first exploration of the frustration, pain, anger, and sometimes violence of Black victims of centuries of racial oppression (Grier & Cobbs, 1968).

Conversely, the history of racism in the United States often omits the levels of resistance and agency that characterized the Black populations during slavery and after. The book *Gabriel's Rebellion: The Virginia Slave Conspiracies of 1800 and 1802* by Douglas R. Egerton uses primary documents and extensive research to tell the stories of strategy, organization, and rebellion by enslaved and literate Black men during the Revolutionary era in U.S history (Egerton, 2003). The book provides a powerful glimpse into the state of chronic fear and anxiety that characterized the enslavement era. It also depicts the hypocrisy of the founding fathers and their tenets of equality in the face of maintaining slavery. This is one of several books including the well-known slave narratives that portrayed the will and determination embodied in enslaved populations. The legal and institutionalized system of oppression minimized by the term *Jim Crow* is not well understood or appreciated by the general public today. This system of segregation and enforced adherence to segregation lasted from the 19th century through the 1960s. Like slavery, this systemic and legally enforced form of oppression could be maintained only through violence and subjugation. In her brilliant exploration of the Jim Crow era in the book *By Hands Now Known: Jim Crow's Legal Executioners*, legal scholar Margaret A. Burnham uses an expansive database exceeding 1,000 cases to portray the complex nuances of state and national laws used to maintain and, in some cases, fight this system. Readers are drawn into the violence of lynching and murders and the horrific consequences in the lives and minds of families and communities (Burnham, 2023).

Violence is an anathema to health and well-being. It is particularly harmful to mental health. It is harmful to the victims of violence and to the perpetrators as well. Most of the existing knowledge about the effects of violence on mental health emerged from studies of veterans engaged in warfare, and most recently, studies of the effects of exposure to trauma and adverse life experiences on child and adult development. During the formative centuries in the United States that were characterized by the violence of racial oppression, little focus or attention was paid to the health and mental health consequences of the normalization of racial violence. The nation was engaged in mass denial of the truth and the cruelty of the institutionalized systems, which grew out of the entrenched belief in a false hierarchy of human value.

Just as Jim Crow enforced segregation and separation in housing, transportation, employment, and medical care, it also resulted in separate and exceedingly unequal mental health care. The deeply held beliefs in racial hierarchy and the rampant permission to dehumanize people of color allowed segregated mental illness asylums to be misused as ways to contain, exploit, and criminalize African Americans. The book *Madness: Race and Insanity in a Jim Crow Asylum* by award-winning journalist Antonia Hylton depicts the racism that characterized mental health treatment for African Americans through the 20th century and links it to the protracted histories of slavery and the Jim Crow era (Hylton, 2024). Hylton tells the story of how the Crownsville Hospital in Maryland was built by Black men who were subsequently institutionalized there for most, if not all of their lives and reminds us of the unjust treatment of people of color. Crownsville became a work farm and holding place for men, women, and children with mental health challenges and for those whose behavior was often arbitrarily deemed unacceptable by persons in the White community. The story is heart-wrenching but should be required reading for understanding the historical basis of inequities and the opportunity for mental health for persons of color in America.

Equity information and data considerations must include an examination and understanding of the effects of centuries of denial of opportunity and unequal treatment, as well as information about the resistance to this imposed on humanity. The data and information that are collected at local, county, and state levels should support and document progress toward redressing and transforming systems and policies needed for ensuring equitable opportunities for well-being.

PROGRESS, INSPIRATION, AND HOPE

Those in the field of social justice and health equity advocacy say, as popularized by Dr. Martin Luther King Jr., "The arc of the moral universe is long, but it bends toward justice." After decades of work in the field of health equity, the arc is clearly bending, but slowly. Racial inequities remain a feature of the U.S. healthcare landscape 20 years after the former Institute of Medicine (now the National Academy of Medicine) published the landmark report, *Unequal Treatment: Confronting Racial and Ethnic Disparities in Health Care* (Smedley et al., 2003). This breakthrough publication unequivocally documented widespread racial and ethnic inequities in the quality of healthcare, even after accounting for access-related factors such as health insurance coverage. And yet, inequities persist.

KFF (formerly known as Kaiser Family Foundation) is an independent source for health policy research, polling, and journalism. KFF's mission is to serve as a nonpartisan source of information for policy makers, the media, the health policy community, and the public.

Therefore, it was not surprising that recent findings by KFF demonstrated that the experiences of people of color within the medical system were characterized by discrimination and perceived negative encounters (see **Figure 22.1**). KFF conducted a nationally representative survey based on responses from more than 6,000 adults, providing new data on individuals' experiences with racism and discrimination and the impacts of these experiences, both broadly and within racial and ethnic groups (Artiga et al., 2023). The good news is that the survey tapped into the voices of the populations directly affected by the racial hierarchy that persists within the nation's healthcare delivery system.

As America seeks to bring equity to communities and advance social justice, it is vital that healthcare, public health policy, advocacy, and budgeting decisions focus on racial equity and healing. For too long, racism has been the root cause of health disparities and inequities that have ravaged populations of color. The work of eliminating healthcare disparities requires data that help to provide a realistic understanding of the historic and contemporary factors that contribute to healthcare inequities. As recently as 1965, Black patients in some states could receive care only in separate and poorly funded medical facilities, where Black physicians were relegated to practice. When President Lyndon B. Johnson signed Medicare into law, more than 7,000 U.S. hospitals instantly became subject to the civil rights regulations set in Title VI. These hospitals could no longer discriminate and receive federal payments for medical services. However, the decades before that were periods of protracted defiance and resistance by the White population to racial and ethnic integration. Mental health treatment facilities, asylums, and institutions also remained segregated, with gross disparities in the quality of care that reflected the dehumanizing and discriminatory culture of the times (Largent, 2018). This dramatic change in 1965 was fully a hundred years after the end of the Civil War. That war ended more than 2 centuries of denial of the humanity of millions of enslaved African Americans. The permission to enslave and deny full human and civil rights was rooted in a cultural belief in a false hierarchy of human value. This belief was certainly embedded in medical and healthcare practices for centuries, creating a healthcare system that was and remains ill equipped to address the increased vulnerability to illness precipitated by myriad social factors known today as the social determinants of health.

Percentage of adults who had a negative healthcare experience in the past three years and it...

	Total	Hispanic	Black	Asian	AI/AN	White
...caused them to switch healthcare providers	18%	18%	23%	17%	26%	17%
...made them less likely to seek care	17%	18%	17%	15%	29%	16%
...caused their health to get worse	11%	10%	13%	8%	22%	10%
Any of the above	25%	26%	30%	21%	39%	24%

Figure 22.1 KFF study results of negative experiences with healthcare providers affecting health and healthcare use.

AI/AN, American Indian/Alaska Native.

Note: Black, Asian, and AI/AN groups include multiracial and single-race adults of Hispanic and non-Hispanic ethnicity. Hispanic group includes those who identify as Hispanic regardless of race. White includes single-race non-Hispanic adults only. Among adults who said they were treated unfairly or with disrespect by a provider, had a negative healthcare experience with a provider, or experienced a language-access challenge when getting or attempting to get healthcare in the past 3 years.

Source: Artiga, S., Hamel, L., Gonzalez-Barrera, A., Montero, A., Hill, L., Presiado, M., Kirzinger, A., & Lopes, L. (2023). *Survey on racism, discrimination and health: Experiences and impacts across racial and ethnic groups.* KFF. https://www.kff.org/racial-equity-and-health-policy/poll-finding/survey-on-racism-discrimination-and-health/

Systemic racism and unconscious bias continue to contribute to poor health outcomes for populations of color, with far too much suffering by individuals and their families, as infants die prematurely, chronic and infectious diseases ravage communities, and many lack health insurance.

The National Collaborative for Health Equity (NCHE) is a nonprofit based in Washington, DC. NCHE, formerly known as the Health Policy Institute, supports many of the programs and initiatives incubated over many years at the Health Policy Institute of the Joint Center for Political and Economics Studies while also working to develop new initiatives to advance the health and racial equity movement and to leverage its 20-plus–year history as a national convener and coalition builder. NCHE equips institutions and leaders from historically marginalized and excluded communities with tools to improve the social, economic, and environmental conditions that shape health. These tools include leadership development, policy analysis, data mining and analysis, and community organizing and mobilization to address a range of issues that are the ultimate determinants of health. It is vital to highlight some of the innovative strategies and research efforts that are happening around the country, which can be a source of inspiration and hope.

Heart disease remains the leading killer and crippler in America (Centers for Disease Control and Prevention [CDC], 2023). Cardiovascular disease disproportionately burdens communities of color as well. Working with other physicians at Brigham and Women's Hospital in Boston, Dr. Michelle E. Morse spearheaded a study determining that Black and Hispanic heart failure patients treated in the hospital's emergency department were disproportionately sent to general admissions rather than the specialty cardiology unit, where there are better patient outcomes (Eberly et al., 2019). In response, her leadership led to the creation of the Healing ARC (acknowledgment, redress, and closure) intervention and framework, a blueprint for race-conscious interventions that can eliminate racism in patient care. To achieve this, they have developed a computerized clinical decision support system (CDSS) to address racial health inequity. This race-conscious CDSS, which will be evaluated prospectively for impact, is designed to address two antiracism goals simultaneously: clinician education through acknowledgment of the racial inequity and redress for Black and Latinx patients (Wispelwey et al., 2022). This creative intervention helps to mitigate the risk of discriminatory treatment in the clinical setting by leveraging technology to reduce the risk of human error and could possibly be adapted for use in mental health clinical situations.

There is an increasing awareness of the need for effective interventions, which is demonstrated by the growing number of local jurisdictions that have declared racism to be a public health crisis or emergency, which is more than 250 as of this writing (American Public Health Association [APHA], 2023). These local efforts were accompanied by a courageous statement in 2021 by the then-new director of the CDC, Dr. Rochelle Walensky: "Racism is a serious public health threat that directly affects the well-being of millions of Americans. As a result, it affects the health of our entire nation" (Wamsley, 2021).

This nation, despite its racialized history and formation, has yet to follow the lead of more than 40 other countries in the world and implement a national Truth and Reconciliation Commission (TRC) effort. However, there has been leadership by the philanthropic sector to create and support local truth efforts. The W. K. Kellogg Foundation (WKKF) launched the TRHT effort in 2016 in funding partnership with several family, local, and regional philanthropic entities. TRHT, although informed by the TRC model, is a unique process designed to reflect, embrace, and address the unprecedented diversity and unparalleled racialized history of the United States. NCHE works with leaders across the country who are committed to improving health outcomes for communities of color by adapting the comprehensive TRHT framework to their ongoing efforts to achieve health equity. The

TRHT framework includes five pillars or areas of focus: narrative change, racial healing and relationship building, separation, law, and economy (see **Figure 22.2**).

In 2021, in partnership with the APHA and de Beaumont Foundation, NCHE curated a suite of briefs using the TRHT framework that documented policies and practices being implemented across the country to address racism and related social determinants of health and well-being. This set of briefs, Healing Through Policy, can be accessed through the NCHE, APHA, and de Beaumont websites. The Healing Through Policy partner organizations have convened a national community of practice composed of selected jurisdictions that have declared racism a public health crisis and are working to identify, plan actions, and disseminate the local steps needed to pass and implement a subset of curated policies and practices from the suite.

As the landmark study, *Unequal Treatment*, the Healing ARC cardiovascular innovation, and the KFF research (all cited previously) indicate, accurate data are required before effective interventions can be designed and implemented. At NCHE, we believe that data have to go beyond stating disparities and move toward shifting a narrative to create expectations of accountability for measurable progress. Brian Smedley, PhD, chief editor of *Unequal Treatment* and senior fellow at the Urban Institute, worked with leading health scholars and researchers to design the Health Opportunity and Equity (HOPE) Initiative, funded by the Robert Wood Johnson Foundation (RWJF). The HOPE Data Initiative tracks 28 indicators of child and adult health outcomes and the key resources that produce opportunities for health and well-being (see **Box 22.1**). What makes the HOPE Data Initiative unique is the "distance to goal" concept or the concept of focusing on the opportunity to achieve health equity (see **Figure 22.3**). State and/or population groups can use the HOPE Indicators as a tool to identify equity gaps, set equity goals, measure distance to goal, and drive equity action. With funding from the John D. and Catherine T. MacArthur Foundation and RWJF, NCHE is working with local jurisdictions in adapting the HOPE national and state-level indicators to support their local priorities and interventions. This community of practice, Leveraging HOPE to Transform Public Health Data Systems, currently includes representatives of 22 local jurisdictions.

Despite meaningful efforts over the past 4 decades, the diversity of the healthcare workforce in the United States is abysmal. As the general population becomes more diverse, this divide is even more consequential, as the KFF survey results indicate. KFF results also emphasize the importance of doctor–patient concordance. One recent study dramatically illustrates the importance of this as it relates to what is perhaps our nation's most persistent disparity—infant mortality (Greenwood et al., 2020). In the United States, Black newborns

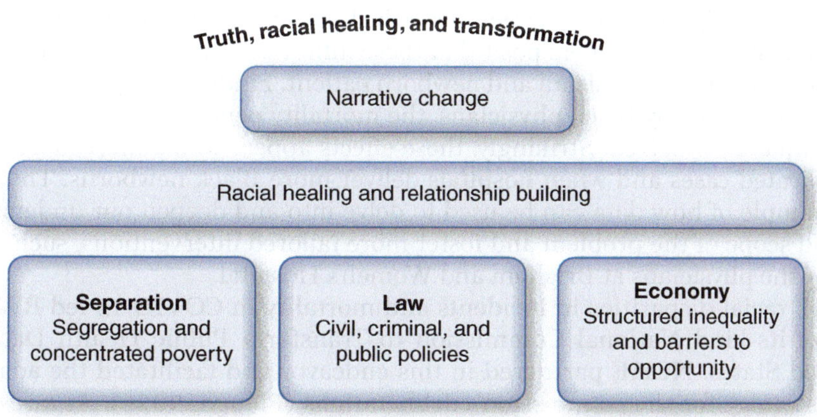

Figure 22.2 Pillars of the Truth, Racial Healing & Transformation framework.

Box 22.1 HOPE DATA: 28 INDICATORS OF HEALTH AND THE BROADER DETERMINANTS OF HEALTH ORGANIZED INTO FIVE DOMAINS

Health Outcomes

Adult Health Status
Mental Health Status
Child Health Status
Premature Mortality
Infant Mortality
Low Birth Weight

Socioeconomic Factors

Livable Income
Affordable Housing
Postsecondary Education
Connected Youth
Preschool Enrollment
Employment

Social Environment

Low Poverty Concentration
Low Murder Rate
Low Assault Rate
Low Rape Rate
Low Robbery Rate

Physical Environment

Homeownership
Housing Quality
Air Quality—Particulate Matter
Low Liquor Store Density
Food Security

Access to Healthcare

Access to Primary Care
Access to Psychiatric Care
Health Insurance Coverage
Affordable Healthcare
Usual Source of Care
Colorectal Cancer Screening

HOPE, Health Opportunity and Equity.

die at 3 times the rate of White newborns. Research examining 1.8 million hospital births in the state of Florida between 1992 and 2015 suggests that newborn–physician racial concordance is associated with a significant improvement in mortality for Black infants. A large body of work highlights disparities in survival rates across Black and White newborns during childbirth. The researchers posit that these differences may be ameliorated by racial concordance between the physician and newborn patient. Findings suggest that when Black newborns are cared for by Black physicians, the mortality penalty they suffer, as compared with White infants, is halved. Strikingly, these effects appear to manifest more strongly in more complicated cases and when hospitals deliver more Black newborns. This study is a powerful example of how data can be used to delve into and deepen our understanding of the scale and scope of the problem and foster more tailored interventions, such as the type described by the physicians at Brigham and Women's Hospital.

The stark racial disparities in incidents and mortality in COVID-19 led RWJF to create a first-of-its-kind National Commission to Transform Public Health Data Systems in the United States. NCHE partnered in this endeavor and facilitated the adaptation of the TRHT strategy for the commission's deliberations (Plough, 2022). As a result, the 17 recommendations for action by multiple sectors are organized around three key themes: (a) center health equity and well-being in narrative change, (b) prioritize equitable

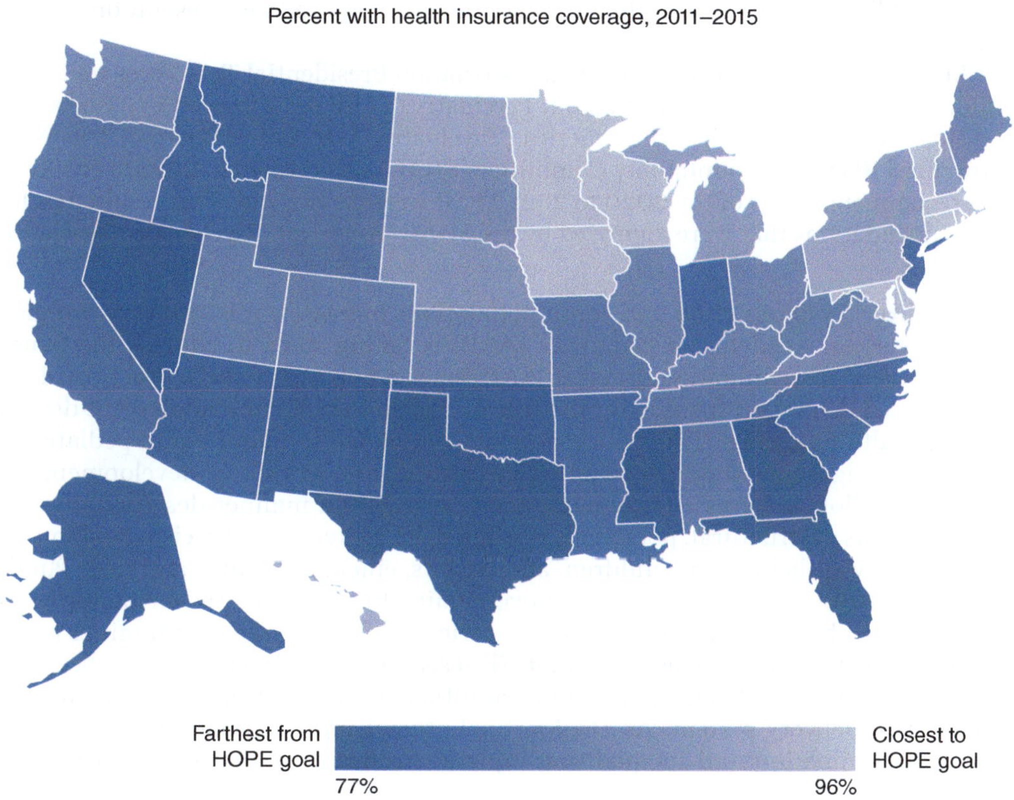

Figure 22.3 HOPE data: National progress to HOPE goal on health insurance coverage.
HOPE, Health Opportunity and Equity.

governance and community engagement, and (c) ensure public health measurement captures and addresses structural racism and other inequities. With continued support from RWJF, the commission's recommendations are influencing federal policy, public health organizations, and jurisdictions across the nation. Additional encouragement comes from the fact that leading health and medical organizations have moved beyond denial of the problem of racial health inequities and have begun the hard work of acknowledging how they have contributed to this problem and are beginning to take meaningful, corrective action. Examples include the following:

- In June 2021, the American Medical Association's (AMA) House of Delegates, representing their peers from all corners of medicine, voted to adopt guidelines addressing systemic racism in medicine, including discrimination, bias and abuse, including expressions of prejudice known as microaggressions. AMA recommended that healthcare organizations and systems use new guidelines to establish institutional policies that promote positive cultural change and ensure a safe, discrimination-free work environment (AMA, 2021).
- In October 2021, the American Psychological Association's (APA) Council of Representatives adopted a resolution because of their role in promoting, perpetuating, and failing to challenge racism, racial discrimination, and human hierarchy in the United States. Recognizing that many existing historical records and narratives have been centered in Whiteness, APA also concluded that it was imperative to capture oral history and the lived experiences of communities of color, so they commissioned

a series of listening sessions and surveys, which also informed their resolution (APA, 2021).

- In June 2020, the American Psychiatric Association Presidential Task Force to Address Structural Racism Throughout Psychiatry (TFSR) was formed by association president Dr. Jeffrey Geller. The American Psychiatric Association Board of Trustees' Structural Racism Accountability Committee (SRAC) was formed in 2021 to ensure the recommendations of the 2020 to 2021 TFSR were carried out. This resulted in 18 recommendations that were approved by the SRAC (American Psychiatric Association, 2023).

As the diversity of our child and youth populations increases, it is also very promising that the American Academy of Pediatrics (AAP) is taking steps to address the issue of racism and racial discrimination. In 2019, AAP issued a policy statement that provided an evidence-based document focused on the role of racism in child and adolescent development and health outcomes. This policy statement intended to better equip pediatricians to proactively engage in strategies to optimize clinical care, workforce development, professional education, systems engagement, and research in a manner designed to reduce the health effects of structural, personally mediated, and internalized racism, and improve the health and well-being of all children, adolescents, emerging adults, and their families (Trent et al., 2019). Achieving the goals of overcoming the legacy of racism and providing opportunities for health and well-being for historically marginalized communities require accelerated efforts. Comprehensively, the KFF research is extremely valuable because it gives the perspective of diverse populations and their lived experiences interacting with the healthcare delivery system. As Dr. Martin Luther King, Jr. admonished us, "Of all forms of discrimination and inequalities, injustice in health is the most shocking and inhumane."

SUMMARY

This chapter discusses three important considerations for centering equity and fairness in efforts to achieve optimal population mental health. The first is a paradigm shift from a focus on pathology and illness to one in which the expectation is mental health, well-being, and equitable opportunities for all population groups to achieve mental health. This requires an honest acknowledgment of historical and contemporary policies and practices that serve as barriers to achieving this goal at best, and as horrific denials of the humanity of marginalized groups at worst.

The second consideration is that the process of uncovering and applying equity-centered data must reflect the authentic voices of groups that have been marginalized by racial hierarchy. The lived experiences as well as the agency of these groups should be expressed and considered a valuable component of the data.

Finally, the context for the data, just as the context for defining expectations for mental health, must be positively oriented and grounded in the expectation of success. *Success* here is defined as the elimination of the false ideology of a hierarchy of human value. This antiquated notion of human value and racial hierarchy must be replaced with an understanding of the interrelated and interconnected as well as interdependent nature of humanity. Ultimately, human beings are relational creatures. Health, mental and physical, is dependent upon loving and nurturing relationships. Centuries of adherence to racial hierarchy can be viewed as centuries of organized lovelessness with destructive effects on human relationships at individual and societal levels.

The longest study of adult human development ever carried out in the United States concluded that strong relationships are the key to happiness and well-being. The book, *The Good Life: Lessons From the World's Longest Study on Happiness*, written by Robert

Waldinger and Marc Schulz, presents the results of the 80-year-long Harvard Study of Adult Development. The authors conclude that relationships are the most important factor for a happy life. Their scientific and empirical research illustrates the primacy of relationships as the key to health and well-being (Waldinger & Schulz, 2023). Strong relationships can be vital factors in mitigating the effects of racism and marginalization and are required for healing polarization and political divides.

The process of overcoming centuries of harm to mental and physical health through adherence to belief systems, policies, and practices of racial hierarchy requires continuous effort and a comprehensive strategy or approach. It also requires a commitment to documenting success and progress to maintain motivation and determination by a critical mass of people. The benefits that are derived from this type of collective effort are measurable. A new report, *The Power of Evidence to Drive America's Progress: A Decade of Results and Potential for the Future*, written by Dr. Christina Ciocca Eller of Harvard University, documents the successful results from bipartisan efforts to design and implement solutions to our nation's most pressing social challenges, such as long-standing disparities and inequities in access to the resources needed for achieving well-being (Eller, 2024). It is a good illustration of the power of documenting progress as part of our comprehensive strategies to create equity and fairness. This report is a road map for the practice of communicating measurable success. Imagine nations, jurisdictions, and states that have committed to ending racism and redressing and repairing the harms that have come from it over time. Imagining or visualizing this reality is the first step to achieving it. The data and information will help to create the narrative required for actualizing this reality.

DISCUSSION QUESTIONS

1. How important is addressing historic racial discrimination to present-day efforts to achieve mental health and well-being?
2. How can we approach mental health in a way that focuses on strengths and resilience rather than deficits, and what might this look like in practice?
3. What is the potential role for leading psychological and medical associations in the work of addressing racism to improve the health of marginalized populations?
4. How important is exposure to chronic stress as an impediment to mental well-being?
5. Why do you think communicating the evidence of progress and success is important in addressing racism as a public health crisis and achieving mental health equity?

REFERENCES

American Medical Association. (2021). *AMA adopts guidelines that confront systemic racism in medicine.* https://www.ama-assn.org/press-center/press-releases/ama-adopts-guidelines-confront-systemic-racism-medicine

American Psychiatric Association. (2023). *Board of trustees approved actions.* https://www.psychiatry.org/psychiatrists/diversity/governance/structural-racism-accountability-committee/board-of-trustees-approved-actions

American Psychological Association. (2021). *Apology to people of color for APA's role in promoting, perpetuating, and failing to challenge racism, racial discrimination, and human hierarchy in U.S.* https://www.apa.org/about/policy/racism-apology

American Public Health Association. (2023). *Racism is a public health crisis.* https://www.apha.org/Topics-and-Issues/Racial-Equity/Racism-Declarations

Artiga, S., Hamel, L., Gonzalez-Barrera, A., Montero, A., Hill, L., Presiado, M., Kirzinger, A., & Lopes, L. (2023, December 5). *Survey on racism, discrimination and health: Experiences and impacts across racial and ethnic groups.* KFF. https://www.kff.org/racial-equity-and-health-policy/poll-finding/survey-on-racism-discrimination-and-health/

Buchanan, L., Bui, Q., & Patel, J. K. (2020). Black Lives Matter may be the largest movement in U.S. history. *The New York Times.* https://www.nytimes.com/interactive/2020/07/03/us/george-floyd-protests-crowd-size.html

Burnham, M. A. (2023). *By hands now known: Jim Crow's legal executioners*. W.W. Norton & Company.

Centers for Disease Control and Prevention. (2023, May 15). *Heart disease facts*. https://www.cdc.gov/heart-disease/data-research/facts-stats/index.html

Compton, M. T., & Shim, R. S. (2015). *Social determinants of mental health*. American Psychiatric Publishing.

Eberly, L. A., Richterman, A., Beckett, A. G., Wispelwey, B., Marsh, R. H., Cleveland Manchanda, E. C., Chang, C. Y., Glynn, R. J., Brooks, K. C., Boxer, R., Kakoza, R., Goldsmith, J., Loscalzo, J., Morse, M., Lewis, E. F., Abel, S., Adams, A., Anaya, J., Andrews, E. H., ..., Zon, R. (2019). Identification of racial inequities in access to specialized inpatient heart failure care at an academic medical center. *Circulation: Heart Failure, 12*(11), e006214. https://doi.org/10.1161/circheartfailure.119.006214

Egerton, D. R. (2003). *Gabriel's Rebellion: The Virginia slave conspiracies of 1800 and 1802*. University of North Carolina Press.

Eller, C. C. (2024). The power of evidence to drive America's progress: A decade of results and potential for the future. *Results for America*. https://results4america.org/the-power-of-evidence-to-drive-americas-progress-a-decade-of-results-and-potential-for-the-future/

Hylton, A. (2024). *Madness: Race and insanity in a Jim Crow asylum*. Legacy Lit.

Greenwood, B. N., Hardeman, R. R., Huang, L., & Sojourner, A. (2020). Physician–patient racial concordance and disparities in birthing mortality for newborns. *National Academy of Sciences of the United States of America, 117*(35), 21194–21200. https://doi.org/10.1073/pnas.1913405117

Grier, W. H., & Cobbs, P. M. (1968). *Black rage*. Basic Books, Inc.

Guidi, J., Lucente, M., Sonino, N., & Fava, G. A. (2021). Allostatic load and its impact on health: A systematic review. *Psychotherapy and Psychosomatics, 90*(1), 11–27. https://doi.org/10.1159/000510696

Largent, E. A. (2018). Public health, racism, and the lasting impact of hospital segregation. *Public Health Reports, 133*(6), 715–720. https://doi.org/10.1177/0033354918795891

Lawrence, J. A., Kawachi, I., White, K., Bassett, M. T., Priest, N., Masunga, J. G., Cory, H. J., Mita, C., & Williams, D. R. (2022). A systematic review and meta-analysis of the everyday discrimination scale and biomarker outcomes. *Psychoneuroendocrinology, 142*, 105772. https://doi.org/10.1016/j.psyneuen.2022.105772

McEwen, B. S., & Stellar, E. (1993). Stress and the individual. Mechanisms leading to disease. *Archives of Internal Medicine, 153*(18), 2093–2101.

Murthy, V. H. (2023). *Together: The healing power of human connection in a sometimes lonely world*. Harper Wave, an imprint of HarperCollinsPublishers.

Plough, A. L. (2022). Charting an equity-centered public health data system. *Big Data, 10*(S1), S1–S2. https://doi.org/10.1089/big.2022.0203

Sapolsky, R. M. (1994). *Why zebras don't get ulcers: A guide to stress, stress related diseases, and coping*. W.H. Freeman.

Smedley, B. D., Stith, A. Y., & Nelson, A. R. (2003). *Unequal treatment: Confronting racial and ethnic disparities in health care*. National Academies Press.

Trent, M., Dooley, D. G., Dougé, J., Section on Adolescent Health, Council on Community Pediatrics, & Committee on Adolescence. (2019). The impact of racism on child and adolescent health. *Pediatrics, 144*(2), e20191765. https://doi.org/10.1542/peds.2019-1765

Waldinger, R., & Schulz, M. (2023). *Good life: Lessons from the world's longest scientific study of happiness*. Simon & Schuster.

Wamsley, L. (2021). *CDC director declares racism a public health threat*. https://www.npr.org/2021/04/08/985524494/cdc-director-declares-racism-a-serious-public-health-threat

Wispelwey, B. P., Marsh, R. H., Wilson, M., Mazimba, S., Heysell, S. K., Aisiku, I. P., Desai, A. S., Georges, C., & Morse, M. E. (2022). Leveraging clinical decision support for racial equity: A sociotechnical innovation. *NEJM Catalyst*. https://catalyst.nejm.org/doi/full/10.1056/CAT.22.0076

World Health Organization. (n.d.). *Constitution of the World Health Organization*. https://www.who.int/about/accountability/governance/constitution

23 INNOVATIVE MODELS FOR MENTAL HEALTH EQUITY

SERGIO AGUILAR-GAXIOLA, PIERLUIGI MANCINI, AND J. LLOYD MICHENER

LEARNING OBJECTIVES

After reading this chapter, readers will be able to:

- Distinguish two types of service delivery: the "waiting mode" and the "seeking mode."
- Describe the ecology of mental health care.
- Discuss the opportunities for innovation in mental health services.
- Identify key elements for advancing equity in mental health care.
- Describe models of innovative mental health care now underway.

INTRODUCTION

Disparities and inequities in mental health among ethnic, racial, and rural populations have been known for decades (Institute of Medicine, 2012). Although some progress is being made on reducing inequities, important mental health gaps persist (Williams & Cooper, 2019). The COVID-19 pandemic further increased inequities in access to and utilization of mental health services. In fact, a recent poll in California found that 52% of those who tried to make a mental health care appointment in the past year had trouble finding a mental health provider who would accept their insurance, and 55% reported unreasonable wait times for mental health treatment (Stremikis, 2024).

The recently released *2023 Update to Equity Action Plan* (U.S. Department of Health and Human Services [HHS], 2024a) outlines new commitments to advance health equity and makes prioritizing the behavioral health of underserved populations one of the priority areas to advance equity. In improving mental health equity, one of the greatest challenges is the need for innovation in models of care. Historically, healthcare, including mental health, has operated in a "waiting mode," in which people seek care after symptoms or signs of illness have developed and reached a concerning level (Aguilar-Gaxiola, 2023). When care is provided, all too often it is not aligned with the language and culture of those seeking help or not provided in a location and manner that are timely and easily accessible, or at a cost that is affordable. The result is inadequate care, loss of trust, and inequities in outcomes.

An alternative approach is a "seeking mode," in which mental health and healthcare groups go to the communities experiencing disparities and inequities, and listen and codesign services with members of the communities, including providing help as or even before symptoms appear (Aguilar-Gaxiola, 2023). In the words of HHS Secretary Xavier Becerra, "Nobody in this country should be left out or left behind because of where they live, their income, education level, or background" (HHS, 2024a). Such a paradigmatic shift to a health/mental health equity approach through meaningful community engagement and provision of services in new ways is underway in communities across the United States (Anaya et al., 2021; The California Endowment, 2020).

THE ECOLOGY OF MENTAL HEALTH CARE

Designing new systems of mental health care requires knowledge of the ecology of mental health care, especially within historically underserved communities (Thornicroft & Tansella, 2003; White et al., 1961).

Ground Zero: Community- and Home-Based Care

For many, mental health care begins outside formal medical settings. In communities and homes, people rely on a blend of traditional practices, home remedies, and advice from within their social networks (Gopalkrishnan, 2018). This layer is influenced by cultural beliefs and traditions, language barriers, and often a mistrust or unfamiliarity with the larger healthcare system (Kopelovich et al., 2021).

Primary Care and Mental Health

As people seek more formal access to health/mental health care, they often begin by seeking to access services from clinicians in their community, and quickly encounter barriers. These can include language barriers, lack of awareness among individuals and community groups about available services, cultural mismatches, and challenges related to healthcare access, coverage, and legal status (Aguilar-Gaxiola et al., 2012). For undocumented residents, fear of deportation or legal repercussions can be a significant deterrent to seeking care (Atkins et al., 2016).

Specialized Care and Referral Systems

When specialized care is needed, people face additional layers of complexity. Navigating referral systems may be daunting because of cultural and linguistic challenges, as well as unfamiliarity with bureaucratic processes (Vega et al., 2001). Moreover, the scarcity of culturally and linguistically responsive providers can lead to miscommunication, misdiagnoses, and misunderstandings, all of which affect the quality of care received (Atkins et al., 2016).

Hospital and Emergency Services

For those who face significant barriers in accessing primary or specialized care, hospitals and emergency department services often become the primary point of contact with the healthcare system. This often results in the use of emergency services for conditions that could have been managed or prevented through earlier intervention (Fleury et al., 2024). Those who require intensive care, such as inpatient services, may face days to months until a bed is available, requiring prolonged stays in emergency departments or hospitals that are not staffed to provide the care needed (Atkins et al., 2016).

Public Health and Policy

At the broadest level, the ecology of mental health care is significantly shaped by public health policies and societal attitudes. Policies that limit access to healthcare, along with social stigma and discrimination, have far-reaching effects on health outcomes (Purtle et al., 2020). Conversely, inclusive policies and community outreach programs can facilitate better access and improved health outcomes (Patel, 2022).

Cultural and Linguistic Responsiveness and Patient-Centered Care

An essential aspect of mental health care is the need for culturally and linguistically competent care (Aguilar-Gaxiola et al., 2012). Healthcare providers must be equipped with the skills and knowledge to understand and respect cultural differences in health beliefs and practices in the communities they serve. This includes language services and patient education strategies that are tailored to the unique needs and characteristics of communities and populations, particularly those that have been historically underserved (Miller et al., 2024).

Mental Health and Social Support

Mental health, and its connection to unmet social needs, is an area that often goes underaddressed in the healthcare system. Many community members, and especially immigrants, experience multiple stressors, including separation from family, adjustment to a new culture, and past traumas (Aguilar-Gaxiola et al., 2022). Further, inadequate safe jobs, housing, transportation, access to food, and interpersonal and community violence powerfully shape mental health needs that are not always amenable to interventions within healthcare systems (Centers for Disease Control and Prevention [CDC], 2011).

Integration of Traditional and Western Medicine

Finally, the ecology of mental health care for members of racially and ethnically diverse communities, and especially immigrants, should acknowledge and integrate the role of traditional medicine. For many, traditional practices are an integral part of their healthcare and of their lives (Vega et al., 1999). A healthcare system that respects and, where possible, incorporates these practices can improve the quality of care and patient satisfaction, as well as patient outcomes (Blignault & Kaur, 2020).

OPPORTUNITIES FOR ADVANCING MENTAL HEALTH EQUITY

In stark contrast to the traditional model of providing services in medical or institutional settings when people need mental health care are new models that begin by engaging with and listening to those in need. These new models also include codesigning services in ways they find helpful and that build on personal and community strengths and values (Aguilar-Gaxiola, 2023). This model of engaging and codesigning has deep roots and increasing recognition, including federal guidance on the *Principles of Community Engagement* (CDC, 2011) and more recent work by the National Academy of Medicine (NAM) on a conceptual model for community engagement and health equity (NAM, 2022).

Key elements of the NAM model are community engagement and the principles of engagement, which together lead to strengthened partnerships, expanded knowledge, improved health, thriving communities, and health equity through transformed systems for health (**Figure 23.1**).

Community engagement is an ongoing, evolving journey of listening attentively to and engaging in multidirectional communication with people about their care and other concerns that matter to them. The process should be engaging, enduring, and equitable to all who participate (Cottler et al., 2025). Building trust is an essential component of meaningful community engagement and requires

- showing up authentically, being honest, and committing to transparency;
- listening;
- following through on commitments; and
- committing to being trustworthy.

The transformative innovation of this model is that it begins with listening to and working with the community to codesign and implement solutions that are culturally and linguistically acceptable and will be trusted, rather than beginning with people who present with problems within a healthcare setting (NAM, 2022).

Once communities are engaged, the range of possible interventions expands beyond those historically used by professional groups and can encompass practices traditionally used in the communities, including photo novellas; caregivers such as doulas, promotors, and community health workers; alternative sites of care, such as schools and mobile vans; and delivery models from social media to digital and online services. Community group engagement may vary depending on the issues and concerns and may include, for instance,

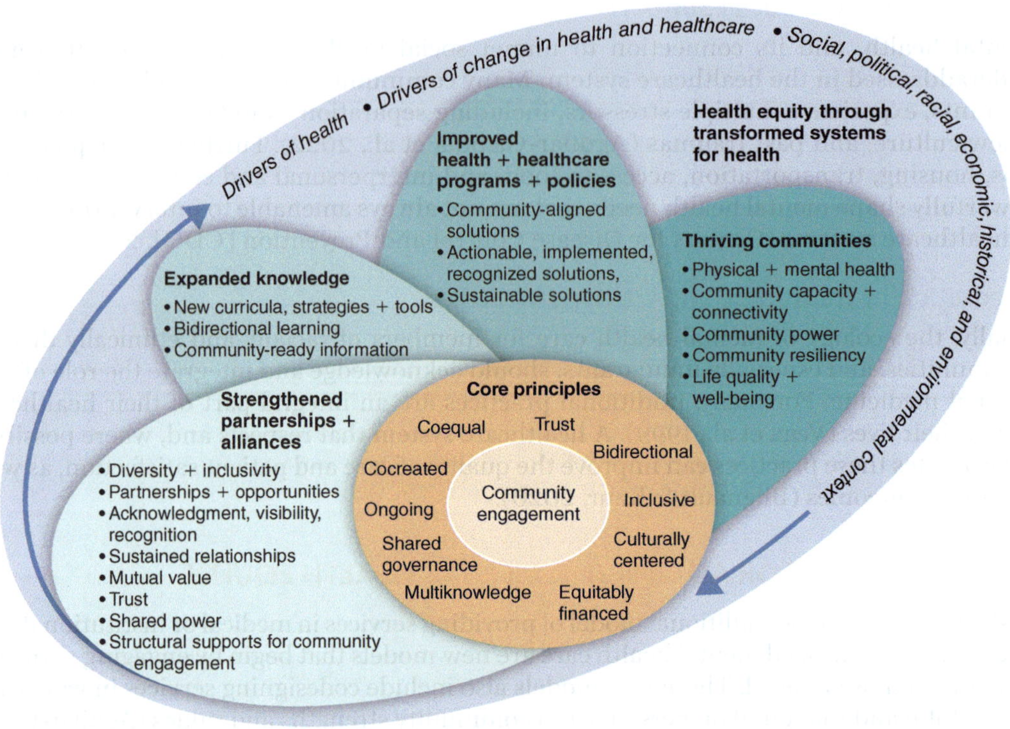

Figure 23.1 A conceptual model to advance health equity through transformed systems for health.
Source: National Academy of Medicine, Organizing Committee for Assessing Meaningful Community Engagement in Health & Health Care Programs & Policies. (2022). *Assessing meaningful community engagement: A conceptual model to advance health equity through transformed systems for health.* NAM Perspectives. https://doi.org/10.31478/202202c. Reproduced with permission from the National Academy of Sciences, Courtesy of The National Academies Press, Washington, DC.

youth groups who design youth- and peer-led services (NAM, 2022). States can have powerful roles in supporting and sustaining community engagement and mental health equity, such as California's Whole Person Care (WPC) Pilots (Tong & Hinton, 2022). WPC is a pilot program that aims to coordinate and integrate physical health, behavioral health, and social services for Medi-Cal (Medicaid) enrollees with complex needs. Federal support also is increasingly available, such as the Centers for Medicare & Medicaid Services Innovation in Behavioral Health Model, which supports interprofessional care teams in community-based behavioral health practices and coordinated behavioral, medical, and health-related social needs (Centers for Medicare & Medicare Services, 2024). Further, cross-federal agency coordination is underway, with the goal of using electronic data to identify health needs, leverage healthcare payment reforms, strengthen community health collaborations, and help trusted healthcare and community organizations provide timely and accurate information to individuals and organizations (NAM, 2024).

An important aspect of these innovations is the shift from single "best practices" that are assumed to be useful for all to a rich mix of services from which people, communities, and behavioral health providers can select and that evolve as needs change, partnerships strengthen, and trust develops (NAM, 2022). Advancing mental health equity requires listening, working together, and sustained partnerships. This is not an easy or quick process, as the following examples demonstrate.

Case Vignette 23.1 SOLANO COUNTY INTERDISCIPLINARY COLLABORATION AND CULTURAL TRANSFORMATION MODEL INNOVATIONS PROJECT

The Solano County (California) Innovations Project Interdisciplinary Collaboration and Cultural Transformation Model (ICCTM) was a multiphase community-initiated innovation project to address the social, environmental, and economic determinants of health for Filipino American, Latinx, and LGBTQ+ communities in Solano County, California (University of California [UC] Davis Health Center for Reducing Health Disparities, 2021). County staff, administrators, community-based organizations, clinicians, community members, and leaders representing their communities codesigned and were active participants in the planning, implementation, evaluation, and dissemination of the project's community-research findings and best practices.

Rooted in community engagement, the ICCTM comprised three phases, aligned with the CDC/National Institutes of Health *Principles of Community Engagement* (CDC, 2011).

- *Phase 1*: Conducting a cultural needs assessment, including key informant interviews, focus groups, community forums, and surveys of community stakeholders, cultural brokers, and leaders representing the populations with whom they shared their lived experiences in accessing and utilizing county mental health services. In this phase, members of the communities were considered the experts and worked to build trusting relationships with organizational and agency partners.
- *Phase 2*: Customizing a training program based on the nationally recognized culturally and linguistically appropriate services (CLAS) standards (HHS, 2024b) required trustworthiness to establish and strengthen a support network among a county, a university, community-based organizations, and members of the three communities of focus.
- *Phase 3*: By working as a collaborative, quality improvement action plans were created and implemented as interventions to transform a delivery-of-care system that is culturally, linguistically, and contextually appropriate to all un/underserved populations. Included was a comprehensive evaluation using a multidirectional communication/feedback approach to continue fine-tuning services and align with the cultural and linguistic needs of the communities of focus.

The ICCTM project had several positive outcomes, including the following: (a) The number of access line callers increased annually for all the communities of focus. (b) The proportion of patients reporting that their services were culturally responsive improved from baseline. Mental health service access calls among Solano County residents also increased (+29%) and were especially high among LGBTQ+ residents (+309%), who had traditionally underutilized services. (c) Members of Solano County's historically underserved communities were less likely to enter the mental health system of care through crisis services and more likely to enter through outpatient care. These trends reflected increased trust toward primary mental health care providers in Solano County and resulted in substantial cost savings. (d) Despite the COVID-19 pandemic, "joy in work" among mental health service providers remained high during the ICCTM project. About 98% of Solano County behavioral health staff reported that their job was meaningful, they felt they were positively influencing people's lives, and they were inspired from working with patients (UC Davis Health Center for Reducing Health Disparities, 2021).

Overall, this community-initiated, outcomes-driven, sustainability-guided project demonstrated that it is possible to address mental health disparities and advance mental health equity in access to care and utilization of services for historically underserved populations. The ICCTM project showed that counties where communities are included as decision-makers investing in transforming services, improving cultural and linguistic responsivity, and practicing high levels of meaningful community engagement are aligned to principles of community engagement. They also are essential to improving access to and utilization of mental health services for the three historically underserved/vulnerable communities of focus. Given the success of this project, the California Mental Health Services Oversight and Accountability Commission, funder of the ICCTM project, approved funding for a statewide learning collaborative to scale up the project's strategies to 161 representatives from 41 counties and public agencies, including the California Department of Health Services, Department of Public Health, and Behavioral Health Directors Association, which showed interest in and commitment to learning from the ICCTM model and possibly implementing it in their respective counties. The statewide learning collaborative included two 1-year-long training cohorts.

Case Vignette 23.2 THE UNIVERSITY OF CALIFORNIA DAVIS DIGITAL HEALTH EQUITY PROJECT

The University of California (UC) Davis Health Digital Health Equity Project (DHE) is a federally funded (Health Resources and Services Administration) project that focuses on bringing health services to where the communities are at the point of need. The goal is to improve access and continuity of care for vulnerable populations in California's Sacramento County and Sacramento Valley, using digital health and partnerships with Federally Qualified Health Centers (FQHCs) and other health organizations. The DHE partnered with the Mobilizing Organizations Via the Equitable Integration of Testing–Treatment through Unified Partnerships (MOVE IT UP^2) project, an innovative service delivery project that sought to increase access to COVID testing and treatment for historically underserved communities, with a focus on Latinx and Latinx farmworkers. The MOVE IT UP^2 project used mobile units that provided rapid testing to connect those who tested positive with on-the-spot, immediate virtual care at two FQHCs, bringing healthcare to where consumers were: at the point of need. This partnership aimed to advance health equity in historically underserved populations, connecting consumers with timely, accessible healthcare. DHE successfully increased test-to-treat services among vulnerable populations by building trust with communities and collaborating with trusted organizations (UC Davis Health Center for Reducing Health Disparities, 2024).

The second phase of DHE is ongoing and provides preventive health screenings for high blood pressure and for depression. The primary goal is to identify individuals who may benefit from remote patient monitoring for hypertension and/or from mental health services for depression. Once individuals are identified, they are connected with an FQHC partner for follow-up and continuity of care. DHE encourages continuity of care by using digital health navigators, who provide guidance and support, helping individuals navigate the complexities of managing high blood pressure and/or accessing mental health services. In our own data collected from Latinx participants in a rural community of the Sacramento Valley, as of November 2024, DHE has demonstrated an extensive reach:

- DHE held more than 150 community screening clinics where people live, work or congregate.
- 805 people have been screened for depression using the Patient Health Questionnaire-9 (PHQ-9):
  - Over 31% of participants had at least mild depressive symptoms (PHQ-9 score ≥5); over 39% did not have health insurance.
- 773 people have been screened for hypertension:
  - More than 270 people were identified as having high blood pressure at the mobile clinics; more than 75 patients (28%) did not have health insurance.

Case Vignette 23.3 THE CLUBHOUSE PROGRAM

In Atlanta, Georgia, the Clubhouse program has emerged as a pioneering approach in the field of adolescent support, demonstrating remarkable success in reducing substance abuse, decreasing involvement with juvenile justice, and improving educational outcomes among at-risk youth. This integrated analysis synthesizes findings from two distinct studies on the Clubhouse and Adolescent Substance Abuse Clubhouse programs highlighting the efficacy of tailored, community-specific interventions. By embracing a holistic and culturally responsive methodology, these programs have facilitated significant mental and academic advancements, underscoring the potential of comprehensive support models in fostering sustainable positive change (Strunz et al., 2015).

Adolescent substance abuse and its consequential impacts on criminal behavior and educational underachievement present significant challenges to societal well-being and individual development (Mulvey et al., 2010). The Clubhouse program, with its multifaceted approach, stands as a beacon of hope, offering a range of services designed to address these issues within diverse cultural and linguistic contexts. The Clubhouse program distinguishes itself through a holistic intervention strategy that encompasses comprehensive counseling, academic reinforcement, employment counseling, social engagement, and physical wellness that are delivered within the community. Designed to meet the unique needs of adolescents, particularly within the Latinx community, the program leverages bilingual and bicultural staff to provide culturally and linguistically responsive services. The integration of recreational amenities and aftercare services further ensures a supportive environment conducive to growth and recovery.

Program evaluation reports a significant decrease in substance abuse among participants, with the Clubhouse achieving a 50% cessation rate of alcohol and drug use shortly after admission. A further 30% of adolescents exhibited decreased substance use within 3 months, illustrating the program's robust impact on mitigating substance abuse behaviors (Strunz et al., 2015).

The intervention's influence extends to a marked reduction in delinquent behaviors, including decreased involvement with the Department of Juvenile Justice by as much as a 78% decrease in recidivism. By addressing the root causes of criminal behavior, the program has been instrumental in steering youth away from criminal activities and gang affiliation and fostering better decision-making and social integration.

A significant facet of the Clubhouse's success lies in its enhancement of educational outcomes. Structured tutoring and GED and SAT preparation courses have bolstered academic performance, leading to an increase in on-time graduations. The tailored support services have resulted in improved school attendance, grades, and higher graduation rates, all of which emphasize the program's comprehensive approach to addressing both psychological and practical needs.

The Clubhouse program exemplifies the efficacy of community-specific, culturally and linguistically responsive interventions delivered in the community to address adolescent substance abuse and its associated challenges. The integration of various support modalities, coupled with a focus on cultural and linguistic relevance, has proven effective in fostering holistic development and sustainable positive change. The longitudinal analysis underscores the program's capacity to empower participants with the skills and resilience necessary for successful adolescence navigation and future prospects.

The Clubhouse stands as a model of evidence-based practice and holistic intervention, demonstrating significant reductions in substance abuse and criminal behavior and improvements in educational attainment. Its success underscores the importance of tailored, comprehensive support services in empowering at-risk youth to overcome challenges and contribute meaningfully to society. As such, the Clubhouse program offers valuable insights into the development of effective adolescent support interventions that can be delivered in the community, paving the way for future initiatives aimed at fostering resilience and positive development among youth populations.

Case Vignette 23.4 DUKE–DURHAM PARTNERSHIPS FOR HEALTH

Improving health in Durham, North Carolina, has been a long-term shared goal of multiple partnerships among communities across Durham and the Duke University Health System (Cook et al., 2010; Michener et al., 2005, 2008). Common to all these initiatives has been the identification of the community as one not well served by current medical groups; multiple meetings in the community to listen to the needs, strengths, and preferences; and extended time for planning and codesigning as a multiple community. Duke and city and county groups worked together on these and included the development of plans for sustainability. The results are programs that are embedded in the community, providing services, including mental health, that the community identified, and in settings that reflect the community they serve. They have been sustained for almost 2 decades while the partnerships formed and lessons learned have been core elements to collaborative response to new challenges, such as COVID-19 (Viera et al., 2021). Examples include the following:

Duke: Southern High School Wellness Center

A school-based wellness center was codesigned with members of the local community, Southern High School and Durham Public Schools leadership, Duke Center for

Child and Family Health, Duke Children's Behavioral Health, Duke Family Medicine and Community Health, and Duke Health.

The goals of the Southern High School Wellness Center are to increase student access to primary care, including mental health; respond to immediate health needs; preempt adverse health and educational outcomes, including student absences from school; and reduce unnecessary use of the emergency department, missed parental work hours, and inadequate care. The wellness center is staffed by a physician assistant, nursing assistant, and family physician and provides urgent as well as ongoing care for chronic conditions and on-site counseling to evaluate and treat emotional health needs, with referrals to clinic-based or community providers if needed. Staff at the center also offer a relationship that children often lack—a continuing relationship with a healthcare provider. After hours care is available evenings, weekends, and school holidays at Duke Family Medicine.

Duke: Walltown Community Clinic

The Walltown Neighborhood Clinic, a joint program of Lincoln Community Health Center and the Duke Division of Community Health, was designed with the help of multiple community members and organizations, including the Walltown Neighborhood Association and the Walltown Neighborhood Ministries, to meet the needs of residents in the Walltown community. The clinic, located in a renovated house in the Walltown neighborhood, is easily accessible to any Durham resident needing care.

The Walltown Neighborhood Clinic staff includes a family physician, physician assistants, nurses, and an office manager. Services are available in English and Spanish and include preventive testing and counseling, well-baby checkups, care for acute illnesses, mental health assessments, and management of chronic health conditions.

LESSONS LEARNED

- Begin with listening and learning.
- Take time to build, establish, and maintain trust.
- Use a health equity lens.
- Share power; codesign or support community leaders and programs.
- Build on what is already present and working.
- Actively look for community assets, strengths, and resilience, and use them.
- Include mental health as a component of holistic health that embraces local culture.
- Plan, design, and implement for sustainability right from the beginning.

SUMMARY

Innovation in mental health care, especially for members of historically underserved communities, is not just possible, but is underway in communities across the United States. These programs are designed and co-led by members of the community, so they incorporate the culture and strengths of the community and include mental health as a core element of a larger, holistic approach to health. Healthcare systems and county and state agencies can help build and sustain these efforts, not by designing programs for the community, but by going to community groups and meetings, listening, and building on programs that are already present and trusted. This is not an easy process, especially for groups that have been focused on professional norms over meeting community needs. The greatest innovation toward advancing mental health equity is going in and listening to the community and building and sustaining community-led programs for health.

DISCUSSION QUESTIONS

1. In your community, which groups have the greatest needs, and what strengths and assets do they possess?
2. Where can members of your community look for advice and guidance on mental health issues?
3. What mental health care programs already exist in your community, and are they operating under the "seeking mode" of service delivery?
4. What are the main barriers to assessing mental health care services for members in your community, and what challenges do providers face in providing culturally and linguistically appropriate services?
5. Are there members of your community who can help mental health care providers begin engaging with the community in meaningful ways?

REFERENCES

Aguilar-Gaxiola, S. (2023). *Innovative models of service delivery: The "waiting" & "seeking" modes.* https://www.linkedin.com/posts/sergio-aguilar-gaxiola-md-phd-38239b17_leadership-message-innovative-service-delivery-activity-7097372102055350273-g8c3/

Aguilar-Gaxiola, S., Loera, G., Méndez, L., & Sala, M., Latino Mental Health Concilio, & Nakamoto, J. (2012). Community-defined solutions for Latino mental health care disparities project, Latino strategic planning workgroup population report. UC Davis. https://health.ucdavis.edu/media-resources/crhd/documents/pdfs/community-defined-solutions-for-latino-mental-health-care-disparities.pdf

Aguilar-Gaxiola, S., Medina-Mora, M. E., & Loera, L. (2022). Mental illness and substance use and migration traumatic exposures during high-risk migration. In S. Galea, C. K. Ettman, & M. H. Zaman (Eds.), *Migration and health* (pp. 98–107). The University of Chicago Press.

Anaya, Y. B., Hernandez, G. D., Hernandez, S. A., & Hayes-Bautista, D. E. (2021). Meeting them where they are on the web: Addressing structural barriers for Latinos in telehealth care. *Journal of the American Medical Informatics Association, 28*(10), 2301–2305. https://doi.org/10.1093/jamia/ocab155

Atkins, M. S., Rusch, D., Mehta, T. G., & Lakind, D. (2016). Future directions for dissemination and implementation science: Aligning ecological theory and public health to close the research to practice gap. *Journal of Clinical Child & Adolescent Psychology, 45*(2), 215–226. https://doi.org/10.1080/15374416.2015.1050724

Blignault, I., & Kaur, A. (2020). Integration of traditional and western treatment approaches in mental health care in Pacific Island countries. *Australasian Psychiatry, 28*(1), 11–15. https://doi.org/10.1177/1039856219859273

The California Endowment. (2020). *Building healthy communities: A decade in review.* https://www.calendow.org/learning/executive-summary/

Centers for Disease Control and Prevention. (2011). *Principles of community engagement.* https://stacks.cdc.gov/view/cdc/11699

Centers for Medicare & Medicare Services. (2024). *Innovation in behavioral health (IBH) model.* https://www.cms.gov/priorities/innovation/innovation-models/innovation-behavioral-health-ibh-model

Cook, J., Michener, J. L., Lyn, M., Lobach, D., & Johnson, F. (2010). Community collaboration to improve care and reduce health disparities. *Health Affairs, 29*(5), 956–958. https://doi.org/10.1377/hlthaff.2010.0094

Cottler, L. B., Prue, C. E., Holliday, C. S., McCloskey, D. J., McDonald, M. E., Cohen, I. P., Aguilar-Gaxiola, S., & Eder, M. (2025, January). Community engagement—Definitions and key concepts. *Principles of community engagement* (3rd ed., pp. 14–36, Chapter 1). Agency for Toxic Substances and Disease Registry. https://hsc.unm.edu/population-health/_documents/principles-of-community-engagement_3rd-edition.pdf

Fleury, M. J., Cao, Z., & Grenier, G. (2024). Emergency department use among patients with mental health problems: Profiles, correlates, and outcomes. *International Journal of Environmental Research and Public Health, 21*(7), 864. https://doi.org/10.3390/ijerph21070864

Gopalkrishnan, N. (2018). Cultural diversity and mental health: Considerations for policy and practice. *Frontiers in Public Health, 6*, 179. https://doi.org/10.3389/fpubh.2018.00179

Institute of Medicine. (2012). *Healthy people 2010: How far have we come in reducing health disparities?* The National Academies Press (pp. 7–30). https://doi.org/10.17226/13383

Kopelovich, S. L., Monroe-DeVita, M., Buck, B. E., Brenner, C., Moser, L., Jarskog, L. F., Harker, S., & Chwastiak, L. A. (2021). Community mental health care delivery during the COVID-19 pandemic: Practical strategies for improving care for people with serious mental illness. *Community Mental Health Journal, 57*, 405-415. https://doi.org/10.1007/s10597-020-00662-z

Michener, J. L., Champagne, M. T., Yaggy, D., Yaggy, S. D., & Krause, K. M. (2005). Making a home in the community for the academic medical center. *Academic Medicine: Journal of the Association of American Medical Colleges, 80*(1), 57–61. https://doi.org/10.1097/00001888-200501000-00014

Michener, J. L., Yaggy, S., Lyn, M., Warburton, S., Champagne, M., Black, M., Cuffe, M., Califf, R., Gilliss, C., Williams, R. S., & Dzau, V. J. (2008). Improving the health of the community: Duke's experience with community engagement. *Academic Medicine: Journal of the Association of American Medical Colleges, 83*(4), 408–413. https://doi.org/10.1097/ACM.0b013e3181668450

Miller, A. B., Davis, S. H., Mulder, L. A., Winer, J. P., Issa, O. M., Cardeli, E., & Ellis, B. H. (2024). Leveraging community-based mental health services to reduce inequities for children and families living in United States who have experienced migration-related trauma. *Psychological Trauma: Theory, Research, Practice, and Policy, 16*(Suppl 2), S426–S434. https://doi.org/10.1037/tra0001392

Mulvey, E. P., Schubert, C. A., & Chasin, L. (2010). Substance use and delinquent behavior among serious adolescent offenders. U.S. Department of Justice (DOJ), *Juvenile Justice Bulletin*, 1–15. https://www.ojp.gov/pdffiles1/ojjdp/232790.pdf

National Academy of Medicine. (2022). Organizing committee for assessing meaningful community engagement in health & health care programs & policies: Assessing meaningful community engagement: A conceptual model to advance health equity through transformed systems for health. *NAM Perspectives*. Commentary, National Academy of Medicine. https://doi.org/10.31478/202202c

National Academy of Medicine. (2024). Collaborative short-term action to advance America's health. https://nam.edu/event/collaborative-action-for-americas-health-short-and-long-term-strategies-across-public-health-health-systems-and-social-services/

Patel, S. (2022). Embedded healthcare policing. *UCLA Law Review, 69*. UCLA School of Law, Public Law Research Paper No. 22-28. Available at SSRN: https://ssrn.com/abstract=4245989

Purtle, J., Nelson, K. L., Counts, N. Z., & Yudell, M. (2020). Population-based approaches to mental health: History, strategies, and evidence. *Annual Review of Public Health, 41*, 201–221. https://doi.org/10.1146/annurev-publhealth-040119-094247

Stremikis, K. (2024). Top five takeaways from CHCF's 2024 California Health Policy Poll. *The CHCF blog*. https://www.chcf.org/blog/top-takeaways-california-health-policy-poll/#related-links-and-downloads

Strunz, E., Jungerman, J., Kinyua, J., & Frew, P. M. (2015). Evaluation of an assertive continuing care program for Hispanic adolescents. *Global Journal of Health Science, 7*(5), 106–116. http://dx.doi.org/10.5539/gjhs.v7n5p106

Thornicroft, G., & Tansella, M. (2003). *What are the arguments for community-based mental health care?* World Health Organization. Regional Office for Europe. https://iris.who.int/handle/10665/363767

Tong, M., & Hinton, E. (2022). *California efforts to address behavioral health and SDOH: A look at whole person care pilots*. https://www.kff.org/mental-health/issue-brief/california-efforts-to-address-behavioral-health-and-sdoh-a-look-at-whole-person-care-pilots/

UC Davis Health Center for Reducing Health Disparities. (2021). *Solano County Interdisciplinary Collaboration and Cultural Transformation Model (ICCTM) innovations project*. https://health.ucdavis.edu/media-resources/crhd/documents/pdfs/icctm-final-report-2021-09-13.pdf

UC Davis Health Center for Reducing Health Disparities. (2024). MOVE IT UP^2—Mobilizing organizations via the equitable integration of testing–treatment through unified partnerships. https://health.ucdavis.edu/crhd/archived-projects/move-it-up

U.S. Department of Health and Human Services. (2024a). *HHS releases 2023 update to equity action plan, outlines new commitments to advance equity*. https://www.hhs.gov/about/news/2024/02/14/hhs-releases-2023-update-equity-action-plan-outlines-new-commitments-advance-equity.html

U.S. Department of Health and Human Services. (2024b). *National culturally and linguistically appropriate services standards* https://thinkculturalhealth.hhs.gov/clas/standards

Vega, W. A., Kolody, B., & Aguilar-Gaxiola, S. A. (2001). Help-seeking for mental health problems among Mexican Americans. *Journal of Immigrant Health, 3*(3), 133–140. https://doi.org/10.1023/A:1011385004913

Vega, W. A., Kolody, B., Aguilar-Gaxiola, S., & Catalano, R. (1999). Gaps in services utilization by Mexican Americans with mental health problems. *American Journal of Psychiatry, 156*(6), 928–934. https://doi.org/10.1176/ajp.156.6.928

Viera, A. J., Barnett, J., Case, M., Epling, C., Halstater, B., Lyn, M., Martinez-Bianchi, V., Ragsdale, J., Railey, K., Said, K., Sawin, G., Spotts, H., Vaughn, J., Weigle, N., & Michener, J. L. (2021). Partnerships to care for our patients and communities during COVID-19. *Journal of the American Board of Family Medicine: JABFM, 34*(5), 1003–1009. https://doi.org/10.3122/jabfm.2021.05.210091

White, K. L., Williams, T. F., & Greenberg, B. G. (1961). The ecology of medical care. *The New England Journal of Medicine, 265*, 885–892. https://doi.org/10.1056/NEJM196111022651805

Williams, D. R., & Cooper, L. A. (2019). Reducing racial inequities in health: Using what we already know to take action. *International Journal of Environmental Research and Public Health, 16*, 606. https://doi.org/10.3390/ijerph16040606

24 ADVANCING MENTAL HEALTH EQUITY THROUGH COMMUNITY ENGAGEMENT

KISHA BRAITHWAITE, EBONI C. WINFORD, SHAAKIRA A. FORD, AND RONJONETTE O'BANNON

LEARNING OBJECTIVES

After reading this chapter, readers will be able to:

- Delineate psychosocial, sociocultural, and environmental contributors to mental health disparities.
- Discern key components of community engagement for diverse communities.
- Elucidate operative aspects of community-engaged participatory research.
- Express the effectiveness of culturally centered prevention and integrated care to help reduce mental health disparities and inequities.
- Demonstrate the roles of effective communication, leadership, and partnership development in supporting the advancement of mental health equity.

INTRODUCTION

It is imperative to critically examine the multisectoral and comprehensive methods that may be used to advance mental health equity. One promising foundational philosophy that should be utilized is community engagement approaches. This is particularly significant for underresourced and vulnerable communities (Andrasik et al., 2021; Mitchell & Chavous, 2021). Healthy People 2030's framework includes a vision in which all people can achieve their full potential for health and well-being across the life span and five overarching goals: (a) attain healthy, thriving lives and well-being free of preventable disease, disability, injury, and premature death; (b) eliminate health disparities, achieve health equity, and attain health literacy to improve the health and well-being of all; (c) create social, physical, and economic environments that promote attaining the full potential for health and well-being for all; (d) promote healthy development, healthy behaviors, and well-being across all life stages; and (e) engage leadership, key constituents, and the public across multiple sectors to take action and design policies that improve the health and well-being of all (U.S. Department of Health and Human Services [HHS], n.d.).

Given the significance of mental health disparities that plague underserved, at-risk, vulnerable, and/or underresourced communities, it is imperious that attention be given to community-engaged strategies that offer connection and ongoing commitment to uplifting quality comprehensive healthcare (Dawes et al., 2023; Gadomski et al., 2010). Addressing the multifaceted mental health needs of ethnically and culturally diverse individuals in the United States is a complex issue that requires inventive community-centered strategies to reduce risk factors and buttress protective factors to promote greater well-being among individuals, families, and communities. With growing diversity concerning various ethnicities and nationalities and with significant changes in the constellation of multiple risk factors that can influence health outcomes, it is important that strategic efforts are delineated that encourage better access to primary care, focused community-based programs, multidisciplinary clinical and translational research methodologies, and mental health policy advocacy initiatives that may improve individuals' longevity and quality of life (Lewis et al., 2023; Williams et al., 2019). The various issues with engaging racial and ethnic minorities into mental health treatment are multifactorial and occur at individual, organizational, and systemic levels.

This chapter focuses on deconstructing some of the key community engagement issues that may impact mental, emotional, and behavioral health elements to consider when working with ethnically, culturally, and linguistically diverse populations. Specifically, the learning objectives provided at the beginning of the chapter provide a framework for understanding the aims to be achieved.

UNDERSTANDING MENTAL HEALTH DISPARITIES AND INEQUITIES

In the aim to reduce mental health disparities to help encourage equity in healthcare for diverse communities, it is important to comprehend some of the unique issues that impact Black, Indigenous, people of color (BIPOC) populations. BIPOC groups have long been a pervasive concern in both theory and practice for healthcare professionals and extensively documented by researchers and advocates (Brave Heart et al., 2016; Garcia et al., 2020). These scholars have emphasized systemic racial and ethnic inequalities that persistently impact the mental and emotional well-being of minoritized communities.

FRAMING HEALTH DISPARITIES AND INEQUITIES

Whereas scientific literature is vast on racial and ethnic disparities, so are the varying definitions and interpretations. The framework for this chapter is posited by Berger and Miller (2010):

> Health disparities are systematic, plausibly avoidable health differences adversely affecting socially disadvantaged groups; they may reflect social disadvantage, but causality need not be established. This thought, grounded in ethical and human rights principles, focuses on the subset of health differences reflecting social injustice, distinguishing health disparities from other health differences.

The Heckler report (1985), published by the HSS Secretary's Task Force on Black and Minority Health, was the first comprehensive analysis of the chronic health issues faced by ethnic and racial minorities, providing a contextual explanation and recommendations to support people of color in the areas of access to care, training of health providers, service quality, and treatment outcomes. More than 3 decades later, social scientists remain committed to examining health disparities from a psychosocial, sociocultural, and environmental perspective. Scholars have defined disparities as racial and ethnic differences that do not arise from variable clinical needs or appropriateness of treatment milieu. These disparities contribute to increased disability, disease, and death among racial and ethnic minority populations (LaVeist et al., 2011).

When defining health inequities, we refer to the World Health Organization's (2018) observation that there are systematic differences in the health status of various population groups that highlight disparities between the health outcomes of White individuals and people of color. These differences include deviations in the span of life, quality of life, and social and emotional well-being. Such inequities have considerable social and economic consequences, affecting individuals and communities for generations, as indicated in **Figure 24.1**.

THE PREVALENCE OF MENTAL HEALTH DISPARITIES

According to the National Institute of Mental Health (2023), one in five adults report living with a mental health disorder. Although the rates of mental health disorders are similar for White and BIPOC groups, the research shows that people of color with mental health disorders are more likely to suffer from long-lasting disabling symptoms. Further research suggests that in the past year, fewer Asian adults, Latinx adults, and Black or African American adults received mental health services for mental health disorders compared with White or multiracial adults. Among the different racial or ethnic groups, Asian adults were the least likely to receive mental health services (Substance Abuse and Mental Health Services Administration, 2022).

Since 2003, the Agency for Healthcare Research and Quality has submitted an annual report summarizing racial and ethnic disparities. These disparities impact access to care, service quality, and healthcare outcomes. Consequently, the 2023 report expanded on the complexities of mental health disparities by highlighting the increase in racial and ethnic diversity in the United States and the negative impact of COVID-19 on already vulnerable populations. For example, among racial and ethnic groups, Native Hawaiian/Pacific Islander (NHPI), Latinx, and Black populations were more likely to die from COVID-19 than other groups. NHPI people were less likely to get infected but more likely to die if infected. Latinx and Black people were more likely to get infected but exhibited similar risks of dying if infected as White people. Native Hawaiian persons were both more likely to get infected and more likely to die if infected.

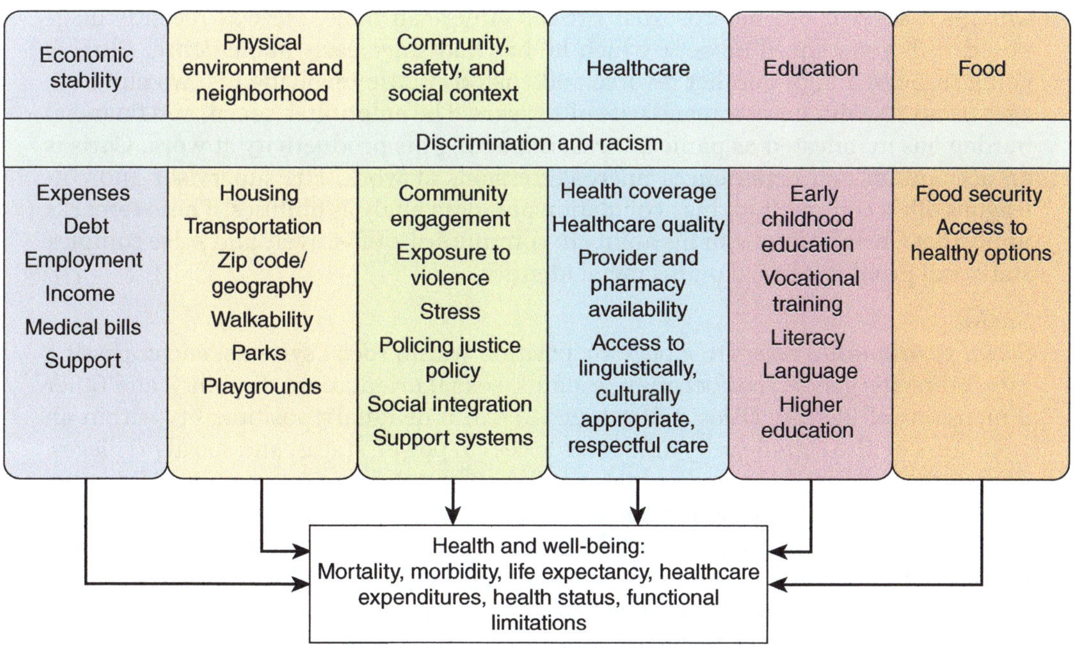

Figure 24.1 Health disparities are driven by social and economic inequities.

Source: Braithwaite, R. L., Akintobi, T. H., Blumenthal, D. S., & Langley, W. M. (2020). *The Morehouse model: How one school of medicine revolutionized community engagement and health equity*. Johns Hopkins University Press.

A BRIEF HISTORY OF THE PERSON-IN-ENVIRONMENT PERSPECTIVE

The disparities in mental health are more acute among racial and ethnic minorities, and this may be explained by the availability of fewer resources compared with White individuals (Yearby, 2020). The person-in-environment (PIE) model is an insightful tool in addressing these disparities. Mary Richmond's work in the early 1900s underscored the link between poverty, societal exclusion, and health inequalities. In 1889, she acknowledged the role of the Charity Organization Societies (COS) in tackling the societal issues brought on by urbanization and industrialization across various U.S. cities. Her engagement with COS led to her advocating for reforms that highlighted the importance of structural influences on resource availability within communities, thereby impacting the health and welfare of disadvantaged populations.

EXPLORING THE UNDERPINNINGS OF THE PERSON-IN-ENVIRONMENT APPROACH

Delineating nuances regarding interactive processes is often complex. There are varying perspectives and approaches to PIE (Debek, 2014; Rogge & Cox, 2001). However, at its core, the PIE perspective is a cornerstone in understanding human behaviors through an individual (micro) and systems (macro) lens. It is imperative to examine case vignettes that represent real-life experiences of individuals that reflect the complex intersectional systemic issues.

Case Vignette 24.1 ANXIETY IN REAL: CHRIS'S STORY

Chris is a 45-year-old heterosexual African American male. He was recently diagnosed with generalized anxiety, which he has had since early adolescence. Chris is going through a high-conflict divorce and custody battle involving his two children, ages 8 and 10, with his estranged wife of 13 years. The emotional, social, and financial burden has manifested as panic attacks, impacting his productivity at work. Chris is an accountant and experiences microaggressions at work. His supervisor and colleagues often comment on his articulation and data analysis abilities. These remarks imply that Chris is unique in his ability to communicate effectively and solve complex statistical problems based on his racial identity.

Social

Social positionality refers to a person's position within social systems, encompassing race, ethnicity, gender, socioeconomic status, sexual orientation, disability, and other dimensions of identity (Ríos & Patel, 2023). An individual's positionality within an environment also significantly influences access to power, status, and social privileges. Therefore, when assessing individuals within social systems, we recognize PIE as a reciprocal integrative–transactional process. As an example, consider the case vignette of Chris. When examining the social underpinnings of an individual's life, we must include aspects of their relational dynamics, support systems, education, employment and job security, and societal messages related to identity. In Chris's case, it is essential to consider the historical and current context of relational interactions with his family.

Research has consistently found that married couples experience better mental health outcomes and greater socioeconomic stability than their unmarried counterparts (DeMaris & Oates, 2022). Yet, African American couples are at greater risk of divorce than either Latinx or White marriages (Bulanda & Brown, 2007). Although there are a variety of factors that contribute to the higher rates of dissolution of African American marriages, sociocultural factors play a significant role in shaping identity and the mental health well-being of individuals following a traumatic event such as divorce (Ngambi et al., 2023).

In contrast to public belief and discourse regarding Black families, many African American communities recognize marriage as a societal status symbol of integrity and stability (duCille, 2018). The ending of Chris's marriage represents the loss of an intimate partner relationship and identity that was connected to the roles and responsibilities established within the union. The uncertainties and losses of the marriage and the engagement with the family court system to maintain fair and equal access to his children can be a source of significant stress (Andreasson & Johansson, 2019). For many African American men, the court systems may be fraught with systemic biases, discrimination, and other inequalities that are demeaning and question their capabilities as fathers. The misconceptions about divorced fathers, particularly men of color, can negatively impact their ability to maintain healthy connections with their children, leading to a prolonged state of mental and emotional turmoil affecting mental health well-being and ability to effectively co-parent (Andreasson & Johansson, 2019; Nielsen, 1999).

Economic

Oppressive frameworks, such as racism and discrimination, underpin the structural inequities that influence racial and ethnic groups' socioeconomic status. In recent years, the cost of microaggressions in the workplace has received increased awareness and acknowledgment from administrators (Fattoracci & King, 2023). Microaggressions are the everyday slights, insults, put-downs, invalidations, and offensive behaviors that people experience in daily interactions with generally well-intentioned individuals who may be unaware that they have engaged in demeaning ways (Sue et al., 2007).

In a 10-part *Washington Post* series, Michelle Singletary discussed common misconceptions involving race and inequality. In it, she speaks directly to White people about overly complimenting Black people for ordinary deeds and how this is harming their overall health. Intentional or not, microaggressions are derogatory and perpetuate stereotypes of racial and ethnic minorities. In the case of Chris, it is vital to remember that Black Americans disproportionately experience microaggressions. In a recent study, the Gallup report shared that across all types of microaggressions, African Americans were more likely than White, Hispanic, and Asian Americans to report experiencing microaggressions. Over time, these microaggressions can accumulate, causing ongoing psychological stress that may impact Chris's mental health, reinforce social marginalization, and potentially negatively affect future earnings and ability to retain his attorney for his ongoing custody case (Hall & Fields, 2015).

Environmental

In recent years, the intersection of environmental issues within the PIE perspective has garnered increasing attention. However, this concerning trend has highlighted bias and stereotypes that perpetuate false narratives regarding racial and ethnic minorities and persons with low-income engagement concerning environmental matters. Researchers have shed light on these misconceptions and stereotypic representations of who can be an environmentalist. For example, it is documented that the groups that are most concerned about the environment are persons identifying as Latinx, Asian American, and African American. Conversely, these racial/ethnic groups are misperceived to be the least concerned about the environment (Pearson et al., 2018; see **Figure 24.2**).

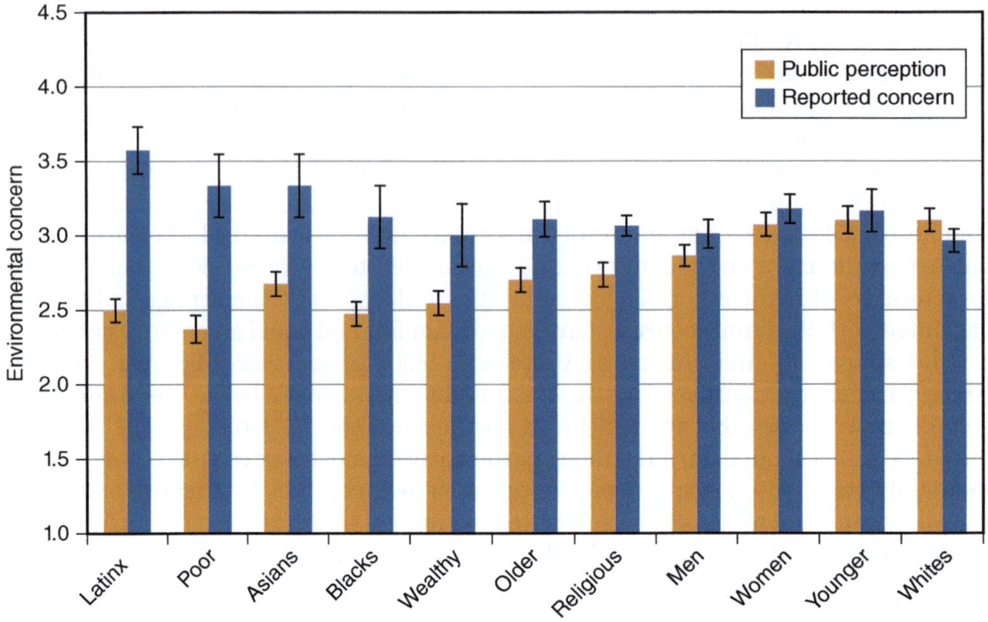

Figure 24.2 Perception and concern reported for the environment across racial and ethnic groups.
Source: Pearson, A. R., Schuldt, J. P., Romero-Canyas, R., Ballew, M. T., & Larson-Konar, D. (2018). Diverse segments of the US public underestimate the environmental concerns of minority and low-income Americans. *Proceedings of the National Academy of Sciences of the United States of America, 115*(49), 12429–12434. https://doi.org/10.1073/pnas.1804698115

These misconceptions not only undermine the environmental consciousness of diverse narratives, but reflect the broader systemic barriers related to health equity. Furthermore, healthcare professionals and policy analysts must expand the discourse related to inclusivity of environmental hazards. Issues concerning climate change and air and water pollution are common environmental threats against our ecosystem and communities (Raihan, 2023). However, people of color and low-income individuals underscore their disproportionate vulnerability to exposure to environmental harm, such as aging infrastructure, community violence, limited access to green spaces, and reduced access to specialized healthcare services (Lewis et al., 2020).

When considering the PIE perspective and environmental factors, it is crucial to recognize that Chris is navigating through multiple life challenges, one of which is a pervasive public health issue: the limited access to mental health care services for racial and ethnic minorities. This limitation is particularly acute for Black men, who are statistically less likely to engage in psychotherapy because of bias within healthcare systems, societal stigma, mistrust surrounding mental health, and cultural norms that may have the same surrounding psychological vulnerability or help-seeking (Turner et al., 2024).

These barriers are compounded when it comes to psychotropic medication. The historical basis of structural racism and African American men's mental health is diagnostically complex. Because of structural racism, Black men are less likely to adhere to recommendations for medication routines that support mental health but are at an increased risk of suicide (Adams & Thorpe, 2023). The reluctance of medication management may stem from a deep-rooted mistrust of medical institutions, which historically have not always acted in the best interest of racial and ethnic minority populations (Richmond et al., 2023). Additionally, cultural beliefs about self-reliance and masculinity may dissuade Black men from accepting such treatments. For Chris, these factors could severely hinder his ability to receive and accept comprehensive mental health care during a period when he is most in need of support (Bauer et al., 2022). This could further increase his risk for long-term disability or other mental health needs.

The PIE perspective provides a comprehensive framework for comprehending, evaluating, and addressing mental health inequities. We analyzed the intersections of identities and lived experiences through the story of Chris, exploring the complex interplay between mental health and people of color in a broader societal context. By advocating for inclusive and equitable policies and practices, we can challenge oppressive systems and institutions.

PRINCIPLES OF COMMUNITY-BASED PARTICIPATORY RESEARCH

The central focus of community-based participatory research (CBPR) is to find equity in collaborations by joining the strengths of researchers and communities to eliminate health disparities and inequities (Gilbert et al., 2023; Suarez-Balcazar et al., 2020). Conducting meaningful scientific research to improve overall health and wellness of individuals, families, and communities has not historically always allowed for positive pathways forward. CBPR, in which researchers and community groups work together as equal partners, acts as a mechanism to include communities in research and to ensure equity in research endeavors. Generally, CBPR is a promising method; yet, adequately engaging a racially and ethnically diverse population requires elements to build trust and "buy-in" (Argyriadis et al., 2022; Varcarolis & Fosbre, 2020). Moreover, CBPR engenders approaches that emphasize community–academic partnerships with shared leadership in the planning, implementation, and evaluation of interventions (Akintobi et al., 2023; Sánchez et al., 2021). In 2008, the National Institutes of Health highlighted CBPR as a core strategy in eliminating disparities (Dankwa-Mullan et al., 2010).

CBPR is an approach to research that is rooted in the principles of equity, justice, and fairness and that aims to ensure that all the partners in a research project obtain what they need from the research project (Akintobi et al., 2018; Yau et al., 2024). The evolution and application of CBPR in communities have led to increased research participation and community ownership. Conceptually, it is anticipated that through using CBPR, outcomes will include not only answering a research question and reaping associated benefits, but also addressing community-identified social, economic, or policy priorities. One of the tenets of CBPR is the principle that researchers who want to conduct effective health research must invest time and resources in building partnerships with community-based organizations or neighborhood residents who are gatekeepers to establishing and maintaining community buy-in, ownership, and sustainability. Ideally, community residents are equal or senior partners throughout the research process (Holden et al., 2016).

Previous meta-analyses and reviews have been conducted to understand CBPR, provide practical recommendations in its use, and evaluate its research value, impact on health status and systems change, and contextual determinants of CBPR success, which include the ability to collaboratively navigate conflict, negotiate, and build consensus (Jones et al., 2020). Among the results of successful partnerships are culturally and contextually tailored research, enhanced participant recruitment, and project sustainability. According to scholars at Yale School of Medicine, community engagement in research has enabled academic researchers to

- increase the validity within the study by improving accuracy of measurements,
- conduct research that can be implemented in partnership with the studied communities, and
- design meaningful and effective community interventions that are culturally and linguistically appropriate for communities.

Also, community engagement in research has enabled community organizations to:

- ask questions that are meaningful to their community members,
- develop and evaluate effective programs for their clients,
- demonstrate effectiveness of their programs for future funding opportunities, and
- increase the legitimacy of their work among funders, policy makers, and other stakeholders.

A useful approach for promoting community engagement are tenets of a social–ecological model (Silberberg & Martinez-Bianchi., 2019), which conceptualize health broadly and focus on multiple factors that might affect health. This framework (see **Figure 24.3**) enables community-engaged partnerships to identify a comprehensive list of factors that contribute to poor health. It also provides the underpinnings of a broad approach to health problems that involves actions at many levels—such as individual, group/community, physical, social, and political environments—that interact with each other to produce and reinforce change. This broad approach to thinking of health, advanced in the 1947 Constitution of the World Health Organization (WHO), includes physical, mental, and social well-being (Parran, 1947).

WHY CULTURALLY CENTERED HEALTHCARE AND DIVERSITY MATTER

History is wrought with examples of the harm caused to minoritized and marginalized individuals as a result of culturally naïve and insensitive healthcare. Some of the most widely known examples include nonconsensual experimentation on enslaved women (e.g., Anarcha, Betsey, and Lucy; Fannie Lou Hamer's "Mississippi Appendectomy"; Ebb Cade's receipt of plutonium injections—the same substance used to create atomic bombs—to explore the

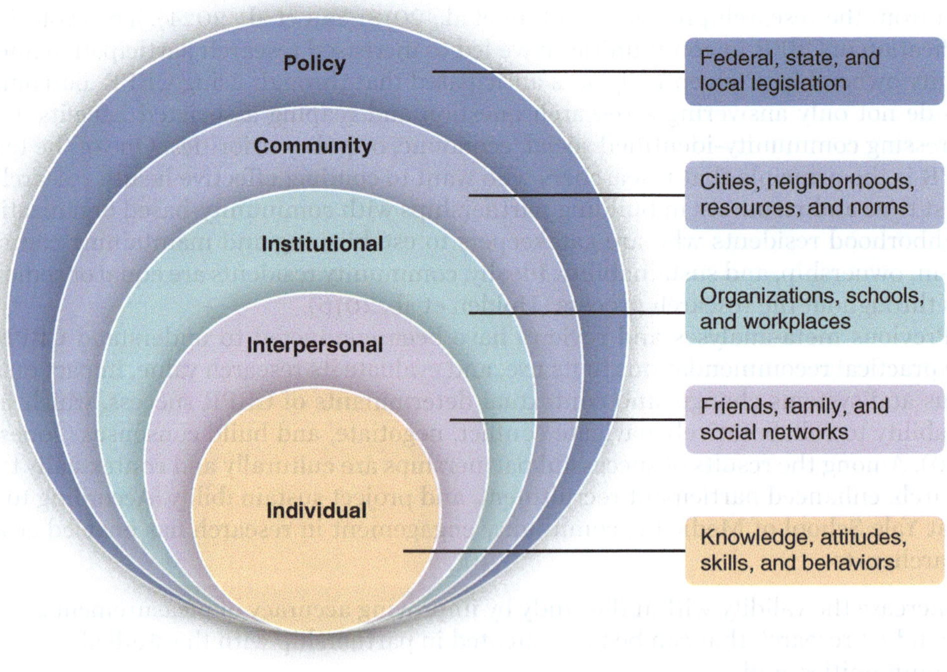

Figure 24.3 Social–ecological model of health.

Source: Bronfenbrenner, U. (1994). Ecological models of human development. In T.N. Postlethwaite & T. Husen (Eds), *International encyclopedia of education* (2nd ed.). Pergamon Press/Elsevier Science.

impact of radiation toxicity on the body; and the use of injectable contraception among Indigenous women despite its use being banned among this group for decades (Clarke, 2021). In more recent years, high-profile examples include Serena Williams and Dr. Susan Moore, Black women who were each ignored when they shared concerns related to their bodies postpartum and in the course of treatment for COVID-19, respectively (Floyd James et al., 2023). Although Williams's requests were ultimately honored and she survived, Dr. Moore's were tragically ignored and resulted in her untimely death. Anecdotal evidence from Latinx people who have delivered children in hospitals indicate that timely and appropriate interpretation often is not available, and that medical providers and staff do not always wait for interpreters to convey providers' intentions before performing intrusive behaviors such as digital cervical dilation checks or vaginal examinations. Further, their requests to labor naturally rather than process with unnecessary medical intervention, such as cesarean sections, are frequently ignored (Hemphill et al., 2023).

In addition to being invalidating, these experiences are harmful, and they represent a resounding concern within healthcare spaces: that the lack of culturally and linguistically oriented care perpetuates historical harms and contributes to ongoing health inequities and disparities. A breadth of studies indicate the importance of cultural humility, sensitivity, and awareness when providing care to clients who have been disenfranchised, minoritized, stigmatized, and marginalized (Cano-Ibáñez et al., 2021; Curtis et al., 2019; Diamond et al., 2019; Lopez et al., 2023). Further research provides evidence that a diverse and ethnically and linguistically representative healthcare workforce also improves health outcomes, access to care, and perceptions of the quality of care they receive (Zephyrin et al., 2023).

Underrepresentation in mental health has been shown to contribute to ongoing mental health stigma, beliefs about causes and consequences of mental health, misdiagnoses, discordant treatment, and a tendency to ignore clients' values, voices, and experience. A survey of 3,000 healthcare workers (Fernandez et al., 2024) revealed that nearly 50% of them had witnessed discrimination against patients based on race, ethnicity, or language, including poor treatment of non–English-speaking patients and labeling as aggressive or belligerent patients who advocate for their care. They reported witnessing greater levels of discrimination in facilities where the majority of patients were Black or Latinx. Further, fewer White healthcare workers perceived racism against patients as a major problem or crisis compared with Black, Latinx, and American Indian and Pacific Islander workers.

Despite overwhelming evidence that healthcare workforces that reflect diversity and represent an institution's patient demographics contribute to improved outcomes and access to care, there are still no universal policies requiring steps to meet this goal. For example, there are no universal educational standards for medical and graduate school training nor are their payment metrics associated with authentic and intentional efforts on the part of healthcare organizations to increase diversity not just on paper, but also in action (Boatright et al. 2023). Adding to this difficulty is the recent overturning of the practice of race-conscious affirmative action for undergraduate admissions by the U.S. Supreme Court—a decision that has created a path for other institutions of higher education to follow. Diversity in healthcare represents a strategy toward achieving health equity in mental and physical health arenas, and barriers across and within multiple ecological layers prohibit the realization of this goal.

LEADERSHIP AND PARTNERSHIP DEVELOPMENT

A special issue of the academic journal *American Psychologist* titled "How Psychologists Can Help Achieve Equity in Health Care: Advancing Innovative Partnerships and Models of Care Delivery" offers an excellent contextual description of how the field of psychology and non-psychology experts can help to reduce mental health disparities (Thurston et al.,

2023). Moreover, it provides useful information and strategies to bolster equity-centered scholarship, practice, and policy. Despite numerous efforts, healthcare equity, or the assurance that everyone should have a fair and just opportunity to attain their best health, eludes our society. Hence, establishment of strong partnerships and leadership development is vital (Jackson-Triche et al., 2020). Community interventions to promote mental health and social equity, which may involve multisector partnerships, emphasize community members as integral to the intervention and/or the delivery of services in community settings (Castillo et. al., 2019).

In the Institute of Medicine's landmark report entitled *The Future of Public Health* (1988), one major issue promoted was that "the need for leaders is too great to leave their emergence to chance" (p. 23). Moreover, we contend that principles espoused in the book *Ethical Leadership: The Quest for Character, Civility and Community* (Fluker, 2009) are essential to progressive, innovative approaches and initiatives to reduce inequities and build healthier communities. In particular, it is critical that leaders adopt leadership principles including (a) insight—the importance of self-awareness, personal biases, and having empathy for others' circumstances; (b) integrity—ethical governance and developing congruence between one's own values and one's actions; (c) synergy—learning the ability to work cooperatively and effectively with others in ways that empower individuals to use their gifts and make contributions that can benefit all parties; (d) sharing the "commitment to action"—developing the motivation to translate knowledge into action and foster buy-in and support, and to become actively involved in individual and collaborative efforts to foster personal and social change; and (e) impact—promoting positive civic engagement and social responsibility through an ethic of service and a concern for justice. In part, it will require focused training in these domains for community leaders to advance health equity.

Examples of model leadership development programs are within the Satcher Health Leadership Institute (SHLI) at the Morehouse School of Medicine (MSM). For example, SHLI's Community Health Leadership Program, Health Policy Leadership Fellowship, Integrated Care Leadership Program, and Smart and Secure Parent Leadership Development Program have established pioneering strategies for preparing diverse community members, postdoctoral health professionals, physician leaders, and parents to tackle the myriad of complex and intricate health issues that plague underserved, vulnerable communities.

Effective and ethical leadership is a critical key to success in the quest for reducing mental health disparities and inequities and building healthier communities. To encourage ethical responsibility for future mental health care providers, researchers, and public health professionals, priority regarding leadership training is key. Leaders must be good learners, continually learning more about themselves, those they lead, and the cause or missions for which they work. Focused initiatives and cross-cultural collaborations will be achieved as we continue to transform the science of ethical decision-making and discovery in research, health promotion, and practice. U.S.-based public health professionals, practitioners, research scientists, policy makers, community leaders, and individual consumers collectively have unique roles as thought leaders in the design, implementation, and evaluation of innovative strategies to promote community health and advance health equity.

STRATEGIC DISSEMINATION OF MENTAL HEALTH PREVENTION MATERIALS

Communication in health may serve several functions: informational, instrumental, social control, and communal (Viswanath, 2006). Strategic dissemination of mental health prevention materials is important to help decrease stigma and reduce mental health disparities. For example, publishing research outcomes in open-access journals, which are more readily available to the academic community and media, is promising. So, too, are research briefings tailored for academic decision-makers, perhaps presented at national conventions, meetings, and forums. Further, infographics and other broadly accessible platforms (e.g., blogs, podcasts, fact sheets) have great potential in the broader dissemination of mental health prevention information. It is also suggested that a user-friendly companion or parallel document for community members be devised.

When communicating about health and mental health, there are several attributes of effective communication that should be taken into consideration. These attributes include the following:

- *Use of nonjudgmental and/or leading statements and declarations*: With verbal and nonverbal communication, it is suggested to avoid broad generalizations about a specific ethnically and culturally diverse population. This includes avoiding the use of personal bias–centered stereotypical commentary.
- *Encourage questioning*: If a particular issue relevant to a dissimilar community is unknown, simply ask about the topic. This approach is more well received than assuming, which may be wrong.
- *Offer plain and nonclinical jargon:* Do not use clinical terms that may be difficult to understand. Break down complex concepts into relatable and understandable terms.
- *Practice active listening*: Use good eye contact and reframe statements given as necessary.
- *Demonstrate cultural respect and reverence*: Learn selected CLAS (culturally and linguistically appropriate services) standards that were developed to address cultural respect and improve the quality of care (Barksdale et al., 2017).
- *Offer language assistance*: This approach is particularly helpful for individuals who have limited English proficiency and/or other communication needs. Inform all individuals of the availability of language assistance services clearly and in their preferred language, both verbally and in writing. Ensure the competence of individuals providing language assistance, recognizing that the use of untrained individuals and/or minors as interpreters should be avoided.
- *Provide easy-to-understand print and multimedia materials and signage*: Work with individual(s) from a target community to ensure that the information is communicated in a way that is readily acceptable.

SUMMARY

This chapter offers information concerning significant psychosocial, sociocultural, and environmental issues that impact mental health and related inequities for BIPOC communities. Further, it provides contextual components of elevating dialogue about the benefits of community engagement, community-based participatory research, and culturally centered care. A multidimensional focus is necessary to help reduce mental health disparities and inequities that align with effective communication, leadership, and partnership development. Although a great deal of meaningful work and systemic level actions that improve functionality are necessary, it is promising that commitments for development, implementation, and evaluation of scientific mental health interventions and prevention strategies are in existence.

DISCUSSION QUESTIONS

1. Considering the cumulative effect of microaggressions on individuals' mental health, what strategies can be used within communities or institutions to mitigate this impact on individuals with minoritized identities?

2. How can the PIE perspective inform the development of culturally sensitive outreach approaches to address multifaceted barriers to mental health care services for BIPOC and other individuals with marginalized identities? What are some examples of outreach strategies that address cultural, social, and environmental factors to improve access to mental health support within diverse communities?
3. What are three ways that cultural insensitivity and language-discordant healthcare interactions negatively affect health outcomes of minoritized or marginalized people?
4. What do you think are the two best strategies for developing and implementing universal graduate and medical education that trains future clinicians to consider racial, ethnic, and linguistic differences in their practice?
5. How are various types of stressors encountered by diverse populations actualized in a multitude of complex ways?
6. What do you believe is the significance of community engagement and partnerships relative to reducing mental health disparities and inequities?

REFERENCES

Adams, L. B., & Thorpe, R. J. (2023). Achieving mental health equity in Black male suicide prevention. *Frontiers in Public Health, 11*, 1113222. https://doi.org/10.3389/fpubh.2023.1113222

Akintobi, T. H., Barrett, R., Hoffman, L., Scott, S., Davis, K., Jones, T., Brown, N. D. V., Fraire, M., Fraire, R., Garner, J., Gruner, A., Hill, J., Meckel, R., Obi, C., Omunga, P., Parham, Q., Rice, T., Samples, O., & Terrill, T. (2023). The community engagement course and action network: Strengthening community and academic research partnerships to advance health equity. *Frontiers in Public Health, 11*, 1114868. https://doi.org/10.3389/fpubh.2023.1114868

Akintobi, T. H., Lockamy, E., Goodin, L., Hernandez, N. D., Slocumb, T., Blumenthal, D., Braithwaite, R., Leeks, L., Rowland, M., Cotton, T., & Hoffman, L. (2018). Processes and outcomes of a community-based participatory research-driven health needs assessment: A tool for moving health disparity reporting to evidence-based action. *Progress in Community Health Partnerships, 12*(1), 139–147. https://doi.org/10.1353/cpr.2018.0029

Andrasik, M. P., Broder, G. B., Wallace, S. E., Chaturvedi, R., Michael, N. L., Bock, S., Beyrer, C., Oseso, L., Aina, J., Lucas, J., Wilson, D. R., Kublin, J. G., & Mensah, G. A. (2021). Increasing Black, Indigenous and people of color participation in clinical trials through community engagement and recruitment goal establishment. *PLoS One, 16*(10), e0258858. https://doi.org/10.1371/journal.pone.0258858

Andreasson, J., & Johansson, T. (2019). Becoming a half-time parent: Fatherhood after divorce. *Journal of Family Studies, 25*(1), 2–17. https://doi.org/10.1080/13229400.2016.1195277

Argyriadis, A., Patelarou, E., Paoullis, P., Patelarou, A., Dimitrakopoulos, I., Zisi, V., Northway, R., Gourni, M., Asimakopoulou, E., Katsarou, D., & Argyriadi, A. (2022). Self-assessment of health professionals' cultural competence: Knowledge, skills, and mental health concepts for optimal health care. *International Journal of Environmental Research and Public Health, 19*(18), 11282. https://doi.org/10.3390/ijerph191811282

Barksdale, C. L., Rodick, W. H., Hopson, R., Kenyon, J., Green, K., & Jacobs, C. G. (2017). Literature review of the national CLAS standards: Policy and practical implications in reducing health disparities. *Journal of Racial and Ethnic Health Disparities, 4*, 632–647. https://doi.org/10.1007/s40615-016-0267-3

Bauer, A. G., Pean, K., Lalwani, T., Julien, L., & Shevorykin, A. (2022). Community needs and recommendations for multilevel mental health interventions among young Black men with previous trauma exposure. *Journal of Consulting and Clinical Psychology, 90*(10), 760–769. https://doi.org/10.1037/ccp0000741

Berger, J. T., & Miller, D. R. (2021). Health disparities, systemic racism, and failures of cultural competence. *The American Journal of Bioethics, 21*(9), 4–10.

Boatright, D., London, M., Soriano, A. J., Westervelt, M., Sanchez, S., Gonzalo, J. D., McDade, W., & Fancher, T. L. (2023). Strategies and best practices to improve diversity, equity, and inclusion among US graduate medical education programs. *JAMA Network Open, 6*(2), e2255110. https://doi.org/10.1001/jamanetworkopen.2022.55110

Brave Heart, M. Y. H., Lewis-Fernández, R., Beals, J., Hasin, D. S., Sugaya, L., Wang, S., Grant, B. F., & Blanco, C. (2016). Psychiatric disorders and mental health treatment in American Indians and Alaska Natives: Results of the national epidemiologic survey on alcohol and related conditions. *Social Psychiatry and Psychiatric Epidemiology, 51*(7), 1033–1046. https://doi.org/10.1007/s00127-016-1225-4

Bulanda, J. R., & Brown, S. L. (2007). Race-ethnic differences in marital quality and divorce. *Social Science Research, 36*(3), 945–967. https://doi.org/10.1016/j.ssresearch.2006.04.001

Cano-Ibáñez, N., Zolfaghari, Y., Amezcua-Prieto, C., & Khan, K. S. (2021). Physician–patient language discordance and poor health outcomes: A systematic scoping review. *Frontiers in Public Health, 9*, 629041. https://doi.org/10.3389/fpubh.2021.629041

Castillo, E. G., Ijadi-Maghsoodi, R., Shadravan, S., Moore, E., Mensah, M. O., 3rd, Docherty, M., Aguilera Nunez, M. G., Barcelo, N., Goodsmith, N., Halpin, L. E., Morton, I., Mango, J., Montero, A. E., Rahmanian Koushkaki, S., Bromley, E., Chung, B., Jones, F., Gabrielian, S., Gelberg, L., Greenberg, J. M., ... Wells, K. B. (2019). Community interventions to promote mental health and social equity. *Current Psychiatry Reports, 21*(5), 35. https://doi.org/10.1007/s11920-019-1017-0

Clarke, E. (2021). Indigenous women and the risk of reproductive healthcare: Forced sterilization, genocide, and contemporary population control. *Journal of Human Rights and Social Work, 6*(2), 144–147. https://doi.org/10.1007/s41134-020-00139-9

Curtis, E., Jones, R., Tipene-Leach, D., Walker, C., Loring, B., Paine, S.-J., & Reid, P. (2019). Why cultural safety rather than cultural competency is required to achieve health equity: A literature review and recommended definition. *International Journal for Equity in Health, 18*(1), 174. https://doi.org/10.1186/s12939-019-1082-3

Dankwa-Mullan, I., Rhee, K. B., Williams, K., Sanchez, I., Sy, F. S., Stinson, N., & Ruffin, J. (2010). The science of eliminating health disparities: Summary and analysis of the NIH summit recommendations. *American Journal of Public Health, 100*(Suppl 1), S12–S18. https://doi.org/10.2105/AJPH.2010.191619

Dawes, D., Holden, K. B., & Williams, D. R. (2023). *Health equity, African Americans, and public health.* APHA Press. https://doi.org/10.2105/9780875533292

Debek, M. (2014). Towards people's experiences and behaviours within their own worlds. The integrative-transactional framework for studying complex people–environment interactions. *Social Space, 8*(2), 1–55.

DeMaris, A., & Oates, G. (2022). The trajectory of subjective well-being: A partial explanation of the marriage advantage. *Journal of Family Issues, 43*(6), 1650–1668. https://doi.org/10.1177/0192513X211030033

Diamond, L., Izquierdo, K., Canfield, D., Matsoukas, K., & Gany, F. (2019). A systematic review of the impact of patient–physician non-English language concordance on quality of care and outcomes. *Journal of General Internal Medicine, 34*(8), 1591–1606. https://doi.org/10.1007/s11606-019-04847-5

duCille, A. (2018). Blacks of the marrying kind: Marriage rites and the right to marry in the time of slavery. *Differences, 29*(2), 21–67. https://doi.org/10.1215/10407391-6999760

Fattoracci, E. S., & King, D. D. (2023). The need for understanding and addressing microaggressions in the workplace. *Perspectives on Psychological Science, 18*(4), 738–742.

Fernandez, H., Ayo-Vaughan, M., Zephyrin, L. C., & Block, R., Jr. (2024). *Revealing disparities: Health care workers' observations of discrimination against patients.* Commonwealth Fund. https://doi.org/10.260999/jjme-gb35

Floyd James, K., Smith, B. E., Robinson, M. N., Thomas Tobin, C. S., Bulles, K. F., & Barkin, J. L. (2023). Factors associated with postpartum maternal functioning in Black women: A secondary analysis. *Journal of Clinical Medicine, 12*(2), 647. https://doi.org/10.3390/jcm12020647

Fluker, W. E. (2009). *Ethical leadership: The quest for character, civility, and community.* 1517 Media. https://doi.org/10.2307/j.ctv13vdfcd

Gadomski, A., Wissow, L. S., Slade, E., & Jenkins, P. (2010). Training clinicians in mental health communication skills: Impact on primary care utilization. *Academic Pediatrics, 10*(5), 346–352. https://doi.org/10.1016/j.acap.2010.06.012

Garcia, M. E., Hinton, L., Gregorich, S. E., Livaudais-Toman, J., Kaplan, C., & Karliner, L. (2020). Unmet mental health need among Chinese and Latino primary care patients: Intersection of ethnicity, gender, and English proficiency. *Journal of General Internal Medicine, 35*, 1245–1251.

Gilbert, K. L., Shaw, M., Siddiqi, A., & Goodman, M. S. (2023). Achieving the health equity agenda through transformative community-engaged strategies. *Preventing Chronic Disease, 20*, E99. https://doi.org/10.5888/pcd20.230077

Hall, J. M., & Fields, B. (2015). "It's killing us!" Narratives of Black adults about microaggression experiences and related health stress. *Global Qualitative Nursing Research, 2*, 233339361559156. https://doi.org/10.1177/2333393615591569

Hemphill, N. O., Crooks, N., Zhang, W., Fitter, F., Erbe, K., Rutherford, J. N., Liese, K. L., Pearson, P., Stewart, K., Kessee, N., Reed, L., Tussing-Humphreys, L., & Koenig, M. D. (2023). Obstetric experiences of young Black mothers: An intersectional perspective. *Social Science & Medicine, 317*, 115604. https://doi.org/10.1016/j.socscimed.2022.115604

Holden, K., Akintobi, T. H., Hopkins, J., Belton, A., McGregor, B., Blanks, S., & Wrenn, G. (2016). Community engaged leadership to advance health equity and build healthier communities. *Social Sciences, 5*(1), 2. https://doi.org/10.3390/socsci5010002

Institute of Medicine Committee for the Study of the Future of Public Health. (1988). *The future of public health.* National Academies Press.

Israel, B. A., Schulz, A. J., Parker, E. A., Becker, A. B., Allen, A. J., III, Ricardo Guzman, J., & Lichtenstein, R. (2008). Critical issues in developing and following community-based participatory research principles. In N. W. M. Minkler (Ed.), *Community-based participatory research for health* (pp. 47–62). Jossey-Bass.

Jackson-Triche, M. E., Unützer, J., & Wells, K. B. (2020). Achieving mental health equity: Collaborative care. *The Psychiatric Clinics of North America, 43*(3), 501–510. https://doi.org/10.1016/j.psc.2020.05.008

Jones, D. E., Lindquist-Grantz, R., & DeJonckheere, M. (2020). A review of mixed methods community-based participatory research applications in mental health. *Journal of Social, Behavioral, and Health Sciences*, *14*(1), 254-288. https://scholarworks.waldenu.edu/cgi/viewcontent.cgi?article=1447&context=jsbhs

LaVeist, T. A., Gaskin, D., & Richard, P. (2011). Estimating the economic burden of racial health inequalities in the United States. *International Journal of Health Services: Planning, Administration, Evaluation*, *41*(2), 231–238. https://doi.org/10.2190/HS.41.2.c

Levine, R. L. (2021). Healthy People 2030: A beacon for addressing health disparities and health equity. *Journal of Public Health Management and Practice*, *27*(Suppl 6), S220–S221. https://doi.org/10.1097/PHH.0000000000001409

Lewis, C. L., Yan, A., Williams, M. Y., Apen, L. V., Crawford, C. L., Morse, L., Valdez, A. M., Alexander, G. R., Grant, E., Valderama-Wallace, C., & Beatty, D. (2023). Health equity: A concept analysis. *Nursing Outlook*, *71*(5), 102032. https://doi.org/10.1016/j.outlook.2023.102032

Lewis, N. A., Bravo, M., Naiman, S., Pearson, A. R., Romero-Canyas, R., Schuldt, J. P., & Song, H. (2020). Using qualitative approaches to improve quantitative inferences in environmental psychology. *MethodsX*, *7*, 100943. https://doi.org/10.1016/j.mex.2020.100943

Lopez, V. A., Thomas, K., Trinh, C., & Nausheen, F. (2023). A case study of the impact of language concordance on patient care, satisfaction, and comfort with sharing sensitive information during medical care. *Journal of Immigrant and Minority Health*, *25*(6), 1261–1269. https://doi.org/10.1007/s10903-023-01463-8

Mitchell, T. D., & Chavous, T. (2021). Centering social justice in the scholarship of community engagement. *Michigan Journal of Community Service Learning*, *27*(1), 1. https://doi.org/10.3998/mjcsloa.3239521.0027.101

National Institute of Mental Health. (2023). *Mental illness.* https://www.nimh.nih.gov/health/statistics/mental-illness

Ngambi, S. N., Ndhlovu, D., & Changala, M. (2023). Popular literature on post-divorce traumatic experiences. *International Journal of Social Science Humanity & Management Research*, *2*(4), 212–217.

Nielsen, L. (1999). Demeaning, demoralizing, and disenfranchising divorced dads: A review of the literature. *Journal of Divorce & Remarriage*, *31*(3–4), 139–177. https://doi.org/10.1300/J087v31n03_08

Parran, T. W. (1947). The World Health Organization. *The Yale Journal of Biology and Medicine*, *19*(4), 401–410.

Pearson, A. R., Schuldt, J. P., Romero-Canyas, R., Ballew, M. T., & Larson-Konar, D. (2018). Diverse segments of the US public underestimate the environmental concerns of minority and low-income Americans. *Proceedings of the National Academy of Sciences of the United States of America*, *115*(49), 12429–12434. https://doi.org/10.1073/pnas.1804698115

Raihan, A. (2023). A review of the global climate change impacts, adaptation strategies, and mitigation options in the socio-economic and environmental sectors. *Journal of Environmental Science and Economics*, *2*(3), 36–58.

Richmond, J., Anderson, A., Cunningham-Erves, J., Ozawa, S., & Wilkins, C. H. (2023). Conceptualizing and measuring trust, mistrust, and distrust: Implications for advancing health equity and building trustworthiness. *Annual Review of Public Health*, *45*(1), 465–484. https://doi.org/10.1146/annurev-publhealth-061022-044737

Ríos, C. D. L., & Patel, L. (2023). Positions, positionality, and relationality in educational research. *International Journal of Qualitative Studies in Education*, 1–12. https://doi.org/10.1080/09518398.2023.2268036

Rogge, M. E., & Cox, M. E. (2001). The person-in-environment perspective in social work journals: A computer-assisted content analysis. *Journal of Social Service Research*, *28*(2), 47–68. https://doi.org/10.1300/J079v28n02_03

Sánchez, V., Sanchez-Youngman, S., Dickson, E., Burgess, E., Haozous, E., Trickett, E., Baker, E., & Wallerstein, N. (2021). CBPR implementation framework for community-academic partnerships. *American Journal of Community Psychology*, *67*(3-4), 284–296. https://doi.org/10.1002/ajcp.12506

Silberberg, M. P., & Martinez-Bianchi, V. M. D. (2019). Community and stakeholder engagement. *Primary Care*, *46*(4), 587–594. https://doi.org/10.1016/j.pop.2019.07.014

Suarez-Balcazar, Y., Francisco, V. T., & Rubén Chávez, N. (2020). Applying community-based participatory approaches to addressing health disparities and promoting health equity. *American Journal of Community Psychology*, *66*(3–4), 217–221. https://doi.org/10.1002/ajcp.12487

Substance Abuse and Mental Health Services Administration. (2022). *Key substance use and mental health indicators in the United States: Results from the 2021 National Survey on Drug Use and Health* (HHS Publication No. PEP22-07-01-005, NSDUH Series H-57). Center for Behavioral Health Statistics and Quality, Substance Abuse and Mental Health Services Administration. https://www.samhsa.gov/data/report/2021-nsduh-annual-national-repo

Sue, D. W., Capodilupo, C. M., Torino, G. C., Bucceri, J. M., Holder, A. M. B., Nadal, K. L., & Esquilin, M. (2007). Racial microaggressions in everyday life: Implications for clinical practice. *American Psychologist*, *62*(4), 271–286. https://doi.org/10.1037/0003-066X.62.4.271

Thurston, I. B., Alegría, M., Hood, K. B., Miller, G. E., Wilton, L., & Holden, K. (2023). How psychologists can help achieve equity in health care—Advancing innovative partnerships and models of care delivery: Introduction to the special issue. *The American Psychologist*, *78*(2), 73–81. https://doi.org/10.1037/amp0001153

Turner, E. A., Douglas, C., & Haseeb, A. (2024). Predictors of seeking mental health treatment in Black men: Therapy fears and expectations about counseling. *Community Mental Health Journal, 60*(2), 385–393. https://doi.org/10.1007/s10597-023-01183-1

U.S. Department of Health and Human Services: Task Force on Black and Minority Health, & Heckler, M. (1985). *Report of the Secretary's Task Force on Black and Minority Health.* U.S. Department of Health and Human Services.

U.S. Department of Health and Human Services. (n.d.). *Healthy people 2030.* https://odphp.health.gov/healthypeople/about/healthy-people-2030-framework

U.S. Department of Health and Human Services. (2010). *Healthy people 2020.* The George Washington University.

Varcarolis, E. M., & Fosbre, C. D. (2020). Essentials of psychiatric mental health nursing-E-book: A communication approach to evidence-based care. Elsevier.

Viswanath, K. (2006). Public communications and its role in reducing and eliminating health disparities. In G. E. Thomas, F. Mitchel, & M. B. Williams (Eds.), *Examining the health disparities research plan of the National Institutes of Health: Unfinished business* (pp. 215-253). National Academies Press.

Williams, D. R., Lawrence, J. A., & Davis, B. A. (2019). Racism and health: Evidence and needed research. *Annual Review of Public Health, 40,* 105-125. https://doi.org/10.1146/annurev-publhealth-040218-043750

World Health Organization. (2018). *Health in all policies as part of the primary health care agenda on multisectorial action* (Publication No. 11). https://iris.who.int/bitstream/handle/10665/326463/WHO-HIS-SDS-2018.59-eng.pdf?sequence=1

Yau, J. H. Y., Wong, E. L. Y., Kanagawa, H. S., Liu, T., Wong, G. H. Y., & Lum, T. Y. S. (2024). Effectiveness of community-based participatory research (CBPR) interventions on mental health outcomes: A systematic review. *Social Science and Medicine, 363,* Article 117491. https://doi.org/10.1016/j.socscimed.2024.117491

Yearby, R. (2020). Structural racism and health disparities: Reconfiguring the social determinants of health framework to include the root cause. *Journal of Law, Medicine, and Ethics, 48*(3), 518–526. https://doi/10.1177/1073110520958876

Zephyrin, L. C., Rodriguez, J., & Rosenbaum, S. (2023, July). The case for diversity in health professions remains powerful. *To the Point.* https://doi.org/10.26099/shph-nr71

25 PREPARING PUBLIC AND BEHAVIORAL HEALTH PROFESSIONALS FOR LEADERSHIP WITH IMPACT

JUAN CARLOS ARAQUE AND EUGENIA L. WEISS

LEARNING OBJECTIVES

After reading this chapter, readers will be able to:

- Understand the importance of leadership in the public and behavioral health professions for improving mental health equity.
- Implement the IDDEA (**I**nnovation, **D**esign, **D**iversity, **E**xecution, and **A**ssessment) Leadership Framework by Araque and Weiss (2024) in their programs and organizations.
- Describe the benefits of designing and implementing a leadership model to improve programming in public and behavioral health organizations.[1]
- Identify the benefits of implementing a leadership model with behavioral professionals who provide services to vulnerable populations.
- Learn about the participants' knowledge and application results during and after their leadership program participation.

INTRODUCTION

Effective and efficient leadership in the public and behavioral health fields is more important today than ever before. According to the 2024 Lyra Health report on the global workforce outlook, 94% of leaders identify mental health benefits as "very important" to employees—more than triple the rate from a few years earlier. The report also highlights how environmental issues (such as the COVID-19 pandemic, wars, and man-made and natural disasters) could greatly affect employees' mental health on both personal and professional levels (Lyra Health, 2023). Thus, leadership in mental health is relevant worldwide. Moreover, we know that most historically marginalized populations continue to be disproportionately impacted by loneliness, isolation, depression, anxiety, and stress because of the lack of access to appropriate education, health, and mental health services (Kujawa et al., 2020).

Although advancements in technology, such as social media and artificial intelligence, have made the world more interconnected, the challenges faced by individuals, organizations, and communities remain as formidable as ever. The dynamic nature of our society

[1] The authors would like to acknowledge the Substance Abuse and Mental Health Services Administration (SAMHSA) and the National Latino Behavioral Health Association (NLBHA) for the successful implementation of the National Executive Leadership Program that incorporated the IDDEA Leadership Framework within the Prevention and Addiction Technology Transfer Centers across the country.

necessitates adapting to and addressing significant issues. Persistent problems such as poverty, discrimination, immigration, homelessness, inequities in physical and mental health access and outcomes, social injustice, and educational disparities persist, demanding innovative and creative solutions. Traditional and isolated approaches within health and human services have proven limited and often fail to bring about lasting social change. A new form of leadership is imperative—one that is purposeful, fueled by passion, and executed with the skills required to motivate individuals and communities toward achieving mental health equity.

The vision for impactful leadership is rooted in the fundamental principle that the well-being of humanity must be the top priority, without compromise. This commitment is comparable to an airline pilot prioritizing the safety of the crew and passengers above all else. Public and behavioral health professionals are crucial in guiding individuals, organizations, and communities to enhance their quality of life. Innovative leaders with a vision toward health equity are integral to crafting a carefully planned path forward, considering the complexities of how individuals and communities function and how they are impacted by systems. Beginning with self-awareness and extending outward to team members, partners, and communities, these leaders connect with the world around them, gaining a profound understanding of needs and resources to craft effective plans.

Leaders in public and behavioral health fields wield significant power and opportunity as change makers. Envisioning, designing, constructing, managing, and evaluating healthy communities requires collaboration with various stakeholders, including government representatives, foundations, corporations, and the public. As "social architects," these leaders are pivotal in shaping and constructing a thriving society (Araque & Weiss, 2019). Building trust and working collaboratively with every community member necessitates a clear leadership approach. Therefore, the social architect's mission includes ensuring the sustainability of effective programs and delivery systems and empowering communities to become self-reliant over time.

THE INNOVATION, DESIGN, DIVERSITY, EXECUTION, AND ASSESSMENT LEADERSHIP FRAMEWORK

To establish a robust vision and achieve desired objectives, effective social architects can use the IDDEA Leadership Framework. This framework has been specifically crafted for the tasks undertaken by public and behavioral health professionals. The early stage of the framework focuses on the crucial nature of recognizing the necessity for addressing social needs. These needs could encompass areas such as education, health disparities and inequities, poverty, homelessness, behavioral and mental health challenges, harassment, discrimination, and inadequate responses to family and community crises. When individuals and communities encounter these social needs, societal reactions often manifest as anger, frustration, divisiveness, and conflict. Typically, this results in negative and punitive energy. However, it becomes evident that redirecting this substantial energy toward innovative solutions can bring people together and yield improved outcomes for those in need (see **Figure 25.1**; Araque & Weiss, 2019).

The IDDEA Leadership Framework encompasses the following five components: innovation, design, diversity, execution, and assessment.

Innovation

Social architects engage in envisioning and designing plans to strengthen organizations and communities. The success of this challenging endeavor relies on identifying innovative strategies to provide public and behavioral health services to those in need, with the ultimate goal of advancing mental health equity. Innovative leaders, guided by a strong ethical and moral compass, emphasize collaborative efforts and establish social networks with stakeholders from diverse disciplines to advance their causes and bring about social change.

Design

The social architect shapes the organizational and social landscape to optimize resource utilization, enhance service delivery, and minimize risks. Throughout the formulation and development of innovations, leaders cultivate positive collaborations and partnerships to design a pathway for implementing improved programs and services. The design element involves understanding how ideas will be implemented and considers factors such as partnerships, financial resources, capacity, and commitment.

Diversity

As social architects develop innovative strategies, they must consider the diversity, equity, and inclusion of stakeholders and populations. Recognizing that a single innovative strategy cannot cater to all groups or have the same impact on everyone, leaders must be culturally proficient. Adaptation to meet the demands of diverse, vulnerable, and historically marginalized populations is crucial. Innovative leaders can identify and allocate resources that are relevant to the unique needs of clients and communities.

Execution

Successful social architects formulate a feasible, realistic, and innovative plan for implementation and management. This new effort, often experimental in nature, undergoes repeated testing. The implementation phase requires direction, strength, and flexibility. Leaders and their teams must exercise various competencies, skills, and abilities that include strategic planning, supervision, financial management, program implementation, and constant adaptation to achieve the desired goals.

Assessment

Successful social architects continuously assess internal and external factors throughout the innovation process. Internally, leaders evaluate their self-capacity, well-being, and

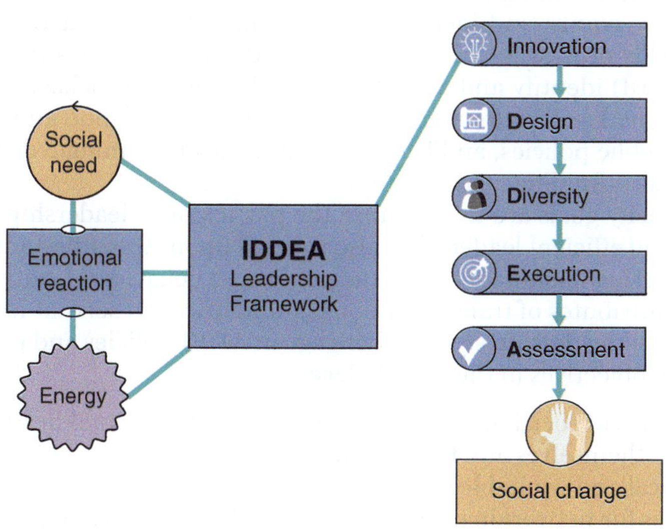

Figure 25.1 The IDDEA Leadership Framework.
IDDEA, innovation, design, diversity, execution, and assessment.

motivation, along with the internal climate of the organization and stakeholder groups. Only the most robust organizational patterns and social arrangements will come to fruition and expand. Externally, leaders use formal and informal evaluation methods to assess the progress of the innovation initiative, eventually determining improved organizational arrangements and social norms. Social architects remain vigilant to societal, political, and environmental forces beyond agency walls, allowing them to more effectively adjust to advance health equity as needed.

NATIONAL EXECUTIVE LEADERSHIP PROGRAM

Background

Thanks to a grant provided by the Substance Abuse and Mental Health Services Administration (SAMHSA), the National Latino Behavioral Health Association (NLBHA) and Weiss Research and Consulting LLC launched the National Executive Leadership Program (ELP) in 2020. The ELP's purpose was to provide executive leadership capacity building to managers and administrators identified by the National Hispanic and Latino Prevention and Addiction Technology Transfer Centers. The goal was to identify and recruit participants (the Fellows) across the United States and territories who would receive formal leadership training and coaching to maximize their leadership potential in behavioral health and integrated health services. The Fellows were public and behavioral health professionals with careers in the health and behavioral health and substance use sectors who have demonstrated potential and interest in executive leadership positions. Annually, between 20 to 25 Fellows were identified to participate in the online (virtual) ELP.

Executive Leadership Program Description

The 10-month ELP focuses on leadership capacity building. In October of every year, NLBHA invites public and behavioral health professionals to apply for the ELP. This is a competitive application process. By December, the 20 to 25 selected Fellows receive a letter to participate, and the first virtual session begins in January of every year. Between January and October, Fellows virtually meet once or twice per month. Sessions can last 2 or 3 hours, depending on the content being covered. At the conclusion of the ELP, each Fellow should be able to (a) demonstrate authentic and transformational leadership skills; (b) formulate antiracial, diversity, equity, and inclusive (ADEI) management practices; (c) understand career-building skills needed for executive-level leadership positions in public and behavioral health fields; (d) identify and analyze essential public and behavioral health practices and policies at the local, state, and federal levels; and (e) define and assess behavioral health practices, public policies, and legislative strategies to eliminate disparities and gaps in healthcare services, funding, and research.

The ELP's capacity goals are to maximize the participants' leadership skills not only to become effective and efficient leaders, but also to build upon strengths and talents to further their executive-level leadership careers in the public and behavioral health professions. The Fellows learn key attributes of transformational, authentic, and servant leadership, become self-reflective in their leadership style, and engage in ADEI policies and practices to accomplish the following objectives in their workplace:

- Become architects of social innovation toward increasing mental health equity.
- Foster talent in themselves and their teams.
- Engage in ethical and equitable practices.
- Learn strategies for networking, collaboration, and communication.
- Deepen skills in project management and budgeting.
- Understand the basics of program evaluation to be able to support organizational engagement.

- Maximize the use of social media and technology.
- Improve professional speaking skills.
- Cultivate mentor and coaching relationships.
- Develop personal branding strategies and a professional vision toward career advancement.
- Create an individual wellness plan to maintain physical, mental, and spiritual health.

Participating Fellows attend 15 interactive virtual training sessions (January–October). The content covered during the virtual training sessions includes introduction of each of the Fellows and orientations of the structure and content of the program; participation in group learning meetings based on each of the IDDEA Leadership Framework components; conversations in group learning circles where Fellows share current managerial and/or leadership challenges at the workplace and facilitators, along with peers, who address these challenges and propose potential solutions; and application of presentation skills whereby the Fellows present their policy briefs and fast-pitch final assignments.

One key feature of the ELP is that each Fellow engages in at least three 45-minute individual coaching sessions with an assigned coach who has an established record and extensive experience in public and behavioral health fields. Finally, a few Fellows are selected to participate in an additional mentoring program. At least once a month, mentors meet with mentees to support them in their leadership development, managerial skills, and career choices.

At the end of the ELP, participants will present a 7-minute fast-pitch (with visual aids, such as a PowerPoint slide deck or infographics) on a social innovation project for addressing public and/or behavioral health issues affecting individuals, families, and communities. The purpose of this assignment is for Fellows to apply the IDDEA Leadership Framework by designing their innovations and implementing them in the near future. Each Fellow applies the following seven steps to prepare and deliver their presentations:

1. *Introduction:* State the selected organizational or community-based problem and a brief background.
2. *Innovation*: State the innovative solution.
3. *Design*: Provide key leadership and management concepts needed to solve the problem identified, including budgeting, partnerships, and the use of technology and social media.
4. *Diversity*: Share ADEI considerations, including new proposed policies and/or practices.
5. *Execution*: State how the innovative solution will solve the identified problem and include a strategic plan outline with vision, mission, goals, objectives, budget, and benchmarks.
6. *Assessment*: Share how to support the well-being of the professionals involved in the proposed innovation and how to assess and evaluate the impact of the solution, program, and/or intervention.
7. Provide a conclusion and the next steps for implementation and sustainability. The fast pitch is presented to the cohort of Fellows, and through the oral presentations, the Fellows receive feedback from peers, instructors, and coaches.

It is inspiring to watch and listen to the Fellows' creative ideas and innovative strategies to implement at their organizations or communities and how they will evaluate them. Their innovations range from proposing new policies and programs to improving delivery systems and client outcomes through the lens of mental health equity by applying the IDDEA Leadership Framework. To date, close to 100 participants have graduated from the ELP. An example of participants' organizations, work titles, and states represented are shown in **Table 25.1**.

Table 25.1 EXECUTIVE LEADERSHIP PROGRAM NATIONAL REPRESENTATION

ORGANIZATION NAME	WORK TITLE	STATE
Servicios de Esperanza LLC	Program Director	CA
La Clínica del Pueblo	Manager of Mental Health Programs	CO
University of Houston College of Pharmacy	Clinical Assistant Professor	TX
St. Martin's Hospitality Center	Director of Clinical Programs	GA
Holistic Cultural and Educational Wellness Center	Program Director	IL
Department of Human Services	Director of TANF Programs	MA
Mental Health & Recovery Services Board	Manager of Treatment Services	MD
University of New Mexico Hospital, Child Psychiatric Center	Licensed Psychologist	NM
Dallas Children's Health	Behavioral Health Care Manager	TX
New Mexico Opioid Response Program	Program Manager	NM
University of New Mexico Hospital, Child Psychiatric Center	Doctor and Associate Professor	NM
Alexandria City Public Schools	Substance Abuse Prevention and Intervention Coordinator	VA
University of Riverside, Department of Psychiatry	Program Director	CA
Sanar Institute	Clinical Director	NJ
Endeavors	Case Management Supervisor	NC
CHESS Health	Program Manager	NC
El Futuro Inc.	Manager of Client Care and Engagement	AZ
Families & Youth Innovation Plus	Senior Director	VI
Clinical Family Health	Behavioral Health Manager	NJ
Esperanza United of St. Paul	Research and Evaluation Manager	MI
Veterans Administration Crisis Line	Social Services Coordinator	FL
Community Outreach Center	Supervisor	OH

Executive Leadership Program Results

The ELP conducts a comprehensive evaluation to gauge the overall program satisfaction and the knowledge and application of the leadership concepts learned throughout the year. A separate survey questionnaire is completed by those participating in the additional mentoring program. The data presented here were collected from Fellows who participated in four cohorts from 2020 to 2023.

First, SAMHSA conducted an overall program satisfaction assessment at the end of each year, which included demographic information (see **Table 25.2**) and overall satisfaction with each of the leadership sessions (see **Table 25.3**). The survey questionnaire in **Table 25.3** uses a 5-point Likert scale (strongly agree/very satisfied = 5, agree/satisfied = 4, neither agree

Table 25.2 EXECUTIVE LEADERSHIP PROGRAM PARTICIPANT DEMOGRAPHICS

GENDER	RACE/ ETHNICITY	EDUCATION	OVERALL QUALITY OF THE LEADERSHIP PROGRAM	BENEFITED MY PROFESSIONAL DEVELOPMENT	I WOULD RECOMMEND THIS PROGRAM TO A COLLEAGUE
Female (70%)	Hispanic/ Latine[a] (97%)	Doctoral degree (20%)	Very satisfied (80%)	Strongly agree (80%)	Yes (100%)
Male (25%)	Caucasian (1%)	Master's degree (60%)	Satisfied (20%)	Agree (20%)	No (0%)
Nonbinary (5%)	Other (1%)	Bachelor's degree (20%)	Dissatisfied (0%)	Disagree (0%)	

[a]We use the singular and plural term *Latine* as a gender-neutral definition that includes Hispanics, Latinos, Latinas, and Latinx individuals, families, and communities.

CHESS, Center for Health Enhancement Systems Studies; TANF, temporary assistance for needy families.

Table 25.3 OVERALL SATISFACTION OF THE EXECUTIVE LEADERSHIP PROGRAM SESSIONS

QUESTION / SESSIONS	INNOVATION	DESIGN	DIVERSITY	EXECUTION	ASSESSMENT
Q1: I felt the information in the Web-based module was up to date, clear, and understandable.	4.75	4.75	4.83	4.75	4.71
Q2: I felt engaged in the Web-based training, and my questions were answered.	4.88	4.88	4.83	4.88	4.75
Q3: I felt like an active participant in the web-based training.	4.50	4.88	4.75	4.88	4.86
Q4: The structure of the Web-based module and information presented was logical and easy to follow.	4.50	4.75	4.50	5.00	4.63
Q5: The Web-based material presented had relevance to behavioral health leadership.	4.88	5.00	4.83	4.88	5.00
Q6: The material presented had relevance to the Hispanic or Latine population.	4.63	4.75	4.83	5.00	4.86
Q7: Overall, I would rate the information and quality of this module:	4.75	4.88	5.00	4.86	4.75

nor disagree/neither satisfied nor dissatisfied = 3, disagree/dissatisfied = 2, strongly disagree/very dissatisfied = 1). The results (high averages) suggest that participants in the ELP experienced a high level of satisfaction during each session.

Additionally, the ELP evaluation assessed the Fellows' knowledge and application of the leadership concepts reviewed and learned in the curricula. Each year, Fellows complete the Executive Leadership Knowledge and Application Survey at the beginning (January) and the end (October) of the ELP. This survey questionnaire took approximately 20 to 25 minutes to complete and asked participants to rate their knowledge and application of the leadership content listed in **Box 25.1**. Participants rated each leadership content through a 5-point Likert scale: 5 (expert), 4 (high knowledge), 3 (knowledge), 2 (some knowledge), 1 (no knowledge). A summary of the pre- and posttest results from each subscale is presented in **Table 25.4**. The results strongly suggest that the ELP made a significant difference in the participants' knowledge and application of leadership concepts.

Box 25.1 EXECUTIVE LEADERSHIP KNOWLEDGE AND APPLICATION SURVEY SUBSCALES CONTENT

Innovation

- Innovation models/approaches can be applied to advance organizational goals
- Use of technology to implement innovative projects in your organization
- Policy and advocacy in behavioral health issues
- Application of patient-centered innovation in your work
- Application of design thinking innovation in your work
- Innovative leadership approaches to accomplish your organizational goals

Design

- Create community collaborative efforts
- Building team member motivation
- Develop networking opportunities
- Effective communication strategies to manage conflict among my team members
- Various approaches to engage my team members in teamwork

Diversity

- Racial disparities in healthcare
- Models relating to cultural competency and cultural proficiency
- Use of inclusive and antidiscriminatory strategies in the workplace
- Strategies to advance positive equity and diversity in the workplace
- Cross-cultural communication

Execution

- Organizational strategic planning methods
- Use of logic models
- Application of process objective and/or outcomes objectives
- Application of managerial models/approaches
- Use of action plans and/or key deliverables
- Managing internal and external conflict

(continued)

Box 25.1 EXECUTIVE LEADERSHIP KNOWLEDGE AND APPLICATION SURVEY SUBSCALES CONTENT (*continued*)

Assessment

- Models of evidence-based practices
- Conducting needs assessments
- Measurement (i.e., reliability and validity)
- Evaluation approaches (e.g., participatory, transformational, utilization-focused)
- Research designs (e.g., correlational, quasi-experimental, experimental)
- Development of logic models
- Models of effective use of evaluation findings

Table 25.4 EXECUTIVE LEADERSHIP PROGRAM KNOWLEDGE AND APPLICATION RESULTS

COHORT		1	2	3	4
	Statistic	**2020**	**2021**	**2022**	**2023**
		M (*SD*)	*M* (*SD*)	*M* (*SD*)	*M* (*SD*)
Innovation	Pretest	2.56 (0.96)	2.25 (0.77)	2.20 (0.60)	2.26 (0.76)
	Posttest	3.67 (0.81)	3.49 (0.55)	3.40 (0.54)	3.50 (0.52)
	p value	*p*<0.001	<0.001	<0.001	<0.001
Design	Pretest	2.77 (0.86)	2.76 (0.76)	2.68 (0.74)	2.42 (0.67)
	Posttest	3.52 (0.77)	3.51 (0.57)	3.70 (0.49)	3.74 (0.51)
	p value	<0.001	<0.001	<0.001	<0.001
Diversity	Pretest	3.18 (1.01)	2.68 (0.68)	2.73 (0.74)	2.55 (0.73)
	Posttest	3.76 (0.78)	3.65 (0.47)	3.62 (0.62)	3.59 (0.53)
	p value	<0.001	<0.001	<0.001	<0.001
Execution	Pretest	2.58 (0.98)	2.31 (0.79)	2.12 (0.77)	2.17 (0.76)
	Posttest	3.65 (0.85)	3.33 (0.67)	3.36 (0.55)	3.58 (0.51)
	p value	<0.001	<0.001	<0.001	<0.001
Assessment	Pretest	2.57 (0.89)	2.56 (0.87)	2.09 (0.89)	2.26 (0.75)
	Posttest	3.74 (0.74)	3.35 (0.61)	3.22 (0.72)	3.56 (0.68)
	p value	<0.001	<0.001	<0.001	<0.001

Note: *p* values were calculated by applying paired *t* tests for each of the five subscales.
M, mean; *SD*, standard deviation.

SUMMARY

Public and behavioral health professionals and their clients can benefit from applying the IDDEA Leadership Framework. We have had the opportunity to witness firsthand when these leadership concepts are applied with intent and coordination. One of our most powerful tools is our ability to create and formulate new ideas to improve our service delivery and programs to improve mental health equity. Once those ideas are clear to us and those around us, we must formulate how they will be implemented and evaluated. Having a clear vision, bringing together the partnerships and resources needed, and assessing our progress can and does greatly increase the likelihood of success.

DISCUSSION QUESTIONS

1. What innovations would you design and implement to improve programs and client outcomes toward achieving mental health equity?
2. How would you incorporate the IDDEA Leadership Framework in your organization?
3. Which ADEI policies and practices do you think would be successful in your organization, and what else is needed to support racial and ethnic minority employees in the workplace?
4. What strategies would you apply to support the leadership development of employees and peers?
5. What areas of your personal leadership development would you like to accomplish in the next year? What steps would you take to achieve them?
6. What can you do to start an executive leadership program in your organization?

REFERENCES

Araque, J. C., & Weiss, E. L. (2019). *Leadership with impact: Preparing health and human service professionals in the age of innovation and diversity*. Oxford University Press.

Kujawa, A., Green, H., Compas, B. E., Dickey, L., & Pegg, S. (2020). Exposure to COVID-19 pandemic stress: Associations with depression and anxiety in emerging adults in the United States. *Depression and Anxiety, 37*(12), 1280–1288. https://doi.org/10.1002/da.23109

Lyra Health. (2023). *2024 Mental health trends in the workforce.* https://www.lyrahealth.com/blog/workforce-mental-health-trends-2024/

26 GLOBAL MENTAL HEALTH AND WELL-BEING

CELESTE M. PHILIP AND SHANEETA M. JOHNSON

LEARNING OBJECTIVES

After reading this chapter, readers will be able to:

- Understand the historical context of global mental health as a relatively new field.
- Describe the interrelatedness of mental and physical health and the importance of supporting community-level factors that promote overall well-being.
- Recognize the importance of collectively supporting mental health and well-being in low- and middle-income countries in a culturally relevant manner.
- Describe the current global initiatives to improve mental health.
- Discuss policies and strategies to overcome barriers in access to mental health and well-being.

INTRODUCTION

Mental health is inextricably linked to physical health, and maintenance of both is crucial to achieve overall well-being for individuals, communities, and nations (Prince et al., 2007). That mind and body would have reciprocal effects on each other in both positive and negative ways is a simple concept with complex consequences that requires a public health framework grounded in well-being to express these connections more fully. The relatively recent reframing of mental health and overall well-being models, such as the World Health Organization's (WHO) *World Mental Health Report: Transforming Mental Health for All* (2022), is significant because it sets the global stage for advancing mental health and well-being in all nations. Importantly, *for all* calls attention to challenges in attaining equity faced in low- and middle-income countries (LMICs) and to individuals everywhere more likely to experience poor mental health due to the intersectionality of identities, environmental and societal factors, and existing health conditions.

WHO defines mental health as

> a state of mental well-being that enables people to cope with the stresses of life, to realize their abilities, to learn well and work well, and to contribute to their communities. Mental health is an integral component of health and well-being and is more than the absence of mental disorder. (WHO, 2022, p. 8; see **Box 26.1**)

It is important to reinforce that mental health exists on a continuum with the goal of achieving equity, or an optimal state of well-being (Patel et al., 2018). In some cultures, use of the term *mental health* connotes a negative condition rather than one of wellness. The continuum concept, therefore, is critical for recognizing that someone with a mental health disorder who has access to effective support and treatment can achieve an optimal state of well-being (WHO, 2022, p. 13).

Box 26.1 MENTAL HEALTH TERMS

- *Mental health*: A state of mental well-being that enables people to cope with the stresses of life, to realize their abilities, to learn well and work well, and to contribute to their communities. Mental health is an integral component of health and well-being and is more than the absence of mental disorder.
- *Mental health condition*: A broad term covering mental disorders and psychosocial disabilities. It also covers other mental states associated with significant distress, impairment in functioning, or risk of self-harm.
- *Mental disorder*: As defined by the *International Classification of Diseases 11th Revision* (ICD-11), a mental disorder is a syndrome characterized by clinically significant disturbance in an individual's cognition, emotional regulation, or behavior that reflects a dysfunction in the psychological, biological, or developmental processes that underlie mental and behavioral functioning. These disturbances are usually associated with distress or impairment in personal, family, social, educational, occupational, or other important areas of functioning.
- *Psychosocial disability*: Aligned with the Convention on the Rights of Persons with Disabilities, psychosocial disability is disability that arises when someone with a long-term mental impairment interacts with various barriers that may hinder their full and effective participation in society on an equal basis with others. Examples of such barriers are discrimination, stigma, and exclusion.

Source: World Health Organization. (2022). *World mental health report: Transforming mental health for all*. https://www.who.int/publications/i/item/9789240049338

Globally, mental health conditions are highly prevalent, with about one in eight people living with a mental disorder (WHO, 2022), which in 2019, amounted to approximately 970 million people. Although the prevalence of various mental disorders differs by age and sex, in both males and females, depressive and anxiety disorders are the most common (WHO, 2022). The impact of the recent COVID-19 global pandemic further exacerbated and demonstrated the worsening of these common mental health conditions in all parts of the world, with major depressive disorders increasing by 28% and anxiety disorders by 26% (COVID-19 Mental Disorders Collaborators, 2021). These devastating effects emphasized the need for more investment in the community-level factors that support residents to thrive and withstand these unpredictable events.

HISTORY OF GLOBAL MENTAL HEALTH

As described by Patel (2012), global mental health as a discipline can be traced back to a 1904 investigation in Java (Kraepelin, 2000). Throughout the 1900s, research advanced understanding and firmly established that mental health disorders were universally experienced in all cultures and discounted the belief that these conditions were only Western or colonial notions (Kleinman, 1988; Littlewood, 1990). Soon thereafter, themes of mental health inequities began to emerge and continue to persist today, with 80% of people with a mental disorder living in LMICs (Rathod et al., 2017).

A 1995 WHO report, *World Mental Health: Problems and Priorities in Low-Income Countries* (Desjarlais et al., 1995), first described the strong associations between mental disorders and factors such as poverty, gender, violence, conflicts, and disasters. Soon after, the WHO (2001) published its landmark *World Health Report 2001, Mental Health: New Understanding, New Hope*, which exposed the enormous public health and economic costs of poor mental health and the lack of needed services and treatment. This report served as one of the earliest global frameworks for countries and produced the following 10 recommendations: (a) provide treatment in primary care; (b) make psychotropic medicines available; (c) provide care in the community; (d) educate the public; (e) involve communities, families, and consumers; (f) establish national policies, programs, and legislation; (g) develop human resources; (h) link with other sectors; (i) monitor community mental health; and (j) support more research.

In May 2012, the World Health Assembly adopted a resolution on the global burden of mental disorders that led to the development of the *Comprehensive Mental Health Action Plan 2013-2030* (WHO, 2021) which also included 10 recommendations that evolved to focus on leadership and governance, community-based care, promotion and prevention, and information systems and research. Although progress has been made in the past few decades, much more work remains to be done at all levels of society, particularly in LMICs with fewer financial resources (WHO, 2022).

DETERMINANTS OF MENTAL HEALTH

Because mental health and physical health are intertwined, determinants of mental health are largely the same social, environmental, and political determinants that influence overall health and well-being (WHO, 2022). Where one lives, learns, works, and plays shapes both mental and physical health over the life course. More simply put, place matters. Fundamental to this public health model is the reality that who lives in what villages or cities is not random (Sorel, 2012). Decisions by elected officials—or political determinants—influence who lives in environments that support health and well-being and who is relegated to less favorable or overtly harmful environments (Dawes, 2020). Factors such as wealth, power, and historical discrimination vary by world region but are consistent drivers of policy decisions that favor some groups and disadvantage others, resulting in centuries of significant and long-standing mental and physical health impacts. Adverse childhood experiences (ACEs), lifelong persistent toxic stress, impacts from climate and weather events, and the damaging effects of displacement due to war and conflict all have unhealthy mental and physical repercussions in the immediate and long term and are related to place and political determinants.

RISKS AND PROTECTIVE FACTORS

Because mental health conditions such as anxiety and depression are more common in people with chronic physical health conditions, people who identify as gender or sexual minorities, people of color, people with disabilities, people involved with criminal justice systems, and people who live in poverty, stigma can be amplified and further complicate accessing care, changing one's environment, and improving well-being (WHO, 2022). These effects are even greater for individuals who identify with more than one of these characteristics (Kern et al., 2020). Thus, the intersectionality of identities is a critical factor that warrants more awareness, understanding, and research on effective interventions. Stigmatizing attitudes violate the fundamental human rights of individuals with mental health conditions. Further, denial of dignity, autonomy, and privacy perpetuates discrimination (American Psychiatric Association [APA], 2024).

Compared with other types of common health conditions, such as heart disease or cancer, that have more overt physical symptoms and outcomes, understanding the science of mental health has lagged. The slower pace of progress has undoubtedly contributed to a mystique and the stigma that has persisted in most societies. This stigma may include the belief that individuals with mental health disorders are dangerous and lead to social isolation and discrimination (WHO, 2022). Furthermore, in 20 countries, suicide attempts are a criminal offense (United for Global Mental Health, 2021).

In many cultures, behaviors to cope with stress include smoking, use of alcohol and/or drugs, eating less healthful foods, and more sedentary lifestyles (Firth et al., 2020). These are the same behaviors that contribute to development and worsening of chronic diseases such as diabetes, heart disease, and hypertension (Firth et al., 2020). Over time, the physiologic changes that result from a multitude of risk factors can cause epigenetic changes within these individuals that worsen health. These small genetic changes can be passed through genes to subsequent generations, thereby increasing risks for both mental and physical ill health (Shonkoff et al., 2012).

To combat these risk factors, teaching self-care skills in early childhood allows children to learn how to deal with difficult situations and emotions. Building on these skills as children grow and attend school helps to build resiliency as they develop and to promote overall well-being (WHO, 2022). Community-level factors such as clean air and water, access to safe green spaces, and healthy foods also protect against or mitigate effects from risk factors (WHO, 2022). These environmental supports may encourage more physical activity, improved nutritional status, and less tobacco, alcohol, and drug use (**Figure 26.1**).

VALUE OF PROMOTION AND PREVENTION

As with any major public health challenge, identifying and mitigating the source or root cause of a health issue is as important as providing appropriate care to those already impacted. As stated by Satcher et al. in *21st Century Global Mental Health* (Sorel, 2012), "interventions in the social determinants of health are the best and most cost-effective way to promote mental health and prevent mental illness" (p. 74). In her well-known cliff analogy, Jones et al. (2009) describes a scenario in which people keep falling off a cliff and the need to expand efforts to assist not only those who have already fallen but those on the way down, and best yet, to address the "structures, policies, practices, norms, and values that differentially distribute resources and risks along the cliff face" (p. 1). *Promotion* and *prevention* are related terms that are often used interchangeably but are different. *Promotion* refers to conditions that support well-being for individuals and communities, whereas *prevention* is noted as an absence of illness (Herrman et al., 2005). Promotion greatly contributes to prevention, but *not* having a particular condition does not equate to wellness.

More challenging community- and societal-level factors, such as poverty, gender and sexual minority biases, and limited access to high-quality educational and employment opportunities, require a wide-ranging, multisectoral approach, which is outlined in the WHO *Comprehensive Mental Health Action Plan 2013-2030* (WHO, 2021). A health in all policies approach, in which each new or existing policy is reviewed to assess or predict potential health impacts, is an important tool that can be used to both promote overall health and well-being and avoid unintended consequences leading to poorer mental and physical health outcomes. Pandemic-driven infrastructure enhancements, such as an increase in community health workers, and policy advancements that resulted in greater utilization of telehealth could serve as sustainable solutions for increasing access to healthcare promotion in a more equitable manner.

CASE VIGNETTES

Globally, case vignettes demonstrate the worldwide impact of mental health and well-being. They also illustrate the need for multidisciplinary and comprehensive access to mental health services.

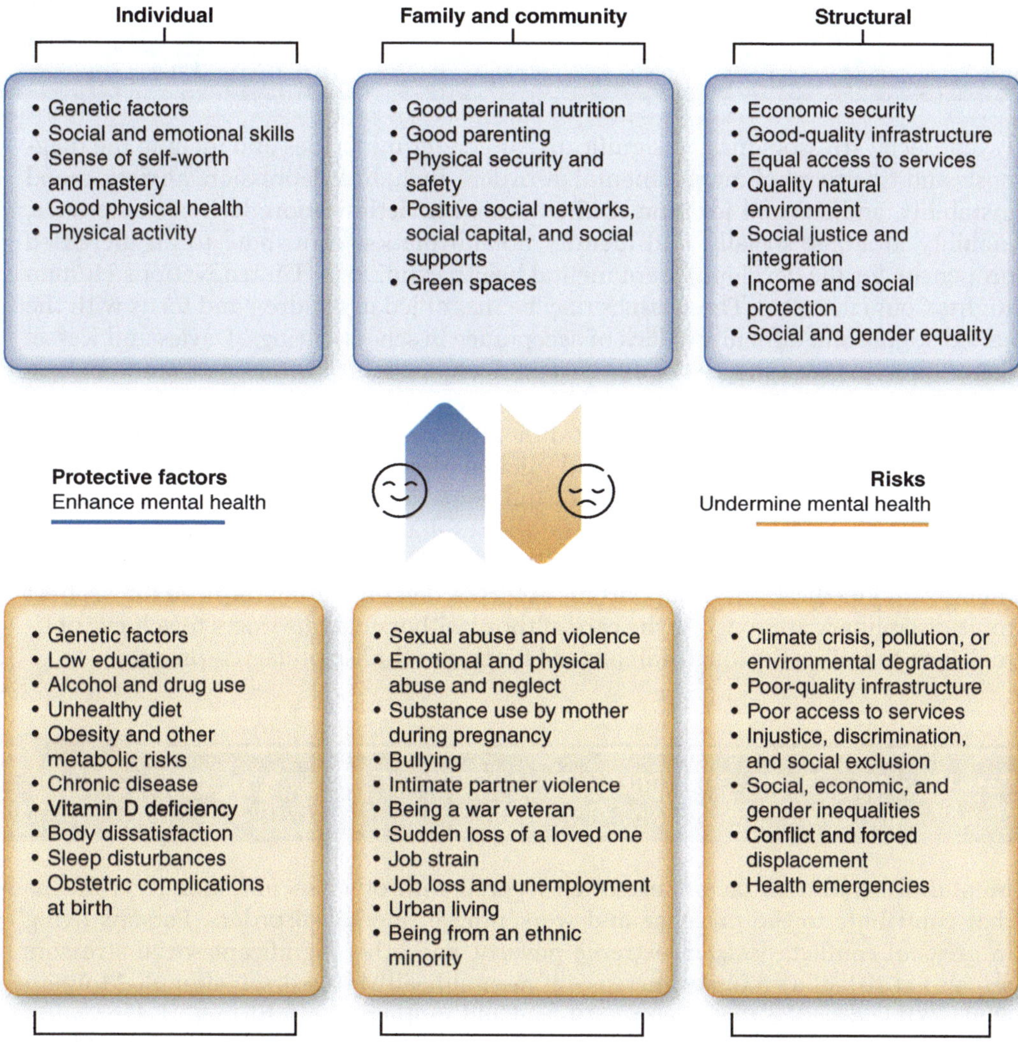

Figure 26.1 Examples of risks and protective factors that determine mental health.
Sources: World Health Organization. (2022). *World mental health report: Transforming mental health for all.* https://www.who.int/publications/i/item/9789240049338"https://www.who.int/publications/i/item/9789240049338

Case Vignette 26.1 PSYCHIATRIC TREATMENT OF A HEALTHCARE WORKER AFTER INFECTION WITH EBOLA VIRUS IN LAGOS, NIGERIA (MOHAMMED ET AL., 2015)

Although the Ebola pandemic had devastating health consequences, the mental health impacts are often overlooked. Mohammed et al. (2015) discuss the case of a young male health worker admitted with a nosocomial Ebola virus infection in Nigeria. The patient demonstrated behavioral symptoms, which also resembled permanent brain injury due to the Ebola virus infection. The psychosocial team was involved in the patient's care, allowing for early treatment and diagnosis. Working in concert with his primary treatment team, the teams successfully treated both physical and mental conditions, allowing the patient to resume work. A multidisciplinary approach to the treatment of mental health conditions, in combination with access to care, is essential in achieving equitable and effective mental health treatment.

Case Vignette 26.2 GENDER MINORITY STRESS, DEPRESSION, AND ANXIETY IN A TRANSGENDER HIGH SCHOOL STUDENT (DAVIES & KESSEL, 2017)

Psychosocial stressors may be significant for gender minorities and include the diagnosis and treatment of myriad mental disorders, including depression, anxiety, mood instability, and suicidal ideation. Difficulties with victimization, lack of acceptance, inability to adjust socially, and identity nonaffirmation contribute to an increased propensity for the development of mental health conditions (United Nations Human Rights Council, 2022). These issues may be magnified in children and teens with the added stigma and difficulty of lack of acceptance in school settings. Davies and Kessel (2017) describe a case report of a 14-year-old adolescent transitioning from female to male and the resultant psychosocial difficulties encountered with a lack of acceptance by peers and family. These significant difficulties resulted in the development of depression, anxiety, mood instability, and suicidal ideation. Additionally, social difficulties such as lack of acceptance at school and home, as well as bullying, contributed to worsening mental health conditions and the resultant impact on his academic progress. The multidisciplinary plan included flexible schedules by the school, psychosocial therapy, and medications to support his progress, demonstrating the need for a robust multidisciplinary approach to the care of those with mental disorders to achieve optimal care, as well as the longitudinal need for this multidisciplinary approach.

Case Vignette 26.3 MAJOR DEPRESSION IN POSTCONFLICT NORTHERN UGANDA (NAKIMULI-MPUNGU ET AL., 2014)

Mental ill-health risk factors are often layered with other socioeconomic problems that contribute to the presence and worsening of mental disorders. Persons living in areas of conflict, disaster, extreme poverty, and other significant social stressors are also at risk of a resultant increase in mental health stressors. Nakimuli-Mpungu et al. (2014) describe the case of a 49-year-old mother with a history of depression and concomitant HIV infection in postconflict northern Uganda. As a result of family violence, the patient experienced increased depression symptoms, isolation, and suicidal ideation, which were compounded by physical illness (HIV infection) and loss of financial independence. Local cultural traditions were carried out to improve the patient's mental health and social circumstances, without change in her symptoms and circumstances. The study demonstrates the need for culturally and socially appropriate mental health care while also highlighting the impact of socioeconomic factors such as isolation from family and possession of work skills to support oneself financially.

Case Vignette 26.4 GROSS NATIONAL HAPPINESS INDEX

The fourth king of Bhutan, King Jigme Singye Wangchuck, first coined the phrase *gross national happiness* in the late 1970s, stating, "Gross national happiness is more important than gross domestic product" (Oxford Poverty and Human Development Initiative, 2022). This framing strengthens the idea that the country's focus should include a holistic view and approach to its progress that accounts for well-being and happiness. Bhutan has created and incorporated the Gross National Happiness (GNH) Index into its policy making and policies, including socioeconomic values such as education, health, and living standards, as well as holistic measures such as culture, community vitality, and psychological well-being.

The index assesses nine domains and 33 indicators to provide an evaluation of the nation's progress. It characterizes the population into four groups: unhappy, narrowly happy, extensively happy, and deeply happy. These results are then used to inform policies to increase happiness and sufficiency (**Figure 26.2**).

The GNH Index has had a significant policy impact and is used by the government to complement existing development measures; prioritize policy areas; track and monitor national progress; align the planning, policies, programs, and projects; and set GNH targets and goals for sectors (Oxford Poverty and Human Development Initiative, 2022).

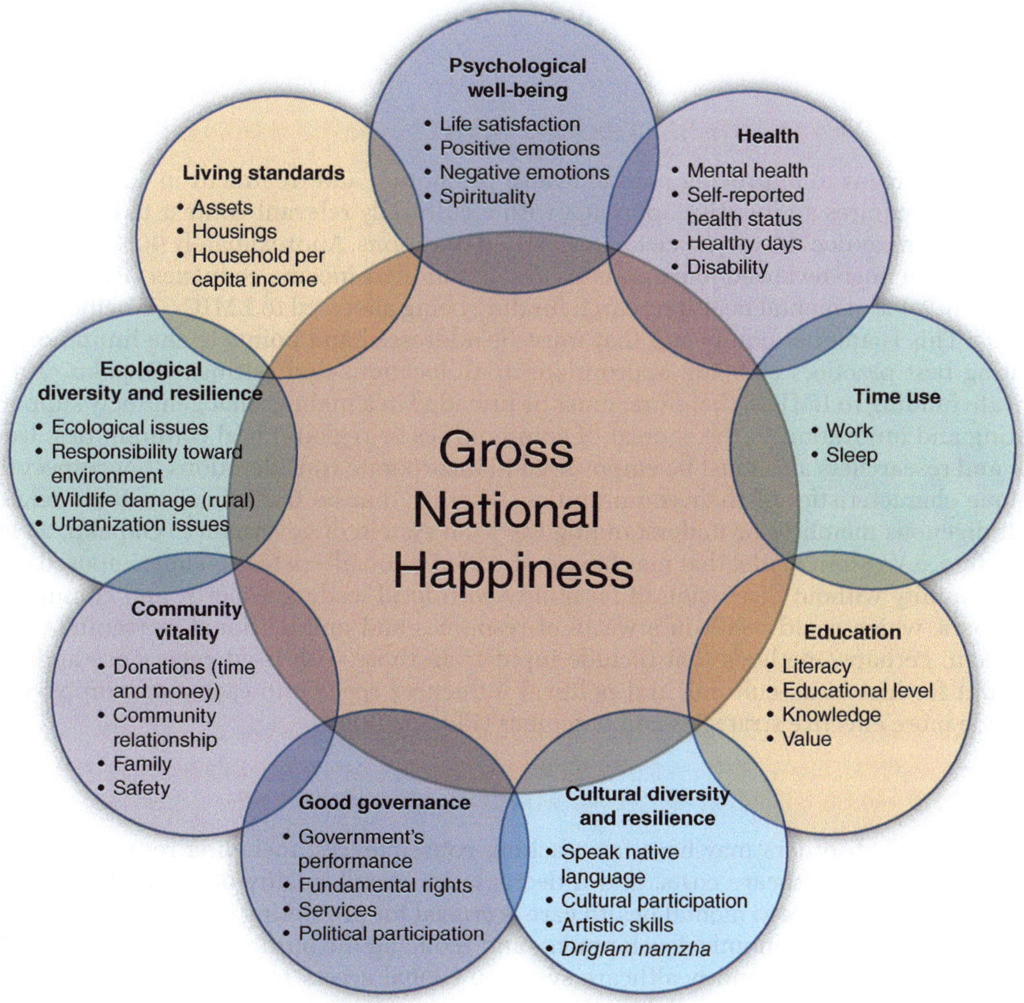

Figure 26.2 **Gross National Happiness Index.**

Source: Oxford Poverty and Human Development Initiative. (n.d.). *Gross national happiness*. https://ophi.org.uk/gross-national-happiness

Case Vignette 26.5 WORLD HEALTH ORGANIZATION INITIATIVES

The WHO's World Mental Health Report, released in 2022 and previously discussed, provides a blueprint for transforming mental health globally. The World Health Assembly adopted the WHO's *Mental Health Action Plan 2013-2020* in 2013, which subsequently was extended until 2030 (WHO, 2021). The plan sets initiatives to promote mental health and well-being, including preventing mental health conditions and achieving universal coverage for mental health.

In 2019, the WHO set forth the *WHO Special Initiative for Mental Health (2019-2023): Universal Health Coverage for Mental Health*, which aimed to provide quality and affordable care for 100 million additional people in 12 priority countries. There were six early adopter countries: Bangladesh, Jordan, Paraguay, the Philippines, Ukraine, and Zimbabwe, all of which joined the initiative in 2020. Argentina, Ghana, and Nepal joined in subsequent years (WHO, 2022). Similarly, the WHO's Mental Health Gap Action Programme was developed to increase services for mental, neurological, and substance use disorders in LMICs (WHO, n.d.).

CHALLENGES TO EQUITABLE GLOBAL MENTAL HEALTH MODELS

The commitment to improving mental health promotion and treatment in LMICs is necessary but requires an iterative approach with a culturally relevant context to be effective. Place matters, as does history, societal norms, and traditions. Approximately 90% of research published in peer-reviewed journals is conducted in high-income countries (Patel, 2007), with only 2.4% of mental health research funding being allocated to LMICs (Woelbert et al., 2020). This is another equity gap that must be addressed and points to the limitations of touting best practices as being appropriate in all locations and settings (Okpaku, 2014). Private funding to LMICs, therefore, must be provided in a manner that genuinely supports testing and innovation in the context of communities or region. Local communities, leaders, and researchers also must be empowered to incorporate considerations that respect the unique characteristics of their communities, whether that be traditional customs related to Indigenous members or understanding the local system of governance (Okpaku, 2014). Too often, a Western model that may have embedded colonial-era bias is superimposed onto a community without discussion of feasibility with local leaders, experts, and community members, which could result in a waste of resources and unintentional worsening of the problem. Perhaps, methods that include input from those with lived experience and that account for historical, cultural, and political influences specific to each community could provide more effective strategies and outcomes (Plough, 2022).

BARRIERS TO EQUITABLE GLOBAL MENTAL HEALTH CARE

Mental health disorders may have far-reaching consequences, including reduced productivity, increased healthcare costs, and a decrease in overall quality of life (WHO, 2022). Ensuring global access to mental health care is crucial for promoting individual well-being, fostering social and economic development, and reducing the burden of mental health disorders on communities and healthcare systems. Global access to mental health care is a pressing need that requires collaborative efforts from governments, healthcare organizations, and communities. Despite the urgent need for mental health care, significant barriers impede equitable access to services. These barriers include stigma and discrimination, lack of awareness of the availability or importance of mental health care, insufficient mental health resources and infrastructure, and limited financial resources (WHO, 2022).

As previously discussed, mental health disorders often are associated with stigma and discrimination, leading to a reluctance to seek help and a lack of understanding and support from society. Stigma may be multiplied in certain diverse cultures in which cultural norms or learned distrust of the healthcare system pose barriers to seeking help (APA, 2024). Fear of judgment and social exclusion often prevents timely intervention, exacerbating symptoms and prolonging suffering. Stigma isolates individuals, limiting their social interactions and support networks. Loneliness and alienation contribute to worsened mental health and hinder recovery. Discrimination in educational and workplace settings perpetuates stigma. Individuals with mental health conditions face challenges in securing employment, advancing their careers, and pursuing education (WHO, 2022). Stigmatized individuals may hesitate to adhere to treatment regimens because of concerns about being labeled or ostracized. Also, research confirms that nonadherence leads to suboptimal health outcomes and increased burden on health systems.

Many individuals, particularly those in low-resource settings, may be unaware of the availability of mental health services or the importance of seeking professional help for mental health conditions. This lack of awareness decreases access to appropriate mental health care and leads to worsened outcomes (Patel et al., 2018).

In many regions, mental health professionals, facilities, and resources to meet the demand for services are still lacking. This shortage is particularly acute in LMICs and is further compounded by the paucity of research in these countries and cultural and other barriers (Collins et al., 2011; Patel et al., 2018). Mental health care may be resource intensive, and individuals from socioeconomically disadvantaged backgrounds may struggle to afford the cost of treatment, even if services are available. Studies have demonstrated lower access to funding for mental health. Ironically, the *Economic Burden of Mental Health Inequities in the United States Report* demonstrated the significant economic benefit of equitable and appropriate treatment of mental health in America and, by extrapolation, globally (Dawes et al., 2022).

Strategies to Promote Global Access to Mental Health Care

To address the barriers to global access to mental health care, several strategies can be implemented, including increasing education and awareness, strengthening mental health infrastructure, addressing government policy, and decreasing access barriers by using technology.

Government Policies and Impact

Mental health is an integral part of overall well-being, yet disparities persist in accessing quality care (Sorel, 2012). Government policies play a pivotal role in determining the availability, affordability, and inclusivity of mental health services. Policies that allocate adequate funding for mental health services, promote mental health parity laws, and prioritize the integration of mental health into primary care settings can significantly improve access to care (WHO, 2022). Additionally, policies aimed at reducing stigma, promoting mental health awareness, and addressing social determinants of mental health, such as poverty and housing instability, can contribute to the overall well-being of the population. Effective government policies can create an environment that supports mental health and fosters the development of comprehensive and accessible mental health care systems.

Effective policies must demonstrate strong leadership and commitment to pursuing equitable policies. Strong government leadership that is informed and proactive is essential for mental health policy formulation and implementation, as well as a commitment to equity that ensures that historically marginalized groups receive quality care (Sorel, 2012).

Engaging relevant stakeholders, such as healthcare providers, nongovernmental organizations, and communities, ensures comprehensive mental health programs, which are critical to ensuring a comprehensive approach to mental health care. This inclusivity of all peoples and their lived experiences amplifies necessary advocacy efforts.

An evidence-based approach to delivery of initiatives to diversify and amplify policy changes is key. Policies must be informed by evidence and address the specific needs and challenges of the communities and individuals. They must also be financially sustainable to promote long-term impact. Finally, policies should uphold human rights, dignity, and autonomy for individuals with mental disorders. They must ensure protection of vulnerable and marginalized groups.

Education and Awareness Campaigns

Education and awareness regarding the prevalence and treatment of mental health are limited. Efforts to raise awareness about mental health disorders and their treatment can help reduce stigma and encourage individuals to seek help (WHO, 2022). However, campaigns should be culturally sensitive and tailored to specific communities, countries, and settings. A survey of teens and young adults found that 90% of these participants were experiencing symptoms of depression and researching their mental health issues online (Rideout et al., 2018).

Strengthening Mental Health Infrastructure

To adequately provide access at the population health level, governments and organizations should invest in developing mental health infrastructure, including training more mental health professionals, establishing accessible facilities, and integrating mental health services into primary care settings. Policies that enforce increased access, funding, infrastructure, and resources are imperative to ensuring adequate access.

Promoting Mental Health Parity Laws

Governments can enact laws that require insurance companies to provide coverage for mental health services that are on par with physical health services. This can help reduce the financial barriers to accessing mental health care. The WHO has implemented its *WHO Special Initiative for Mental Health (2019-2023): Universal Health Coverage for Mental Health* to improve access to mental health services and urge governments to provide these services as part of universal health coverage (WHO, 2019).

Using Technology

As observed during the COVID-19 pandemic, telehealth and online mental health platforms can help bridge the gap in access to care, particularly in remote areas and/or for individuals with limited mobility. Investment in maintaining and updating this infrastructure could support long-term investments in mental and physical health promotion and treatment (WHO, 2022).

SUMMARY

The journey toward achieving equitable mental health worldwide has been marked by both progress and persistent challenges. This chapter explores critical aspects of global mental health and well-being, delving into historical context, interconnectedness with physical health, barriers, and strategies. Mental health and physical health are intertwined. Addressing mental health positively impacts physical health outcomes and vice versa. Chronic stress, anxiety, and depression contribute to cardiovascular diseases, immune dysfunction, and other physical conditions (Prince et al., 2007).

The evolution of mental health disorders and treatment spans centuries, from ancient rituals to modern evidence-based interventions. Understanding this trajectory helps to emphasize the strides made in destigmatizing mental health conditions. However, barriers to achieving mental health and well-being persist, including stigma, resource scarcity, cultural and social barriers, equitable access, and inequitable policies. Education and awareness to promote mental health literacy, reduce stigma, and empower individuals to seek help must be increased. Global and local initiatives to address this significant burden of disease and achieve mental well-being are underway and need to be more robust to ensure that all people and populations have access to quality, culturally relevant global mental health care to make progress toward equitable global mental health.

DISCUSSION QUESTIONS

1. What do you think are the most prevalent reasons that global mental health as a field seemingly has been slow to emerge?
2. What are existing limitations but future opportunities to buttress both mental and physical health within communities?
3. What is a compelling reason for a coordinated global effort to improve mental health and well-being in LMICs, and what are some of the pitfalls?
4. What barriers are present at the individual, community, cultural, and political levels, and how can these be addressed?
5. What are some policies that should be considered to increase equity in mental health and well-being?

REFERENCES

American Psychiatric Association. (2024). *Stigma, prejudice and discrimination against people with mental illness.* https://www.psychiatry.org/patients-families/stigma-and-discrimination

Collins, P. Y., Patel, V., Joestl, S. S., March, D., Insel, T. R., Daar, A. S., Scientific Advisory Board and the Executive Committee of the Grand Challenges on Global Mental Health, Anderson, W., Dhansay, M. A., Phillips, A., Shurin, S., Walport, M., Ewart, W., Savill, S. J., Bordin, I. A., Costello, E. J., Durkin, M., Fairburn, C., Glass, R. I., Hall, W., ... Stein, D. J. (2011). Grand challenges in global mental health. *Nature, 475*(7354), 27–30. https://doi.org/10.1038/475027a

COVID-19 Mental Disorders Collaborators. (2021). Global prevalence and burden of depressive and anxiety disorders in 204 countries and territories in 2020 due to the COVID-19 pandemic. *The Lancet, 398*(10312), 1700–1712. https://doi.org/10.1016/S0140-6736(21)02143-7

Davies, R. D., & Kessel, B. (2017). Gender minority stress, depression, and anxiety in a transgender high school student. *The American Journal of Psychiatry, 174*(12), 1151–1152. https://doi.org/10.1176/appi.ajp.2017.17040439. PMID: 29191036.

Dawes, D. (2020). *The political determinants of health.* Johns Hopkins University Press.

Dawes, D. Bhatt, J., Dunlap, N., Amador, C., Gebreyes, K., & Rush, B. (2022). *The economic burden of mental health inequities in the United States report.* https://www2.deloitte.com/us/en/insights/industry/health-care/economic-burden-mental-health-inequities.html

Desjarlais, R., Eisenberg, L., Good, B., & Kleinman, A. (1995). *World mental health: Problems and priorities in low-income countries.* Oxford University Press.

Firth, J., Solmi, M., Wootton, R. E., Vancampfort, D., Schuch, F. B., Hoare, E., Gilbody, S., Torous, J., Teasdale, S. B., Jackson, S. E., Smith, L., Eaton, M., Jacka, F. N., Veronese, N., Marx, W., Ashdown-Franks, G., Siskind, D., Sarris, J., Rosenbaum, S., Carvalho, A. F., & Stubbs, B. (2020). A meta-review of "lifestyle psychiatry": The role of exercise, smoking, diet and sleep in the prevention and treatment of mental disorders. *World Psychiatry, 19*(3), 360–380. https://doi.org/10.1002/wps.20773

Herrman, H., Moodie, R., Saxena, S., University of Melbourne, Victorian Health Promotion Foundation, & World Health Organization, Department Of Mental Health and Substance Abuse. (2005). *Promoting mental health: Concepts, emerging evidence, practice.* World Health Organization. https://www.loc.gov/item/2021763240/

Jones, C. P., Jones, C. Y., Perry, G., Barclay, G., & Jones, C. A. (2009). Addressing the social determinants of children's health: A cliff analogy. *Journal of Health Care for the Poor and Underserved, 20*(4 Suppl), 1–12. https://doi.org.10.1353/hpu.0.0228

Kern, M., Duinhof, E., Walsh, S., Cosma, A., Moreno-Maldonado, C., Molcho, M., Currie, C., & Stevens, G. (2020). Intersectionality and adolescent mental well-being: A cross-nationally comparative analysis of the interplay between immigration background, socioeconomic status and gender. *Journal of Adolescent Health, 66*(6S), S12–S20. https://doi.org/10.1016/j.jadohealth.2020.02.013

Kleinman, A. (1988). *Rethinking psychiatry: Cultural category to personal experience*. Free Press.

Kraepelin, E. (2000). Comparative psychiatry. In R. Littlewood & S. Dein (Eds.), *Cultural psychiatry and medical anthropology: An introduction and reader* (pp. 38–42). Athlone Press. [Originally published 1904]

Littlewood, R. (1990). From categories to contexts: A decade of the "new cross-cultural psychiatry." *The British Journal of Psychiatry, 156*, 308–327. https://doi.org/10.1192/bjp.156.3.308

Mohammed, A., Sheikh, T. L., Gidado, S., Abdus-Salam, I. A., Adeyemi, J., Olayinka, A., Ohuabunwo, C., Victor, O. O., Nguku, P., Rasheed, E. A., Doherty, F., Waziri, N., Shuaib, F., Joseph, B. O., Bomai, I. M., & Oyemakinde, A. (2015). Psychiatric treatment of a health care worker during the Ebola outbreak in Sierra Leone. *Psychiatric Services (Washington, D.C.), 66*(11), 1166–1168. https://doi.org/10.1176/appi.ajp.2014.14121576

Nakimuli-Mpungu, E., Odokonyero, R., Laker, J., & Alderman, S. (2014). Major depression in postconflict northern Uganda: A case report. *The American Journal of Psychiatry, 171*(9), 925–928. https://doi.org/10.1176/appi.ajp.2014.14020261

Okpaku, S. O. (Ed.). (2014). *Essentials of global mental health*. Cambridge University Press. https://doi.org/10.1017/CBO9781139136341

Oxford Poverty and Human Development Initiative. (2022). *Gross national happiness index*. https://ophi.org.uk/policy/bhutan-gnh-index/#:~:text=The%20GNH%20Index%20value%20increased,2010%20to%200.781%20in%202022

Patel, V. (2007). Closing the 10/90 divide in global mental health research. *Acta Psychiatrica Scandinavica, 115*(4), 257–259. https://doi.org/10.1111/j.1600-0447.2007.01012.x

Patel, V. (2012). Global mental health: From science to action. *Harvard Review of Psychiatry, 20*(1), 6–12. https://doi.org/10.3109/10673229.2012.649108

Patel, V., Saxena, S., Lund, C., Thornicroft, G., Baingana, F., Bolton, P., Chisholm, D., Collins, P. Y., Cooper, J. L., Eaton, J., Herrman, H., Herzallah, M. M., Huang, Y., Jordans, M. J. D., Kleinman, A., Medina-Mora, M. E., Morgan, E., Niaz, U., Omigbodun, O., Prince, M., Rahman, A., ..., UnÜtzer, J. (2018). The Lancet Commission on Global Mental Health and Sustainable Development. *Lancet (London, England), 392*(10157), 1553–1598. https://doi.org/10.1016/S0140-6736(18)31612-X

Plough, A. (Ed.). (2022). *Necessary conversations: Understanding racism as a barrier to achieving health equity*. Oxford University Press.

Prince, M., Patel, V., Saxena, S., Maj, M., Maselko, J., Phillips, M. R., & Rahman, A. (2007). No health without mental health. *The Lancet, 370*(9590), 859–877. https://doi.org/10.1016/S0140-6736(07)61238-0

Rathod, S., Pinninti, N., Irfan, M., Gorczynski, P., Rathod, P., Gega, L., & Naeem, F. (2017). Mental health service provision in low- and middle-income countries. *Health Services Insights, 10*, 1178632917694350. https://doi.org/10.1177/1178632917694350

Rideout, V., Fox, S., & Well Being Trust. (2018). Digital health practices, social media use, and mental well-being among teens and young adults in the U.S. *Articles, Abstracts, and Reports, 1093*. https://digitalcommons.providence.org/publications/1093

Shonkoff, J., Garner, A., the Committee on Psychosocial Aspects of Child and Family Health, Committee on Early Childhood, Adoption, and Dependent Care, and Section on Developmental and Behavioral Pediatrics, Siegel, B., Dobbins, M., Earls, M., McGuinn, L., Pascoe, J., Wood, D. (2012). The lifelong effects of early childhood adversity and toxic stress. *Pediatrics, 129*(1), e232–e246. https://doi.org/10.1542/peds.2011-2663

Sorel, E. (Ed.). (2012). *21st century global mental health*. Jones & Bartlett Learning.

United for Global Health. (2021). *Decriminalising suicide: Saving lives, reducing stigma*. https://unitedgmh.org/knowledge-hub/decriminalising-suicide-saving-lives-reducing-stigma-latest-report/.

United Nations Human Rights Council Fiftieth Session. (2022, June 13-July 8). *Agenda item 3 promotion and protection of all human rights, civil, political, economic, social and cultural rights, including the right to development*. https://docs.un.org/en/A/hrc/res/50/10

Woelbert, E., White, R., Lundell-Smith, K., Grant, J., & Kemmer, D. (2020). The inequities of mental health research (IAMHRF). *Digital Science*, Section 7, pp. 14–26. https://doi.org/10.6084/m9.figshare.13055897.v2

World Health Organization. (n.d.). *Mental health gap action programme (mhGAP)*. https://www.who.int/team/mental-health-and-substance-use/treatment-care/mental-health-gap-action-programme

World Health Organization. (2001). *The world health report, 2001, mental health: New understanding, new hope*. https://iris.who.int/handle/10665/42390

World Health Organization. (2019). *The WHO special initiative for mental health (2019–2023): Universal health coverage for mental health*. https://iris.who.int/handle/10665/310981

World Health Organization. (2021, September). *Comprehensive mental health action plan 2013–2030*. https://www.who.int/publications/i/item/9789240031029

World Health Organization. (2022). *World mental health report: Transforming mental health for all*. https://www.who.int/publications/i/item/9789240049338

27 MENTAL HEALTH SYSTEM TRANSFORMATION AND FUTURE CONSIDERATIONS

OCTAVIO N. MARTINEZ, JR. AND FAZAL KHAN

LEARNING OBJECTIVES

After reading this chapter, the reader will be able to:

- Discuss how systemic and structural racism impact health and mental health.
- Describe how healthcare providers can achieve cultural humility.
- Analyze ethical issues in artificial intelligence (AI) and machine learning, such as biased data sets and prediction errors, that affect mental health care.
- Discuss how race-based variables in diagnostic tools can perpetuate disparities in health outcomes.
- Recommend approaches to create inclusive, fair, and equity-focused AI systems in healthcare.

INTRODUCTION

Mental health equity has emerged as a critical focus in the field of public health and the behavioral sciences, addressing the profound disparities in mental health outcomes and access to care across diverse populations (American Psychiatric Association, 2020; "Cultivating Mental Health Equity," 2023). This chapter explores the multifaceted challenges and potential solutions in achieving mental health equity, emphasizing the need for systemic transformation and innovative approaches that are evidence based. Mental health disparities are deeply rooted in complex societal structures, including systemic racism, socioeconomic inequalities, and cultural barriers (Bhugra et al., 2018). These factors contribute to significant differences in the prevalence of mental health disorders, access to quality care, and treatment outcomes among various demographic groups. Recognizing these disparities is crucial for developing effective strategies to promote mental health equity (Kola et al., 2021).

A critical aspect of addressing mental health inequity is acknowledging and confronting implicit biases and structural racism within the healthcare system. Research has shown that these factors may lead to misdiagnosis, inadequate treatment, and poorer outcomes for marginalized communities (Liang et al., 2016). For instance, studies have revealed that Black patients are more likely to be misdiagnosed with schizophrenia by White psychiatrists, highlighting the urgent need for cultural humility and bias awareness in mental health practice (Gara et al., 2019). Shifting toward community-centered approaches is also essential in promoting mental health equity. This involves engaging with diverse communities, understanding their unique needs and perspectives, and developing culturally competent interventions (Alegría et al., 2018). By prioritizing community voices and experiences, mental health systems can better address the specific challenges faced by underserved populations and create more effective, tailored solutions.

Emerging technologies, particularly artificial intelligence (AI) and telehealth, offer promising avenues for improving access to mental health care (Khan, 2024). These innovations have the potential to bridge geographical gaps, reduce costs, and provide personalized interventions. However, it is crucial to approach these technologies with caution, because they also carry the risk of perpetuating and even amplifying existing biases if not implemented thoughtfully (Khan, 2023). The development of AI systems in mental health must prioritize transparency, explain-ability, and ethical oversight. This includes creating more inclusive data sets that represent diverse populations, implementing rigorous evaluation processes, and ensuring that AI-driven solutions do not exacerbate existing disparities (Khan, 2023).

As we delve deeper into the complexities of mental health equity throughout this chapter, we will explore evidence-based strategies, policy recommendations, and innovative approaches to transform mental health systems and promote equitable outcomes for all individuals, regardless of their background or circumstances.

HISTORICAL CONTEXT OF RACE

Throughout history, humanity has differentiated itself on a cultural basis, by language, symbols, norms, values, rituals, and so forth (Marks, 2007). Only recently, within the past 4 centuries, has the concept of race entered as a distinct differentiating variable (Smedley & Smedley, 2005). This construct was a new ideology about what makes humans different. This approach to structuring society had never existed before (Smedley & Smedley, 2005). There are no genetic or biological bases for the race categories we are all familiar with, despite the fact that it was "science" that developed racial classifications. The roots for race evolved over time to justify unfair, inequitable suppression of one group in order for another group to maintain power and privilege. Long before the construct of race became solidified, the English had a long history of separating themselves. For example, they treated the Irish as alien "others." This English attitude toward the Irish set precedence on how they would treat others in the New World (Encyclopedia Britannica, n.d.-a).

The concept took a while to take hold in the colonies. For the first 6 to 7 decades of colonial history, the social position of Africans and their descendants was not particularly impacted by the ideology of inequality or inferiority (Encyclopedia Britannica, n.d.-a). However, as human slavery took on greater economic value and the American colonies instituted a system of permanent slavery for Africans, categorization of humans became an imperative (Encyclopedia Britannica, n.d.-a; Smedley & Smedley, 2005). It was the Age of Enlightenment. Western European societies were embracing philosophies promoting liberty, justice, brotherhood, and equality, but slavery was antithetical to these philosophies (Smedley & Smedley, 2005). According to historian Philip D. Morgan, "The only effective way to justify slavery was to exclude its victims from the community of man" (Encyclopedia Britannica, n.d.-a). Africans were demoted to nonhuman status, and grotesque descriptions were publicized to instill fear and loathing (Encyclopedia Britannica, n.d.-a; Smedley & Smedley, 2005)

In the 1800s, the Swedish botanist Carolus Linnaeus and the German physiologist Johann Friedrich Blumenbach provided the models, racial terms, and categories we use today. Linnaeus introduced the scientific term *Homo sapiens* and listed four major subdivisions: *H. americanus*, *H. africanus*, *H. europaeus*, and *H. asiaticus*. He also had two additional categories: *H. monstrosus* and *H. ferus*. Blumenbach divided humankind differently. He developed five "varieties": American, Malay, Ethiopian, Mongolian, and Caucasian (Encyclopedia Britannica, n.d.-a; Smedley & Smedley, 2005, p. 21). Over time, the concept of race has promoted the narrative that Black individuals and other minoritized people are inherently and genetically inferior (Bryant et al., 2022). Contributing to this narrative has been the role that medicine has played, despite the fact that racial distinctions are not genetically discrete, not reliably measured, and not scientifically meaningful (Smedley & Smedley, 2005). See **Table 27.1** for historical examples of racialized distinctions.

Table 27.1 HISTORICAL EXAMPLES OF RACIAL DISTINCTIONS BY PHYSICIANS

Charles White (1728–1813)	Manchester, England, physician	Described racial categories in physical terms; identified differences in the head, feet, arms, complexion, skin color, hair texture, and susceptibility to disease.
Samuel Adolphus Cartwright (1793–1863)	American southern physician	Identified "drapetomania"; claimed it caused enslaved Africans to run away and argued the treatment was keeping Black people in submission and could be cured by whippings; also discovered "dysaesthesia aethiopica," a disease in Black people that was distinguished by reduced intellectual ability, laziness, and partial insensitivity of the skin.
Samuel George Morton (1799–1851)	Philadelphia physician	Founder of the field of craniometry; concluded that Black individuals had smaller brains and therefore were less intelligent.
James Marion Sims (1813–1883)	American surgeon	Father of modern gynecology; developed vesicovaginal fistula repair through experimentation on enslaved Black women, without anesthesia, partly because of the belief that Black people did not feel as much pain as White people.

Source: Bailey, Z. D., Feldman, J. M., & Bassett, M. T. (2021). How structural racism works—Racist policies as a root cause of U.S. racial health inequities. *The New England Journal of Medicine, 384*(8), 768–773. https://doi.org/10.1056/NEJMms2025396

SYSTEMIC AND STRUCTURAL RACISM

Scientifically, it has taken about two and a half centuries to overcome Linnaeus's mistaken belief that the human species comes taxonomically organized into a few large, natural groups and to understand that human variation is mostly cultural and polymorphic (Marks, 2007). However, sociopolitically, the concept of race has proven more difficult to undo. Discriminatory behavior has been normalized through structural racism, codified in laws, regulations, and social mores. Law, including the political process, is the tool used to structure American systems (Yearby, 2020). Historical records show that the Virginia Assembly, between 1660 and 1690, began to pass laws and establish practices that sanctioned differential treatment to purposely separate Europeans from Indians and Africans. And by 1723, even free African Americans were prohibited from voting and exercising their civil rights. Part of the dehumanization of Africans was the emphasis on the slave as property, and many of the laws and court decisions at the time reflected that the property rights of a slave owner superseded the human rights of a slave. Through the Emancipation Proclamation, issued on January 1, 1863, by President Abraham Lincoln, and the 13th Amendment to the U.S. Constitution in 1865, slavery was ended, but the ideology of separateness was not. The Black Codes, which had their roots in the "slave codes" that arose in 1865 and 1866 helped legitimize the social philosophy of racism (Encyclopedia Britannica, n.d.-b). By the mid-19th century, the characterization of Africans had become central to the ideology of separateness and transformed social policy. Race became the causal agent of human difference in the courts, statehouses, assemblies, churches, and other American institutions. In addition, the U.S. Supreme Court decisions, such as the *Dred Scott* case of 1857 (Negroes were not and could not be citizens of the United States) and *Plessy v. Ferguson* of 1896 (permitted "separate but equal" facilities), along with the Jim Crow laws of the South, solidified the sociopolitical use of the construct of race as we entered the 20th century (Encyclopedia Britannica, n.d.-a).

It is important to recognize that racism is not simply the result of individual prejudice, but is fueled by wealth, greed, and power. Laws, rules, and practices were implemented by government at all levels and embedded in the economic system to secure a steady supply of cheap labor: the formerly enslaved (Bailey et al., 2021; Encyclopedia Britannica, n.d.-b). The political process, statutes, regulations, policies, advisory opinions, cases, and budgetary decisions, and how laws were enforced, all contributed to what we now refer to as systemic and structural racism (Yearby, 2020). Systemic racism emphasizes the involvement of whole systems, such as the political, legal, criminal justice, economic, healthcare, and educational systems. *Structural racism* refers to the role of the systems' support structures (i.e., the laws, policies, institutional practices, and norms; Braveman et al., 2022). These forms of racism are so penetrating and embedded in our society that they are often assumed to reflect the natural, inevitable order, and unless called out and intentionally addressed, are self-perpetuating (Braveman et al., 2022). Systemic and structural racism impacts inequitably the allocation and access to resources. It functions to devalue and disempower racialized and minoritized groups for the benefit of the so-called "superior" group (Yearby et al., 2022, p. 187).

The resulting lack of political power also impacts health by ensuring poor access to key drivers, resources, and opportunities to be healthy, which we now recognize as the social determinants of health. In fact, systemic and structural racism produces differential conditions between Whites and racialized and/or minoritized groups, resulting in health disparities and health inequities (O'Kane et al., 2021; Yearby, 2020). Opportunities denied include access to good jobs with benefits, fair treatment by the criminal justice system, safe neighborhoods, well-resourced schools, access to healthy food, and high-quality healthcare (Braveman et al., 2022). Daniel Dawes highlights that the political determinants disproportionately influence and impact the social determinants of health and have been the main drivers for the state of health and the alarming inequities in health, especially as they relate to minoritized communities. He states in his book *The Political Determinants of Health* that "Political determinants of health involve the systematic process of structuring relationships, distributing resources, and administering power, operating simultaneously in ways that mutually reinforce or influence one another to shape opportunities that either advance health equity or exacerbate health inequities" (Dawes, 2020, pp. 44–45).

FRAMEWORK FOR HEALTHCARE QUALITY

Many in our society struggle to accept that racism is present and the cause of health disparities and inequities in the U.S. healthcare system; however, a significant body of research has made it clear that although we have made progress as a society, systemic and structural racism continues to affect the health and mental health of many of our communities. In 2003, the Institute of Medicine (IOM; now known as the National Academy of Medicine) released the report *Unequal Treatment: Confronting Racial and Ethnic Disparities in Health Care* (IOM, 2003). The IOM committee, made up of distinguished researchers, scientists, and physicians, reviewed more than 100 studies and concluded that bias, prejudice, and stereotyping contributed to widespread differences in healthcare by race and ethnicity (Bailey et al., 2021). This was a seminal report that added additional understanding to the quality of the U.S. healthcare system. Two years earlier, in 2001, the IOM, in the report *Crossing the Quality Chasm: A New Health System for the 21st Century*, put forth a framework for improving the quality of healthcare. The framework includes six domains. Healthcare should be safe—avoiding harm to people from the care that is intended to help them; effective—providing services based on scientific knowledge to all who could benefit and refraining from providing services to those not likely to benefit; person-centered—providing care that is respectful of and responsive to individual preferences, needs, and values and ensuring that patient values guide all clinical decisions; timely—reducing waits and sometimes harmful delays for both those who receive and those who give care; efficient—avoiding waste, including waste of equipment, supplies, ideas, and energy; and equitable—providing care that does not vary in quality because of personal characteristics such as gender, ethnicity, geographic location, and socioeconomic status (Agency for Healthcare Research and Quality, n.d.; McGuire & Miranda, 2008; O'Kane et al., 2021).

Yet, despite understanding that inequitable health care is low-quality care, and identifying the factors needed to achieve health and mental health equity, disparities and inequities continue (O'Kane et al., 2021) One in five U.S. adults report experiencing discrimination in our healthcare system, especially if one is from a racial or ethnic group (O'Kane et al., 2021). Unfortunately, this is not surprising given that modern American medicine has historical roots in scientific racism and is structured to advantage the White population and disadvantage racialized and minoritized populations (Bailey et al., 2021; Yearby et al., 2022). The notion of race as a biological determinant, despite the evidence that race is not a reliable proxy for genetic difference, continues, and some physicians still use race-adjusted algorithms to perform patient risk assessments and guide clinical care, resulting in false diagnostic conclusions (Bryant et al., 2022; O'Kane et al., 2021). In research, it has contributed to negative stereotypes and the ongoing stigmatization of racialized and minoritized groups (Bryant et al., 2022). Given how embedded systemic and structural racism is in our healthcare system, it is imperative that we "enhance our understanding of how the social phenotype known as race functions in society to preferentially advantage and value White lives, cultural ideals, and norms over those of other racial and ethnic groups" (Bryant et al., 2022, p. 93). If we do not, we will continue to have poor health and mental health outcomes. That is why health and mental health equity must be a priority and should be the most urgent and crucial concern for the fields of medicine and science (O'Kane et al., 2021). Without an explicit focus on health and mental health equity, health and mental health disparities and inequities will continue, and the U.S. healthcare system will remain an inequitable healthcare system (O'Kane et al., 2021).

To that end, although it is the 21st century, daunting challenges remain in collecting accurate and comprehensive health service data and analytics on all of our community members. An equitable healthcare system will not emerge unless health and mental health equity is an explicit outcome prioritized, identified, measured, and analyzed by the system (O'Kane et al., 2021). To paraphrase the British physicist and mathematician William Thompson Kelvin, what is not measured cannot be improved. Comprehensive data are needed to drive improvement (O'Kane et al., 2021). For example, the absence of standardized data categories, the lack of patient trust, the reluctance of providers to collect data, and the lack of disaggregated data have all contributed to making underrepresented, racialized, and minoritized individuals invisible when policies are developed, resources are allocated, and programs are designed and implemented (Braveman et al., 2022; O'Kane et al., 2021). Improvement will require cultural change, system and process changes, and regulatory enforcement (O'Kane et al., 2021). Additionally, we must expand diversity and inclusion as they relate to the health and mental health workforce and align and increase the quality of healthcare interactions between the healthcare system and all the populations it serves (O'Kane et al., 2021). This includes addressing the quality and the makeup of leadership. Every aspect of performance in healthcare organizations (be they private, public, nonprofit, or academic) is influenced by the organization's leadership. Effective and diverse leadership that understands the history of systemic and structural racism, values the six domains of healthcare quality, practices cultural and linguistic humility, and reflects the communities served is needed (O'Kane et al., 2021).

IMPLICIT BIAS AND CULTURAL HUMILITY

The challenge for us comes in understanding and operationalizing an essential component that addresses systemic and structural racism, and that is cultural humility. To accomplish this, we first must understand bias. There are two types: explicit bias and implicit bias. Explicit bias or conscious bias is where an individual is clear about their feelings, attitudes, and related behaviors. Explicit bias is done with intent and may be characterized by negative behaviors expressed verbally and/or physically. Implicit bias, or subconscious bias, operates outside the individual's awareness (National Center for Cultural Competence, n.d.). It may lead to a negative evaluation of a person based on characteristics such as race, ethnicity, or gender, despite one's explicit belief in wanting to treat everyone equally (FitzGerald & Hurst, 2017; see **Box 27.1** for examples of bias). Biases can change over time as the environment changes and as an individual matures and gains insight into their belief system. The brain does have the ability to adapt (National Academies of Sciences, Engineering, and Medicine [NASEM], 2021).

However, it is also human nature to rationalize our subconscious when confronted with our biases and stereotypes. We develop explanations that act as barriers to addressing the inequity we have created, participated in, or benefited from. We tend to take a narrow focus on the individual. It is their fault because they just didn't try hard enough or are not smart enough. We do not take or are not aware of the historical context and its impact on the current situation, and/or we believe the myth of the zero-sum game, that is, my gain is your loss or more importantly perhaps, your gain is my loss. In this calculus, there is no win–win scenario (Harris & Strakowski, 2024; NASEM, 2021).

For healthcare leaders, including health and mental health providers, to improve health and mental health equity, we must understand our biases and stereotypes. This is no trivial matter and is challenging because evidence indicates that healthcare professionals exhibit the same levels of implicit bias as the general population. A major difference is that healthcare providers' biases impact diagnosis, treatment, and the quality of care (FitzGerald & Hurst, 2017). Healthcare studies have found a significant positive relationship between level of implicit bias and lower quality of care (FitzGerald & Hurst, 2017; O'Kane et al., 2021). Implicit bias reinforces systemic and structural racism and helps to perpetuate health and mental health disparities and inequities (O'Kane et al., 2021).

Therefore, understanding how biases and stereotypes are formed and how they influence behavior and decision-making gives one better insight into the human condition, be it positive or negative, and provides the basis for transformation of the health and mental health system for the betterment of all. To mitigate implicit bias and its impact on the quality of healthcare, we need to focus on changing policies and procedures at the systems level, at the structural level, and at the individual level.

Box 27.1 EXAMPLES OF IMPLICIT BIAS IN VARIOUS SECTORS

- *Criminal justice system*: Black faces are more likely to be associated with a weapon.
- *Education*: Black students are more harshly disciplined.
- *Healthcare*: Black Americans more likely to be misdiagnosed with schizophrenia.
- *Workplace*: Résumés that appear to be "White" are more likely to receive a callback.

Source: National Academies of Sciences, Engineering, and Medicine. (2021). *The science of implicit bias: Implications for law and policy, proceedings of a workshop in brief*. The National Academies Press. https://doi.org/10.17226/26191

This is where cultural humility plays a consequential role. Cultural humility is a lifelong commitment to self-evaluation and self-critique. For health and mental health providers, it increases their ability to recognize and respond with self-reflection, relationship building, and community engagement to the ways health and mental health outcomes are influenced by socioeconomic, cultural, political, and economic forces. It includes self-reflection to understand one's implicit biases, learning to recognize and understand the systemic and structural influences on individual health and mental health, the clinical encounter, and the world beyond the four walls of the clinic (Gottlieb, 2023). There are specific action steps that healthcare providers can take to achieve cultural humility (see **Box 27.2**).

Box 27.2 COMPETENCIES IN CROSS-CULTURAL HEALTHCARE

- Assess and describe your own cultural and spiritual/religious values, and discuss the effect of those values on your healthcare beliefs and behavior.
- Identify and understand the heterogeneity within categories and groups of individuals and their families.
- Assess the client's position on the continuum of acculturation in relation to their preferences, perceptions, and definitions, and their explanatory models of physical and mental health and illness, their health literacy, and their health behaviors.
- Demonstrate interviewing skills that promote culturally appropriate decision-making and mutual respect between healthcare providers and their clients and their families in patient-centered care throughout the continuum of their lives, including end-of-life care.
- Communicate effectively and elicit information from individuals of all kinds of backgrounds and their families, particularly those who speak little or no English, with appropriate use of interpreter services and information technology.
- Learn and explain the importance of cultural and historical experiences (e.g., historical trauma from racism and discrimination, real and perceived), and describe their effect on the client's help-seeking behaviors and their access and utilization of healthcare services, including emergency preparedness.
- Communicate with individuals and their families using oral and written strategies mindful of health literacy levels and abilities.
- Identify available resources within individuals, their families, and their respective communities for promoting and maintaining one's physical, mental, and spiritual health, and support those resources in a respectful way.
- Maintain up-to-date knowledge on health and mental health disparities and inequities across the life span and the effect of ethnicity and culture on physical and mental health care of individuals.
- Advocate for adoption of policies and practices that facilitate cultural humility, providing sensitive and proficient healthcare within patient-centered medical homes, institutions, organizations, and professions.

Source: Stanford Geriatric Education Center. (n.d.). *Ethnogeriatric competencies*. https://sgec.stanford.edu/competencies.html

A COMMUNITY-CENTERED APPROACH

The Framework for Healthcare Quality emphasizes the importance of a person-centered approach to achieving quality care, but equally important to achieving quality care and inherently health and mental health equity is a community-centered approach. The IOM's *Unequal Treatment* report recommended community-based care approaches to reducing disparities (O'Kane et al., 2021). Also, in 2021, the National Commission to Transform Public Health Data Systems recommended that community engagement be prioritized to help create a more equity-centered data network (Pokam Tchuisseu et al., 2021). Authentic community engagement and partnership are essential to addressing the determinants of health and mental health. Engaging with communities and community organizations is a powerful method to address systemic and structural racism and health and mental health disparities and inequities (O'Kane et al., 2021). Additionally, a community-centered approach will help build one of the most important core values we have as humans: trust. With trust, innovative programs and research with the community can become reality, such as collaborating with community to cocreate screening tools, interventions, and measurement approaches (Magnan, 2021). When building relationships with community, regardless of whether it is through academia, researchers, or policy makers, it is critical that sufficient time is taken and that certain principles of community engagement are followed. See **Box 27.3** for a list of principles of community engagement. This work requires one to become familiar with the different types of community engagement models and take to heart the core values of respect, justice, integrity, ethics, fairness, empathy, honesty, and transparency (Harris & Strakowski, 2024).

TRANSFORMING CLINICAL ALGORITHMS IN MENTAL HEALTH: A FRAMEWORK FOR ADVANCING HEALTH EQUITY

This section explores the urgent need to reevaluate clinical algorithms in mental health care through an equity lens. It introduces a framework for assessing and transforming these tools to ensure fairer and more inclusive outcomes. By analyzing current algorithmic biases and

Box 27.3 PRINCIPLES OF COMMUNITY ENGAGEMENT

- Understand the history of the community.
- Recognize and acknowledge the cumulative impact of stressful experiences and environments on community members.
- Recognize the role and impact of privilege.
- Create a safe environment for public participation.
- Do not blame individuals or groups for their disadvantaged status.
- Strengthen the social fabric of the neighborhoods that make up the community.
- Include all age groups.
- Work across multiple sectors.
- Focus on community determinants through a health equity lens.
- Measure and track the impact of social policies.
- Build on the strengths and assets of the community.

Source: Harris, S. S., & Strakowski, S. M. (Eds.). (2024). *Redesigning the US mental health care system*. Oxford University Press.

their implications for health disparities, this section offers methodological approaches for evaluation and provides policy recommendations for systematic change. Existing evidence highlights how clinical algorithms, if left unchecked, can perpetuate health inequities because of embedded racial, cultural, and socioeconomic biases. To address this, a structured approach to their reform is essential.

The U.S. healthcare system's growing reliance on clinical algorithms for decision-making underscores the importance of addressing equity and bias in these tools. Although algorithms aim to standardize care and improve outcomes, emerging research has shown how they can inadvertently encode and amplify existing health disparities. For instance, one widely used healthcare algorithm was found to assign Black patients as being healthier than equally ill White patients because it used healthcare costs as a proxy for medical need (Obermeyeret al., 2019). This approach resulted in over half of Black patients being excluded from receiving additional care. Reformulating this algorithm to remove cost-based assumptions effectively mitigated the bias, demonstrating that such tools must be critically examined and recalibrated to achieve equitable outcomes (Obermeyer et al., 2019). This issue is particularly pressing in mental health care, where disparities in access, diagnosis, and treatment outcomes for marginalized populations are already well documented.

BACKGROUND: HEALTH ALGORITHMS IN ACTION

The Vaginal Birth After Cesarean (VBAC) Calculator exemplifies how clinical algorithms can institutionalize bias through race-based corrections (Vyas et al., 2020). This tool excluded variables such as marital status and insurance type despite their known correlation with VBAC success, and instead incorporated race as a correction factor. By underestimating VBAC success rates for non-White women, the algorithm reinforced disparities in maternal health outcomes. This is particularly troubling given the higher rates of cesarean deliveries and maternal mortality among Black women in the United States (Vyas et al. 2020). The use of race as a variable in medical algorithms reflects a failure to adopt a more nuanced understanding of race as a social construct rather than a biological determinant (Cerdeña et al., 2022). Transitioning toward race-conscious practices that address social determinants of health and inequities is critical to fostering more equitable maternal and mental health outcomes.

Diagnostic tools such as the Patient Health Questionnaire-9 (PHQ-9) also reveal significant cultural biases in mental health care (Levis et al., 2019). This widely used screening tool often fails to capture culturally specific expressions of depression, such as the physical symptoms more commonly reported in some Asian populations (Yeung & Chang, 2002). As a result, depression may be underdiagnosed or improperly treated in these groups. Addressing such gaps requires reevaluating diagnostic tools to incorporate culturally competent frameworks that reflect the diverse ways mental health conditions manifest across populations.

ADVANCING EQUITY THROUGH CULTURALLY COMPETENT ARTIFICIAL INTELLIGENCE

Machine learning and AI hold immense potential for personalized mental health care but face significant challenges due to biased data, underrepresentation of minority groups, and systemic inequities (Char et al., 2018; Gianfrancesco et al., 2018). For example, predictive models often perform poorly for underserved populations because they are trained on data sets that lack diversity, leading to inaccurate predictions and perpetuating disparities (Chen et al., 2019). Studies have found disparities in error rates across race, gender, and socioeconomic status in clinical prediction models, highlighting the need for more inclusive data and rigorous testing (Obermeyer et al., 2019; Rajkomar et al., 2018).

To address this algorithmic bias and health inequities in AI-driven clinical tools, algorithms should include diverse data, capture social determinants of health, and be tested for discriminatory behavior (Gianfrancesco et al., 2018; Rajkomar et al., 2018). Studies using ICU and psychiatric clinical notes have revealed disparities in prediction errors across race, gender, and insurance types, with significant differences in error rates linked to systemic biases in data (Char et al., 2018; Obermeyer et al., 2019). Continuous human oversight, interdisciplinary collaboration, and a focus on clinically meaningful outcomes are essential to ensure fairness and reduce biases (Chen et al., 2018). AI and machine learning offer promise for personalized care but risk amplifying existing biases if trained on incomplete or biased data (Char et al., 2018). Ultimately, machine learning must aim to enhance care for all patients without amplifying existing healthcare disparities (**Table 27.2**).

THE ROLE OF GOVERNMENT AND STAKEHOLDERS

To systematically address bias in clinical algorithms, a comprehensive framework for evaluation and transformation is necessary. This framework must include a thorough review of the historical contexts in which biases have influenced the development of existing algorithms, followed by rigorous technical evaluations. Statistical validation across diverse subpopulations is critical for identifying and addressing disparities in algorithmic performance. Policy implementation should then focus on developing guidelines and standardized methods that promote equity in algorithm design and deployment.

Key stakeholders, including federal agencies such as the U.S. Department of Health and Human Services (HHS), the National Institute of Standards and Technology (NIST), and the Centers for Medicare & Medicaid Services (CMS) must play a central role in ensuring compliance and incentivizing equitable practices.

Engaging community health leaders and integrating the lived experiences of marginalized populations are equally essential to ensure that these frameworks address systemic disparities effectively. The private sector also has a responsibility to collaborate with regulators and communities to advance equity in AI systems. However, relying solely on industry self-regulation risks prioritizing profit over fairness. Public accountability and oversight are critical to aligning technological innovation with societal needs.

Table 27.2 HEALTH ALGORITHMS: KEY ISSUES AND RECOMMENDATIONS

ASPECT	ISSUE	SOLUTION/RECOMMENDATION
VBAC Calculator	Excluded marital status and insurance type as variables Included race as a correction factor, reinforcing disparities for non-White women	Transition toward race-conscious practices. Address SDOH and inequities.
PHQ-9	Cultural biases: fails to capture culturally specific expressions of depression Example: Physical symptoms reported by Asian populations are often missed.	Incorporate culturally competent frameworks in diagnostic tools.
AI and machine learning	Biased data and underrepresentation of minority groups Higher prediction error rates for underserved populations Example: ICU and psychiatric prediction disparities based on race and gender.	Use diverse data sets and rigorous testing, and capture SDOH. Continuous human oversight and interdisciplinary collaboration. Ensure fairness and clinically meaningful outcomes.

AI, artificial intelligence; PHQ-9, Patient Health Questionnaire-9; SDOH, social determinants of health; VBAC, vaginal birth after cesarean.

CRITICALLY ASSESSING ARTIFICIAL INTELLIGENCE IN MENTAL HEALTH

AI and telehealth technologies offer unprecedented opportunities to expand access and improve the quality of mental health care. However, these benefits come with significant challenges, including risks of bias, privacy concerns, and the potential loss of human-centered care. Addressing these challenges requires designing AI systems that are transparent and explainable, ensuring that their decision-making processes allow for scrutiny and correction of biases. Inclusive data practices are equally vital, because collecting diverse and representative data sets improves the accuracy and equity of these systems. Regular audits and evaluations are necessary to detect and mitigate biases in algorithmic performance, particularly across demographic groups. Engaging with affected communities and stakeholders in the development and deployment of AI technologies ensures that these tools align with the needs and values of the populations they are meant to serve. In parallel, robust regulatory frameworks must enforce standards for fairness, accountability, and transparency to guide the ethical use of AI in mental health care.

Transforming clinical algorithms in mental health care requires a systemic, equity-focused approach that prioritizes fairness, inclusivity, and accountability. From redesigning existing tools to developing rigorous frameworks for evaluation, the healthcare system must actively work to dismantle embedded biases and promote equitable outcomes. Achieving this goal demands collaboration among technologists, policy makers, healthcare providers, and community leaders, with a shared commitment to addressing the structural determinants of health. With thoughtful implementation, clinical algorithms and AI systems have the potential to revolutionize mental health care—ensuring that advancements benefit all individuals regardless of their race, ethnicity, or socioeconomic status.

MENTAL HEALTH CARE ACCESS CHALLENGES AND THE POTENTIAL ROLE OF ARTIFICIAL INTELLIGENCE AND TELEHEALTH

The United States is grappling with a profound crisis in mental health care access that affects both urban and rural areas, underscoring systemic barriers that impede vulnerable populations from receiving timely, affordable, and comprehensive mental health services (Jacoby & Li, 2022; Khan, 2024). Given that the shortage of medical professionals is unlikely to improve, this crisis calls for innovative solutions that leverage telehealth technologies and regulatory reforms to address these persistent challenges and promote equitable access to care. As we delve deeper into this issue, it becomes clear that a multifaceted approach is necessary to overcome the complex obstacles hindering mental health care delivery across diverse geographic and socioeconomic landscapes.

THE CURRENT MENTAL HEALTH CARE LANDSCAPE

Mental health care access in the United States is marked by deep inequities and systemic inadequacies that have far-reaching consequences for individuals, families, and communities. The disparities in access and quality of care between urban and rural areas are particularly stark, reflecting broader patterns of healthcare inequality across the nation.

In rural regions, the scarcity of mental health providers is particularly acute. According to the Health Resources and Services Administration (HRSA), nearly 20% of Americans live in rural areas, but only 10% of licensed mental health professionals practice in these communities (Nielsen et al., 2017). This disparity leaves rural residents with limited access to care, exacerbating psychological vulnerabilities and unmet mental health needs (Morales et al., 2020). Research has shown that suicide rates in rural areas (18.3–20.5 per 100,000 residents) are significantly higher than in urban areas (10.9–12.5 per 100,000 residents), highlighting the urgent need for improved mental health services in these communities

(Centers for Disease Control and Prevention, 2024). Rural residents often face additional barriers, such as long travel distances to reach mental health providers, limited public transportation options, lack of anonymity in seeking mental health services in small communities, and cultural stigma surrounding mental health issues (Jacoby & Li, 2022).

In urban areas, where resources might seem more abundant, barriers such as high costs, prolonged wait times, and limited availability of specialized services constrain access (Jacoby & Li, 2022). Despite a higher concentration of providers, structural challenges—ranging from socioeconomic disparities to fragmented service delivery systems—undermine the mental health care infrastructure in these settings. Urban residents, particularly those in low-income neighborhoods, face unique challenges, including overcrowded mental health facilities with long waiting lists, high costs of care often prohibitive for uninsured or underinsured individuals, cultural and linguistic barriers for diverse urban populations, and lack of coordination between mental health services and other social services (KFF, 2023; **Table 27.3**).

TELEHEALTH AND THE IMPACT OF THE COVID-19 PANDEMIC

The COVID-19 pandemic highlighted these systemic deficiencies, bringing unprecedented strain to the mental health care system while simultaneously demonstrating the transformative potential of telehealth technologies. During the pandemic, telehealth utilization surged dramatically, with significant increases in telehealth utilization as federal and state agencies, along with private insurers, waived most existing regulations related to the use of this modality (Khan, 2024). Patient satisfaction surveys revealed that a large majority of respondents found virtual care effective and expressed a preference for its continued availability post pandemic. These findings underscore the opportunity to leverage telehealth's capabilities to address access disparities across the urban–rural divide.

Table 27.3 RURAL VERSUS URBAN MENTAL HEALTH DISPARITIES

FACTOR	RURAL AREAS	URBAN AREAS
Population distribution	Nearly 20% of Americans live in rural areas.	Majority live in urban areas
Mental health provider availability	Only 10% of licensed mental health professionals	Higher availability of licensed providers
Suicide rates	18.3–20.5 per 100,000 residents	10.9–12.5 per 100,000 residents
Access to care	Limited access due to fewer providers	Greater access to care
Travel distance	Long distances to mental health providers	Shorter distances to providers
Transportation options	Limited public transportation	Better public transportation infrastructure
Anonymity in seeking care	Low (small communities reduce anonymity)	Higher (easier to maintain anonymity)
Cultural stigma	Greater stigma surrounding mental health issues	Comparatively lower stigma

BARRIERS TO MENTAL HEALTH CARE ACCESS

Several interrelated systemic barriers impede the realization of a comprehensive and equitable mental health care system. Understanding these barriers is crucial for developing effective solutions. Particularly for telehealth, state-based licensing regulations are a significant obstacle, creating artificial geographic boundaries that restrict mental health professionals' ability to serve patients across state lines. These frameworks, rooted in an era of localized practice, are ill-suited for the demands of a digitized and interconnected healthcare landscape. Scope-of-practice limitations further constrain access by preventing advanced practice providers, such as psychiatric nurse practitioners, from utilizing their full training and expertise. Although numerous studies demonstrate that nurse practitioners provide care on par with physicians in terms of quality and outcomes, restrictive policies in many states deny them full practice authority, limiting their ability to address provider shortages effectively. Rural and economically marginalized urban communities face compounded barriers due to geographic and economic constraints. In rural areas, some counties have only a single mental health provider serving populations exceeding 3,500 residents, far below the recommended ratios for adequate care access (Zhang et al., 2020). Urban centers, despite a greater density of providers, grapple with affordability and systemic inequities that disproportionately affect marginalized populations.

A FRAMEWORK FOR REFORM

To address these systemic barriers, a comprehensive reform strategy centered on telehealth regulations and scope of practice and licensing should be considered. Doing so could create a more flexible, efficient, and accessible mental health care system. Mutual recognition of mental health professional licenses across state lines, specifically for telehealth services, would create a more flexible and efficient system (Khan, 2024). This reform would enable licensed providers to deliver virtual care nationwide while preserving the ability of state licensing boards to regulate in-person practice and medical providers in their state. Expanding the scope of practice for mental health professionals through a competency-based framework could alleviate workforce shortages and enhance access. By prioritizing demonstrated competencies over traditional professional hierarchies, psychiatric nurse practitioners and other advanced practice providers could deliver care at the highest levels of their training. Integrating AI-based diagnostic tools further amplifies the potential of mental health care delivery. AI can assist in early detection of mental health conditions, personalized treatment recommendations, and continuous monitoring of patient progress. However, as discussed in the previous section of this chapter, AI-based therapeutic systems are not a panacea, and efforts to address biased algorithms and lack of diversity in data sets are essential from an equity vantage point.

MEASURING THE IMPACT OF POLICY INNOVATIONS: THE ROLE OF LEGAL EPIDEMIOLOGY

The reforms discussed previously hold the potential to transform the mental health care landscape by increasing access for underserved populations, alleviating provider shortages, and reducing costs through more efficient service delivery. Rural communities could benefit from access to a broader range of mental health professionals through telehealth, reduced travel times and associated costs for mental health care, and increased availability of specialized mental health services previously unavailable locally. Urban areas could see improvements such as reduced wait times for mental health appointments; greater choice of providers, leading to better patient–provider matches; and improved integration of mental health services with primary care. In addition, the reforms could lead to cost savings through reduced emergency department visits for mental health crises, earlier intervention and prevention of severe mental health conditions, and more efficient use of provider time through telehealth and AI-assisted diagnostics.

Although evidence-based research and sound policy rationale support the aforementioned predictions, policy makers cannot be confident that these innovations are effective without measuring their actual impact. To measure the impact of these policy innovations, legal epidemiology offers powerful tools that can provide valuable insights into how regulatory shifts affect healthcare delivery and patient outcomes (Thompson et al., 2020).

LEGAL EPIDEMIOLOGY BASICS

To assess the effectiveness of these reforms, legal epidemiologists would first conduct a systematic collection and coding of relevant laws and regulations across different jurisdictions. This process, known as legal mapping, could capture important features of telehealth policies, such as licensing requirements, reimbursement rules, and privacy protections (Lane & Stergachis, 2024). Researchers can then employ quasi-experimental or observational research methods to analyze the effects of policy changes. For example, they might use interrupted time series analysis to examine changes in telehealth utilization rates before and after the implementation of new regulations. Difference-in-difference estimation could be used to compare outcomes between jurisdictions that adopted more permissive telehealth policies and those that maintained stricter regulations.

To fully understand the impact of policy changes, a combination of quantitative analysis and qualitative research methods could be used. This might involve interviewing healthcare providers, patients, and policy makers to gain insights into how regulatory changes affect clinical practice, patient access, and health outcomes. Researchers would examine outcomes such as changes in healthcare utilization patterns, patient satisfaction, health disparities, and clinical outcomes for specific conditions. They could also assess the economic impacts of telehealth policy changes, including effects on healthcare costs and provider reimbursement.

Health law policy scholars have made the argument that the mental health care access crisis demands bold, technology-enabled policy solutions (Khan, 2024). By reimagining licensing and scope-of-practice regulations, the United States can create a more equitable, accessible, and responsive mental health care ecosystem. These reforms, grounded in evidence and driven by strategic incentives, offer a pathway to address the diverse needs of urban and rural communities alike, fostering a system that prioritizes accessibility, quality, and equity. Through the adoption of such measures and rigorous evaluation using legal epidemiology, the nation has the opportunity to not only address current deficiencies but also build a future-oriented mental health care infrastructure capable of meeting the challenges of a growing and diverse population. As we move forward, it is crucial to maintain a focus on patient-centered care, cultural competence, and cultural humility, and ongoing evaluation of reform impacts to ensure that these changes truly benefit those in need of mental health services across all communities.

SUMMARY

Transforming mental health systems to address inequities requires a comprehensive and multifaceted approach that targets the root causes of disparities and ensures sustained, meaningful change. This begins with a deep understanding of implicit biases that permeate the healthcare system, including biases embedded in provider practices, institutional policies, and even technological innovations such as AI. Recognizing and addressing these biases are fundamental to dismantling the systemic barriers that disproportionately affect marginalized populations.

In tandem with addressing implicit biases, tackling structural racism must remain a cornerstone of this transformation. Structural racism manifests in unequal access to care, disparities in funding, and systemic underrepresentation of minority voices in decision-making processes. Meaningful progress requires embedding equity into the very fabric of mental health systems—through equitable resource allocation, culturally tailored interventions, and the inclusion of diverse perspectives at every level of planning and implementation.

Community partnerships are another vital pillar in this effort. True transformation cannot occur without the active involvement of the communities most affected by mental health inequities. Engaging these communities as equal partners ensures that interventions are not only culturally competent but also responsive to the unique needs and challenges faced by different populations. Such partnerships foster trust, build accountability, and create sustainable pathways for change.

Technology, particularly AI and telehealth, offers significant opportunities to address gaps in mental health care. However, leveraging technology responsibly is critical to ensure that advancements do not exacerbate existing inequities. Transparent AI systems, developed using inclusive data sets that reflect the diversity of patient populations, can help reduce bias and improve the accuracy and fairness of mental health assessments and interventions. At the same time, regulatory oversight must be robust, ensuring that AI and telehealth systems are held to the highest standards of safety, efficacy, and ethical use.

Strong regulatory frameworks also play an essential role in safeguarding against unintended consequences. Such frameworks must address issues such as data privacy, algorithmic bias, and unequal access to technological tools. Policies must ensure that the benefits of AI and telehealth are distributed equitably, with particular attention to rural and underserved communities that often face additional barriers to accessing mental health services.

Beyond technological and policy considerations, it is imperative to adopt a holistic and systems-based approach to mental health care. This includes integrating mental health with primary care, expanding access to affordable services, and fostering interdisciplinary collaboration among healthcare professionals. It also requires ongoing investment in mental health research, workforce development, and community education to address stigma and promote understanding of mental health as a critical component of overall well-being.

Finally, creating a more equitable mental health care system demands accountability and adaptability. Continuous monitoring and evaluation of interventions, coupled with a willingness to refine approaches based on emerging evidence, will be essential to achieving long-term success. The challenges we face are complex, but they are not insurmountable. By embracing innovation, fostering inclusivity, and prioritizing equity, we can build a mental health system that serves all individuals—regardless of their background, location, or socioeconomic status.

In conclusion, addressing mental health inequities is not just a matter of improving systems or leveraging technology—it is a moral and societal imperative. Mental health is foundational to human flourishing, and access to high-quality mental health care should be a universal right, not a privilege. By committing to systemic transformation, we can create a future where everyone has the opportunity to thrive mentally, emotionally, and socially, paving the way for healthier, more equitable communities worldwide.

DISCUSSION QUESTIONS

1. How does implicit bias impact healthcare providers? What strategies can be implemented to address these biases at systemic and individual levels?
2. Is it possible for the U.S. healthcare system to provide quality care to all without addressing health and mental health equity?
3. Why is community engagement crucial for transforming mental health systems to achieve equity? Discuss how culturally tailored interventions can build trust and address the specific needs of marginalized populations.
4. How can clinical tools, such as the PHQ-9 or other mental health algorithms, be redesigned to reflect cultural competence and equity? What steps can policy makers, clinicians, and technologists take to evaluate and reduce biases in these tools?
5. Although AI and telehealth present opportunities to improve access to mental health care, how can we ensure that these technologies do not reinforce existing inequities? What role do inclusive data and transparency play in achieving equitable outcomes?

ACKNOWLEGMENTS

The authors acknowledge Clarissa Moreno for her review.

REFERENCES

Agency for Healthcare Research and Quality. (n.d.). *Six domains of healthcare quality.* https://www.ahrq.gov/talkingquality/measures/six-domains.html

Alegría, M., Nakash, O., & NeMoyer, A. (2018). Increasing equity in access to mental health care: A critical first step in improving service quality. *World Psychiatry, 17*(1), 43–44. https://doi.org/10.1002/wps.20486

American Psychiatric Association. (2020). *Social (in)justice and mental health.* American Psychiatric Association Publishing.

Bailey, Z. D., Feldman, J. M., & Bassett, M. T. (2021). How structural racism works—Racist policies as a root cause of U.S. racial health inequities. *The New England Journal of Medicine, 384*(8), 768–773. https://doi.org/10.1056/NEJMms2025396

Bhugra, D., Bhui, K., & Shan Wong, S. Y. (2018). Health equity. In D. Bhugra, Bhui, K., & Shan Wong, S. Y. (Eds.), *Oxford textbook of public mental health.* Oxford University Press. https://doi.org/10.1093/med/9780198792994.003.0013

Braveman, P. A., Arkin, E., Proctor, D., Kauh, T., Holm, N. (2022). Systemic and structural racism: Definitions, examples, health damages, and approaches to dismantling. *Health Affairs, 41*(2), 171–178. https://doi.org/10.1377/hlthaff.2021.01394

Bryant, B. E., Jordan, A., & Clark, U. S. (2022). Race as a social construct in psychiatry research and practice. *JAMA Psychiatry, 79*(2), 93–94. https://doi.org/10.1001/jamapsychiatry.2021.2877

Cerdeña, J. P., Plaisime, M. V., & Tsai, J. (2022). From race-based to race-conscious medicine: How anti-racist uprisings call us to act. *The Lancet, 396*(10257), 1125–1128. https://doi.org/10.1016/S0140-6736(20)32076-6

Centers for Disease Control and Prevention. (2024). *Suicide disparities: Rural and urban differences.* Retrieved from https://www.cdc.gov/suicide/disparities/

Char, D. S., Shah, N. H., & Magnus, D. (2018). Implementing machine learning in health care—Addressing ethical challenges. *New England Journal of Medicine, 378*(11), 981–983. https://doi.org/10.1056/NEJMp1714229

Chen, I. Y., Szolovits, P., & Ghassemi, M. (2019). Can AI help reduce disparities in general medical and mental health care? *AMA Journal of Ethics, 21*(2), E167–E179.

Cultivating mental health equity, one page at a time. (2023). *Nature Mental Health, 1*(1), 1–2. https://doi.org/10.1038/s44220-023-00015-1

Dawes, D. E. (2020). *The political determinants of health.* Johns Hopkins University Press.

Encyclopedia Britannica. (n.d.-a). *Race: History, ideology, science.* https://britannica.com/topic/race-human/The-history-of-the-idea-of-race

Encyclopedia Britannica. (n.d.-b). *Black codes: Definition, U.S. history, and examples.* https://britannica.com/topic/Black-Codes

FitzGerald, C., & Hurst, S. (2017). Implicit bias in healthcare professionals: A systematic review. *BMC Medical Ethics, 18,* 19. https://doi.org/10.1186/s12910-017-0179-8

Gara, M.A., Minsky, S., Silverstein, S.M., Miskimen, T., & Strakowski, S. M. (2019). A naturalistic study of racial disparities in diagnosis at an outpatient behavior health clinic. *Psychiatric Services, 70*(2), 130–135. https://doi.org/10.1176/appi.ps.201800223

Gianfrancesco, M. A., Tamang, S., Yazdany, J., & Schmajuk, G. (2018). Potential biases in machine learning algorithms using electronic health record data. *JAMA Internal Medicine, 178*(11), 1544–1547. https://doi.org/10.1001/jamainternmed.2018.3763

Gottlieb, M. (2023, January 12). What is cultural humility? 3 Principles for social workers. *The New Social Worker.* https://www.socialworker.com/feature-articles/practice/what-is-cultural-humility-3-principles-for-social-workers/

Harris, S. S., & Strakowski, S. M. (Eds.). (2024). *Redesigning the US mental health care system.* Oxford University Press.

Institute of Medicine. (2003). *Unequal treatment: Confronting racial and ethnic disparities in health care.* The National Academies Press. https://doi.org/10.17226/12875

Jacoby, A., & Li, Y. (2022). Mental health care access and individual help-seeking during the COVID-19 pandemic. *Community Mental Health Journal, 58*(8), 1572–1583. https://doi.org/10.1007/s10597-022-00973-3

KFF. (2023, January 27). *Access and coverage for mental health care: Findings from the 2022 KFF women's health survey.* https://www.kff.org/mental-health/

Khan, F. (2023). Regulating the revolution: A legal roadmap to optimizing AI in healthcare. *Minnesota Journal of Law, Science & Technology, 25,* 49.

Khan, F. (2024). From pixels to prescriptions: The case for national telehealth licensing and AI-enhanced care. *Indiana Law Review, 57,* 581–611.

Kola, L., Kohrt, B. A., Acharya, B., Mutamba, B. B., Kieling, C., Kumar, M., Sunkel, C., Zhang, W., & Hanlon, C. (2021). The path to global equity in mental health care in the context of COVID-19. *The Lancet, 398*(10312), 1670–1672. https://doi.org/10.1016/S0140-6736(21)02233-9

Lane, J., & Stergachis, A. (2024). Combining legal epidemiology and implementation science to improve global access to medicines: Challenges and opportunities. *Frontiers in Health Services, 3,* 1291183. https://doi.org/10.3389/frhs.2023.1291183

Levis, B., Benedetti, A., & Thombs, B. D. (2019). Accuracy of Patient Health Questionnaire-9 (PHQ-9) for screening to detect major depression: Individual participant data meta-analysis. *BMJ, 365,* l1476. https://doi.org/10.1136/bmj.l1476

Liang, J., Matheson, B. E., & Douglas, J. M. (2016). Mental health diagnostic considerations in racial/ethnic minority youth. *Journal of Child and Family Studies, 25*(6), 1926–1940. https://doi.org/10.1007/s10826-015-0351-z

Magnan, S. (2017). Social determinants of health 101 for health care: Five plus five. *NAM Perspectives.* https://nam.edu/perspectives/social-determinants-of-health-101-for-health-care-five-plus-five/

Marks, J. (2007). Long shadow of Linnaeus's human taxonomy. *Nature, 447,* 28. https://doi.org/10.1038/447028a

McGuire, T. G., & Miranda, J. (2008). Racial and ethnic disparities in mental health care: Evidence and policy implications. *Health Affairs, 27*(2), 393–403. https://doi.org/10.1377/hlthaff.27.2.393

Morales, D., Barksdale, C., & Beckel-Mitchener, A. (2020). A call to action to address rural mental health disparities. *Journal of Clinical and Translational Science, 4*(5), 463–467. https://doi.org/10.1017/cts.2020.42

National Academies of Sciences, Engineering, and Medicine. (2021). *The science of implicit bias: Implications for law and policy: Proceedings of a workshop in brief.* The National Academies Press. https://doi.org/10.17226/26191

National Center for Cultural Competence. (2024, December 8). *Two types of bias.* https://nccc.georgetown.edu/bias/module-3/1.php

Nielsen, M., D'Agostino, D., & Gregory, P. (2017). Addressing rural health challenges head on. *Missouri Medicine, 114*(5), 363–366.

Obermeyer, Z., Powers, B., Vogeli, C., & Mullainathan, S. (2019). Dissecting racial bias in an algorithm used to manage the health of populations. *Science, 366,* 447–453. https://doi.org/10.1126/science.aax2342

O'Kane, M., Agrawal, S., Binder, L., Dzau, V., Gandhi, T. K., Harrington, R., Mate, K., McGann, P., Meyers, D., Rosen, P., Schreiber, M., & Schummers, D. (2021). An equity agenda for the field of health care quality improvement [Discussion paper]. *NAM perspectives.* National Academy of Medicine. https://doi.org/10.31478/202109b

Pokam Tchuisseu, Y., Jacobs, J., Chhean, E., Thoumi, A., Tewarson, H., & Hockenberry, S. (2021). *Achieving progress toward health equity using race and ethnicity data: State strategies and lessons learned.* National Academy of State Health Policy, Duke-Margolis Center for Health Policy, National Governors Association Center for Best Practices.

Rajkomar, A., Hardt, M., Howell, M. D., Corrado, G., & Chin, M. H. (2018). Ensuring fairness in machine learning to advance health equity. *Annals of Internal Medicine, 169*(12), 866–872. https://doi.org/10.7326/M18-1990

Smedley, A., & Smedley, B. D. (2005). Race as biology is fiction, racism as a social problem is real. *American Psychologist, 60*(1), 16–26. https://doi.org/10.1037/0003-066X.60.1.16

Thompson, B. L., Cloud, L. K., & Gable, L. (2020). Advancing legal epidemiology: An introduction. *Journal of Public Health Management and Practice, 26*(Suppl 2), S1–S3. https://doi.org/10.1097/PHH.0000000000001119

Vyas, D. A., Eisenstein, L. G., & Jones, D. S. (2020). Hidden in plain sight—Reconsidering the use of race correction in clinical algorithms. *New England Journal of Medicine, 383*(9), 874–882. https://doi.org/10.1056/NEJMms2004740

Yearby, R. (2020). Structural racism and health disparities: Reconfiguring the social determinants of health framework to include the root cause. *Journal of Law, Medicine & Ethics, 48*, 518–526. https://doi.org/10.1177/1073110520958876

Yearby, R., Clark, B., & Figueroa, J. F. (2022). Structural racism in historical and modern US health care policy. *Health Affairs, 41*(2), 187–194. https://doi.org/10.1377/hlthaff.2021.01466

Yeung, A., & Chang, D. (2002). Adjustment disorder: Intergenerational conflict in a Chinese immigrant family. *Culture, Medicine and Psychiatry, 26*(4), 509–525. https://doi.org/10.1176/foc.4.1.10

Index